RHEOLOGICAL MEASUREMENT

RHEOLOGICAL MEASUREMENT

Edited by

A. A. COLLYER

Department of Applied Physics
Sheffield City Polytechnic, Sheffield, UK

and

D. W. CLEGG

Department of Metallurgy and Materials Science,
University of Nottingham, Nottingham, UK

ELSEVIER APPLIED SCIENCE
LONDON and NEW YORK

CHEMISTRY

0285 0989

ELSEVIER APPLIED SCIENCE PUBLISHERS LTD
Crown House, Linton Road, Barking, Essex IG11 8JU, England

Sole Distributor in the USA and Canada
ELSEVIER SCIENCE PUBLISHING CO., INC.
52 Vanderbilt Avenue, New York, NY 10017, USA

WITH 29 TABLES AND 198 ILLUSTRATIONS

© 1988 ELSEVIER APPLIED SCIENCE PUBLISHERS LTD

British Library Cataloguing in Publication Data

Rheological measurement.
1. Rheometry
I. Collyer, A. A.   II. Clegg, D. W.
531'.11

ISBN 1-85166-196-4

Library of Congress Cataloging-in-Publication Data

Rheological measurement/edited by A. A. Collyer and D. W.
Clegg.
   p. cm.
   Bibliography: p.
   Includes index.
   ISBN 1-85166-196-4
   1. Rheology, 2. Rheometers, I. Collyer, A. A. II. Clegg,
D. W.
   QC189.5.R49   1988
   681'.2–dc19   88-2064
                                                         CIP

Typeset at the Alden Press, London, Northampton, Oxford
Printed in Great Britain at the University Press, Cambridge

Preface

In many cases rheological measurements are carried out in the simplest of geometries, but the interpretation involved in obtaining the rheological parameters of the test fluids from these measurements is surprisingly complex. The purpose of this book is to emphasise the points on which most workers in the field agree, and to let the authors deal with the contentious points according to their own beliefs and experience. This work represents a summary of the current thought on rheological measurement by experts in the various techniques.

When making measurements and obtaining from them parameters that describe the flow behaviour of the test fluids, it is essential that the experimentalist understands the underlying theory and shortcomings of the measurement technique, that he is aware of the likely microstructure of the fluid, and that from this he can appreciate how the fluid and the measuring system will interact with each other. It is this interaction that gives both the required rheological parameters of the fluids and the artefacts that confuse the issue.

This book covers the main rheological measurement techniques from capillary, slit and stretching flows to rotational and oscillatory rheometry in various geometries including sliding plate measurements. These topics are backed up by chapters on more practical aspects, such as commercial instruments, and on computer control and data acquisition. The chapters deal with the basic methods, how the measurements are taken, and what assumptions and interpretations are made to obtain valid data on the test fluids.

Another group of chapters, on die swell, shear heating and hole pressure measurement, build on the more commonplace techniques and enable the experimentalist to correct his data or to use further methods to obtain the rheological parameters of the test fluids. The chapter on flow visualisation techniques illustrates the need to use other techniques to assist the rheological measurement.

The final two chapters concentrate on the test fluids themselves rather than on techniques. One deals with the macroscopic flow behaviour of blends and complex fluids, and the other chapter examines the ways in which mathematical models of two-phase fluids can be derived from assumptions made on the fluid microstructure.

Rheology is a vast and exciting subject and can scarcely be covered in one book, albeit a large one. In this book it has been the aim to concentrate on the basic techniques and the physical principles underlying them, with some discussion of multiphase fluids, which are a large class of fluids of industrial interest and importance.

The work is of considerable importance and relevance to all establishments in which rheological work is carried out, be the materials polymeric, biological, slurries, food or other complex fluids. Materials scientists, engineers or technologists in industry, research laboratories or in academic institutions should find the book valuable in providing an up-to-date review of current thought from experts in the field of rheology from different parts of the world.

A. A. COLLYER and D.W. CLEGG

Contents

List of Contributors

F. S. BAKER
Royal Ordnance Explosives Division, Sewardstone Road, Waltham Abbey, Essex EN9 1AY, UK

D. BARTHES-BIESEL
Division de Biomécanique et Instrumentation Médicale, UA CNRS 858, UTC/Département de Génie Biologique, BP 233, 60206 Compiègne Cedex, France

D. V. BOGER
Department of Chemical Engineering, University of Melbourne, Parkville, Victoria 3052, Australia

G. J. BROWNSEY
AFRC Institute of Food Research, Colney Lane, Norwich, NR4 7UA, UK

R. E. CARTER
Royal Ordnance Explosives Division, Sewardstone Road, Waltham Abbey, Essex EN9 1AY, UK

J. M. DEALY
Department of Chemical Engineering, McGill University, 3480 University Street, Montreal PQ, Canada H3A 2A7

G. H. FRANCE
Department of Applied Physics, Sheffield City Polytechnic, Pond Street, Sheffield S1 1WB, UK

A. J. GIACOMIN
Department of Mechanical Engineering, Texas A & M University, College Station, Texas 77843, USA

A. G. GIBSON
Department of Materials Science and Engineering, University of Liverpool, PO Box 147, Liverpool L69 3BX, UK

R. K. GUPTA
Department of Chemical Engineering, State University of New York at Buffalo, Clifford C. Furnas Hall, Buffalo, New York 14260, USA

CHANG DAE HAN
Department of Chemical Engineering and Polymer Research Institute, Polytechnic University, 333 Jay Street, Brooklyn, New York 11201, USA

A. S. LODGE
Rheology Research Center, University of Wisconsin, 1500 Johnson Drive, Madison, Wisconsin 53706, USA

M. E. MACKAY
Department of Chemical Engineering, University of Queensland, St Lucia, Queensland 4067, Australia

M. R. MACKLEY
Department of Chemical Engineering, University of Cambridge, Pembroke Street, Cambridge CB2 3RA, UK

GÉRARD MARIN
Laboratoire de Physique des Matériaux Industriels, Université de Pau et des Pays de l'Adour, Avenue de l'Université, 64000 Pau, France

ROBERT L. POWELL
Department of Chemical Engineering, University of California, Davis, California 95616, USA

G. J. PRIVETT
Royal Ordnance Explosives Division, Sewardstone Road, Waltham Abbey, Essex EN9 1AY, UK

T. SRIDHAR
Department of Chemical Engineering, Monash University, Clayton, Victoria 3168, Australia

ROGER I. TANNER
Department of Mechanical Engineering, University of Sydney, Sydney, New South Wales 2006, Australia

L. A. UTRACKI
National Research Council of Canada, Industrial Materials Research Institute, 75 de Mortagne Boulevard, Boucherville, Quebec, Canada J4B 6Y4

R. C. WARREN
Weapons Systems Research Laboratory, Defence Research Centre, Salisbury, GPO Box 2151, Adelaide, South Australia 5001, Australia

Chapter 1

Capillary Rheometry

M. R. MACKLEY

Department of Chemical Engineering, University of Cambridge, UK

1.1. INTRODUCTION

This chapter outlines the important physical aspects of the flow of fluids, especially polymeric fluids, within capillaries. The problem appears deceptively simple in that, if a steady viscometric flow is assumed within the

1

constant circular section tubing, it is generally very easy to derive equations from elementary constitutive equations which yield the velocity profile and pressure drop within the pipe. We shall discover that for polymer melts the flows are experimentally observed to be far from being viscometric within the capillary section; however, in spite of this, the 'classic' viscometric pressure drop equations are usually adequate for most engineering calculations, although of dubious merit for detailed characterisation of rheologically complex fluids.

Capillary rheometry is used as a method of characterising a test fluid's rheological properties. It also represents a particular case of the slightly more general problem of understanding the way in which fluids flow within a duct of variable cross section. This latter problem of course represents the heart of all extrusion processing which incorporates continuous extrusion such as the manufacture of plastic pipes, batch extrusion such as the flow of toothpaste out of a tube, blow moulding for the production of polymer film, and injection moulding of complex shapes. The current trend is towards increasingly diverse and sophisticated rheological fluids being processed faster within more complex geometrical dies, and consequently there is now a real need to understand fully both general duct flow and, in particular, capillary flow.

If it were possible to have an indefinitely long capillary section many of the problems associated with capillary rheometry would be removed. In reality the capillary section will have a beginning and an end. In terms of rheometry the entry region is very important, whilst the exit region has less influence on pressure drop measurements. The exit region does of course have profound significance for polymer processing because die swell and instabilities emanating from the exit are usually the two factors that control the maximum output of an extrusion process. In this chapter we choose not to examine exit effects too deeply but concentrate our attention on the capillary and entry region.

1.2. PHYSICAL ASPECTS

In this section we outline the main variables with which we will be concerned. It is important when dealing with unusual or novel fluids to check that the base assumptions applied to the analysis are valid for the particular fluid under test.

1.2.1. Geometrical Constraints

The primary geometric parameters shown in Fig. 1.1 are the L_0/D_0 ratio of the capillary section, the entrance contraction ratio D_1/D_0, and the entrance angle ϕ of the capillary. Typically we might expect D_0 to vary from say 100 μm to 5 mm and L_0/D_0 ratios from 0 to 500. Entrance contractions D_1/D_0 vary from about 2 to about 200 and the entrance angle is usually 90° but can vary between say 15° and 90°.

When dealing with structured fluids and composite fluids the ratio D_0/l_f may be important, where l_f is the largest length scale associated with the structured fluid. In general the precision of circular holes is good and this together with surface finish and/or wall material composition will probably not influence measurements greatly.

1.2.2. External Fluid Boundary Condition

Desirably the choice is between a constant volumetric flow within the capillary or a constant pressure drop. Most capillary rheometers work on the basis of a constant velocity piston driving fluid from the reservoir to the capillary. Fluid pressure is measured either using a force transducer on the piston or a side entry pressure transducer upstream of the capillary entrance. The disadvantage of the piston force transducer is that piston friction and reservoir wall viscosity must be taken into account. The force divided by the piston cross-sectional area gives a measure of the mean upstream hydrostatic pressure in the reservoir. Side transducers usually present problems in ensuring a flush mounting on the inside convex face

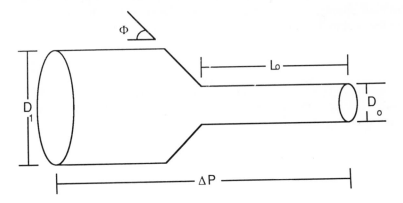

Fig. 1.1. Schematic diagram of duct geometrical parameters.

of the reservoir wall. The side transducer measures the normal force at the reservoir wall.

It is possible in principle to run a capillary rheometer at a constant pressure drop, where measurement of the volumetric flow can be obtained from continuous weight measurements of the extruding fluid; however, when working in this mode it is often difficult to run the fluid in a stable manner over a wide range of pressures.

1.2.3. Fluid/Solid Boundary Conditions

The fluid/solid boundary conditions are every bit as important as the constitutive equation of the fluid. It is usual to assume that the velocity of the fluid is zero at the wall, and this is generally the case for Newtonian fluids. The zero slip condition is also true for most but not all situations for flowing molten polymers. However, when one comes to examine e.g. structured fluids, composite fluids and some foodstuffs, the possibility of wall slip becomes a reality with very serious consequences in the rheological interpretation of data.

1.2.4. Inertia

The Reynolds number (Re) of capillary flow is usually but not always sufficiently low for inertia effects to be ignored, which means that creeping flow solutions are generally appropriate.

1.2.5. Temperature

Viscosity is a thermally activated process[1] and consequently the rheology of a fluid is very dependent on temperature. Accurate temperature control of fluid conditions is essential and there is the possibility that shear heating at the wall may influence results at high extrusion rates for high viscosity fluids, as discussed in Chapter 5.

1.2.6. Pressure

Absolute pressure also influences fluid viscosity[1] and Cogswell[2] for example considers that pressure can have a significant effect on polymer melt rheology.

1.2.7. Bulk Fluid Properties

Apart from the fluid/solid boundary conditions the bulk fluid properties represent the most difficult and intriguing aspect of fluid rheology. Firstly, the question of incompressibility should be considered. Generally, fluids that are dominantly viscous are incompressible, but viscoelastic fluids can show significant compressibility effects.[2] The question of composition uniformity may also be important as polymer fluids can in principle segregate with different molecular weight components in different regions of the flow. When polymer solutions are processed there is the possibility of different polymer concentrations in different regions of the flow, and in particular there may be a depletion or enhancement[3] of polymer concentration at or near the solid wall.

The constitutive equation of the fluid is of course the aspect of central importance in terms of the correct description of flow behaviour. Popular equations used in an engineering context are:

(1) Newtonian fluid

$$\tau(t) = \eta\dot{\gamma}(t) \tag{1.1}$$

where τ is the shear stress, $\dot{\gamma}$ the shear rate and η the viscosity.

(2) Bingham plastic fluid

$$\tau(t) = \tau_y + \eta\dot{\gamma}(t) \qquad (\tau > \tau_y)$$
$$\dot{\gamma} = 0 \qquad (\tau \leqslant \tau_y) \tag{1.2}$$

where τ_y is the yield stress of the fluid.

(3) Power law fluid

$$\tau(y) = K\dot{\gamma}(t)^n \tag{1.3}$$

where K and n are constants.

(4) Cox equation

$$\tau(t) = \left(\eta_\infty + \frac{\eta_0 - \eta_\infty}{1 + \alpha\dot{\gamma}(t)^n}\right)\dot{\gamma}(t) \tag{1.4}$$

where η_0 and η_∞ are limiting viscosities at low and high shear rates respectively and α and n are constants.

In all these equations the shear stress τ at a particular position or (equivalent) time depends only on the strain rate at that particular position or time. The fluid does not have a memory of the past. Polymer fluids in particular do remember where they have come from and consequently their past deformation history does matter; thus the correct way to describe a polymer fluid should have a constitutive equation that takes past deformation histories into account. Constitutive equations of the following form generally cover this point:

$$\sigma_{ij}(t) \;=\; \int_{-\infty}^{t} G(t - t') f(\gamma_{kl}(t'), \dot{\gamma}_{kl}(t')) \, \mathrm{d}t' \qquad (1.5)$$

where the stress components σ_{ij} at a current time t can be expressed in terms of the past strain $\gamma_{kl}(t')$ and/or strain rate $\dot{\gamma}_{kl}(t')$ components at time t'. The relaxation modulus term $G(t - t')$ is a measure of the material's fading memory. Various forms of the type of equation given above have been proposed[4-6] but we defer further discussion of this point to a later section.

1.3. VISCOMETRIC CAPILLARY FLOW FOR SIMPLE CONSTITUTIVE EQUATIONS

If we make a number of sweeping assumptions about capillary flow it is straightforward to arrive at expressions for the pressure drop of the fluid flowing within the capillary. We shall see that by measuring the pressure drop ΔP as a function of flow rate Q it is possible to fit the data to a Newtonian fluid, a power law fluid or express the flow in terms of an apparent viscosity. In this section we make no attempt to consider generalised constitutive equations.

The necessary base assumptions are that

  (a) fluid velocity is zero at wall;
  (b) fluid streamlines are parallel to wall and there is no circumferential motion;
  (c) hydrostatic pressure is uniform across any radial section of capillary;
  (d) flow is viscometric, i.e. does not change with time;
  (e) entrance and exit effects are ignored.

1.3.1. Creeping Flow Solution for a Newtonian Fluid
From a force balance carried out on an element shown in Fig. 1.2:

$$\tau 2\pi r \, \mathrm{d}x - \frac{\mathrm{d}P}{\mathrm{d}x} \, \mathrm{d}x \, \pi r^2 \;=\; 0$$

$$\tau \;=\; \frac{r}{2} \frac{\mathrm{d}P}{\mathrm{d}x} \qquad (1.6)$$

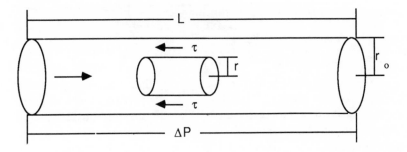

Fig. 1.2. Schematic diagram of element for force balance in a circular duct.

Constitutive equation

$$\tau = \eta \frac{du}{dr} \qquad (1.7)$$

Combination of eqns (1.6) and (1.7) and integration with boundary conditions $u = 0$, $r = r_0$ gives

$$u = \frac{\Delta P}{4L\eta} (r_0^2 - r^2) \qquad (1.8)$$

which yields the familiar parabolic profile. The shear rate is given by

$$\dot{\gamma} = \frac{du}{dr} = -\frac{\Delta P}{2L\eta} r \qquad (1.9)$$

This reveals an important result in that the shear rate varies from zero at the centre of the capillary to a maximum at the wall. In many ways this exposes a fundamental weakness of capillary rheometry in that the shear rates and shear stress are not uniform for the fluid under test.

By integration of eqn (1.8), the pressure drop can be expressed as a function of flow rate Q:

$$\Delta P = \frac{8\eta L}{\pi r_0^4} Q \qquad (1.10)$$

1.3.2. Creeping Flow Solution for a Power Law Fluid
Replacement of eqn (1.7) by

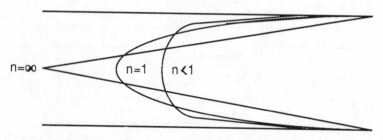

Fig. 1.3. Schematic diagram of transverse velocity profiles for a power law fluid with $n = \infty$, $n = 1$ and $n < 1$.

$$\tau = K\left(\frac{du}{dr}\right)^n \tag{1.11}$$

yields

$$u = \left(\frac{\Delta P}{2LK}\right)^{1/n} \frac{n}{n+1} \left(r_0^{(n+1)/n} - r^{(n+1)/n}\right) \tag{1.12}$$

which gives velocity profiles of the form shown in Fig. 1.3 and a pressure equation given by

$$\Delta P = 2LK\left(\frac{(3n+1)}{\pi n r_0^{(3n+1)/n}}\right)^n Q^n \tag{1.13}$$

Molten polymers are often modelled using a power law fluid equation. Typically the power law index might vary between $n = 1.0$ and 0.3, decreasing with increasing molecular weight. The power law model has often been adequate in describing capillary data which have been obtained over perhaps up to two decades in wall shear rate from say 10 to $1000\,\text{s}^{-1}$. If shear rates outside this range are examined the two-parameter power law model usually becomes increasingly inadequate, particularly at the lower shear rates.

1.3.3. Creeping Flow Solution for a Bingham Plastic Fluid

Replacement of eqn (1.7) by

$$\tau = \tau_y + \eta\frac{du}{dr} \qquad (\tau > \tau_y) \tag{1.14}$$

(Care should be taken to ensure the sign of τ_y is such that the yield stress

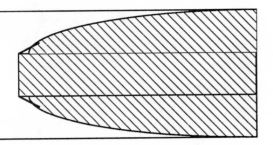

Fig. 1.4. Schematic diagram of transverse velocity profile for a Bingham plastic fluid.

τ_y opposes the fluid motion) and integration yields

$$u = \frac{1}{\eta}\left[\frac{\Delta P}{4L}\left(r_0^2 - r^2\right) - \tau_y\left(r_0 - r\right)\right] \qquad (1.15)$$

for $r > r_1$ where $r_1 = 2\tau_y L/\Delta P$.

The form of the velocity profile is shown schematically in Fig. 1.4 where the new feature of plug flow within the capillary core becomes apparent. Unlike the previous Newtonian and power law cases, it is not easy to express the pressure drop as a simple function of Q.

1.3.4. Apparent Viscosity

The term apparent viscosity can mean different things to different people.[7] Usually apparent viscosity $\eta_a(\dot{\gamma})$ is defined as

$$\tau = \eta_a(\dot{\gamma}) \times \dot{\gamma} \qquad (1.16)$$

The apparent viscosity can be determined if the quantities τ and $\dot{\gamma}$ can be determined at the same position. By considering events at the capillary wall, eqn (1.6) gives

$$\tau_0 = \frac{r_0 \Delta P}{2L} \qquad (1.17)$$

The shear rate at the wall $\dot{\gamma}$ can be determined by following the so-called Rabinowitsch correction procedure:[7]

$$Q = 2\pi \int_0^{r_0} ru(r)\,dr = 2\pi \left\{\left[\frac{r^2}{2}u(r)\right]_0^{r_0} - \int_0^{r_0} \frac{r^2}{2}\,du\right\}$$

M. R. Mackley

when $r = r_0$, $u = 0$

$$\therefore Q = -\pi \int_0^{r_0} r^2 \frac{\mathrm{d}u}{\mathrm{d}r}\,\mathrm{d}r$$

Now $r = r_0 \tau/\tau_w$

$$\therefore Q = -\frac{\pi r_0^3}{\tau_w^3} \int_0^{\tau_w} \dot{\gamma} \tau^2\,\mathrm{d}\tau$$

which yields

$$\frac{1}{\pi r_0^3}\left(\tau_w^3 \frac{\mathrm{d}Q}{\mathrm{d}\tau_w} + 3\tau_w^2 Q\right) = -\dot{\gamma}_w \tau_w^2$$

or using eqn (1.6)

$$-\dot{\gamma}_w = \frac{1}{\pi r_0^3}\left(3Q + \Delta P \frac{\mathrm{d}(Q)}{\mathrm{d}(\Delta P)}\right) \tag{1.18}$$

Hence, if ΔP is known as a function of Q, both τ_w and $\dot{\gamma}_w$ can be determined from eqns (1.17) and (1.18), and the apparent viscosity can be determined

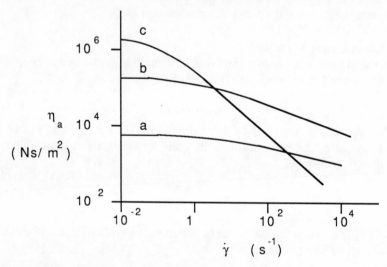

Fig. 1.5. Typical flow curves of apparent viscosity as a function of shear rate for a molten polymer. Curves a, b, c show the effect of increasing molecular weight (c represents the highest molecular weight).

from

$$\tau_w = \eta_a(\dot\gamma)\dot\gamma_w \tag{1.19}$$

For most polymeric systems η_a has a typical form as shown in Fig. 1.5 where η_a is usually a decreasing function of $\dot\gamma$.

1.4. ENTRY FLOW CORRECTIONS

In order to eliminate the pressure drop due to the entry region of the capillary it is usual to make the so-called Bagley correction.[7] This simply involves making measurements of the pressure drop for different L/r_0 ratios at chosen values of wall shear rate. Curves of the form shown in Fig. 1.6 are obtained. Bagley assumed that the entry pressure drop was equivalent to an 'added length' of capillary given by Nr_0. Thus

$$\tau_w = \frac{\Delta P r_0}{2(L + Nr_0)}$$

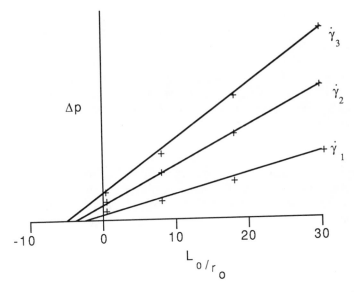

Fig. 1.6. Schematic diagram showing the Bagley plot for entry pressure drop.

or

$$\Delta P = 2\tau_w \left(\frac{L}{r_0} + N \right) \qquad (1.20)$$

When $\Delta P = 0$ the negative intercept on Fig. 1.6 yields the value of N. This is a somewhat unsatisfactory correction as N is usually a function of flow rate, geometry and temperature for most non-Newtonian fluids. Modern piston rheometers of the type manufactured for example by Rosand[8] use a double barrel system with one barrel having a zero L/r_0 die and the other having a finite value. The entry pressure for the test conditions can then be immediately eliminated and the 'true' capillary pressure drop determined. It is not possible to derive reliable analytic expressions that accurately describe entry pressure drops, and consequently the experimental route for eliminating this term seems currently to be the most satisfactory approach. As we shall see in the next section, it is now however possible numerically to compute entry pressure drops for Newtonian fluids, power law fluids and some viscoelastic fluids.

1.5. NUMERICAL SIMULATION OF CAPILLARY FLOW

Commercial software packages such as Fluent[9] and Polyflow[10] are now available for the numerical simulation of flows within constrained boundaries. The solvers work using either a finite difference or a finite element scheme and can solve the full Navier–Stokes equations for Newtonian fluids. Fluent for example uses finite differences and solves velocities and pressures iteratively using a primitive variable method. The velocity and pressure profiles for a Newtonian fluid flowing within a circular section duct are shown in Figs 1.7–1.9. These profiles were obtained using Fluent with a 60×30 finite difference mesh in the axial plane of the duct; details of the flow are given in the captions.

Figure 1.7(a) shows the streamlines of the flow into a circular section duct where the tube entry Reynolds number Re is 400. The transverse velocity profiles in Fig. 1.7(b) show the expected fluid acceleration into the constriction and the development of the velocity profiles within the capillary section. At this Reynolds number the velocity profile can be seen to be evolving with distance along the capillary and, even at the final profile shown, the profile is not fully parabolic. The slow development of the parabolic profile is also reflected in Fig. 1.7(c) which is the centre line axial velocity along the duct. Following the fluid's acceleration into the throat

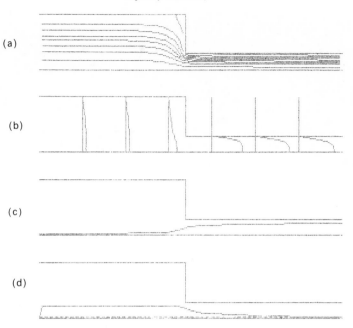

Fig. 1.7. 'Fluent' numerical simulation of the flow of a Newtonian fluid in a cylindrical duct: $D_1 = 0.04\,$m, $D_2 = 0.013\,$m; length of duct $= 0.12\,$m; entry velocity $= 0.01\,$m/s; viscosity $\eta = 10^{-3}\,$Ns/m^2. (a) Corresponds to streamline contours in upper half of duct; (b) corresponds to normalised transverse velocity profiles along duct; (c) corresponds to normalised centre line velocity profile along duct; (d) corresponds to normalised centre line pressure profile along duct.

it can be seen that the velocity is still changing within the capillary section. The flow is therefore not viscometric within the capillary and the pressure profile shown in Fig. 1.7(d) reflects this in that the pressure change within the capillary section does not decrease linearly along the capillary section. The simulation successfully predicts the whole pressure profile including entry pressure changes.

In Fig. 1.8 the entry Reynolds number has been reduced to 0·4. The streamline contours look similar to those of Fig. 1.7 but the velocity profile contours are now essentially uniform within the capillary section. The flow is now viscometric from, say, one half capillary diameter downstream of the throat. The centre line velocity profile within the capillary section shown in Fig. 1.8(c) is now constant and the pressure change within this section linear as shown in Fig. 1.8(d). A further reduction in Reynolds

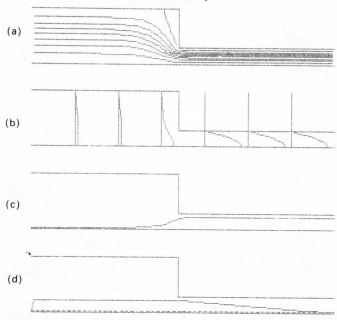

(a)

(b)

(c)

(d)

Fig. 1.8. Details as for Fig. 1.7 except viscosity $\eta = 1\cdot0\,\mathrm{Ns/m^2}$.

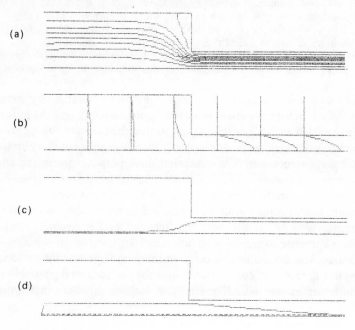

(a)

(b)

(c)

(d)

Fig. 1.9. Details as for Fig. 1.7 except viscosity $\eta = 10^3\,\mathrm{Ns/m^2}$.

number to 4×10^{-4} given in Fig. 1.9 shows no further change in the normalised velocity and pressure profiles.

From the curves described above it can be seen that apparently accurate velocity and pressure profile information can be obtained from simulations together with entry pressure drop values which are not available from any reliable analytic expression. In our laboratory we have recently tested these simulations against corresponding experiments and found them to yield good agreement, and consequently it is clear that a combination of reliable experimental capillary measurements together with numerical simulations can provide a powerful combined approach to understanding capillary rheometry.

Fluent is also able to solve for power law fluids in a generalised inertia flow. The contours and profiles obtained for the same boundary conditions discussed previously are given in Fig. 1.10 for a fluid where the power law index $n = 0.5$ and the power law constant $K = 0.001$. It can be seen that in this case the velocity profile within the capillary section is much flatter than in the Newtonian case. In addition, the flow rapidly approaches its viscometric state within the capillary section.

1.6. EXPERIMENTALLY OBSERVED VELOCITY AND STRESS FIELDS

In addition to experimental pressure profile measurements it is possible to make direct measurements of velocity fields within capillaries and in some cases stress fields also. The circular sections associated with capillaries often make optical measurements difficult, and most rheo-optic measurements are usually carried out in pseudo-two-dimensional slit geometries.[11,12] The author has been involved on a long-term programme examining the way in which molten polymers flow within slits,[13-15] and some of the results that have been obtained will be described in this section. In general, molten polymers are sufficiently optically transparent to allow both laser velocimetry and flow birefringence techniques to be used. Thus it is possible to obtain both the velocity and the stress distributions for polymer flowing into and within slits. These techniques are discussed fully in Chapter 14.

Figure 1.11 shows the flow birefringence of molten polyethylene flowing into a wineglass shaped slit.[15] The slit is 1 mm in width and the extinction bands seen within the flowing melt correspond to different levels of principal stress difference, which progressively increase up to the throat of the slit. The principal stress difference is a maximum at the edge of the throat, with a small variation across the throat; there will of course be an entry pressure drop associated with this stress build-up. Within the slit there is

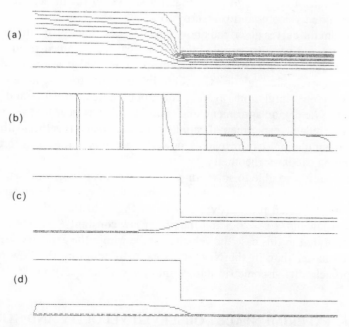

Fig. 1.10. Conditions as for Fig. 1.7 but for a power law fluid: $K = 0.001$, $n = 0.5$.

a rapid change in the stress profile. Shear stresses develop at the side of the slit and the observation that the fringes run essentially parallel to the slit at the wall implies that the shear stress at the wall is, for the case shown, uniform along the length of the slit. It is this observation that makes capillary or equivalently slit rheometry meaningful because, apart from numerical simulations, it is usual to assume a constant shear stress at the wall.

The centre line behaviour of the stress distribution is interesting in that it shows behaviour far from that of viscometric flow. At the throat the centre line stress is a maximum. As the fluid enters the throat the material is essentially convected down the centre line without further deformation. If the fluid was Newtonian the stress would therefore rapidly decay and the flow become viscometric. Molten polymers are viscoelastic and take a finite time to relax after deformation. We therefore see a centre line stress relaxation taking place within the slit where stress generated in the entry section relaxes in the central region of the slit. This observation has important consequences in terms of exit effects such as die swell and

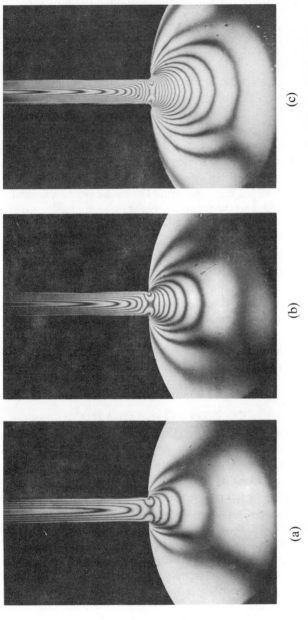

(a) (b) (c)

Fig. 1.11. Flow birefringence photographs of high density polyethylene (Rigidex type 006-60) at $T = 170°C$ flowing into a 1 mm width slit. Maximum centre line entry velocity gradient $\dot{e}_m$ given by (a) $3\cdot6\,\text{s}^{-1}$, (b) $14\,\text{s}^{-1}$, (c) $22\,\text{s}^{-1}$.[15]

overall levels of molecular orientation, although perhaps surprisingly it does not significantly influence capillary or slit pressure drop measurements.

Velocity profiles corresponding to stress fields already shown are given in Figs. 1.12 and 1.13.[14] Figure 1.12 shows a centre line velocity profile and Fig. 1.13 shows transverse velocity profiles within the slit section.

The velocity profiles show results strikingly similar in form to the results of the numerical simulations. The centre line velocity profile, with the exception of an observed experimental high flow rate velocity overshoot, bears a very close resemblance to a power law entry flow. The transverse profiles within the slit section also fit a power law profile well, and in addition it can be noted that the transverse profile within the slit almost immediately takes up a uniform form. Thus we have now seen that both the wall shear stress and shear rate are constant along the length of the slit section.

Our general findings have been that velocity fields model reasonably closely to that predicted by a power law constitutive equation in the whole field of observation. In the entry region and along the centre of the flow, modelling of the time dependent stress field can only be achieved if full viscoelastic behaviour is taken into account. However, of important significance to capillary rheometry wall shear stresses, corresponding pressure drops can be modelled certainly to a first approximation using power law modelling. Wall behaviour in the parallel section of the die represents a large-strain essentially time independent deformation.

1.7. CONSTITUTIVE EQUATIONS

The choice of constitutive equation depends on the level of sophistication and the precision required from any calculation. It has been indicated that, for the case of molten polymers, power law modelling will prove adequate for many engineering calculations including capillary flow. However, if detailed rheological characterisation and/or stress field predictions are needed, a greater level of information content is required. This is reflected in the evolution of the way in which rheological properties of molten polymers have been measured. Initially a single parameter melt flow index was used; subsequently more complete apparent viscosity η_a vs. apparent shear rate data $\dot{\gamma}_a$ was obtained; and recently the emergence of reliable small-strain oscillatory rheometers has led to polymer characterisation measurements using storage modulus G', loss modulus G'' and complex viscosity η^*. Empirically the apparent viscosity and the complex viscosity are linked for most polymers by the Cox–Merz rule[16] where

$$\eta^*(\omega) = \eta_a(\dot{\gamma}_a) \tag{1.21}$$

where $\omega = \dot{\gamma}_a$ and ω is the angular frequency of the small-strain oscillatory motion.

In many ways this is a remarkable correlation, as it directly links the small-strain, time dependent behaviour of the polymer with the large-strain time independent capillary shear stress.

If complete characterisation and/or rheological stress field predictions are required, the full consequences of viscoelastic behaviour must be faced. In addition, effects such as die swell and melt instabilities test constitutive equations to their highest level, and modelling using approximate constitutive equations will almost certainly give misleading results.

Molten polymers remember their past deformation history and consequently it is reasonable to express the stress at some current time t in terms of the past deformation history:[15]

$$\sigma_{ij}(t) = \int_{-\infty}^{t} G(t - t')\dot{\gamma}_{ij}(t')\, dt' \tag{1.22}$$

In eqn (1.22) the stress is expressed in terms of a relaxation modulus $G(t - t')$ and past deformation rate $\dot{\gamma}_{ij}$. In the form written, the equation is not 'objective'; in order to make it objective, $\dot{\gamma}_{ij}(t')$ can be expressed as a corotational deformation tensor Γ_{ij} as described by Bird *et al.*[5] Using small-strain linear viscoelastic oscillatory measurements, it is possible to obtain experimentally $G(t - t')$, the relaxation modulus for a polymer,[15] and test the equation's validity against experimental results.

The predictions of molecular theories, and in particular those of Doi and Edwards,[6] have resulted in the testing of constitutive equations of the following form:

$$\sigma_{ij}(t) = \int_{-\infty}^{t} \mu(t - t')h(\gamma)c^{-1}(tt')\, dt' \tag{1.23}$$

In this equation $\mu(t - t')$ is the polymer memory function which is equivalent to the relaxation modulus cited in eqn (1.22). c^{-1} is a measure of the past strain deformation and currently the Finger tensor deformation is favoured, given by

$$c^{-1}(tt') = E^{-1}(tt')E^{-1}(tt')^{T} \tag{1.24}$$

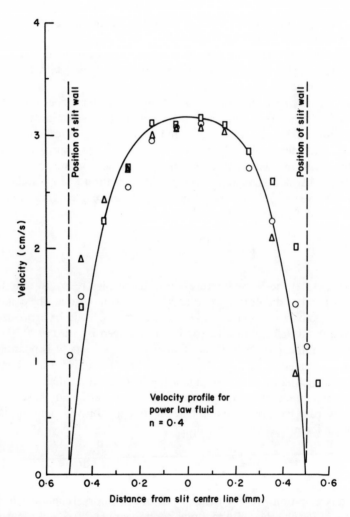

Fig. 1.12. Transverse velocity profiles across a 1 mm slit for high density polyethylene (Rigidex type 006-60) at $T = 210°C$. Distance downstream from throat: Δ 0·1 mm, $\square$ 2·0 mm, $\circ$ 6·0 mm. The continuous curve represents the velocity profile of a power law fluid with power law index $n = 0·4$.[14]

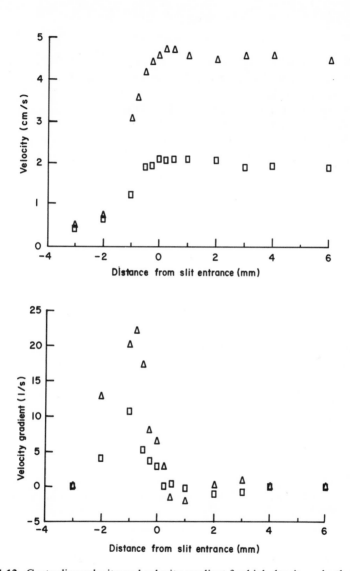

Fig. 1.13. Centre line velocity and velocity gradient for high density polyethylene (Rigidex type 006-60) at 170°C flowing into a slit. Throat position at 0 mm. Maximum entry velocity gradient $\dot{e}_m$: $\square$ $14 \, \text{s}^{-1}$, $\triangle$ $22 \, \text{s}^{-1}$.[14]

with the deformation strain tensor E^{-1} given by

$$E^{-1}(tt') = \frac{\partial x}{\partial x'} \qquad (1.25)$$

where x' denotes the deformed configuration coordinates. The term $h(\gamma)$ is termed a damping function which is a polymer-property dependent term (see e.g. Larson[17]).

For monodisperse polymers the Doi–Edwards constitutive equation predicts both the form of the memory function and the form of $h(\gamma)c^{-1}$ which is replaced by their universal Q tensor. From experiments carried out in this laboratory by Mead,[18] it has been found that for polydisperse polymer the form of the experimentally determined memory function is required rather than that predicted by Doi and Edwards. The Q tensor performs well in many parts of the flow but needs refinement in regions where the product of the deformation rate and largest polymer relaxation time is high.

Equations of the type (1.23) can predict for example the Cox–Merz rule, and steady shear behaviour, and hence can be directly related to capillary rheometry. However, the full richness of time dependent molten polymer behaviour is not seen using average pressure drop measurements from capillary data. Consequently oscillatory measurements, step strain experiments or flow birefringence observations of constrained flows are required to characterise the polymer fully. Given the correct characterisation of the material, there then remains the not insignificant problem of numerically predicting behaviour in complex flow geometries such as capillaries with entrances and exits.

1.8. CONCLUSION

The future of capillary rheometry is assured in that it represents a relatively simple experimental technique which bears a close resemblance to most commercial extrusion processes. As a precision rheological tool for characterising polymers, results from capillary rheometry must be treated with care. Certainly it is a necessary condition that the rheological modelling chosen should be able to predict capillary behaviour. However, as has been indicated in previous sections, the full time dependent behaviour of the fluid may reveal more information about fluid properties which, in terms of capillary rheometry, would require a detailed study of the capillary entry flow behaviour and centre line stress relaxation within the capillary.

At present there is no one universal instrument for fluid rheological characterisation. However, in the opinion of this author the capillary rheometer combined with an oscillatory, variable frequency and strain device does offer a viable set of experimental equipment for most fluid characterisation.

REFERENCES

1. D. Tabor, *Gas, Liquids and Solids*, Cambridge University Press, 1979.
2. F. N. Cogswell, *Polymer Melt Rheology*, George Goodwin Ltd, in assoc. with Plastics and Rubber Institute, London, 1981.
3. P. J. Barham, R. A. M. Hikmet, K. A. Narh and A. Keller, *Colloid Polym. Sci.,* 1986, **264**, 507.
4. A. S. Lodge, *Elastic Liquids*, Academic Press, London, 1964.
5. R. B. Bird, R. C. Armstrong and O. Hassager, *Dynamics of Polymeric Liquids —II*, Wiley, New York, 1977.
6. M. Doi and S. F. Edwards, *The Theory of Polymer Dynamics*, Clarendon Press, Oxford, 1986.
7. J. A. Brydson, *Flow Properties of Polymer Melts*, George Goodwin (in association with Plastics and Rubber Institute), 1981.
8. Rosand Precision Ltd, Welwyn Garden City, Herts, UK.
9. Creare, Box 71, Hanover, New Hampshire 03755, USA.
10. M. C. Crochet, Department of Applied Mathematics, University of Louvain la Neuve, Belgium.
11. D. V. Boger, *Advances in Transport Processes*, vol. 2, Wiley, 1982, pp. 43–105.
12. J. L. S. Wales, *The Application of Flow Birefringence to Rheological Studies of Polymer Melts*, Delft University Press, 1976.
13. N. Checker, M. R. Mackley and D. W. Mead, *Phil. Trans. Roy. Soc.,* 1983, **A308**, 451–77.
14. M. R. Mackley and I. P. T. Moore, *J. Non-Newtonian Fluid Mech.,* 1986, **21**, 337–58.
15. S. T. E. Aldhouse, M. R. Mackley and I. P. T. Moore, *J. Non-Newtonian Fluid Mech.,* 1986, **21**, 359–76.
16. W. P. Cox and E. H. Merz, *J. Polym. Sci.,* 1958, **28**, 619.
17. R. G. Larson and V. A. Valesano, *J. Rheol.,* 1986, **30**, 1093–108.
18. D. W. Mead, PhD Thesis, Cambridge University, 1988.

Chapter 2

Slit Rheometry

CHANG DAE HAN

Department of Chemical Engineering and Polymer Research Institute, Polytechnic University, Brooklyn, New York, USA

NOTATION

S_{zz}	wall normal stress in flow direction
N_1	first normal stress difference
P_{Exit}	exit pressure
$-\partial S_{zz}/\partial z$	gradient of wall normal stress
$-\partial p/\partial z$	pressure gradient
λ	characteristic time of fluid
$\dot{\gamma}$	shear rate
σ_{12}	shear stress
w	width of slit die
h	height of slit die
$\dot{\gamma}_w, \dot{\gamma}$	wall shear rate
σ_w, σ	wall shear stress
Q	volumetric flow rate

n	slope of log σ_w versus log $(6Q/wh^2)$ plot
η	fluid viscosity
η_0	zero-shear viscosity
n	constant in eqn (2.6)
A, b	constants in eqn (2.7)
W_e	Weissenberg number
N_D	Deborah number
t_f	time for fluid to pass through exit region
L_{ex}	exit length
$\langle V \rangle$	Average flow velocity in slit die
$\bar{M}_w$	Weight-average molecular weight
ρ	fluid density
R	universal gas constant
T	Kelvin temperature
C_p	specific heat in eqn (2.11)
k	thermal conductivity in eqn (2.11)
k_0, b	constants in eqn (2.12)
T_0	reference temperature in eqn (2.12)
$\dot{\gamma}_0$	shear rate at which non-Newtonian behavior commences (eqn (2.12))

2.1. INTRODUCTION

The slit die has long been used to determine the viscosity of fluids. Experimentally, pressure drops are measured along the fully developed region of the die as a function of flow rate. Wall shear stress is calculated from the pressure gradient and shear rate from the volumetric flow rate. Finally, the viscosity is determined by the ratio of shear stress to shear rate.

However, it is a relatively new approach to use a slit die to determine the first normal stress difference, in addition to the viscosity of viscoelastic polymeric melts.[1,2] In such an endeavor, the wall normal stress (S_{zz}), commonly referred to as 'pressure', is measured in the fully developed region along the die axis z (see Fig. 2.1), as a function of volumetric flow rate under isothermal conditions, and then the first normal stress difference (N_1) is determined by extrapolating the S_{zz} to the exit plane of the die, commonly referred to as 'exit pressure' (P_{Exit}). There are a number of things that one must be aware of when using such an experimental technique.

First, one must make sure that the profile of S_{zz} is *linear* with respect to

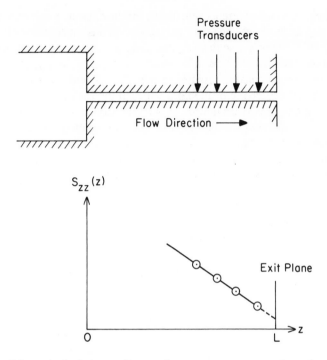

Fig. 2.1. Schematic depicting wall normal stress measurements along the axis of a slit die.

z, to ensure that the flow is fully developed in the region where the values of S_{zz} are measured. Note that when flow is fully developed, the gradient of wall normal stress, $-\partial S_{zz}/\partial z$, is equal to the pressure gradient, $-\partial p/\partial z$.[2] Today, it is a well documented fact that the establishment of a *linear* pressure profile is a necessary condition, although not a sufficient one, to achieve fully developed flow of viscoelastic fluids. If this necessary condition is not satisfied, regardless of its origin, physical or experimental, one should *not* proceed to determine the rheological properties of viscoelastic fluids. Assuming that pressure transducers are calibrated within acceptable accuracy, *nonlinear* pressure profiles may be observed in situations where (1) the die is not sufficiently long, (2) pressure measurements are taken at positions which include the entrance region, and (3) appreciable viscous shear heating occurs.

The length of a die required to achieve fully developed flow varies not only with the type of fluid (i.e. the characteristic time λ of a fluid) but also with shear rate $\dot{\gamma}$. For viscoelastic fluids, the entrance length increases with increasing $\lambda\dot{\gamma}$. It should be noted that when viscous shear heating becomes appreciable (i.e. very viscous polymer melts at high shear rates) there is a chance for the fluid to have a temperature variation along the die axis, giving rise to *nonlinear* pressure profiles, i.e. $-\partial p/\partial z \neq$ constant. This means that the viscosity of the fluid varies along the die axis. Under such circumstances, the determination of the viscosity of a fluid using a theory based on isothermal conditions is of no rheological significance. Some investigators[3,4] have encountered such situations, but unfortunately they went ahead and used the data to calculate the viscosity. The critical value of $\dot{\gamma}$ (or shear stress σ_{12}) at which viscous shear heating becomes significant in a slit die can be estimated by solving the equations of motion and heat transfer, which includes the term that represents viscous heat dissipation.

Secondly, one must make sure that an extrapolation of S_{zz} to the exit plane of the die can be justified for all intents and purposes. The validity of extrapolation would depend on the type of fluid (i.e. the characteristic time of a fluid, λ) and shear rate $\dot{\gamma}$. Therefore one should not generalize as to whether the extrapolation is valid or not, based on measurements of S_{zz} for dilute polymer solutions that have small λ values or for viscoelastic molten polymers at very low shear rates (or low shear stresses). Even if one were in a situation where the extrapolation was justifiable (to be discussed below), one would have to take measurements of S_{zz} at a sufficiently large number of positions along the die axis. One must use at least three pressure transducers or, ideally, as many pressure transducers as practically possible, so that the quality of data might be improved. Some investigators[5] have used only *two* pressure transducers and determined values of P_{Exit}, using an extrapolation procedure. Such a practice should never have been used, because of the inherent errors associated with the pressure transducer itself and measurements with it (e.g. balancing the zero position of the transducer); pressure readings can never be free from errors. If only two pressure transducers were used, there would be no other way but to draw a straight line between the two data points, which is tantamount to a claim that any error associated with the pressure measurements was negligible.

2.2. THEORY

Consider the flow in a long slit die with pressure transducers mounted far away from its entrance along the die axis, as shown schematically in Fig.

2.1. Let us assume that the width (w) of the die cross section is very large compared to its height (h) (i.e. $w \gg h$). It has been amply demonstrated that viscoelastic molten polymers, which exhibit appreciable extrudate swell, give rise to measurable quantities of P_{Exit}, which increases with increasing shear rate or shear stress.[1,2] Figure 2.2 gives representative results of such an experimental observation.

It can be shown, using experimental results such as those in Fig. 2.2, that the shear stress at the wall σ_w may be determined from

$$\sigma_w = -\left(\frac{\partial p}{\partial z}\right)\frac{h}{2} \tag{2.1}$$

where $-\partial p/\partial z$ is the pressure gradient. Also, shear rate at the wall $\dot{\gamma}_w$ can be determined from

$$\dot{\gamma}_w = \left(\frac{2n + 1}{3n}\right)\frac{6Q}{wh^2} \tag{2.2}$$

where Q is the volumetric flow rate and n is the slope of the log σ_w versus log ($6Q/wh^2$) plot. For convenience hereafter we shall drop the subscript w from both σ_w and $\dot{\gamma}_w$. We can then determine the viscosity of the fluid η from the definition $\eta = \sigma/\dot{\gamma}$.

Assuming that the extrapolation procedure is valid, Han[1] and Davis *et al.*[6] derived the following expression which relates the first normal stress difference N_1 to exit pressure P_{Exit} in a slit die:

$$N_1 = P_{Exit}\left(1 + \frac{d \ln P_{Exit}}{d \ln \sigma}\right) \tag{2.3}$$

It should be mentioned that in the derivation of eqn (2.3) the effect of inertia was assumed negligibly small, which is certainly valid for molten polymers. As will be discussed below, it should be emphasized that the use of eqn (2.3) is valid for viscoelastic molten polymers at sufficiently large values of σ. In other words, the extrapolation procedure, and thus the use of eqn (2.3), may not be justifiable for dilute polymer solutions and for molten polymers at low values of σ which exhibit little or no extrudate swell. The critical value of σ at and above which eqn (2.3) may be used will be discussed below.

Chang Dae Han

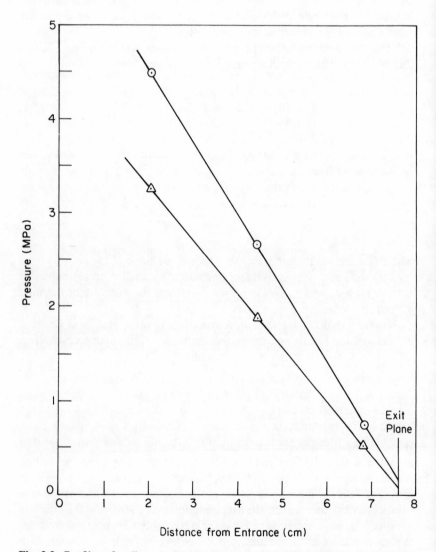

Fig. 2.2. Profiles of wall normal stress along the axis of a slit die for low-density polyethylene at 200 °C: ⊙ $214.8\,s^{-1}$; △ $161.2\,s^{-1}$.

2.3. METHOD

In using the 'exit pressure' method there are a number of design considerations that must be taken into account: (1) pressure transducers must be mounted at positions far away from the entrance region; (2) the number of pressure transducers must be at least three and preferably more (ideally as many as practically possible); (3) the distance between the melt discharge from either an extruder or a pump and the entrance of the die must be sufficiently long, so that the stresses in the melt can relax completely before entering the die; (4) for a slit die, the width to height ratio (w/h) of the die must be sufficiently large, so that the isovels of the melt stream are parallel to the long side of the die cross section; (5) for a slit die, the dimension of the width (w) of the die cross section must be much larger than the diameter of the tip of the pressure transducer, so that the isovels of the melt stream are parallel to the surface of the tip of the pressure transducer; and (6) the ratio of the reservoir diameter to the slit height (h) must be sufficiently large, so that the natural streamlines of the melt in the reservoir section are not disturbed by the wall of the reservoir as the polymer melt approaches the die entrance. The rheological implications of each of these design considerations are documented in a monograph by Han.[2] If any of these design criteria is *not* met, measurements of S_{zz} can give rise to erroneous results in rheological properties, especially in P_{Exit}.

There are also some operational considerations that must be taken into account, in order to obtain reliable and meaningful results for S_{zz}, especially for P_{Exit}. It should be mentioned that, since P_{Exit} is obtained from an extrapolation of S_{zz} measured along the die axis to the exit plane of the die, a small variation in S_{zz} can have a large influence on the value of P_{Exit}. In this regard it is worth emphasizing that, even after the pressure transducers have been carefully calibrated within acceptable accuracy, one must be extremely careful in determining the zero position of each pressure transducer before measurements begin. More often than not the zero position of a pressure transducer is shifted during measurement and thus gives rise to pressure readings larger than, or smaller than, the true values. If this happens, one might obtain *negative* values of P_{Exit}. One of the most serious things that one often overlooks is the fact that an adjustment of the zero position of a pressure tranducer must be made with a minimum influence of the stresses in the polymer melt residing in the flow channel. It should be remembered that complete relaxation of the stress in a viscoelastic polymer melt may require a long time after stopping the melt flow through the die. In other words, a slight off-set of the zero position of a pressure transducer can bring about spurious readings of S_{zz}, yielding inaccurate values of P_{Exit}.

2.4. DISCUSSION

2.4.1. Correlations of P_{Exit} and N_1 with σ

Figure 2.3 gives plots of log P_{Exit} versus log σ for low-density polyethylene (LDPE) (Rexene PE143, El Paso Polyolefin Company) at two temperatures, 200 and 220 °C. These data were obtained using a slit die of 2·54 cm width and 0·127 cm height. Using the data in Fig. 2.3, values of N_1

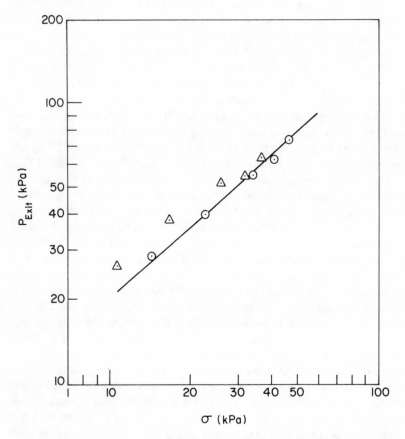

Fig. 2.3. Log P_{Exit} versus log σ for low-density polyethylene: ⊙ 200 °C; △ 220 °C.

were calculated with the aid of eqn (2.3) and the results are plotted in Fig. 2.4. For comparison purposes, values of N_1 obtained from a cone-and-plate rheometer (the Model 16 Weissenberg Rheogoniometer) are also plotted in Fig. 2.4. It is seen in Fig. 2.4 that the data obtained with the slit die are consistent with those obtained with the cone-and-plate rheometer.

Note, however, in Fig. 2.4 that the values of N_1 determined from P_{Exit}

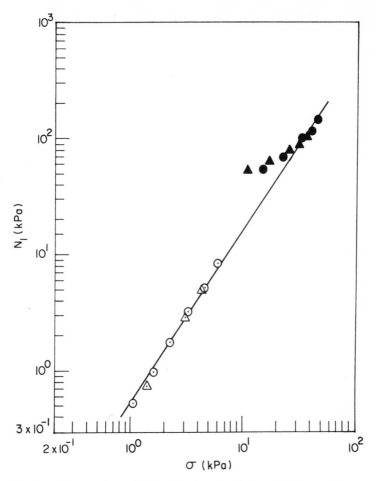

Fig. 2.4. Log N_1 versus log σ for low-density polyethylene. (a) From exit pressure data: ● 200°C; ▲ 220°C. (b) From a cone-and-plate rheometer: ⊙ 200°C; △ 220°C

start to deviate from the linear correlation between log N_1 and log σ as the value of σ becomes lower than about 25 kPa, suggesting that the exit pressure data must be taken at shear stresses greater than a certan critical value. Log N_1 versus log σ plots are given in Fig. 2.5 for polystyrene (Styron 678, Dow Chemical Company) at 200 and 220 °C, in Fig. 2.6 for high-density polyethylene (Amoco 33-360B, Amoco Chemical Company) at 180 and 200 °C, and in Fig. 2.7 for polypropylene (Profax 6423,

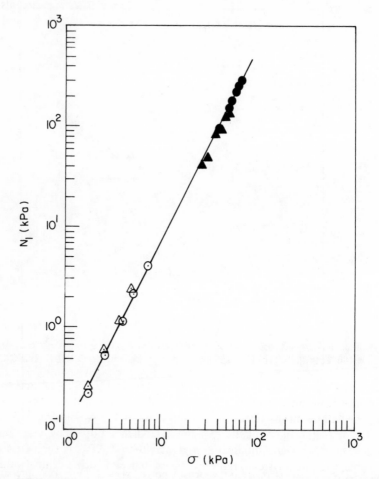

Fig. 2.5. Log N_1 versus log σ for polystyrene. (a) From exit pressure data: ● 200 °C; ▲ 220 °C. (b) From a cone-and-plate rheometer: ⊙ 200 °C; △ 220 °C.

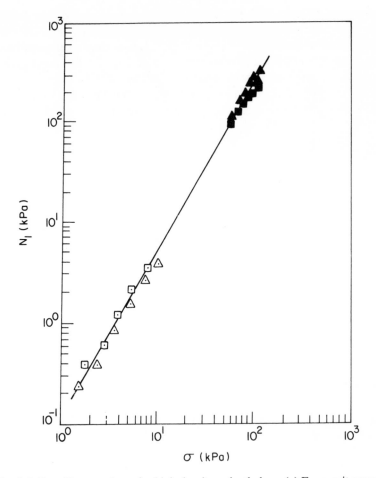

Fig. 2.6. Log N_1 versus log σ for high-density polyethylene. (a) From exit pressure data: ● 180°C; ■ 200°C. (b) From a cone-and-plate rheometer: ⊙ 180°C; ▢ 200°C.

Hercules Corporation) at 200 and 220 °C. Note in Figs. 2.5–2.7 that the N_1 values determined from P_{Exit} were obtained at σ greater than 30 kPa and that they all lie on the linear correlation between log N_1 and log σ. As a matter of fact, *almost* all the exit pressure data reported by Han and co-workers[1,2,13-24] were obtained at σ greater than 25 kPa, as summarised in Table 2.1. The physical origin for the existence of such a critical value of σ will be elaborated below, when discussing some practical limitations of the exit pressure method.

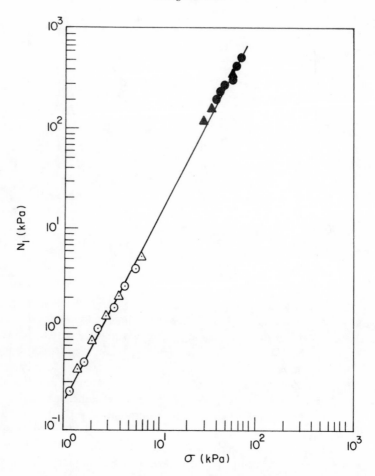

Fig. 2.7. Log N_1 versus log σ for polypropylene. (a) From exit pressure data: ●
200 °C; ▲ 220 °C. (b) From a cone-and-plate rheometer: ⊙ 200 °C; △ 220 °C.

It is significant to note in Figs. 2.4–2.7 that logarithmic plots of N_1
versus σ show *virtually* no temperature dependence. It has been reported
that the dynamic storage modulus (G') of viscoelastic polymer melts, when
plotted against the dynamic loss modulus (G'') on logarithmic coordinates,
also gives rise to correlations that become *virtually* independent of temperature.[7-11] Han and Jhon[12] have offered a theoretical interpretation of
the existence of such correlations, based on molecular theories.

TABLE 2.1
Materials and the Lower Limits of Shear Stress and Exit Pressure Used in Studies by Han and Co-workers

Material	Temp. (°C)	σ (kPa)	P_{Exit} (psig)	Ref.
LDPE, HDPE, PP, PS, PMMA	200	> 25	> 7	1
HDPE, PP	180	> 65	> 10	13
HDPE, LDPE	200	> 62	> 20	14
PS	200–240	> 30	> 5	15
HDPE, PP	200–240	> 60	> 5	16
HDPE, PP	200	> 50	> 5	17
LDPE, HDPE, PS	200	> 25	> 5	18
HDPE, LDPE	154	> 40	> 8	19
HDPE, PS	200–240	> 30	> 15	20
LDPE, HDPE	160–200	> 25	> 6	21
LDPE, HDPE, PS	200–240	> 25	> 10	22
LDPE, HDPE, PP, PS, PMMA	180–230	> 40	> 5	23
LDPE	180–220	> 35	> 5	24

There are practical limitations to each of the various rheological techniques. The use of a cone-and-plate rheometer is limited to low shear stresses (say below 20 kPa) for viscoelastic polymeric liquids, because at higher shear stresses the flow becomes unstable due to the onset of secondary flow, giving rise to erratic outputs of torque and normal force. On the other hand, the use of a slit rheometer, whose principles are described above, has limitations in that data must be taken at sufficiently high shear stresses (say above 25 kPa), so that the extrapolation procedure is valid. More of this will be elaborated on below. In this sense, the exit pressure method may be considered as high shear-stress rheometry. When a viscous molten polymer is forced to flow through a slit or capillary die, viscous shear heating can become significant at and above a certain critical value of shear stress or shear rate. Such a critical value varies with the chemical structure of polymers, so a generalization is not possible. Therefore slit rheometry is limited to shear stresses or shear rates below which viscous shear heating can be neglected.

Using finite element analysis, Tuna and Finlayson[25] determined the following relationship between P_{Exit} and N_1 in a slit die:

$$P_{Exit}/\sigma = 0.28 N_1/\sigma + 0.30 \qquad (2.4)$$

on the basis of a convected Maxwell model. It should be mentioned that the convected Maxwell model predicts that the viscosity η is independent of shear rate $\dot{\gamma}$ and first normal stress difference N_1 is proportional to $\dot{\gamma}^2$. Therefore, in predicting the flow behavior in steady shearing flow, the convected Maxwell model used by Tuna and Finlayson is not different from the second-order fluid, which was also used by Reddy and Tanner[26] who obtained the following expression:

$$P_{\text{Exit}}/\sigma = 0.26 N_1/\sigma + 0.31 \qquad (2.5)$$

In other words, eqns (2.4) and (2.5) were derived based on a constitutive equation of state that is not able to describe the shear-thinning behavior of polymeric liquids.

On the other hand, the polymer melts that give rise to a measurable exit pressure, over the particular range of shear stresses considered, also exhibit shear-thinning behavior, as may be seen in Fig. 2.8. It has been observed that, when the exit pressure is measured over a range of shear rates or shear stresses where shear-thinning behavior is absent, the magnitude of P_{Exit} is too small to be of any rheological significance and/or the extent of exit disturbances is very large, greatly affecting the accuracy of the P_{Exit} values determined. Therefore any attempt to make a quantitative

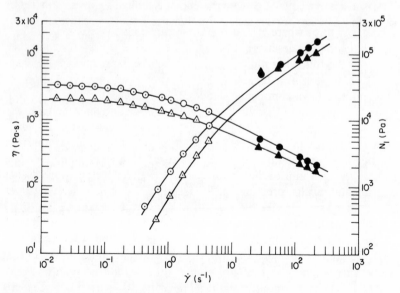

Fig. 2.8. Log η versus log $\dot{\gamma}$, and log N_1 versus log $\dot{\gamma}$, for a low-density polyethylene. (a) From exit pressure data: ● 200 °C; ▲ 220 °C. (b) From a cone-and-plate rheometer: ○ 200 °C; △ 220 °C.

comparison between experimental results of P_{Exit} obtained at $\sigma > 25\,kPa$ and computational results based on eqn (2.4) or eqn (2.5) is of no rheological significance.

In spite of the fact that the convected Maxwell model used by Tuna and Finlayson[25] has some serious deficiencies, it is clear from their computational results that finite element analysis predicts positive exit pressure in a slit die, which is consistent with the experimental results presented in Fig. 2.2 and the earlier experimental results by Han and co-workers,[1,2,13–24] but contradicts the experimental results of Lodge and de Vargas[5] who reported *negative* values of exit pressure, using only *two* pressure transducers.

Using finite element analysis, Vlachopoulos and Mitsoulis[27] also have calculated P_{Exit} and N_1 in steady shearing flow of a viscoelastic polystyrene in a slit die. They used the following empirical expressions:

$$\eta(\dot{\gamma}) = \eta_0[1 + (\lambda\dot{\gamma})^2]^{(n-1)/2} \tag{2.6}$$

to relate viscosity η to shear rate $\dot{\gamma}$, where η_0 is the zero-shear viscosity, λ is a characteristic time of the fluid and n is a constant, and

$$N_1 = A\sigma^b \tag{2.7}$$

to relate N_1 to σ, where A and b are constants, characteristic of a fluid. Note that eqn (2.6) describes shear-thinning behavior. For computations, they used the following numerical values for the parameters: $\eta_0 = 9500$ Pa.s; $\lambda = 1\cdot148\,s$; $n = 0\cdot5$; $A = 3\cdot47 \times 10^{-3}\,Pa^{1-b}$; and $b = 1\cdot66$, as representative for a commercial grade of polystyrene.

Vlachopoulos and Mitsoulis[27] concluded that the difference between the N_1 value obtained from their finite element analysis and the N_1 value calculated using eqn (2.3) *decreased* rapidly as σ increased, as summarized in Table 2.2. It is seen in Table 2.2 that, at $\sigma = 28\cdot2\,kPa$, the difference between the two approaches is only 2%. Their conclusion supports the experimental results, presented above (see Figs 2.4–2.7), that at σ values greater than, say, 25 kPa the exit disturbance can be considered to be negligibly small for all intents and purposes. Thus the exit pressure method may be used to determine N_1 at shear stresses greater than, say, 25 kPa. It can therefore be concluded that the exit pressure data reported by Lodge and de Vargas[5] and also by Baird *et al.*,[28] for σ values less than or equal to 13 kPa, may have contained significant exit disturbances and hence their results may be subject to error.

At this juncture it is worth pointing out that, instead of shear rate, shear stress should be used to specify the upper operating limit of a rheometer.

TABLE 2.2

Comparison of N_1 Values for Polystyrene Predicted by Eqn (2.3) with Those
Calculated Using Finite Element Analysis (FEA) of Vlachopoulos and Mitsoulis[27]

σ (kPa)	N_1 (kPa) from eqn (2.3)	P_{Exit} (kPa)	N_1 (kPa) from FEA	Error (%)
5·2	5·115	3·0	8·18	37·0
15·5	31·350	13·8	34·50	9·0
20·0	47·870	20·6	51·80	7·6
28·2	84·670	34·6	86·90	2·6
35·5	124·080	49·3	126·70	2·0
43·5	173·870	68·5	173·70	−0·1
51·8	232·340	89·7	231·00	−0·6

When specifying shear stress, one does not have to distinguish how viscous
a fluid is, i.e. whether the fluid under consideration is a dilute polymer
solution or a molten polymer. On the other hand, when specifying shear
rate, the upper operating limit of a rheometer varies with the type of fluid
to be investigated.

2.4.2. Extent of Flow Disturbance Near the Die Exit

The exit pressure method assumes that flow is fully developed at the exit
plane or that the extent of flow disturbances at the exit plane is negligibly
small for all intents and purposes. The subject of flow disturbances near
the exit plane of a die has been discussed by a number of investigators[29–32]
who conducted experiments either with dilute polymer solutions or with
polymer melts at very low shear rates or low shear stresses. Using flow
birefringence, Han and Drexler[33] investigated exit disturbance for a
molten polyethylene and concluded that the extent of exit disturbances,
decreases with increasing shear rate. However, there is a practical limitation to the use of flow birefringence in determining the exit disturbances
at high shear stresses. Specifically, the flow birefringence technique does
not allow one to observe isochromatic fringe patterns in a slit die at shear
stresses greater than about 15 kPa. The reason is that, as shear stress is
increased, the number of isochromatic fringe patterns in a slit die increases
very rapidly, making it almost impossible to distinguish the fringe
patterns. On the other hand, today there exists no rigorous theory that
predicts a critical value of shear rate or shear stress above which exit
disturbances may be considered negligible for all intents and purposes.

Using finite element analysis, Tuna and Finlayson[25] showed that for
Weissenberg number (W_e) of 0.6, which corresponded to a shear rate $\dot{\gamma}$ of

$0.4 \, s^{-1}$, a velocity rearrangement occurred as the fluid approached the die exit, but the velocity profiles remained *more* fully developed as the value of W_e *increased*. In their study, W_e was defined by $\lambda \dot{\gamma}$, where λ is a characteristic time of the fluid. It should be noted that the value of $\dot{\gamma} = 0.4$ corresponds to the situation where a viscoelastic polymer melt does not yet begin fully to exhibit shear-thinning behavior. Apparently, owing to numerical instabilities encountered, Tuna and Finlayson could not carry out computations at higher values of W_e, comparable to the values where significant exit pressure may be observed experimentally (i.e. $\dot{\gamma}$ values in the order of $100 \, s^{-1}$). Very recently, similar computational results have been reported by Vlachopoulos and Mitsoulis[27] who also used finite element analysis. They too encountered numerical instabilities for values of W_e greater than 2.4. Nevertheless, their computational results point out that the extent of exit disturbances *decreases* with *increasing* W_e (i.e. as the amount of energy stored in the fluid increases).

Let us now consider the flow of a viscoelastic fluid in a slit die, including the exit region, as shown schematically in Fig. 2.9. As noted above, the exit pressure method assumes that the flow remains laminar and fully developed at the exit plane. The extent to which this assumption is valid or invalid can be discussed using the concept of the Deborah number (N_D), the ratio of the material time to the process time, first introduced by Reiner.[34] In the situation under consideration (see Fig. 2.9), N_D can be represented by

$$N_D = \lambda/t_f \qquad (2.8)$$

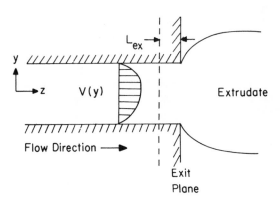

Fig. 2.9. Schematic depicting the flow in the exit region of a slit die.

where λ is the characteristic time of a fluid and t_f is the time required for the fluid to travel through the exit region. The t_f, in turn, can be expressed by $t_f = L_{ex}/\langle V \rangle$, where L_{ex} is the exit length and $\langle V \rangle$ is the average velocity of a fluid in the slit die. According to Reiner,[34] a fluid will behave more like an elastic solid when the value of N_D becomes much larger than unity. In the context of the variables defined above, we can state that when λ is much larger than t_f the fluid behaves more like an elastic solid, and thus the extent of exit disturbances will be negligible. On the other hand, when λ is much smaller than t_f the extent of exit disturbances may become significant, making the exit pressure method inapplicable.

In order to gain some physical insights into eqn (2.8) to determine the situations where the extent of exit disturbances may be negligible, we have calculated the values of N_D for low-density polyethylene (LDPE), corresponding to the flow conditions that appear in Figs 2.3 and 2.4. The results are summarized in Table 2.3. In calculating the values of N_D in Table 2.3, we have used the following numerical values for the various parameters involved: (1) the average velocity $\langle V \rangle$ was calculated from the expression

$$\langle V \rangle = \dot{\gamma}[3n/(2n + 1)](h/6) \tag{2.9}$$

where $h = 1.77$ mm and $n = 0.5$; (2) λ was estimated using the expression $\lambda = \eta_0 \bar{M}_w/\rho RT$, where η_0 is the zero-shear viscosity which is 3052 Pa.s at 200 °C and 2025 Pa.s at 220 °C, $\bar{M}_w$ is the weight-average molecular weight which is 1.41×10^5, ρ is the density of LDPE in the molten state which

TABLE 2.3
Deborah Number for the LDPE in the Exit Region of a Slit Die

	$\dot{\gamma}$ (s^{-1})	σ (kPa)	$\langle V \rangle$ (ms^{-1})	N_D
At 200 °C	28·24	14·87	$6·248 \times 10^{-3}$	0·54
	56·84	22·77	$1·882 \times 10^{-2}$	1·62
	115·11	33·98	$2·547 \times 10^{-2}$	2·20
	161·22	40·92	$3·567 \times 10^{-2}$	3·08
	214·84	46·76	$4·753 \times 10^{-2}$	4·10
At 220 °C	27·29	10·79	$6·038 \times 10^{-3}$	0·33
	54·94	16·94	$1·215 \times 10^{-2}$	0·67
	111·26	26·10	$2·462 \times 10^{-2}$	1·35
	155·84	31·95	$3·448 \times 10^{-2}$	1·89
	207·66	37·04	$4·594 \times 10^{-2}$	2·53

Note that λ is 0·1528 s at 200 °C and 0·0973 s at 220 °C.

is $716\,\mathrm{kg\,m^{-3}}$, R is the universal gas constant, $8 \cdot 314\,\mathrm{J\,mol^{-1}\,K^{-1}}$, and T is the absolute temperature; and (3) the value of L_{ex} was chosen to be the same as the slit height h, i.e. $L_{ex}/h = 1$. Experimental studies[29–32] have indicated that the L_{ex}/h ratio in a slit die is about $1 \cdot 0$ or less for dilute polymer solutions or Newtonian liquids. It should be pointed out, however, that L_{ex}/h should depend on the type of fluid and shear rate $\dot{\gamma}$. There is evidence (experimental and theoretical) suggesting that, at the same value of $\dot{\gamma}$, L_{ex}/h is much smaller for viscoelastic polymer melts than for Newtonian liquids and dilute polymer solutions, and that L_{ex}/h decreases with increasing $\lambda\dot{\gamma}$. Therefore, $L_{ex}/h = 1$ used in our calculations may be considered to be a very conservative value for the viscoelastic LDPE melt under consideration.

It is of great interest to observe in Table 2.3 that N_D is less than $1 \cdot 0$ at low shear stresses and steadily increases (exceeding $1 \cdot 0$) with increasing shear stress, and that a definite relationship appears to exist between the value of N_D and a critical value of shear stress σ at which the exit pressure data deviate from the linear log N_1 versus log σ correlation, given in Fig. 2.4. In other words, a shear stress σ of about 25 kPa, below which the data points in Fig. 2.4 deviate from the linear log N_1 versus log σ correlation, corresponds to a value of N_D slightly larger than $1 \cdot 0$. It should be emphasized at this point that the intent here is not to determine an exact value of N_D at which exit disturbances can be considered to be negligible, but to indicate that whether the extent of exit disturbances may be considered to be negligibly small or not can, for all intents and purposes, be decided upon by using the dimensionless quantity N_D. It is also clear from Table 2.3 that shear rate is not correlatable to N_D, but shear stress is, insofar as determining the flow conditions under which the extent of exit disturbances may be considered to be negligible.

Note that the seemingly low values of N_D in Table 2.3 stem from the fact that the LDPE melt considered had relatively small values of λ, i.e. $\lambda = 0 \cdot 153$ s at 200 °C and $0 \cdot 0973$ s at 220°C. It should be remembered that the value of λ, which was defined as $\lambda = \eta_0 \bar{M}_w / \rho RT$ from the molecular point of view, depends on the chemical structure (via η_0) of the polymer, the molecular weight $\bar{M}_w$ and density ρ of the polymer, and the temperature T under consideration. At very small values of λ (say $0 \cdot 01$– $0 \cdot 001$ s), which are characteristic of dilute polymer solutions and very weakly elastic polymer melts, e.g. nylon, polycarbonate, and poly(ethylene terephthalate), the values of N_D that are calculated using eqn (2.8) can be much smaller than $1 \cdot 0$ even at large values of σ. This suggests to us that, for dilute polymer solutions and very weakly elastic polymer melts, the extent of exit disturbances may never become negligible, even at large values of σ.

It can therefore be concluded that, for all intents and purposes, the extent of exit disturbances may be considered to be negligible for strongly viscoelastic polymer melts at high shear stresses (say $\sigma > 25$ kPa), justifying the extrapolation procedure for obtaining P_{Exit} and thus making the exit pressure method valid. However, this conclusion cannot be extended to dilute polymer solutions and very weakly elastic polymer melts. This then indicates that one cannot and must not make a sweeping generalization of the validity or invalidity of the exit pressure method based on information of the extent of exit disturbances observed for dilute polymer solutions or Newtonian liquids, as Carreau *et al.*[35] have done. Moreover, the use of the extrapolation procedure of Han and co-workers[1,2,13-24] in strongly viscoelastic molten polymers at high shear stresses ($\sigma > 25$ kPa) (see Table 2.1) has been criticized by Boger and Denn.[36] On the basis of the numerical computations performed by Vlachopoulos and Mitsoulis[27] (see Table 2.2) and the argument presented above using the concept of the Deborah number (see Table 2.3), we can now conclude that the argument of Boger and Denn made against the exit pressure data of Han and co-workers[1,2,13-24] is dubious.

2.4.3. Extent of Viscous Shear Heating

For very viscous polymer melts, one may encounter situations where the extent of viscous shear heating is sufficiently large, which would create *non-isothermal* flow conditions. If this happens, the viscosity of the fluid will decrease along the die axis, thus causing pressure gradients to become *nonlinear*. Under such circumstances, one should not use measurements of S_{zz} to determine η and N_1. It should be remembered that eqns (2.1) and (2.3) are valid *only* when the pressure gradient $-\partial p/\partial z$ is constant. In the past, some investigators[3,4,37,38] reported nonlinear pressure profiles and yet went ahead and calculated η and P_{Exit} from such data. We must conclude that such results are of *no* rheological significance.

The upper limit of shear stress (or shear rate) at which the extent of viscous shear heating becomes significant, making the exit pressure method inapplicable, can be predicted theoretically, by solving the equations of motion and heat transfer. For slit flow, one must solve the following equations in rectangular coordinates (x, y, z):

$$\frac{\partial}{\partial y}\left(\eta \frac{\partial v_z}{\partial y}\right) = \frac{\partial p}{\partial z} \tag{2.10}$$

$$\rho C_p v_z \frac{\partial T}{\partial z} = k \frac{\partial^2 T}{\partial y^2} + \eta \left(\frac{\partial v_z}{\partial y}\right)^2 \tag{2.11}$$

where ρ is the density, C_p is the specific heat, k is the thermal conductivity, and η is the viscosity.

For non-Newtonian viscoelastic fluids, one must express η in terms of velocity gradients. For fully developed flow, it is reasonable to use the following form of the truncated power law relationship:

$$\eta(T, \dot{\gamma}) = \begin{cases} k_0 \exp\left[-b(T - T_0)\right] & \text{for } \dot{\gamma} \leqslant \dot{\gamma}_0 \\ k_0 \exp\left[-b(T - T_0)\right](\dot{\gamma}/\dot{\gamma}_0)^{(n-1)} & \text{for } \dot{\gamma} > \dot{\gamma}_0 \end{cases} \tag{2.12}$$

where $\dot{\gamma}$ is shear rate, T_0 is a reference temperature, and $\dot{\gamma}_0$ is the value of shear rate at which η deviates from Newtonian behavior. If viscous shear heating is significant, the solution of eqns (2.10) and (2.11) will yield temperature profiles that vary with both y and z.

For the LDPE used to generate the information on η and N_1 given in Figs 2.4 and 2.8, we have estimated the temperature rise due to viscous shear heating, by numerically solving eqns (2.10) and (2.11) with the aid of eqn (2.12). Our computational results indicate that (1) at $\dot{\gamma} = 400\,\text{s}^{-1}$, which corresponds to $\sigma = 54\cdot8\,\text{kPa}$, the average temperature of the LDPE melt at the exit plane of the die (with $7\cdot62\,\text{cm}$ die length) would have risen from 200 to $200\cdot6\,°\text{C}$, and (2) at $\dot{\gamma} = 600\,\text{s}^{-1}$, which corresponds to $\sigma = 67\cdot1\,\text{kPa}$, the average temperature of the LDPE melt at the die exit plane would have risen from 200 to $200\cdot9\,°\text{C}$. Note in Table 2.3 that the maximum value of σ used in Fig. 2.4 is $46\cdot76\,\text{kPa}$. Therefore we can conclude for all intents and purposes that the exit pressure data in Fig. 2.4 have negligible effect of viscous shear heating. It should be noted that, as the shear rate or shear stress is increased continuously, one may reach a point where the extent of viscous shear heating can no longer be neglected, i.e. there exists an upper limit of shear rate or shear stress at which a slit rheometer may no longer be useful for generating the rheological properties of polymer melts under isothermal conditions. It should be emphasized, however, that such an upper limit of shear rate or shear stress would depend upon the viscosity and thus the structure of the polymer.

Therefore a generalization of the value of the upper limit is not possible for all fluids. Chapter 5 deals more fully with the subject of viscous heating.

2.5. CONCLUDING REMARKS

The rotational method using a cone-and-plate rheometer is considered as low shear-stress rheometry, while the exit pressure method using a slit or capillary rheometer can be considered as high shear-stress rheometry. The exit pressure method using a slit die allows one to determine η and N_1 for viscoelastic polymer melts at high stresses (say for σ greater than 25 kPa), where the exit disturbances can be neglected. This is precisely the reason why *almost* all the exit pressure data reported by Han and co-workers[1,2,13-24] were taken at σ greater than 25 kPa (see Table 2.1). On the other hand, at low shear stresses the extent of exit disturbances may become significant enough to make the exit pressure method inapplicable. Therefore the exit pressure data reported by Lodge and de Vargas[5] and Baird *et al.*[28] for low-density polyethylene and polystyrene melts at low shear stresses ($\sigma \leqslant 13$ kPa) in a slit die may have been appreciably affected by exit disturbances, and hence the accuracy of their results is questionable. Furthermore, based on the argument presented above using the concept of the Deborah number, the use of dilute polymer solutions or very weakly elastic polymer melts can give rise to significant exit disturbances, making the exit pressure method inapplicable. It can therefore be concluded that the argument made by Boger and Denn[36] against the exit pressure data obtained for strongly viscoelastic polymer melts at high σ (say greater than 25 kPa) is inapplicable.

An additional limitation on the exit pressure method is that, at very large values of σ, viscous shear heating can become significant, making the exit pressure method inapplicable. When viscous shear heating becomes significant, nonlinear pressure profiles may be observed along the die axis. Thus the data taken under such flow conditions should not be used to determine exit pressures. Therefore the accuracy of exit pressure data based on nonlinear pressure profiles, reported by Laun[3] and Rauwendaal and Fernandez,[4] remains very questionable.

It is concluded that the exit pressure method using a slit die can give rise to reliable rheological information on η and N_1 over a limited range of σ for viscoelastic molten polymers, such that σ is large enough to make the exit disturbances negligible and yet low enough not to cause significant viscous shear heating. However, such a limited range of shear stress seems to lie within the region where many polymer processing operations are practiced in industry.

The use of a slit die allows one to determine η and N_1 for multiphase polymer systems, including heterogeneous polymer blends, particulate-filled polymer melts, and polymer melts containing volatile organic solvents.[39] The use of a slit die allows one to mount pressure transducers flush with the die wall, so that dead spaces created by pressure-tap holes can be avoided. This consideration is important in situations where one must deal with particulate-filled polymer melts or polymers that may easily undergo thermal degradation or cross-linking reactions in stagnant pressure-tap holes.

A cone-and-plate rheometer is not suitable for determining the rheological properties of polymeric liquids containing volatile solvents at temperatures higher than the boiling point of the solvent. However, the use of a slit rheometer allows one, at least, to determine the viscosities of such mixtures, as long as the measurements of wall normal stress are taken in the region where phase separation does not occur (i.e. as long as the pressure gradient is constant). Indeed, Han and Ma[40,41] have used a slit rheometer to measure the viscosities of mixtures of polystyrene and a fluorocarbon blowing agent, and mixtures of low-density polyethylene and a fluorocarbon blowing agent, at temperatures above the boiling points of the fluorocarbon blowing agents. It was reported by Han and Ma[40,41] that, as the mixture of molten polymer and volatile solvent approaches the die exit, phase separation may occur, yielding nonlinear pressure profiles near the die exit. In such situations it is not possible to obtain any accurate rheological information near the die exit. However, one can overcome this difficulty by installing an environmental chamber at the exit of the die and then pressurizing the chamber to such an extent that phase separation inside the die can be precluded. As long as phase separation does not occur inside the die, giving rise to linear pressure profiles, the exit pressure method can be used to determine η and N_1 for mixtures of a molten polymer and a volatile solvent.

REFERENCES

1. C. D. Han, *Trans. Soc. Rheol.,* 1974, **18**, 163.
2. C. D. Han, *Rheology in Polymer Processing*, Academic Press, New York, 1976, Ch. 5.
3. H. M. Laun, *Rheol. Acta,* 1983, **22**, 171.

4. C. Rauwendaal and F. Fernandez, *Polym. Eng. Sci.*, 1985, **25**, 765.
5. A. S. Lodge and L. de Vargas, *Rheol. Acta*, 1983, **22**, 151.
6. J. M. Davis, J. F. Hutton and K. Walters, *J. Phys. (D)*, 1973, **6**, 2259.
7. C. D. Han and K. W. Lem, *Polym. Eng. Rev.*, 1983, **2**, 135.
8. H. K. Chuang and C. D. Han, *J. Appl. Polym. Sci.*, 1984, **29**, 2205.
9. C. D. Han and H. K. Chuang, *J. Appl. Polym. Sci.*, 1985, **30**, 2431.
10. C. D. Han and H. K. Chuang, *J. Appl. Polym. Sci.*, 1985, **30**, 4431.
11. C. D. Han, Y. J. Ma and S. G. Chu, *J. Appl. Polym. Sci.*, 1986, **32**, 5597.
12. C. D. Han and M. S. Jhon, *J. Appl. Polym. Sci.*, 1986, **32**, 3809.
13. C. D. Han, M. Charles and W. Philippoff, *Trans. Soc. Rheol.*, 1970, **14**, 393.
14. C. D. Han, T. C. Yu and K. U. Kim, *J. Appl. Polym. Sci.*, 1971, **15**, 1149.
15. C. D. Han and T. C. Yu, *Rheol. Acta*, 1971, **10**, 398.
16. C. D. Han, *J. Appl. Polym. Sci.*, 1971, **15**, 2567.
17. C. D. Han, *A.I.Ch.E.J.*, 1972, **18**, 116.
18. C. D. Han, *J. Appl. Polym. Sci.*, 1973, **17**, 1289.
19. C. D. Han, *J. Appl. Polym. Sci.*, 1973, **17**, 1403.
20. C. D. Han and Y. W. Kim, *Trans. Soc. Rheol.*, 1975, **19**, 245.
21. C. D. Han and C. A. Villamizar, *J. Appl. Polym. Sci.*, 1978, **22**, 1677.
22. C. D. Han and R. Shetty, *Polym. Eng. Sci.*, 1978, **18**, 180.
23. C. D. Han, Y. J. Kim and H. K. Chuang, *Polym. Eng. Rev.*, 1933, **3**, 1.
24. C. D. Han, Y. J. Kim, K. H. Chuang and T. H. Kwack, *J. Appl. Polym. Sci.*, 1983, **28**, 3435.
25. N. Y. Tuna and B. A. Finlayson, *J. Rheol.*, 1984, **28**, 79.
26. K. R. Reddy and R. I. Tanner, *Trans. Soc. Rheol.*, 1978, **22**, 661.
27. J. Vlachopoulos and E. Mitsoulis, *Polym. Eng. Rev.*, 1985, **5**, 173.
28. D. G. Baird, M. D. Read and R. D. Pike, *Polym. Eng. Sci.*, 1986, **26**, 225.
29. W. R. Schowalter and R. C. Allen, *Trans. Soc. Rheol.*, 1975, **19**, 129.
30. J. R. Clermont, J. M. Pierrard and O. Scrivener, *J. Non-Newt. Fluid Mech.*, 1976, **1**, 175.
31. B. A. Whipple and C. T. Hill, *A.I.Ch.E.J.*, 1978, **24**, 664.
32. M. Gottlieb and R. B. Bird, *Ind. Eng. Chem. Fund.*, 1979, **18**, 357.
33. C. D. Han and L. H. Drexler, *Trans. Soc. Rheol.*, 1973, **17**, 659.
34. M. Reiner, *Phys. Today*, 1964, January, 62.
35. P. J. Carreau, L. Choplin and J. R. Clermont, *Polym. Eng. Sci.*, 1985, **25**, 669.
36. D. V. Boger and M. M. Denn, *J. Non-Newt. Fluid Mech.*, 1980, **6**, 163.
37. J. L. Leblanc, *Polymer*, 1976, **17**, 235.
38. N.Y. Tuna and B.A. Finlayson, *J. Rheol.*, 1988, **32**, 285.
39. C. D. Han, *Multiphase Flow in Polymer Processing*, Academic Press, New York, 1981.
40. C. D. Han and C. Y. Ma, *J. Appl. Polym. Sci.*, 1983, **28**, 831.
41. C. D. Han and C. Y. Ma, *J. Appl. Polym. Sci.*, 1983, **28**, 851.

Chapter 3

Converging Dies

A. G. GIBSON

Department of Materials Science and Engineering, University of Liverpool, UK

NOTATION

Subscripts 0 and 1 refer to die entry and exit respectively.

R radial distance in cylindrical coordinates; die or capillary radius

x axial distance from die cone apex

L capillary length

r, θ, ϕ spherical coordinates, based on die cone apex

α die semi-angle; $\breve{\alpha}$, value for minimum pressure

a surface area of spherical shell

b	radius of spherical shell in exit region
V	volume of truncated spherical exit region
β	angle subtended at axis by die exit at distance b
Re	Reynolds number
ρ	density
v	velocity; v_r, r-direction component; $\bar{v}$, mean value
σ	elongating stress
τ	shear stress
$\dot{\varepsilon}$	elongational strain rate
$\dot{\gamma}$	shear strain rate; $\dot{\gamma}_A$, apparent wall shear rate at the die exit or in the capillary
A, n	extensional power law constants
B, m	shear power law constants
λ	extensional viscosity or anisotropic extensional viscosity; λ_A, apparent ($n = 1$) value. Subscripts $\parallel$ and $\perp$ refer to directions parallel and perpendicular to anisotropic reference direction. λ_{Res} refers to resin phase only
η	shear viscosity or anisotropic shear viscosity; η_{Res} resin phase shear viscosity; η_A apparent ($m = 1$) shear viscosity
a_{ij}	coefficients in the reciprocal viscosity tensor
P	reservoir hydrostatic pressure
P_{Ent}, P_{Cap}	contributions of entry flow and capillary flow towards total pressure
$P_{S_{Ent}}, P_{E_{Ent}}$	contributions of shear dissipation and extensional dissipation towards P_{Ent}
P'_{Ent}	contribution of exit transition region
$\check{P}_{Ent}$	minimum value
P^*	dimensionless pressure
p	hydrostatic pressure
Q	volume flow rate
V_f, l, d	volume fraction; length and diameter of reinforcement

3.1. INTRODUCTION

Although the flow behaviour of non-Newtonian fluids in channels of constant cross-section is well understood, and there are established models to describe it, the same is not yet true of flow in convergences where the extensional strain rate becomes significant compared to the wall shear rate. Various methods of describing the convergent flow behaviour of polymeric liquids in dies and in other regimes have formed the basis of recent reviews[1-3] (see also Chapter 8).

In rheological measurements involving flow through a converging die into a capillary, the usual procedure is to eliminate the pressure drops which occur in the convergence and at the die exit by using the Bagley plot procedure described in Chapter 1. The entrance effect, which is a measure of the energy dissipated in extensional and shear flow in that region, is usually large compared with the exit effect. Orifice entry pressure data, obtained by extrapolating the Bagley plot to zero die length, contain useful information which can be used to calculate pressure drops at convergences of known geometry. Although the theory relating entry pressure to flow properties is still imperfect, the entry pressure data can nevertheless be used to obtain good estimates of extensional viscosity in a strain rate regime where other techniques do not work well.

Although many industrially processed fluids exhibit anomalous behaviour in convergent flow, polymer moulding materials are one of the most important classes. The relationships described in this chapter are particularly applicable to polymer melts and solutions but could also refer to a range of other fluids, including concentrated fibre suspensions and some liquid crystal polymer systems.

In the context of polymer processing, important examples of flow resembling that in a convergent die include flow at the exit of an extruder into a choke or die, flow into fibre spinnerets or into film dies, flow in the nozzles of injection moulding machines, and mould flow involving changes in runner cross-section or flow through gates.

A number of simplifying assumptions will be made in this chapter. 'Creeping flow' will be assumed; that is, Reynolds numbers will be taken to be low enough for inertia effects to be neglected in comparison to viscous forces. The Reynolds number for a fluid flowing in a convergent die may be taken to be

$$\mathrm{Re} \;=\; \frac{2\rho \bar{v}_r R_1}{\eta} \;=\; \frac{2\rho Q}{\pi R_1 \eta} \tag{3.1}$$

The results of Sutterby[4] show that inertia effects begin to have a significant effect on the velocity field at Re values greater than about 1, so this assumption is reasonable for the majority of polymer processes, although there may be small errors at the highest shear rates attainable in injection moulding.

As mentioned above, in addition to the pressure drop at the die entry, the Bagley ends effect contains a contribution due to the die exit pressure loss. The exit loss, which has been discussed extensively elsewhere (e.g. by Han[5]), is often related to the elastic properties of polymer melts. Although this is an important effect, it generally represents only a small proportion of the overall pressure drop, so it will be neglected here.

It is recognised that both the extensional and shear response of polymeric liquids contain elastic effects, some of the deformation in the die entry and capillary being recoverable. However, in the flow laws used here, no stipulation will be made regarding the relative proportions of viscous and elastic strains. There may be virtue in the argument advanced by Cogswell[3] and other workers that, for fairly large ratios of reservoir to die radius, the elastic strain value saturates at a relatively small proportion of the total strain.

Several types of constitutive equation have been used to represent polymer flow behaviour, taking into account effects such as shear-thinning and strain history. These models, which have been reviewed by Han[5] usually describe the response to flow in terms of the invariants of the strain rate and strain tensors. Although they can describe important viscoelastic effects, they generally treat the material as being isotropic in its response to strain and strain rate, despite abundant evidence, such as the results of flow-induced birefringence measurements, that high levels of material anisotropy can occur in extensional flow. Another disadvantage of the more complex forms of flow model is the amount of experimentation required to measure all the constants needed to describe a material. Given the large number of commercially available polymer compounds and the urgent need for data banks of flow properties obtained under realistic conditions, it is necessary to re-examine the possibility of using simple constitutive relationships containing the minimum number of constants.

The simplest realistic way of describing the flow of a polymer melt with any degree of generality is to assume that extensional flow and shear flow behaviour are each governed by power law relationships of the form

$$\sigma = A\dot{\varepsilon}^n \tag{3.2}$$

$$\tau = B\dot{\gamma}^m \tag{3.3}$$

The extensional and shear viscosities at a particular strain rate will therefore be given by

$$\lambda = \frac{\sigma}{\dot{\varepsilon}} = A\dot{\varepsilon}^{n-1} \tag{3.4}$$

$$\eta = \frac{\tau}{\dot{\gamma}} = B\dot{\gamma}^{m-1} \qquad (3.5)$$

The fact that λ and η are independent and are not constrained by the relationship $\lambda = 3\eta$, which would apply for an incompressible Newtonian fluid, has certain implications which will be discussed later, the main one being that the fluid is anisotropic. Equations (3.2)–(3.5) are not invariant with respect to direction within the fluid: eqns (3.2) and (3.4) only apply to extension in the principal orientation direction of the fluid, and eqns (3.3) and (3.5) only apply to shear where the velocity vector is parallel to that direction.

Although the assumption of power law behaviour implies that the log viscosity vs. log strain rate plot is linear, it does enable behaviour to be modelled fairly accurately over a particular range of strain rates. It may be necessary in some circumstances to use different sets of power law constants for different strain rate regions. An alternative and somewhat less accurate approach, which avoids the non-linearities inherent in the power law model, is to assume that $n = m = 1$ and use the simplified expressions obtained to calculate 'apparent' values of extensional and shear viscosity, λ_A and η_A (λ is preferred to η_E because of the numerous subscripts used later). The subscript, A, distinguishes these quantities from those defined in eqns (3.4) and (3.5).

Finally, viscous heating and pressure effects will be neglected. It was earlier concluded that flow data could generally be corrected for viscous heating by applying a 'mean temperature' correction.[6,7] The loss of accuracy encountered by omitting this correction is not usually too great —particularly when the data are to be used in flow calculations for situations also involving a temperature rise. Pressure effects can also be significant[8] and may be corrected for. The results as presented here have not been corrected for either of these effects, but the application of the corrections would not alter their significance.

3.2. BEHAVIOUR OF POLYMER MELTS, SOLUTIONS AND FIBRE SUSPENSIONS

Figure 3.1 illustrates schematically the way in which shear and extensional viscosity of a polymer melt or solution may vary with strain rate. The shear viscosity shows the well known Newtonian region at low shear rates,

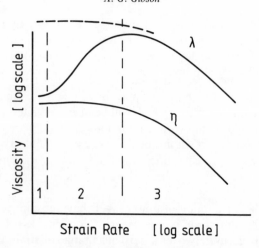

Fig. 3.1. Schematic illustration of the variation of extensional viscosity and shear viscosity with strain rate for polymer melts or solutions. The dashed curve shows extensional viscosity behaviour of a fibre suspension.

followed by a transition to power law behaviour at high shear rates, corresponding to the onset of molecular orientation and the break-up of entanglements. Many of the more important industrial processes operate in the power law region.

The probable form of extensional behaviour, shown for the unfilled resin, was suggested by Lamonte and Han[9] amongst others and has been discussed by Han.[5] There is not yet a universally accepted explanation for the shape of this relationship. At sufficiently low strain rates, the fluid is Newtonian with $\lambda/\eta = 3$. However, with increasing stretch rate, the level of molecular orientation in the stretch direction increases, giving increased resistance to extensional deformation, so the extensional viscosity increases. Eventually a maximum level of molecular extension is achieved, then the extensional viscosity begins to fall in a similar manner to the shear viscosity. This fall, which is not observed with all polymer systems, may be associated with the break-up of entanglements.

There are therefore three principal regions of materials behaviour:

(1) Newtonian at low strain rates
(2) Shear thinning, but extension thickening at intermediate strain rates
(3) Shear thinning and extension thinning at high strain rates

Flows concerned with polymer extrusion often involve strain rates in the range 50–1000 s^{-1}. These may correspond to either of regions (2) or (3), depending on the material. Injection moulding, which involves higher strain rates in the region 500–10 000 s^{-1}, usually corresponds to region (3). Under processing conditions it is not unusual to encounter values of λ/η, the Trouton ratio, in the range 30–1000. This implies a considerably greater resistance to extensional flow compared with the Newtonian case.

With some systems the high strain rate region of extensional flow may not be observable due to the onset of melt fracture.

Where fluids contain suspended fibres, high Trouton ratios can result solely from the fibre alignment which occurs at convergences. Batchelor[10] proposed the following equation to describe the extensional viscosity of a suspension of aligned fibres in terms of the shear viscosity of the fluid:

$$\lambda = \eta_{\text{Res}} \left(3 + \frac{4V_{\text{f}}(l/d)^2}{3 \ln (c/V_{\text{f}})} \right) \tag{3.6}$$

Although Batchelor only claimed validity for this at relatively low fibre volume fractions, the author's own results suggest that it may be used with fitted values of c in the range 0·907–3·628 for volume fractions up to about 0·3. In the case of polymer moulding materials containing fibres, both molecular orientation and fibre orientation effects can occur simultaneously to give high Trouton ratios. The fibre orientation effect will be strain, rather than strain rate dependent, so this effect will persist even at low strain rates, as shown in Fig. 3.1. The Batchelor model can be modified to take into account the case where the fluid has a high extensional viscosity:

$$\lambda = \lambda_{\text{Res}}(1 - V_{\text{f}}) + V_{\text{f}}\eta_{\text{Res}} \left(\frac{4(l/d)^2}{3 \ln (c/V_{\text{f}})} \right) \tag{3.7}$$

With some polymer moulding materials containing fibres, the molecular orientation and fibre orientation effects may be of similar magnitude at processing strain rates. In this case, as was observed with polypropylene,[8] the addition of fibres produces little apparent change in flow properties.

3.3. CAPILLARY FLOW EXPERIMENTS

The procedure for investigating shear flow properties of non-Newtonian fluids using a capillary rheometer involves measurement of a flow rate and a pressure drop, as discussed in Chapter 1. In instruments of the piston–cylinder type, the flow rate is easily measured from the piston displacement, provided that leakage past the piston is negligible, and the pressure drop can be obtained from the piston load, provided that friction is negligible. In some circumstances it is necessary to use a pressure transducer to measure the upstream reservoir pressure. The location of transducers requires careful consideration if meaningful results are to be obtained. Ideally the transducer should be situated far enough upstream of the converging die for it to be unaffected by the die entry flow pattern. If the fluid is already beginning to converge at the point of pressure measurement, the stress may not be hydrostatic and it will be unclear what the transducer is actually measuring. It is also desirable that the velocity upstream is as low as possible to minimise the normal stress effects. This requires the ratio of reservoir to capillary diameter to be as large as practicable.

Workers may be tempted to place transducers within the conical region of convergent dies, or even at the point where the cone ends and the capillary begins, with the aim of eliminating the die entry pressure drop. This is not advisable, as there is a considerable difference between the axial and transverse stresses in these regions, so the pressure is not purely hydrostatic. Location of transducers within the capillary itself is not advisable, as the quantity measured here would be the sum of the hydrostatic pressure and the normal stress due to the Weissenberg effect. Although normal stress effects can, in principle, be measured by using transducers situated at different points along the capillary, the technique is cumbersome and prone to error with small diameter capillaries. A slit die geometry is more appropriate for this type of experiment. The Han rheometer (Chapter 2), which is equipped with a slit die rather than a capillary, makes use of this principle to measure both shear viscosity and normal stress difference. In short, the most useful place to situate a transducer for routine capillary flow measurements is at a point a reasonable distance upstream from the die.

A wide range of laboratory equipment is now available for capillary rheometry, as discussed in Chapter 7. Several different means of applying pressure to the reservoir are used, including weights, gas pressure and the use of screw-driven testing machines. One feature of most laboratory rheometers is their relatively small size. Many have a barrel diameter of the order of 10 mm, enabling them to produce data from quite small quantities of material and minimising the time required for thermal equilibration. Laboratory rheometers also have disadvantages: the process history which they impose on the material differs from that in real processes, there being no shearing and homogenisation prior to entry into the die. Moreover, the scale of the flow regime is much smaller than that in the real equipment. The latter effect may be important with filled and reinforced materials because of the possibility of size effects when the capillary dimensions are comparable to the length of the reinforcement. For these reasons there is current interest in applying instrumentation to full scale processing equipment to obtain rheological data.

Figure 3.2 shows instrumentation for capillary rheometry using an injection moulding machine. Flow rate is measured by a displacement tranducer attached to the carriage of the machine. Pressure drop is measured by the transducer shown. This type of experimental arrangement has been used to obtain flow data under injection moulding conditions on DMC,[6,7,11] unfilled and glass reinforced polypropylene,[12] and unfilled and glass reinforced nylon 66.[13,14] Equipment of similar design has been used by other workers with polypropylene.[8]

In addition to the advantage of making rheological measurements under the same conditions as the process to which they relate, there are other advantages to this technique. The low cost of microprocessor-based data capture equipment enables existing moulding machines to be converted for rheometry at a lower cost than that of laboratory rheometry equipment. Since instrumentation need not impair the use of a moulding machine for its original purpose, there is interest in using on-line rheometry as a routine quality and process control technique. Instrumental moulding machines also have some disadvantages compared with

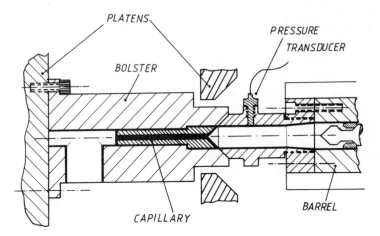

Fig. 3.2. Rheometer head for use with an injection moulding machine.

laboratory scale equipment: the quantity of material required for measurements is much larger and, because there is less control over the temperature of the material being tested, the reproducibility of data is not quite so good.

3.4. TREATMENT OF CAPILLARY FLOW DATA

The pressure drop when a power law fluid flows in a cylindrical capillary is given by the well known expression

$$P_{Cap} = \frac{2BL}{R_1^{(1+3m)}} \left(\frac{1 + 3m}{\pi m} \right)^m Q^m = \frac{2BL}{R_1} \left(\frac{1 + 3m}{4m} \right)^m \dot{\gamma}_A^m \quad (3.8)$$

The quantity $\dot{\gamma}_A$ is the apparent Newtonian wall shear rate, which is given by

$$\dot{\gamma}_A = \frac{4Q}{\pi R_1^3} \quad (3.9)$$

When $m = 1$, the Newtonian case, eqn (3.8) reduces to the Hagen–Poiseuille equation:

$$P_{Cap} = \frac{8\eta_A LQ}{\pi R_1^4} \quad (3.10)$$

Ignoring exit losses, the total pressure drop in a capillary flow experiment is given by

$$P = P_{Ent} + P_{Cap} \quad (3.11)$$

where P_{Ent} corresponds to pressure losses in the convergent part of the die.

The usual practice is to eliminate the entry pressure loss by performing measurements with a range of dies of different length, but having the same diameter and entry geometry. A plot of total pressure against die length to radius ratio, the Bagley plot, is then made, as shown in Fig. 3.3. The entry pressure drop, determined from the intercept of this graph is then subtracted from the total measured pressure drop to give the capillary pressure drop. This procedure must always be performed if accurate values of the flow parameters are required (see Chapter 1).

One short-cut method has been proposed[15] which can be used if the Bagley plots are known to be linear. Only two sets of measurements are

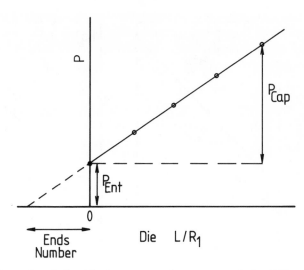

Fig. 3.3. Schematic relationship between total pressure and die L/R_1 ratio at constant flow rate (Bagley plot).

taken: one with an orifice die which can be taken as having zero length, and another with a capillary die having a high length/radius ratio. The orifice die pressure is taken to be equal to the Bagley correction and subtracted from the capillary die pressure. Some double-barrelled rheometers have been made to enable both measurements to be made simultaneously.

Experimenters are warned against a dubious procedure which is often used—that of performing measurements with a die of very large aspect ratio and assuming that the ends correction is small enough to be ignored. This frequently gives invalid results, particularly at the high strain rates involved in injection moulding. Although the ends correction may well be small for Newtonian fluids, it is seldom small enough to be neglected with polymeric liquids having a high Trouton ratio.

As an example of the behaviour of polymer moulding compounds at fairly high shear rates, Fig. 3.4 shows results obtained on unfilled and glass reinforced polypropylene melts. These show that, rather than being a small correction, the ends effect can often represent a significant proportion of the total pressure drop. The data in Fig. 3.4 show the similarity in flow behaviour between unreinforced and short fibre reinforced polypropylenes. It should, however, be noted that the polypropylene resins

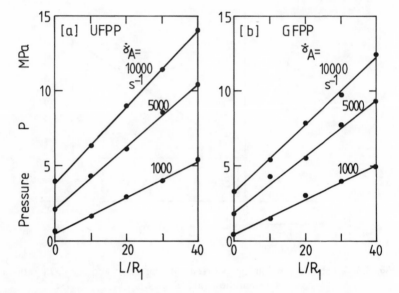

Fig. 3.4. Total pressure vs. die L/R_1 ratio at different values of shear rate for (a) UFPP, an unfilled injection moulding grade of polypropylene (ICI GWM 101), and (b) GFPP, a polypropylene grade containing 30% wt of glass (ICI HW60 GR30); die entry angle 45 °; die radius 2 mm; temperature 240 °C.

were not the same in each case, the resin in the glass reinforced material having a somewhat lower molecular weight.

The ends correction can be expressed either as a pressure, or as an 'ends number' corresponding to the negative intercept of the plot on the horizontal axis. The ends number is the length of capillary, expressed in capillary radii, which would give a pressure drop equivalent to the entry effect.

Although the numerical value of the Bagley correction is usually discarded after the correction has been made, it contains useful information on extensional flow behaviour, which could in principle be used to calculate the pressure drop for flow in convergences.

Routine rheological measurements are generally made using dies of just one cone semi-angle, often 90 ° (flat entry) or 45 °. It would, of course, be necessary to propose a model for entry flow if results obtained at one die angle are to be used to predict flow behaviour at other die angles. Possible models will be discussed later in this chapter. However, if measurements of the entry effect are made using dies of several different entry angles, these data alone, without the use of further theory, could be used to calculate the pressure drop in a convergence of any arbitrary geometry, for a particular value of die angle.

To characterise entry flow it is useful to define a dimensionless entry pressure, P^*, given by

$$P^* = \frac{P_{Ent}}{\eta \dot{\gamma}_A} \tag{3.12}$$

The material entry flow behaviour can then be described by a plot of P^* against die angle. An example of this is shown in Fig. 3.5, which contains data from three different types of nylon 66 moulding compound. The Bagley plots in Fig. 3.5(a) indicate that unfilled nylon 66 melt shows a relatively small entry pressure for a polymeric material. Adding short glass fibres increases both the shear viscosity and the entry pressure. The 'long fibre' material, which contains 10 mm glass fibres, shows a substantially larger entry effect. The large entry effect with the LF material is also

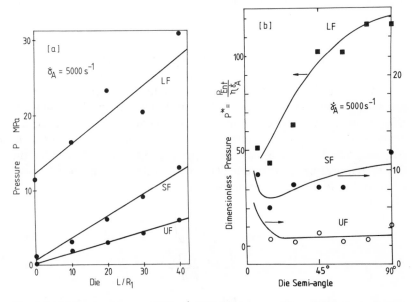

Fig. 3.5. (a) Bagley plots at $5000\,s^{-1}$ ($45°$ die entry angle), and (b) dimensionless entry pressure vs. die angle at the same shear rate, for three grades of nylon 66 moulding material at $285°C$: UF, unfilled (ICI Maranyl A100); SF, filled with 50% wt of conventional short glass fibres (ICI Maranyl A690); LF, filled with 50% wt of 10 mm long glass fibres (ICI Verton). Die bore radius 2 mm.

apparent in the dimensionless pressure plot of Fig. 3.5(b). The shape of the pressure vs. die angle plot is clearly different for the three materials.

The entry pressure for any given convergence angle can be found, using a rearranged version of eqn (3.12). This approach should give accurate results provided that the value of $\dot{\gamma}_A$ is in the same region as that in which P^* was determined, and provided also that

$$1 \gg \frac{R_1^3}{R_0^3}$$

The rearranged form of eqn (3.12) can be modified to deal with convergences where the exit/entrance ratio is not small enough to satisfy this, by observing the form of relationships discussed later in the chapter, such as eqn (3.21) or eqn (3.38). This gives

$$P_{Ent} = P^* \eta \dot{\gamma}_A \left(1 - \frac{R_1^3}{R_0^3} \right) \tag{3.13}$$

The dimensionless entry pressure, P^*, can be shown to be numerically equal to half the Bagley ends number.

3.5. FLOW IN CONVERGENCES OF SHALLOW ANGLE

Provided that the convergence angle is shallow enough to allow the extensional component of flow to be neglected, the problem may be treated simply as a case of laminar flow in a conduit of slowly changing cross-section. Consider the thin section, of thickness dx and radius R, perpendicular to the die axis shown in Fig. 3.6. From eqn (3.8), the differential pressure drop due to shear flow in this element, being equivalent to that in a tube of length $-dx$ and radius R, is

$$dP_{Ent} = 2B \left(\frac{1 + 3m}{\pi m} \right)^m Q^m \frac{dx}{R^{1+3m}}$$

$$= \frac{2B}{\tan \alpha} \left(\frac{1 + 3m}{\pi m} \right)^m Q^m \frac{dR}{R^{1+3m}} \tag{3.14}$$

since $R/x = \tan \alpha$ and $dx = dR/\tan \alpha$. This can then be integrated from R_0 to R_1, giving

$$P_{Ent} = \frac{2B}{3m \tan \alpha} \left(\frac{1 + 3m}{4m} \right)^m \dot{\gamma}_A^m \left(1 - \left(\frac{R_1}{R_0} \right)^{3m} \right) \tag{3.15}$$

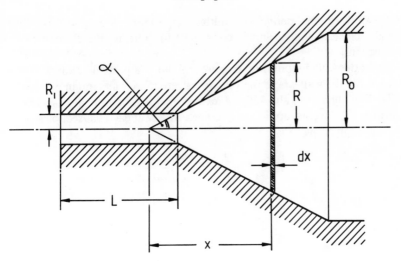

Fig. 3.6. Die entry flow geometry and nomenclature in cylindrical coordinates.

For $m = 1$ this reduces to

$$P_{\text{Ent}} = \frac{2\eta_A \dot{\gamma}_A}{3 \tan \alpha} \left(1 - \frac{R_1^3}{R_0^3} \right) \tag{3.16}$$

3.6. COGSWELL'S MODEL

Methods of treating the problem of conical die flow have been reviewed by Forsyth[2] and by Cogswell[3] and are mentioned in Chapter 8. The majority of models give expressions for the entry pressure drop which contain two terms, corresponding to shear flow and extensional flow:

$$P_{\text{Ent}} = P_{S_{\text{Ent}}} + P_{E_{\text{Ent}}} \tag{3.17}$$

Cogswell[16] considered the forces on an element as in Fig. 3.6 and derived expressions for $P_{S_{\text{Ent}}}$ and $P_{E_{\text{Ent}}}$ by assuming that the velocity profile at each flat section in the die was similar to that in a parallel-sided capillary of the same radius. This assumption is the same as that which led to eqn (3.14), so the shear contribution is given by

$$P_{S_{\text{Ent}}} = \frac{2B}{3m \tan \alpha} \left(\frac{1 + 3m}{4m} \right)^m \dot{\gamma}_A^m \left(1 - \left(\frac{R_1}{R_0} \right)^{3m} \right) \tag{3.18}$$

[Cogswell's original derivation omitted the term $((1 + 3m)/4m)^m$ which is usually close to unity. This is equivalent to omitting the Rabinowitsch correction.]

The extensional strain rate in a conical die at a particular value of x is zero at the die wall where the velocity is zero, and a maximum on the die axis. The average value of the extensional strain rate also increases towards the die cone apex. The average velocity at each flat section within the die is given by

$$\bar{v} = \frac{Q}{\pi R^2} = \frac{Q}{\pi x^2 \tan^2 \alpha}$$

Therefore the average strain rate at each section is

$$\bar{\dot{\varepsilon}} = -\frac{d\bar{v}_r}{dx} = \frac{2Q}{\pi x^3 \tan^2 \alpha} = \frac{2Q \tan \alpha}{\pi R^3} \tag{3.19}$$

This expression is independent of the form of the velocity profile. The differential contribution of the extensional energy dissipation within each thin element to the overall pressure drop is

$$dP_{E_{Ent}} = \sigma d\varepsilon = A\bar{\dot{\varepsilon}}^n d\varepsilon = -2A \left(\frac{2Q \tan \alpha}{\pi R^3} \right)^n \frac{dR}{R}$$

so

$$P_{E_{Ent}} = -2A \int_{R_0}^{R_1} \left(\frac{2Q \tan \alpha}{\pi} \right)^n \frac{dR}{R^{1+3n}}$$

$$\therefore P_{E_{Ent}} = \frac{2A}{3n} \left(\frac{\tan \alpha}{2} \right)^n \dot{\gamma}_A^n \left(1 - \left(\frac{R_1}{R_0} \right)^{3n} \right) \tag{3.20}$$

For $n = 1$, the case originally considered by Cogswell, this reduces to

$$P_{E_{Ent}} = \frac{\lambda_A \tan \alpha}{3} \dot{\gamma}_A \left(1 - \frac{R_1^3}{R_0^3} \right) \tag{3.21}$$

In many cases the ratio R_1/R_0 is small enough to allow the last term in eqns (3.18), (3.20) and (3.21) to be taken as unity.

It is interesting to note that the shear contribution to the entry pressure, which varies inversely with $\tan \alpha$, is only really significant at low die angles and decreases rapidly with increasing die angle. For many polymeric liquids the shear contribution at die angles of 30° and above is only a small percentage of the total entry pressure. In contrast to the shear component, the predicted extensional term is directly proportional to tan α, so it increases almost linearly at low die angles, going to infinity at $90°$. Although the Cogswell equations are only claimed to be accurate at low die angles, they describe behaviour reasonably well up to angles of about $45°$. Within this region they provide a means of calculating extensional viscosity from die entry pressure data. The procedure for doing this from raw data would be as follows:

(i) Use a Bagley plot to evaluate the true capillary pressure drop, and hence find the shear flow parameters, B and m.

(ii) From the Bagley plot, obtain the die entry pressure.

(iii) Use the shear flow parameters found above to calculate the shear contribution to the entry pressure from eqn (3.18) and subtract this from the entry pressure to leave only the extensional flow contribution.

(iv) Use eqn (3.20) or (3.21) to evaluate the extensional flow parameters.

Assuming that $1 \gg (R_1/R_0)^{3n}$ in eqn (3.20), then using eqns (3.4) and (3.19) to substitute for A and $\dot{\varepsilon}_1$ gives, on re-arranging:[6]

$$\lambda = \frac{3n\, P_{E_{Ent}}}{\dot{\gamma}_A \tan \alpha} \tag{3.22}$$

This allows the extensional viscosity, λ, to be evaluated. Alternatively, an apparent viscosity, λ_A, can be evaluated by treating eqn (3.21) in a similar fashion:

$$\lambda_A = \frac{3 P_{E_{Ent}}}{\dot{\gamma}_A \tan \alpha} \tag{3.23}$$

A source of possible confusion arises here. It can be seen that eqns (3.22) and (3.23) are identical, apart from a factor of n, so

$$\lambda = n\lambda_A \tag{3.24}$$

It is therefore necessary, when discussing extensional viscosity data obtained from this type of experiment, to state whether the quantity is λ, obtained from the power law definition of viscosity, or λ_A, the apparent value obtained from the simplified expression with $n = 1$. The problem is analogous to the one of whether or not to apply the Rabinowitsch correction to capillary shear flow data, although the possible errors are greater in the present case.

Figure 3.7 shows the dimensionless pressure vs. die angle relationship predicted by Cogswell's model with $n = m = 1$, for various values of the Trouton ratio.

Figure 3.8 shows apparent shear and extensional viscosities for dough moulding compounds containing fibres of different lengths, evaluated from the results of convergent die measurements with the instrumented injection moulding machine described earlier. The high values of Trouton ratio, in excess of 100, are worth noting, as is the fact that increasing fibre length strongly affects the extensional viscosity but not the shear viscosity. It should be borne in mind that these viscosity values apply to a highly

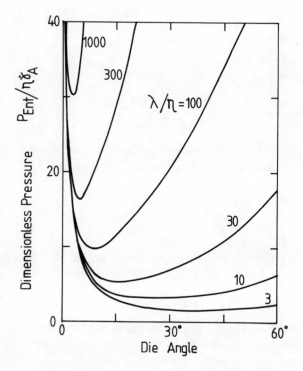

Fig. 3.7. Dimensionless entry pressure, P^*_{Ent}, from Cogswell's model vs. die angle for different values of the Trouton ratio.

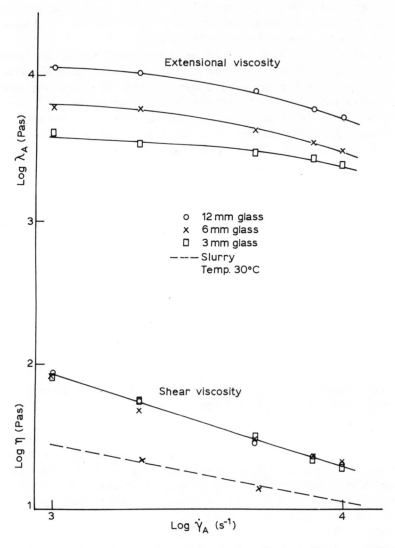

Fig. 3.8. Apparent shear and extensional viscosities of dough moulding compounds containing 20% wt of glass fibres of different lengths. Slurry without glass contains 1·65:1 wt ratio of calcium carbonate filler to resin. The resin phase consists of isophthalic polyester resin and LP40 PVA low profile additive, 2:1 wt.

oriented fibrous material, so the shear viscosity will not necessarily be the same as that of a similar material with random orientation. Considering the high level of fibre alignment and the fact that shear is taking place parallel to the fibre orientation direction, it is not surprising that shear viscosity is virtually unaffected by fibre length.

It can be seen from Fig. 3.7 that with the Cogswell model there is an optimum die angle for minimum entry pressure. Below this angle, shear flow dissipation dominates and, above it, extensional flow is the most important factor affecting the pressure. The optimum can be found, either by differentiating the expression for total entry pressure with respect to die angle and putting the differential equal to zero, or by observing that at the optimum angle the shear and pressure contributions are equal. For $m = n = 1$ this gives the optimum die angle as

$$\check{\alpha} = \tan^{-1} \sqrt{\frac{2\eta_A}{\lambda_A}} \tag{3.25}$$

and the entry pressure as

$$\check{P}_{Ent} = \frac{2}{3} \dot{\gamma}_A \sqrt{2\lambda_A \eta_A} \tag{3.26}$$

In many cases the optimum angle is too low to be of use in rheometry or process design. In many practical convergences the extensional contribution to the pressure drop will outweigh that due to shear.

In a previous discussion on freely convergent flow into flat entry dies,[16] an expression for the entry pressure was derived by assuming that, at any point in the die, the material would converge at an angle which would minimise the pressure, as outlined above. Unfortunately, the resulting expression, eqn (3) of reference 16, gives extensional viscosity values for 90° dies which disagree with those obtained at low die angles using the version of Cogswell's model outlined here (eqns (3.18) and (3.21)). The model used in ref. 16 for flat entry dies may not be appropriate, one possible reason being that the boundary conditions applied to the edge of the convergent region in its derivation are not representative of the actual situation in flat entry flows.

3.7. A CONVERGENT DIE MODEL USING SPHERICAL COORDINATES

To describe entry flow behaviour over the full range of possible die semi-angles up to 90°, models based on spherical coordinates have some advantages over those based on cylindrical coordinates. Some of the many models of this type which have been proposed are reviewed in references 2 and 3. Oka, for instance, presented a treatment which satisfies equilibrium and continuity for both Newtonian[17] and power law[18] fluids. Metzner and Metzner[19] derived a model based on sink flow. Gibson and Williamson[7] compared the predictions of a similar model, based on spherically convergent flow, with those of the Cogswell model, using each to describe die entry pressures for DMC over a range of die angles.

3.7.1. Fluid Anisotropy

The significance of the anisotropy of flow properties that can arise as a result of molecular orientation or the orientation of suspended fibres has not been widely discussed.

The value of 3 for the Trouton ratio of a Newtonian fluid is obtained by assuming that it is both isotropic and incompressible. If a fluid has a Trouton ratio greater than 3 it cannot therefore be both isotropic and incompressible. The fluids discussed here are, to a good approximation, incompressible, so it follows that they must be anisotropic in their behaviour.

For the fluids considered here, a cylindrical form of anisotropy will be assumed, flow properties being invariant with respect to rotation about some symmetry or reference axis within the flowing material. The solid analogue of such a fluid would be a material possessing transverse isotropy or fibre symmetry. The principal characteristic of fluids having molecular or fibre orientation of this type is that their resistance to extensional deformation parallel to the reference axis is higher than that of a Newtonian fluid. In other words, there is a high extensional viscosity in the orientation direction. Tensile deformation transverse to the symmetry axis and shear deformation are governed by lower viscosity values.

Looking again at the analogy between the flow of anisotropic fluids and the elastic behaviour of anisotropic solids, it is possible to write down a relationship for flow behaviour of the liquid system by replacing strain with strain rate in the well known tensor relationships which govern a solid material's response to stress. The familiar relationship for the strain response of a transversely isotropic solid, given e.g. in reference 20, can therefore be modified to give the analogous relationship for a transversely isotropic fluid:

$$
\begin{Bmatrix} \dot{\varepsilon}_1 \\ \dot{\varepsilon}_2 \\ \dot{\varepsilon}_3 \\ \dot{\gamma}_{23} \\ \dot{\gamma}_{31} \\ \dot{\gamma}_{12} \end{Bmatrix} = \begin{bmatrix} a_{11} & a_{12} & a_{13} & 0 & 0 & 0 \\ a_{12} & a_{11} & a_{13} & 0 & 0 & 0 \\ a_{13} & a_{13} & a_{33} & 0 & 0 & 0 \\ 0 & 0 & 0 & a_{44} & 0 & 0 \\ 0 & 0 & 0 & 0 & a_{44} & 0 \\ 0 & 0 & 0 & 0 & 0 & 2(a_{11} - a_{12}) \end{bmatrix} \begin{Bmatrix} \sigma_1 \\ \sigma_2 \\ \sigma_3 \\ \tau_{23} \\ \tau_{31} \\ \tau_{12} \end{Bmatrix} \quad (3.27)
$$

This notation takes the 3-axis as the symmetry axis. There are five independent constants, representing reciprocal viscosities. These are analogous to the compliance constants found in the solid case. The nine constants in the top left-hand corner determine the extensional response to direct stresses. The three diagonal terms on the right are reciprocal shear viscosities. In contrast to the solid case, the material will be assumed to deform at constant volume, so

$$ \dot{\varepsilon}_1 + \dot{\varepsilon}_2 + \dot{\varepsilon}_3 = 0 $$

Hence

$$ (a_{11}\sigma_1 + a_{12}\sigma_2 + \sigma_{13}\sigma_3) $$
$$ + (a_{12}\sigma_1 + a_{11}\sigma_2 + a_{13}\sigma_3) + (a_{13}\sigma_1 + a_{13}\sigma_2 + a_{33}\sigma_3) = 0 $$

so

$$ (\sigma_1 + \sigma_2)(a_{11} + a_{12} + a_{13}) = -\sigma_3(2a_{13} + a_{33}) $$

In order to maintain volume constancy under all stress conditions, this leads to a further two relationships between constants, since

$$ a_{11} + a_{12} + a_{13} = 0 \quad \text{and} \quad 2a_{13} + a_{33} = 0 $$

The total number of constants required is therefore three. It is worth pointing out that, in contrast to the solid case, where the matrix of compliance constants can be inverted to give a matrix of stiffness constants, this cannot be done here as the stiffness terms are infinite for an incompressible material.

Of the three constants, a_{33} and a_{11} represent reciprocal extensional viscosities parallel and perpendicular to the reference axis, and a_{44} is a reciprocal shear viscosity.

Making use of the relationships between constants, the strain rate response can be rewritten:

$$
\begin{Bmatrix}
\dot{\varepsilon}_1 \\
\dot{\varepsilon}_2 \\
\dot{\varepsilon}_3 \\
\dot{\gamma}_{23} \\
\dot{\gamma}_{31} \\
\dot{\gamma}_{12}
\end{Bmatrix}
=
\begin{bmatrix}
1/\lambda_\perp & (1/2\lambda_\parallel - 1/\lambda_\perp) & -1/2\lambda_\parallel & 0 & 0 & 0 \\
(1/2\lambda_\parallel - 1/\lambda_\perp) & 1/\lambda_\perp & -1/2\lambda_\parallel & 0 & 0 & 0 \\
-1/2\lambda_\parallel & -1/2\lambda_\parallel & 1/\lambda_\parallel & 0 & 0 & 0 \\
0 & 0 & 0 & 1/\eta & 0 & 0 \\
0 & 0 & 0 & 0 & 1/\eta & 0 \\
0 & 0 & 0 & 0 & 0 & 4/\lambda_\perp - 1/\lambda_\parallel
\end{bmatrix}
$$

$$
\times
\begin{Bmatrix}
\sigma_1 \\
\sigma_2 \\
\sigma_3 \\
\tau_{23} \\
\tau_{31} \\
\tau_{12}
\end{Bmatrix}
\tag{3.28}
$$

When, as in the present case, deformation is symmetric about the 3-axis, the transverse extensional viscosity, $\lambda_\perp$, need not be known, so just two constants, $\lambda_\parallel$ and η, are needed to describe behaviour.

Of course the axis of anisotropy of the flowing fluid will change direction as the fluid flows through the convergence. However, the simplifying assumption will be made that the fluid axis (the 3-direction mentioned above) coincides with the r-axis of the spherical coordinate system used to model die flow, shown in Fig. 3.9.

If the assumption is made that the two die stresses σ_1 and σ_2 are equal, then there is just one relationship between tensile stresses and strain rates, ε_θ and ε_ϕ being equal. Equation (3.28) gives

$$
\dot{\varepsilon}_r = \frac{1}{\lambda_\parallel} (\sigma_r - \sigma_\theta) \tag{3.29}
$$

It is now possible to write down all the components of the stress tensor for this problem:

$$
\sigma_r = -p + \frac{2\lambda}{3} \frac{\partial v_r}{\partial r}
$$

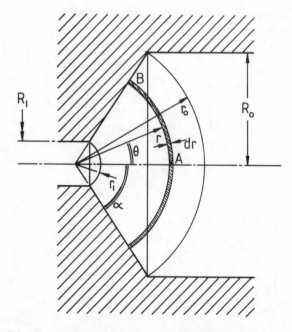

Fig. 3.9. Die entry geometry and nomenclature using spherical coordinates.

$$\sigma_\theta = -p + \frac{2\lambda}{3}\frac{v_r}{r}$$

$$\sigma_\phi = \sigma_\theta \qquad\qquad (3.30)$$

$$\tau_{r\theta} = \frac{\eta}{r}\frac{\partial v_r}{\partial \theta}$$

$$\tau_{\phi r} = \tau_{\theta\phi} = 0$$

This set of equations is identical to those which would apply in the Newtonian case, except that the Newtonian viscosity terms have been replaced by anisotropic values. For brevity, the subscript has been omitted from λ. It should be understood that, although no special subscripts have been given to λ and η, they now refer to an anisotropic fluid, so they do not have the same meaning as they did in the Newtonian case.

It will be assumed that, in the conical part of the die, the streamlines are straight lines converging on the die apex, so $v_\theta = v_\phi = 0$. To satisfy continuity, the velocity component v_r must therefore be given by

$$v_r = \frac{kf(\theta)}{r^2} \qquad (3.31)$$

where k is a constant and $f(\theta)$ is a function of angle. Since the flow rate is given by

$$Q = \int_0^\alpha 2\pi r^2 v_r \sin\theta \, d\theta = \int_0^\alpha 2\pi k f(\theta) \sin\theta \, d\theta$$

$$= 2\pi k I_1$$

where

$$I_1 = \int_0^\alpha f(\theta) \sin\theta \, d\theta \qquad (3.32)$$

the constant, k, can be eliminated, and

$$v_r = \frac{Qf(\theta)}{2\pi I_1 r^2} \qquad (3.33)$$

If the fluid under consideration were Newtonian, it would be appropriate to use the Navier–Stokes equation, expressed in spherical coordinates, to derive a solution to the problem which satisfies equilibrium. The r-direction Navier–Stokes equation (neglecting inertia terms) would be

$$\frac{\partial p}{\partial r} = \eta \left(\frac{1}{r} \frac{\partial^2}{\partial r^2} (rv_r) - \frac{2v_r}{r^2} + \frac{1}{r^2} \frac{\partial^2 v_r}{\partial \theta^2} + \frac{\cot\theta}{r^2} \frac{\partial v_r}{\partial \theta} \right) \qquad (3.34)$$

It will be recalled that the Navier–Stokes equations for the creeping flow case are obtained by substituting the appropriate stress expressions into the equilibrium equations. In eqn (3.34) the first two terms on the right arise from extensional stresses, while the second two arise from shear stresses. If the stress equations for the anisotropic fluid being considered here (eqns (3.30)) are substituted into the equilibrium equations, the expressions which result are analogous and similar in form to the Navier–Stokes equations. The difference is that in the extensional terms the Newtonian viscosity is replaced by $\lambda/3$ and in the shear terms the meaning of the shear viscosity is changed as described above. This gives

$$\frac{\partial p}{\partial r} = \frac{\lambda}{3} \left(\frac{1}{r} \frac{\partial^2}{\partial r^2} (rv_r) - \frac{2v_r}{r^2} \right) + \frac{\eta}{r^2} \left(\frac{\partial^2 v_r}{\partial \theta^2} + \cot\theta \frac{\partial v_r}{\partial \theta} \right) \qquad (3.35)$$

Unlike the Navier–Stokes equations, this relationship only applies when the reference axis of the anisotropic fluid coincides with the r-direction of the coordinate system. Substituting for v in eqn (3.35) gives

$$\frac{\partial p}{\partial r} = \frac{\eta Q}{2\pi I_1 r^4} (f''(\theta) + \cot \theta \cdot f'(\theta)) \qquad (3.36)$$

It is interesting to note that the extensional terms in eqn (3.35) have cancelled out, leaving only the shear terms.

The die entry and exit boundary conditions for this problem will be formulated in terms of the direct stress, σ_r, rather than pressure, so p will be eliminated from eqn (3.36). Rearranging the σ_r stress equation in (3.30) gives

$$\frac{\partial p}{\partial r} = -\frac{\partial \sigma_r}{\partial r} + \frac{2\lambda}{3} \frac{\partial^2 v_r}{\partial r^2}$$

Substituting for $\partial p / \partial r$ in eqn (3.36) gives

$$-\frac{\partial \sigma_r}{\partial r} = -\frac{2\lambda}{3} \frac{\partial^2 v_r}{\partial r^2} + \frac{\eta Q}{2\pi I_1 r^4} (f''(\theta) + \cot \theta \cdot f'(\theta))$$

$$\therefore \frac{\partial \sigma_r}{\partial r} = \frac{2Q}{\pi I_1 r^4} \left(\lambda f(\theta) - \frac{\eta}{4} (f''(\theta) + \cot \theta \cdot f'(\theta)) \right)$$

which, on integration, gives

$$\sigma_r = \frac{-2Q}{3\pi I_1 r^3} \left[\lambda f(\theta) - \frac{\eta}{4} (f''(\theta) + \cot \theta \cdot f'(\theta)) \right] + C(\theta)$$

If the exit condition is that $\sigma_r = 0$ when $r = r_1$, then the constant of integration can be found, and the value of σ_r at the die entry, σ_{r_0}, will be

$$\sigma_{r_0} = \frac{-2Q}{3\pi I_1} \left[\lambda f(\theta) - \frac{\eta}{4} (f''(\theta) + \cot \theta \cdot f'(\theta)) \right] \left(\frac{1}{r_1^3} - \frac{1}{r_0^3} \right)$$

$$= \frac{-2Q}{3\pi I_1 r_1^3} \left[\lambda f(\theta) - \frac{\eta}{4} (f''(\theta) + \cot \theta \cdot f'(\theta)) \right] \left(1 - \frac{r_1^3}{r_0^3} \right)$$

$$= \frac{-2Q \sin^3 \alpha}{3\pi I_1 R_1^3} \left[\lambda f(\theta) - \frac{\eta}{4} (f''(\theta) + \cot \theta \cdot f'(\theta)) \right] \left(1 - \frac{R_1^3}{R_0^3} \right)$$

$$= \frac{-\dot{\gamma}_A \sin^3 \alpha}{6 I_1} \left[\lambda f(\theta) - \frac{\eta}{4} (f''(\theta) + \cot \theta \cdot f'(\theta)) \right] \left(1 - \frac{R_1^3}{R_0^3} \right)$$

The average value of σ_r over the surface of the spherical shell at the die entry can then be equated to the hydrostatic pressure, $-P$, in the reservoir, so

$$P_{\text{Ent}} = \frac{-\int_0^\alpha \sigma_{r_0} \sin \theta \cdot d\theta}{\int_0^\alpha \sin \theta \cdot d\theta} = \frac{\dot{\gamma}_A \sin^3 \alpha}{6I_1(1 - \cos \alpha)}$$

$$\times \int_0^\alpha \left[\lambda f(\theta) - \frac{\eta}{4} (f''(\theta) + \cot \theta \cdot f'(\theta)) \right] \sin \theta \cdot d\theta$$

$$\times \left(1 - \frac{R_1^3}{R_0^3} \right) = \frac{\dot{\gamma}_A \sin^3 \alpha}{6I_1(1 - \cos \alpha)} [\lambda I_1 - \frac{\eta}{4} I_2]$$

$$\times \left(1 - \frac{R_1^3}{R_0^3} \right)$$

where

$$I_2 = \int_0^\alpha (f''(\theta) + \cot \theta \cdot f'(\theta)) \sin \theta \cdot d\theta$$

It is informative to split the solution into the separate components due to shear and extension:

$$P_{S_{\text{Ent}}} = \frac{-\eta \dot{\gamma}_A \sin^3 \alpha I_2}{24 I_1 (1 - \cos \alpha)} \left(1 - \frac{R_1^3}{R_0^3} \right) \tag{3.37}$$

$$= \frac{-\eta \dot{\gamma}_A \sin \alpha (1 + \cos \alpha) I_2}{24 I_1} \left(1 - \frac{R_1^3}{R_0^3} \right)$$

and

$$P_{E_{\text{Ent}}} = \frac{\lambda \dot{\gamma}_A \sin \alpha (1 + \cos \alpha)}{6} \left(1 - \frac{R_1^3}{R_0^3} \right) \tag{3.38}$$

The effect of different forms of velocity profile can now be considered. As with the solution described in the previous section, the form of eqn (3.38) for the extensional component does not depend on the shape assumed for the velocity profile. In fact it is identical to the expression proposed by Metzner and Metzner for sink flow.[19] Although choosing different types of velocity profile will not affect the extensional component, it will affect the shear component.

The simplest velocity profile is a flat one with $f(\theta)$ constant. This corresponds to spherically convergent sink flow with slip at the die walls. Since $f'(\theta) = f''(\theta) = 0$, there is no shear dissipation so the total entry pressure is given by eqn (3.38).

In this case, eqn (3.36) implies that flow takes place without a change in hydrostatic pressure as the material passes through the die entry. The ability of an energy-dissipating flow to occur without a hydrostatic pressure drop has troubled some rheologists. However, reassurance can be gained by observing that the stress state in the die entry is not a purely hydrostatic one. The r-component of stress, which is the component doing work on the fluid, varies considerably through the die. The boundary conditions at the die entry and exit are more correctly expressed in terms of σ_r rather than pressure. For instance, at the exit ($r = r_1$) of an orifice die, it is σ_r which is zero, not p. p will have a finite value, even at the exit, since the fluid there will be exerting a stress, σ_θ, on the wall.

A velocity profile of more practical interest than the one described above is that where

$$f(\theta) = \cos^2\theta - \cos^2\alpha$$

This satisfies the condition of zero velocity at the die wall and reduces to a parabolic profile at low die angles. Profiles equivalent to this have been derived or suggested by Oka,[17] Harrison[21] and Bond[22] amongst others.

Evaluating I_1 gives

$$I_1 = \frac{1}{3}(1 - \cos\alpha)^2(1 + 2\cos\alpha)$$

so

$$v_r = \frac{3Q(\cos^2\theta - \cos^2\alpha)}{2\pi r^2(1 - \cos\alpha)^2(1 + 2\cos\alpha)}$$

$$= \frac{3Q(1 + \cos\alpha)\left(1 - \dfrac{\sin^2\theta}{\sin^2\alpha}\right)}{2\pi r^2(1 + 2\cos\alpha)} \tag{3.39}$$

Evaluating I_2 gives

$$I_2 = 2\cos\alpha(\cos\alpha + 1)(\cos\alpha - 1)$$

so in this case the shear component, $P_{S_{Ent}}$, is given by

$$P_{S_{Ent}} = \frac{\eta\dot{\gamma}_A \sin\alpha \cos\alpha(1 + \cos\alpha)^2}{4(1 - \cos\alpha)(1 + 2\cos\alpha)}\left(1 - \frac{R_1^3}{R_0^3}\right) \tag{3.40}$$

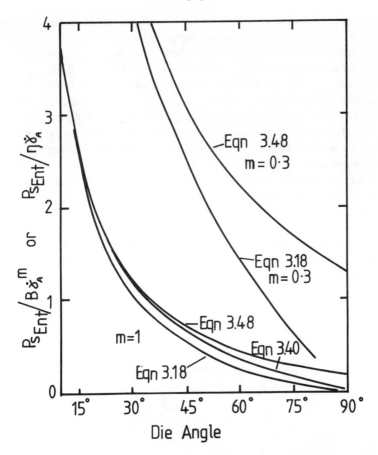

Fig. 3.10. Shear flow contribution to entry pressure, expressed in dimensionless form vs. die angle. Comparison of three models: Cogswell's (eqn. (3.18)); equilibrium model (eqn. (3.40)); and full power law model using spherical coordinates (eqn. (3.48)).

Figure 3.10 compares the shear component from Cogswell's treatment (eqn (3.18)) with that given by eqn (3.40), assuming that $R_1^3/R_0^3 \ll 1$. The agreement between the two theories is encouraging. At low die angles, both become asymptotic to the same expression, giving

$$\lim_{\alpha \to 0} P_{S_{Ent}} = \frac{2\eta\dot{\gamma}_A}{3\alpha} \quad \text{for} \quad \frac{R_1^3}{R_0^3} \ll 1$$

Both expressions for $P_{S_{Ent}}$ therefore approach the solution for flow in a tube of constant radius at low die angles.

Figure 3.11 shows a comparison between Cogswell's model for the extensional component, $P_{E_{Ent}}$ with $n = 1$ (eqn (3.21)), and the present model (eqn (3.38)). As might be expected, both agree at low die angles. Equation (3.38) has the advantage that it gives a finite value of pressure for a flat entry die. However, it gives poor agreement with experimental results above die angles of about $40°$ and has in the past been rejected for this reason.[6] The behaviour of a wide range of different viscous liquids can be fitted equally well by Cogswell's model or eqn (3.38) at low die angles, but none of these real liquids shows the maximum at $60°$ predicted by eqn (3.38). Moreover, experimental pressures in the range of die angles between $60°$ and $90°$ are invariably higher than those predicted by the model in the form so far described.

The reason for the inaccuracy of eqn (3.38) at large die angles, as previously pointed out,[3] is that no allowance has been made for the pressure drop between the spherical exit boundary at $r = r_1$ and the entrance to the capillary. The discrepancy which results from ignoring this is greatest at larger die angles where the convergent regime continues for some distance beyond the spherical exit boundary. To refine the model, it

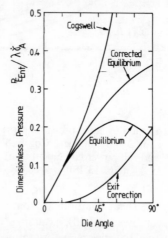

Fig. 3.11. Extensional flow contribution to entry pressure, expressed in dimensionless form vs. die angle. Comparison of Cogswell's model (eqn (3.21)), the equilibrium model in spherical coordinates (eqn (3.38)), and the equilibrium model corrected for the extra pressure drop between the exit boundary and the capillary entrance (eqn (3.38) + eqn (3.46)). The correction term (eqn (3.46)) is also shown.

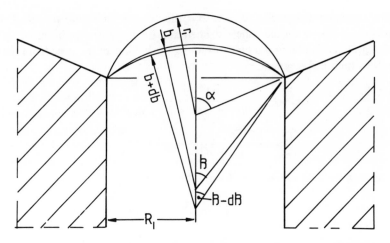

Fig. 3.12. Geometry of the exit of the convergence, showing nomenclature used to derive the extra pressure drop between the spherical exit boundary and the capillary entrance.

is necessary therefore to determine the extra pressure, P'_{Ent}, due to flow in the region shown in Fig. 3.12.

Consider the crescent-shaped element between spherical shells of radii b and $b + db$ as shown in Fig. 3.12. The surface area, a, of the shell of radius b subtending angle β at the axis is

$$a = 2\pi b^2(1 - \cos \beta) = \frac{2\pi R_1^2(1 - \cos \beta)}{\sin^2 \beta}$$

$$= \frac{2\pi R_1^2}{1 + \cos \beta}$$

Only the extensional contribution to the pressure drop will be considered. The differential reservoir pressure drop due to the material flowing between the two shells can be found from the work rate, since

$$dP'_{Ent} = \lambda \dot{\varepsilon} \, d\varepsilon \tag{3.41}$$

Neglecting the losses due to shear can be justified on the grounds that in most cases these are only significant at low die angles.

The effective change in strain of the material crossing the element can be found from the change in cross-sectional area, since

$$d\varepsilon = \frac{da}{a} = \frac{\sin \beta}{1 + \cos \beta} \, d\beta \tag{3.42}$$

The volume of material, dV, within the crescent must be found. The volume, V, between the spherical shell and the flat entrance boundary of the capillary can be found by subtracting the volume of the cone from that of the spherical segment:

$$
\begin{aligned}
V &= \frac{2\pi R_1^3}{3 \sin \beta (1 + \cos \beta)} - \frac{\pi R_1^3 \cos \beta}{3 \sin \beta} \\
&= \frac{\pi R_1^3 (2 - \cos \beta - \cos^2 \beta)}{3 \sin \beta (1 + \cos \beta)}
\end{aligned}
\tag{3.43}
$$

This can be differentiated and simplified to give

$$
dV = \frac{\pi R_1^3}{(1 + \cos \beta)^2} \, d\beta
\tag{3.44}
$$

The effective residence time, dt, of the fluid in the element is

$$
dt = \frac{dV}{Q} = \frac{\pi R_1^3}{Q(1 + \cos \beta)^2} \, d\beta
\tag{3.45}
$$

So the effective strain rate can be found, since

$$
\begin{aligned}
\dot{\varepsilon} = \frac{d\varepsilon}{dt} &= \frac{\sin \beta}{1 + \cos \beta} \, d\beta \, \frac{Q(1 + \cos \beta)^2}{\pi R_1^3 \, d\beta} \\
&= \frac{Q \sin \beta}{\pi R_1^3} (1 + \cos \beta)
\end{aligned}
$$

Substituting for $\dot{\varepsilon}$ and $d\varepsilon$ in eqn (3.41) gives

$$
dP'_{\text{Ent}} = \frac{\lambda Q \sin^2 \beta \cdot d\beta}{\pi R_1^3}
$$

So the total pressure loss, P'_{Ent}, due to flow in the transition regime between the spherical exit boundary and the actual die exit can be found by integration:

$$
P'_{\text{Ent}} = \frac{\lambda Q}{\pi R_1^3} \int_{\beta = 0}^{\beta = \alpha} \sin^2 \beta \, d\beta
$$

$$
\therefore \ P'_{\text{Ent}} = \frac{\lambda \dot{\gamma}_A}{8} \left(\alpha - \frac{\sin 2\alpha}{2} \right)
\tag{3.46}
$$

The total entry pressure drop in a convergent die is therefore given by

$$P_{Ent} = \dot{\gamma}_A \left[\left(\frac{\eta \sin \alpha \cos \alpha (1 + \cos \alpha)^2}{4(1 - \cos \alpha)(1 + 2 \cos \alpha)} + \frac{\lambda \sin \alpha (1 + \cos \alpha)}{6} \right) \right.$$

$$\left. \times \left(1 - \frac{R_1^3}{R_0^3} \right) + \frac{\lambda}{8} \left(\alpha - \frac{\sin 2\alpha}{2} \right) \right] \qquad (3.47)$$

The exit pressure correction and the total extensional contribution are shown in Fig. 3.11. The exit correction is only significant at die angles above about $45°$.

However, for a $90°$ die it represents a substantial proportion of the total pressure, so the correction is essential if the model is to be accurate over the full range of die angles.

Equation (3.47) can only apply strictly when $n = m = 1$. However, with most polymer fluids it may be employed to a good approximation over limited ranges of strain rate, using 'apparent' viscosity values, as discussed previously. A more widely applicable treatment would require the assumption of power law behaviour. Such a treatment, which has great flexibility and which involves only a little extra computation, will be presented in the next section, using an approach slightly different from that adopted here.

3.8. ENTRY FLOW OF ANISOTROPIC POWER LAW FLUIDS

Unfortunately the equilibrium method used in the previous section to derive the shear and extensional components in the entry region cannot be easily extended to take in power law behaviour without resorting to numerical methods. This route was taken by Oka and Takami.[18]

An energy method, which is more flexible for fluids with a non-linear stress–strain rate response, will be used here to calculate both the shear and extensional components in the main entry region. Consider the spherical shell of radius r and thickness dr shown in Fig. 3.9. Assume, for the purpose of calculating the shear component, that the velocity profile over this shell is the same as in a parallel-sided tube of radius, $r\alpha$, equal to the length of the circular arc AB shown. The differential contribution of this shell to the shear dissipation will be given by the relationship for the pressure drop of a power law fluid flowing in a cylindrical capillary, eqn (3.8), with dr for the capillary length and $r\alpha$ for the radius, so

$$dP_{S_{Ent}} = \frac{2B \, dr}{(r\alpha)^{1 + 3m}} \left(\frac{1 + 3m}{\pi m} \right)^m Q^m$$

Integrating this in the region between the spherical entry and exit shells at $r = r_0$ and $r = r_1$ gives

$$P_{S_{Ent}} = \frac{2B}{3m\alpha^{1+3m}} \left(\frac{1 + 3m}{\pi m}\right)^m \left(\frac{Q}{r_1^3}\right)^m \left(1 - \left(\frac{r_1}{r_0}\right)^{3m}\right)$$

so

$$P_{S_{Ent}} = \frac{2B \sin^{3m}\alpha}{3m\alpha^{1+3m}} \left(\frac{1 + 3m}{4m}\right)^m \dot{\gamma}_A^m \left(1 - \left(\frac{R_1}{R_0}\right)^{3m}\right) \quad (3.48)$$

Values of $P_{S_{Ent}}$ from eqn (3.48) are compared in Fig. 3.10 with those of Cogswell's model, eqn (3.18), and the model derived in the last section, eqn (3.37). All three models become identical at low die angles, and for $m = 1$ they agree well over the complete range of die angles. At the lower m value of 0.3, there is some divergence between eqns (3.18) and (3.48) at higher die angles, but this is unlikely to affect the overall accuracy of the model since the shear component will normally be only a small part of the total pressure in this region. No special advantages are claimed for eqn (3.48) over Cogswell's model, except that it is based on the same coordinate system and assumptions as the rest of the model proposed in this section. Its use is therefore more consistent.

The average velocity, $\bar{v}_r$, of material crossing a spherical shell of radius r is

$$\bar{v}_r = \frac{Q}{a} = \frac{Q}{2\pi r^2(1 - \cos\alpha)}$$

so the effective elongational strain rate will be

$$\bar{\dot{\varepsilon}}_r = -\frac{\partial \bar{v}_r}{\partial r} = \frac{Q}{\pi r^3(1 - \cos\alpha)} = \frac{Q \sin^3\alpha}{\pi R^3(1 - \cos\alpha)}$$

The effective die exit elongational strain rate will therefore be

$$\bar{\dot{\varepsilon}}_1 = \frac{Q}{\pi R_1^3} \sin\alpha(1 + \cos\alpha) = \frac{\dot{\gamma}_A \sin\alpha(1 + \cos\alpha)}{4}$$

The differential contribution towards the extensional pressure drop of the material flowing in the spherical element will be given by

$$dP_{E_{Ent}} = \sigma \cdot d\varepsilon = -2A\bar{\dot{\varepsilon}}^n \cdot \frac{dr}{r}$$

$$\therefore \ dP_{E_{Ent}} \ = \ -2A \left(\frac{Q}{\pi r^3 (1 \ - \ \cos \alpha)} \right)^n \frac{dr}{r}$$

$$= \ -2A \left(\frac{Q}{\pi(1 \ - \ \cos \alpha)} \right)^n \frac{dr}{r^{3n+1}}$$

Integrating between the two spherical boundaries gives

$$P_{E_{Ent}} \ = \ \frac{2A}{3n} \left(\frac{Q}{\pi(1 \ - \ \cos \alpha)} \right)^n \left(\frac{1}{r_1^{3n}} \ - \ \frac{1}{r_0^{3n}} \right)$$

$$= \ \frac{2A}{3n} \left(\frac{Q}{\pi(1 \ - \ \cos \alpha) r_1^3} \right)^n \left(1 \ - \ \left(\frac{r_1}{r_0} \right)^{3n} \right)$$

$$= \ \frac{2A \dot{\gamma}_A^n}{3n} \left(\frac{\sin \alpha \ (1 \ + \ \cos \alpha)}{4} \right)^n \left(1 \ - \ \left(\frac{R_1}{R_0} \right)^{3n} \right) \quad (3.49)$$

The fact that this reduces to eqn (3.38) when $n \ = \ 1$ lends support both to this model and to the one in the previous section. No particular velocity profile has been assumed here, the strain rate being taken as an average effective value over the spherical surface.

Applying a similar approach to that used above for the region between the spherical exit boundary and the capillary entrance, this time assuming power law extensional behaviour gives

$$dP'_{Ent} \ = \ A \dot{\varepsilon}^n \ d\varepsilon$$

$$= \ A \left(\frac{Q}{\pi R_1^3} \sin \beta (1 \ + \ \cos \beta) \right)^n \frac{\sin \beta \cdot d\beta}{1 \ + \ \cos \beta}$$

$$\therefore \ P'_{Ent} \ = \ A \left(\frac{Q}{\pi R_1^3} \right)^n \int_0^\alpha \sin^{n+1} \beta (1 \ + \ \cos \beta)^{n-1} \ d\beta$$

$$\therefore \ P'_{Ent} \ = \ \frac{A \dot{\gamma}_A^n}{4^n} \Phi(n, \ \alpha) \quad (3.50)$$

where

$$\Phi(n, \ \alpha) \ = \ \int_0^\alpha \sin^{n+1} \beta (1 \ + \ \cos \beta)^{n-1} \ d\beta$$

TABLE 3.1

Values of Φ Obtained by Use of the Die Exit Effect Integral,

$$\Phi(n, \alpha) = \int_0^\alpha \sin^{n+1} \beta (1 + \cos \beta)^{n-1} \, d\beta$$

for a Range of n Values and Die Angles

n	$30°$	$45°$	$60°$	$75°$	$90°$
0·1	0·0660	0·1558	0·2882	0·4677	0·7003
0·2	0·0629	0·1535	0·2892	0·4730	0·7080
0·3	0·0601	0·1515	0·2904	0·4787	0·7162
0·4	0·0575	0·1497	0·2920	0·4848	0·7249
0·5	0·0550	0·1481	0·2939	0·4913	0.7339
0·6	0·0528	0·1467	0·2961	0·4983	0·7434
0·7	0·0507	0·1455	0·2985	0·5055	0·7533
0·8	0·0488	0·1444	0·3011	0·5132	0·7636
0·9	0·0470	0·1435	0·3040	0·5212	0·7743
1·0	0.0453	0·1427	0·3071	0·5295	0·7854
1·2	0·0422	0·1414	0·3139	0·5472	0·8087
1·4	0·0394	0·1406	0·3215	0·5662	0·8334
1·6	0·0370	0·1401	0·3299	0·5865	0·8597
1·8	0·0348	0·1399	0·3391	0.6082	0·8874
2·0	0·0328	0·1399	0·3490	0·6313	0·9167

Although this can only be integrated analytically when $n = 1$, Φ can be evaluated numerically for any required value of n. Values of Φ obtained in this way are given in Table 3.1 for the range of n values and die angles of practical interest. Interpolation may be used for n values and die angles within the range shown without undue loss of accuracy. The total extensional pressure dissipation for a power law fluid is therefore

$$P_{E_{Ent}} = A\dot{\gamma}_A^n \left[\frac{2}{3n} \left(\frac{\sin \alpha (1 + \cos \alpha)}{4} \right)^n \left(1 - \left(\frac{R_1}{R_0} \right)^{3n} \right) + \frac{\Phi(n, \alpha)}{4^n} \right] \quad (3.51)$$

so the total overall pressure drop will be given by the sum of eqns (3.48) and (3.51). The behaviour of eqn (3.51) as a function of die angle and power law index is shown in Fig. 3.13 for the case where $(R_1/R_0)^{3n} \ll 1$. The expression has been plotted in terms of the dimensionless power law quantity $nP_{E_{Ent}}/A\dot{\gamma}_A^n$. To illustrate the significance of the dissipation in the transition zone, the solution without this component, eqn (3.49), has also been shown. It can be seen that, to a good approximation, the transition zone dissipation can be neglected for die angles below about 45°. At higher die angles, however, the effect is significant and the Φ term must be included.

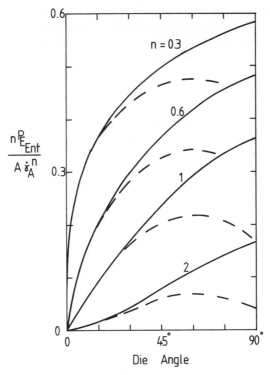

Fig. 3.13. Extensional flow contribution to entry pressure for power law model in spherical coordinates, expressed in dimensionless form vs. die angle, for different values of the index, n. The full line represents the total value of $P_{E_{Ent}}$ (eqn (3.51)). The dashed line is the value without the exit correction (eqn (3.49)).

One important effect, which is a result of the change of strain rate with die angle, is that the shape of the pressure versus die angle relationship changes with the n value of the material. At low n values, in the extension-thinning region, the entry pressure varies very little over quite a wide range of die angles. If n differs substantially from 1, therefore, the full power law treatment may well be desirable to obtain the greatest accuracy.

It was mentioned earlier that the approach adopted here makes no attempt to model the recirculation zones, often seen with non-Newtonian fluids at large die angles. However, it has been pointed out that the main form of dissipation at large die angles is extensional and that the extensional dissipation is not a strong function of the velocity field. It may be expected therefore that the entry pressure for large angle dies, in particular

90 ° dies, is given reasonably accurately by eqns (3.48) and (3.51) irrespective of whether or not recirculation zones form. In other words, although recirculation zones sometimes constitute a very visible feature of the flow pattern, they are second-order effects as far as pressure drop is concerned, being primarily associated with shear energy dissipation, which itself is only a small part of the total energy loss in the die entry.

Another argument in support of this assertion is concerned with any possible transition from constrained flow at low die angles to unconstrained flow at angles near to 90 °. In the majority of cases, the flow field up to moderate die angles may be taken to be of the constrained type, where streamlines are strongly influenced by die geometry. If recirculation zones, involving unconstrained flow, form at large die angles this implies that, at some intermediate angle, there must be a transition from constrained to unconstrained flow, as shown schematically in Fig. 3.14. Such a transition would only take place if the pressure drop for the unconstrained case were lower than the pressure drop for constrained flow. If the difference in pressure between the two types of flow were significant, this would produce a change in the slope of the pressure vs. die angle plot. If the slope of the plot for the unconstrained case were negative, as is possible, this could even result in a negative slope at large die angles. If no

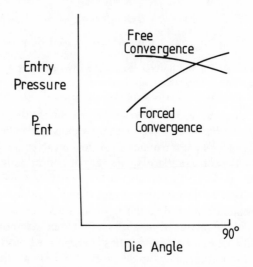

Fig. 3.14. Schematic illustration of possible transition from constrained to freely convergent flow.

such slope change is seen in the experimental pressure vs. die angle plot, or if it is so small as to be masked by experimental scatter, it is probably safe to assume that the pressure difference between the two types of flow regime is small, in which case eqns (3.48) and (3.51) are sufficiently accurate. No convincing evidence of a slope difference has been observed by the author in materials examined so far. Nevertheless, it is advisable to examine data obtained over a range of die angles and to check that the shape of the relationship is the same as shown in Fig. 3.13 for the appropriate n value.

If entry flow data are to be collected for accurate evaluation of the extensional power law constants, the best experimental die angle range to use is 20–45°. In this range, the die angle is generally large enough for the shear component to be either a small correction or negligible. In most instances the transition zone pressure drop will be low, so the numerically determined factor, Φ, may often be negligible. Finally, both the power law version of Cogswell's equation (eqn (3.20)) and eqn (3.51) give similar results in this region.

In the next section the use of the full power law model to treat experimental data will be demonstrated. Equations (3.48) and (3.51) will be used to treat capillary flow data for unfilled and glass reinforced polypropylene.

3.9. USE OF POWER LAW EQUATIONS TO TREAT CAPILLARY FLOW DATA OVER A RANGE OF DIE ANGLES

Capillary flow data in the form of Bagley plots, obtained with a 45° die, were shown in Fig. 3.4 for two injection moulding grades of polypropylene. From these results the true capillary pressure drops were found and log-log plots of P_{Cap} vs. $\dot{\gamma}_A$ were made in the normal way. The power law shear constants, m and B, found from the slope and intercept are shown in Table 3.2 for the two materials.

In addition to the results obtained at 45°, a series of measurements of entry pressure was made for each material, using orifice dies with a wide range of entry angles. These results are shown in Fig. 3.15. Although these data again show the surprising similarity in behaviour between the unfilled and glass reinforced grades of material, it should once again be emphasised that the viscosity of the base resin used in the reinforced material was rather lower than that of the unfilled polymer. The pressure drop due to shear dissipation in the die entry was calculated for each point using eqn (3.48) with the appropriate B and m values and subtracted from the

TABLE 3.2
Flow Parameters For a Range of Reinforced and Unreinforced Moulding Materials
(The numerical values of A and B correspond to strain rates in s^{-1} and stresses in Pa. The extensional and shear viscosity values are both at a strain rate of 1000 s^{-1}.)

Material	Temp (°C)	A	n	B	m	Extensional Viscosity (Pa.s) at 1000 s^{-1}	Shear Viscosity (Pa.s) at 1000 s^{-1}
ICI Maranyl A690 (50% glass in Nylon 66)	285	3819	0·766	376	0·683	761	42
ICI Maranyl A100 (unfilled Nylon 66)	285	355·9	0·901	62·1	0·810	179	16·7
ICI Verton RF-700-10 (50% long glass in Nylon 66) 10 mm unidirectional pellets)	285	221 000	0·555	1418	0·572	10 244	73·6
ICI HW60 GR30 (30% glass in polypropylene)	240	10 000	0·678	6224	0·301	1081	49·8
ICI GWM101 (unfilled polypropylene)	240	2800	0·914	4771	0·343	1546	51
DMC (dough moulding compound, unthickened, containing 14 wt% glass)	30	119 466	0·610	2332	0456	8077	54·4

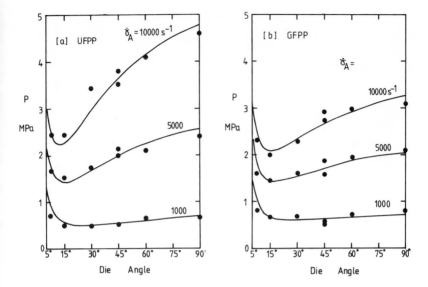

Fig. 3.15. Entry pressure vs. die angle for polypropylene compounds: (a) UFPP and (b) GFPP as described in Fig. 3.4. Die bore radius 2 mm; temperature 240 °C.

measured entry pressure, leaving the pressure drop due to extension only.

From eqn (3.51) it can be seen that a log-log plot of

$$\frac{P_{E_{Ent}}}{\left[\dfrac{2}{3n}\left(\dfrac{\sin \alpha(1 + \cos \alpha)}{4}\right)^n\left(1 - \left(\dfrac{R_1}{R_0}\right)^{3n}\right) + \dfrac{\Phi(n_1\alpha)}{4^n}\right]}$$

versus $\dot\gamma_A$ will have a slope of n and an intercept of log A. Figure 3.16 shows log-log plots of this type. Making these plots requires an iterative process, as the vertical axis is a function of n. An initial estimate of n could be found from a log-log plot of $P_{E_{Ent}}$ vs. $\dot\gamma_A$, or the initial trial value could simply be taken as unity. In the example shown here, the n values which gave the best fit were converged upon after only two trials. The values of A and n obtained from Fig. 3.16 are given in Table 3.2 for the polypropylene materials, along with a range of other materials studied.

To demonstrate the ability of the power law model to fit the range of data, eqns (3.48) and (3.51) were used to calculate the total entry pressure. The calculated solutions, using the four experimentally determined

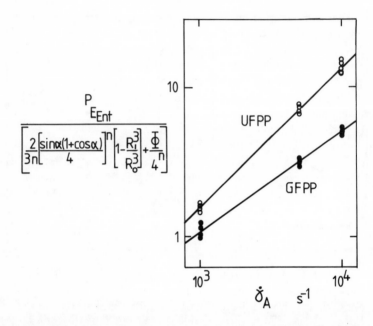

Fig. 3.16. Log-log plots, based on eqn (3.51), containing all the die angle data for UFPP and GFPP. These plots were used to determine A and n.

constants, are shown as continuous curves, plotted through the polypropylene entry pressure data in Fig. 3.15. The power law model also gives a good fit to the data mentioned earlier on nylon 66 compounds. The continuous curves in Fig. 3.5(b) were calculated using the same procedure.

The values of the four flow constants are given in Table 3.2 for six commercially significant moulding materials. All of these materials have a high ratio of extensional viscosity to shear viscosity, the highest being in the case of long fibre reinforced materials such as long glass/nylon and DMC.

3.10. DESIGN OF INJECTION MOULD GATING

In addition to the determination of flow parameters, eqns (3.48) and (3.51) can, of course, be used to calculate the pressure drop in convergences during processing. Although the solutions discussed here only apply strictly to the case of conical dies and channels of circular cross-section, they can be adapted, without much loss of accuracy, to the case of non-circular sections and even cases where the section changes through the convergence. For instance, it is quite common, in the design of gates for injection moulds, to have a convergence which begins with the round or trapezoidal cross-section of the runner and converges to another cross-sectional shape. Provided that the elongational strain in the direction of flow is the predominant strain component, it is often reasonable to treat the convergence as being equivalent to a conical die of the same entry and exit cross-sectional area.

This approach has met with some success in designing injection mould gate and runner systems for a given pressure drop or flow rate, for instance in multi-cavity tools containing cavities of different volumes, where it is desirable for all the cavities to reach the point of complete filling at the same instant.

3.11. CONCLUSIONS

(1) Entry pressure values contain useful information on extensional flow behaviour, which often cannot be generated by other means.

(2) Behaviour can be modelled over a moderate range of strain rates, using only two constants: shear viscosity and extensional viscosity. When extensional viscosity is strain rate dependent, it is necessary to distinguish between λ and λ_A as they differ by a factor of n.

(3) When the Trouton ratio is greater than 3, the flowing fluid is anisotropic, both morphologically and in its response to viscous stresses. Three constants are needed to describe the viscous response of an incompressible anisotropic fluid whose properties are invariant with respect to rotation about the reference axis. Only two of these viscosity constants are needed for flow in conical dies if the fluid reference axis is assumed to coincide with the r direction in spherical coordinates based on the die cone apex.

(4) Energy dissipation arises from both shear and elongational deformations in the die entry. The shear component decreases rapidly with increasing die angle and may often be negligible at moderate die angles. The extensional component increases with die angle and is relatively insensitive to the form of the velocity profile within the die. The model proposed here only describes the pressure drop in constrained convergence. It does not describe or predict the formation of recirculation zones. However, accuracy of the predicted pressure drop is not expected to be strongly affected by the existence or otherwise of recirculation zones.

(5) When modelling entry flow behaviour using a spherical exit boundary, it is necessary to take into account the energy dissipation in the transition region between the spherical exit boundary and the capillary entrance. This effect becomes very significant at die angles above about $45°$.

(6) The most effective treatment of entry flow data involves the assumption of power law behaviour for both shear and extensional flow. The power law constants can be readily computed from the results of capillary flow experiments. The model proposed is able to describe the convergent die flow behaviour of a wide range of polymeric materials at all die angles over a range of flow rates.

REFERENCES

1. J. W. Hill and J. A. Cucolo, *J. Macromol. Sci., Rev. Macromol. Chem.*, 1976, **C14**(1), 107.
2. T. H. Forsyth, *Polym. Plast. Technol. Eng.*, 1976, **6**(1), 101.
3. F. N. Cogswell, *J. Non-Newtonian Fluid Mech.*, 1978, **4**, 23.
4. J. L. Sutterby, *Appl. Sci. Res.*, 1965, **A15**, 241.
5. C. D. Han, *Rheology in Polymer Processing*, Academic Press, New York, 1976.
6. A. G. Gibson and G. A. Williamson, *Polym. Eng. Sci.*, 1985, **25**(15), 968.
7. A. G. Gibson and G. A. Williamson, *Polym. Eng. Sci.*, 1985, **25**(15), 980.
8. R. J. Crowson, A. J. Scott and D. W. Saunders, *Polym. Eng. Sci.*, 1981, **21**, 748.
9. R. R. Lamonte and C. D. Han, *J. Appl. Polym. Sci.*, 1972, **16**, 3285.
10. G. K. Batchelor, *J. Fluid Mech.*, 1971, **46**, 813.
11. G. A. Williamson and A. G. Gibson, *Plast. Rubber Process. Appl.*, 1984, **4**(3), 203.
12. A. G. Gibson, A. N. McClelland, G. Cuff and C. R. Gore, *Developments in the Science and Technology of Composite Materials*, Proc. 1st European Conf. on Composite Materials, Bordeaux, France, 24–27 September, 1985, AEMC, Bordeaux, p. 511.
13. A. G. Gibson and A. N. McClelland, *Fibre Reinforced Composites*, University of Liverpool, 8–10 April 1986, Inst. Mech. Engrs, London, paper 32, p. 99.
14. A. G. Gibson and A. N. McClelland, ICCM6/ECCM2 Conference, Imperial College, London, 20–24 July, 1987.
15. F. N. Cogswell, *Polymer Melt Rheology*, George Godwin/Plastics and Rubber Institute, London, 1981.
16. F. N. Cogswell, *Polym. Eng. Sci.*, 1972, **12**, 64.
17. S. Oka, *J. Phys. Soc. Japan*, 1964, **19**(8), 1481.
18. S. Oka and A. Takami, *Japan J. Appl. Phys.*, 1967, **6**, 423.
19. A. B. Metzner and A. P. Metzner, *Rheol. Acta*, 1970, **9**(2), 174.
20. R. M. Jones, *Mechanics of Composite Materials*, Scripta Book Company, Washington DC, and McGraw-Hill, New York, 1975.
21. W. J. Harrison, *Proc. Cambridge Phil. Soc.*, 1916, **19**, 307.
22. W. N. Bond, *Phil. Mag.*, 1925, **50**, 1958.

Chapter 4

Recoverable Elastic Strain and Swelling Ratio

Roger I. Tanner

Department of Mechanical Engineering, University of Sydney,
New South Wales, Australia

NOTATION

a	constant
$\mathbf{C}^{-1}$	strain tensor
d	recoil distance
D	die diameter
D_∞	final diameter of extrudate
$\mathbf{D}$	rate of strain tensor
$\mathbf{F}_0, \mathbf{F}_1$	deformation gradients
G	modulus
h	thickness
h_f	final sheet half-thickness
h_i	see Fig. 4.2

93

i   unit vector along x-direction
I   unit tensor
L die length
L   velocity gradient
m stretching parameter (eqn (4.34))
n shear-thinning (power law) index
N_1 first normal stress difference
p pressure
P pressure gradient
R_i, R_0 inside and outside radii
R   material tensor
S_R recoverable shear (eqn (4.1))
s parameter $= (t - t')$
t, t' times
t   traction vector (Fig. 4.5)
U potential
v   velocity vector
$\bar{w}$ mean speed in tube
W potential function
W_e Weissenberg number ($\lambda \dot{\gamma}_w$)
x   present position vector
x*   position vector
y coordinate
β neo-Leonov parameter (eqn. (4.31))
γ shear strain
γ_∞ recoil strain
$\dot{\gamma}$ shear rate
$\dot{\gamma}_m$ mean shear rate in die ($8\bar{w}/D$ for tube)
$\Delta/\Delta t$ (upper) convected derivative symbol (eqn (4.25))
ε PTT parameter (eqn (4.27))
$\dot{\varepsilon}$ elongational rate of strain
η viscosity
η_E Trouton or elongation viscosity
λ relaxation time
Λ ratio of lengths, sideways swelling
μ rigidity
ξ PTT parameter (eqn (4.27))
σ shear stress

σ stress tensor
τ extra stress tensor (eqn (4.23))
ϕ Leonov function
χ swelling ratio ($= D_f/D$)

4.1. DEFINITION OF RECOVERABLE ELASTIC STRAIN AND SWELLING RATIO

If a viscoelastic body is in a stressed state, then relaxation of all constraints will cause it to assume a different configuration in the final unstressed condition. Thus one sees a general elastic recovery. The term 'recoverable strain' is usually used more restrictively. Suppose a sample is undergoing a steady shear flow at shear rate $\dot{\gamma}$, where the first normal stress difference is N_1 and the shear stress is σ. If the shear stress is annihilated at $t = 0$, and the normal force constraints are maintained, then the sample will recoil in shear. Suppose the bottom plate defining the shear sample ($z = 0$) is fixed, and the top layer of fluid ($z = h$) recoils through a distance d; the sample thickness is maintained at h always, so the elastic recoil is constrained.[1] For a Lodge-type rubber-elastic liquid,[1] we can show that

$$S_R \equiv \frac{d}{h} = \gamma_\infty = \frac{1}{2}\frac{N_1}{\sigma} \qquad (4.1)$$

The quantity S_R is called the recoverable elastic strain, and for the Lodge model eqn (4.1) is a connection between an elastic property and the viscometric functions. There is evidence[2] that there are real fluids where eqn (4.1) applies, but the connection with the true recoverable shear strain γ_∞ is not exact and will not always be useful. In this chapter we take S_R to be *defined* by $N_1/2\sigma$ and call it the recoverable shear (equivalent to 'recoverable elastic strain'). Note that the factor 2 in this definition is absent in the recoil of solid elastic bodies.[1]

The definition of swelling ratio is taken here to be the ratio $\chi = D_f/D$, where D_f is the final equilibrium extrudate diameter (at the extrudate temperature) and D is the die diameter (Fig. 4.1). There is some influence of temperature variation (across the sample radius) on the swelling, and also die length is important. Thus, we shall assume that the die length is effectively infinite (in practice $L/D > 50$) and also that the flow is isothermal at whatever inlet temperature is relevant. Non-isothermal effects are discussed elsewhere.[3] It is known[4] that some slow changes in D_f can occur

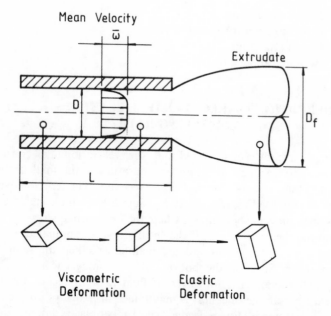

Fig. 4.1. Elastic recovery swelling mechanism.

during cooling (these are supposed to be allowed for in any comparison with experimental measurements); we shall mainly be concerned with swelling which takes place immediately on exit. Gravity, surface tension and Reynolds number (inertia) effects produce only small effects[3] on molten polymer swelling and are ignored here. Briefly, gravity will act like a draw force, reducing swelling (or, if negative, increasing it); surface tension and inertia reduce swelling. We shall assume the material is incompressible and of a single, homogeneous phase to begin with. Under these restrictions, the swelling ratio is just a function of the material rheology and the mean speed of flow ($\bar{w}$) via a Weissenberg number. We now consider various possible mechanisms of swelling.

4.2. ELASTIC THEORY OF SWELLING

One possible swelling mechanism is based on the elastic strain recovery[1] (Fig. 4.1) of a particle of material when released from stress.

To explain the basic idea we may consider the diagram (Fig. 4.1) showing the trajectory of a 'particle' of fluid as it emerges from the die, passing from a stressed viscometric state to an unstressed state. Lodge[1] has shown how such a sheared piece of material exhibits elastic recovery and sideways swelling when released from stress suddenly. We assume that the exit from the tube is sudden and an instantaneous elastic strain takes place which unloads the fluid. (It is more accurate to regard the present calculation as the short-term response to the sudden abolition of the walls in a shear flow.) We shall calculate the instantaneous recovery after shearing two illustrate the mechanism.

As a constitutive equation we assume a KBKZ form:[3]

$$\sigma = -p\mathbf{I} + \int_{-\infty}^{t} U'\mathbf{C}^{-1}\mathrm{d}t' \tag{4.2}$$

where $U' = \partial U/\partial I_{c-1}$ is a function of $(t - t')$ and $I_{c-1} (\equiv \operatorname{tr} \mathbf{C}^{-1})$. Here σ is the stress tensor, p is the pressure, $\mathbf{I}$ is the unit tensor, and $\mathbf{C}^{-1}$ is the Finger strain tensor relating the configuration at time t' (before time t) to that at time t (the present time).[3] We thus ignore the second normal stress difference.

Suppose that the material is undergoing a simple shearing up until $t = 0$, and then is released from constraint. Thus, for $t < 0$, $\mathbf{v} = \dot{\gamma}y\mathbf{i}$, where $\mathbf{v}$ is the velocity vector, $\dot{\gamma}$ is the shear rate, and $\mathbf{i}$ is a unit vector in the x (flow direction); the shear direction is y.

We have, in a viscometric flow

$$\sigma_{xx} - \sigma_{yy} = N_1 = \dot{\gamma}^2 \int_0^{\infty} U's^2\mathrm{d}s$$

$$\sigma_{xy} = \dot{\gamma} \int_0^{\infty} u'\,s\mathrm{d}s \tag{4.3}$$

where $s = t - t'$, and N_1 is the first normal stress difference.

In the present problem the kinematic history consists of a jump strain from the present time $t = 0^+$ to a time $t = 0^-$, then a viscometric history. Let the (unknown) jump strain be described by a deformation gradient $\mathbf{F}_0$. Then the deformation gradient can be written

$$\mathbf{F} = \mathbf{F}^{(v)}\mathbf{F}_0 \tag{4.4}$$

where $\mathbf{F}^{(v)}$ is a viscometric history. Suppose there is a deformed state $\mathbf{x}^*$ just before the jump strain. Then we can write

$$\mathbf{F}^{(v)} = \frac{\partial \mathbf{r}}{\partial \mathbf{x}^*}, \qquad \mathbf{F}_0 = \frac{\partial \mathbf{x}^*}{\partial \mathbf{x}} \tag{4.5}$$

where $\mathbf{r}$ is the particle position at time t'; $\mathbf{x}^*$ is the particle position after the jump ($t = 0^-$) and $\mathbf{x}$ is the current particle position ($t > 0$). Then if $s = -t'$ we have

$$\mathbf{F}^{(\mathrm{v})} = \begin{bmatrix} 1 & -\dot{\gamma}s & 0 \\ 0 & 1 & 0 \\ 0 & 0 & 1 \end{bmatrix} \tag{4.6}$$

For $t' > 0$ we have $\mathbf{F} = \mathbf{I}$, and for $t' < 0^-$ we have $\mathbf{F} = \mathbf{F}^{(\mathrm{v})}\mathbf{F}_0$. Now consider the material for $t > 0$, when the deviatoric stress tensor is zero, but the pressure is non-zero. Then

$$p\mathbf{I} = \int_{-\infty}^{t} U'(\mathbf{F}_0^{\mathrm{T}}\mathbf{F}^{(\mathrm{v})\mathrm{T}}\mathbf{F}^{(\mathrm{v})}\mathbf{F}_0)^{-1}\mathrm{d}t' \tag{4.7}$$

or since $\mathbf{F}_0$ is a constant matrix

$$p\mathbf{F}_0\mathbf{F}_0^{\mathrm{T}} = \int_0^\infty U'\mathbf{C}^{(\mathrm{v})-1}\mathrm{d}s \tag{4.8}$$

where U' is now a function of $\mathrm{tr}(\mathbf{F}_0^{-1}\mathbf{C}^{(\mathrm{v})-1}\mathbf{F}_0^{-\mathrm{T}})$ and s; $\mathbf{C}^{(\mathrm{v})} = \mathbf{F}^{(\mathrm{v})\mathrm{T}}\mathbf{F}^{(\mathrm{v})}$.

To begin with, suppose U' is independent of $\mathrm{tr}\,\mathbf{C}^{-1}$, as in the Lodge rubber-like fluid.[1] Then

$$p\mathbf{F}_0\mathbf{F}_0^{\mathrm{T}} = \begin{bmatrix} G + N_1 & \sigma & 0 \\ \sigma & G & 0 \\ 0 & 0 & G \end{bmatrix} \tag{4.9}$$

where

$$\dot{\gamma}^n \int_0^\infty s^n U' \mathrm{d}s = G, \sigma, N_1 \tag{4.10}$$

for $n = 0, 1, 2$ respectively; G is a modulus, σ is the shear stress in the shear flow, and N_1 is the first normal stress difference. Now the strain matrix $\mathbf{F}_0\mathbf{F}_0^{\mathrm{T}}$ must be volume-preserving, so its determinant must be unity. Taking the determinant of (4.9), we get

$$p^3 = G(G^2 + N_1 G - \sigma^2) \tag{4.11}$$

as a condition on the residual pressure p. The jump strain $\mathbf{F}_0$ is constructed from an elastic displacement field

$$x^* = x/\Lambda^2 + \gamma y$$
$$y^* = \Lambda y \qquad (4.12)$$
$$z^* = \Lambda z$$

where Λ is a sideways expansion and γ is a shear so that

$$\mathbf{F}_0 = \begin{bmatrix} \Lambda^{-2} & \gamma & 0 \\ 0 & \Lambda & 0 \\ 0 & 0 & \Lambda \end{bmatrix} \qquad (4.13)$$

Substituting in (4.9) gives three relations

$$p(\Lambda^{-4} + \gamma^2) = G + N_1$$
$$p\gamma\Lambda = \sigma \qquad (4.14)$$
$$p\Lambda^2 = G$$

Eliminating γ and p from these gives the result for $1/\Lambda$, the sideways swelling:

$$\frac{1}{\Lambda} = \left(1 + \frac{N_1}{G} - \frac{\sigma^2}{G^2}\right)^{1/6} \qquad (4.15)$$

For a single relaxation time

$$\frac{1}{\Lambda} = \left[1 + \left(\frac{N_1}{2\sigma}\right)^2\right]^{1/6} \qquad (4.16)$$

which evaluates the sideways swelling in terms of quantities measurable in viscometric flow. Lodge *et al.*[5] have investigated the response for multiple relaxation times; the result is more complex.

One can apply similar methods to the flow through a tube. If the tube is suddenly removed, then elastic recoil takes place as above. One can calculate the resulting swelling as[6]

$$\chi = \frac{D_f}{D} = \left[1 + \frac{1}{8}\left(\frac{N_1}{\sigma}\right)^2_w\right]^{1/6} \qquad (4.17)$$

or in the plane flow case

$$\chi = \frac{h_f}{h_0} = \left[1 + \frac{1}{12}\left(\frac{N_1}{\sigma}\right)^2_w\right]^{1/4} \qquad (4.18)$$

where N_1/σ is evaluated at the tube or channel wall.

The formulae above agree with some experiments on polymer melts.[7] Huang and White[8] have considered the case where N_1 is proportional to σ^a, where a is a constant, and have replaced the coefficients 8 and 12 in the above formulae by $4a$ and $4(2a - 1)$ respectively, so as to improve the fit of their experimental data.

This mechanism of swelling, though plausible, inadequately describes the kinematics of swelling. For example, where N_1/σ is largest, one expects, from eqn (4.16), the largest local swelling. In fact, as inspection of Fig. 4.1 shows, this must in reality occur on the centreline, where N_1/σ is zero. Pearson and Trottnow[9] have attempted to rectify this problem; their result is not very different in kind from eqn (4.17).

We have now deduced a connection between swelling and $\frac{1}{2}(N_1/\tau)_w$, the recoverable elastic strain at the wall of the die. However, the restrictions on the derivation (single time constant, special constitutive model) and some unsatisfactory features of the kinematics mean that we must look further for the complete explanation of swelling. We now consider an inelastic swelling mechanism.

4.3. INELASTIC THEORY OF SWELLING

There are swellings of extrudates which cannot be explained by the above mechanism. In a *Newtonian* fluid whose viscosity depends on temperature, large swellings can take place when the viscosity near the centreline is lower than that at the outside.[10] It has been proposed that a two-fluid model be used to explain such swellings; Fig. 4.2 shows a sketch of the proposed system. By making a force balance we obtain[11]

$$\chi^2 = \frac{\eta_0}{\eta_i}\left[1 - \left(\frac{R_i}{R_0}\right)^2\left(1 - \frac{\eta_i}{\eta_0}\right)\right] \qquad (4.19)$$

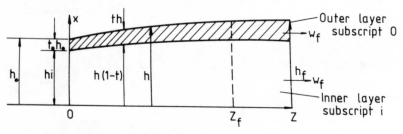

Fig. 4.2. Plane two-layer extrusion; inelastic swelling mechanism.

in the axisymmetric case, and

$$\chi = 1 + \left(\frac{\eta_o}{\eta_i} - 1\right)\left(\frac{h_o - h_i}{h_o}\right) \qquad (4.20)$$

in the plane case.

Here the subscripts (i, o) refer to the inner and outer layers respectively. As an example, if the outer layer has double the viscosity of the inner layer, and $R_i/R_0 = 0.8$, then the axisymmetric and plane formulae give respectively $\chi = 1.166$ and 1.2, relative to the Newtonian case. The Newtonian swelling ratio[3] is about 1.13. Hence the total swelling for the axisymmetric case is about 1.30, by adding 0.13 to the result of eqn (4.19). This idea seems to give a reasonable correlation with numerical calculations but it does contain empiricism. Hence we now consider a more basic approach based on numerical computation of swelling.

4.4. COMPUTATION OF SWELLING FOR VARIOUS RHEOLOGICAL MODELS

In view of the uncertainty of the connection between recoverable shear and swelling, we now present some solutions generated by computation which should better enable us to pin down the causes of swelling. We will first record the equations to be solved and discuss the type of constitutive equation to be used. The methods of computation are discussed elsewhere.[3,12,13]

The flows considered here are assumed to be steady, isothermal, creeping and incompressible. Under these conditions the momentum and continuity equations take the form

$$\mathbf{\nabla} \cdot \boldsymbol{\sigma} = \mathbf{0} \qquad (4.21)$$

$$\mathbf{\nabla} \cdot \mathbf{v} = 0 \qquad (4.22)$$

where $\boldsymbol{\sigma}$ is the total stress tensor, $\mathbf{v}$ is the velocity vector and $\mathbf{0}$ represents the null vector.

The stress tensor in a viscoelastic fluid can be written in the general form

$$\boldsymbol{\sigma} = -p\mathbf{I} + 2\eta_s\mathbf{D} + \boldsymbol{\tau} \qquad (4.23)$$

where p represents the pressure, $\mathbf{I}$ is the unit tensor, η_s is the viscosity of a Newtonian solvent, $\mathbf{D}$ is the rate-of-strain tensor and $\boldsymbol{\tau}$ is the extra stress tensor. The constitutive equations governing the extra stress will be of the type (for a single relaxation mode)

$$\lambda \frac{\Delta \tau}{\Delta t} + \mathbf{R} = 0 \qquad (4.24)$$

where $\Delta\tau/\Delta t$ indicates the upper convected derivative of the extra stress tensor, λ is the relaxation time and $\mathbf{R}$ depends on the particular model chosen. The (upper) convected derivative is given by

$$\frac{\Delta \tau}{\Delta t} = \frac{\partial \tau}{\partial t} + \mathbf{v} \cdot \nabla \tau - \mathbf{L}\tau - \tau \mathbf{L}^{\mathrm{T}} \qquad (4.25)$$

where $\mathbf{L}$ is the velocity gradient tensor. (Components L_{ij} of $\mathbf{L}$ are $\partial v_i/\partial x_j$.) The following models are considered:

Maxwell/Oldroyd-B Model
In this case we define a constant molecular-contributed viscosity, η_m, and choose

$$\mathbf{R} = \tau - 2\eta_m \mathbf{D} \qquad (4.26)$$

The Oldroyd-B model arises if a non-zero value of η_s is adopted in eqn (4.23). In this work we have chosen $\eta_m/\eta_s = 8$.[14]

Phan-Thien–Tanner Model (PTT)
The model proposed by Phan-Thien and Tanner[3] is obtained by choosing

$$\mathbf{R} = \left(1 + \varepsilon \frac{\lambda}{\eta_m} \operatorname{tr}(\tau)\right)\tau + \lambda\xi(\mathbf{D}\tau + \tau\mathbf{D}) - 2\eta_m \mathbf{D} \qquad (4.27)$$

In this model η_m is again constant (in this case the zero-shear-rate viscosity of the model) and $\operatorname{tr}(\tau)$ represents the trace of τ. The parameters[†] ε and ξ are of the order $0\cdot01$ and $0\cdot1$ respectively. The elongational behaviour of the model is largely determined by ε, while ξ affects the shear behaviour (given that ε is small). The values $\varepsilon = 0\cdot01$ and $\xi = 0\cdot1$ were adopted for use with the PTT model.

Unfortunately the PTT model does not behave realistically in steady shear flow. One finds that the shear component of τ approaches zero at high rates of shear. The effect of this can be avoided in an *ad hoc* manner by ensuring that the term η_s in eqn (4.23) is non-zero, so that the total shear stress contains a Newtonian component. It is easily shown that if ε is of order $0\cdot01$ then the total shear stress grows monotonically with the shear

---

[†]The parameter ε used in this chapter is not a strain, it is here just a number; $\dot{\varepsilon}$ however is a tensile strain rate, in accord with the usual notation.

rate when $\eta_m/\eta_s \leqslant 8$. In the present work we have chosen $\eta_m/\eta_s = 8$. However, this alteration has a detrimental effect on the behaviour of the recoverable shear, S_R. If the recoverable shear is plotted against shear rate, one finds that a maximum occurs at a finite value of the shear rate. Thus, the relative significance of the first normal stress difference decreases at higher values of the shear rate. A more pleasing solution to this problem was recently suggested by Phan-Thien.[13] The 'modified PTT model' is obtained by writing

$$\mathbf{R} = \left(1 + \varepsilon\frac{\lambda}{\eta_0}\operatorname{tr}(\tau)\right)\tau + \lambda\xi(\mathbf{D}\tau + \tau\mathbf{D}) - 2\eta_m(\dot{\gamma})\mathbf{D} \qquad (4.28)$$

where $\dot{\gamma} = \sqrt{[2\operatorname{tr}(\mathbf{D}^2)]}$ and

$$\eta_m(\dot{\gamma}) = \eta_0\frac{1 + \xi(2 - \xi)\lambda^2\dot{\gamma}^2}{(1 + \Gamma^2\dot{\gamma}^2)^{(1-n)/2}} \qquad (4.29)$$

In the present paper we set $\Gamma = \lambda$; often it is useful to set $\Gamma > \lambda$. For given ε and ξ, the parameter $0 < n \leqslant 1$ provides control of the steady shear behaviour. The values $\varepsilon = 0.01$ and $\xi = 0$ were adopted for use with the modified PTT model.

In this chapter the original Phan-Thien–Tanner model, eqn (4.27), will be referred to as PTT, while the modified PTT model, eqn (4.28), will be represented as MPTT.

Leonov Model
The Leonov model[15] is obtained by choosing

$$\mathbf{R} = \frac{1}{2}\phi\left[\frac{1}{2\mu}\tau\tau - 2\mu\mathbf{I} + \frac{1}{3}\tau\left(2\mu\operatorname{tr}(\tau^{-1}) - \frac{1}{2\mu}\operatorname{tr}(\tau)\right)\right] \qquad (4.30)$$

where μ is a rheological parameter ($2\lambda\mu$ = zero shear rate viscosity of the model) and $\phi = 1$. Although the Leonov model fits steady shear data extremely well, it is incapable of representing elongational flow realistically; the steady Trouton viscosity is virtually independent of strain rate. Larson[16] recently suggested a modification to the model which allows the elongational behaviour to be altered without greatly affecting the shear behaviour. In this modification the parameter ϕ in eqn (4.30) is replaced by a function of the form

$$\phi = \left(1 + \frac{2\beta}{\pi}\arctan(0.05W/\mu)\right)^{-1} \qquad (4.31)$$

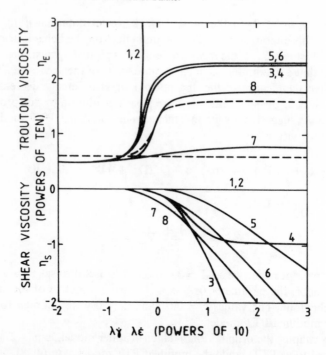

Fig. 4.3. Steady shear viscosity and Trouton viscosity as a function of the dimensionless shear rate, $\lambda\dot{\gamma}$, or elongational strain rate, $\lambda\dot{\varepsilon}$: (1) Maxwell ($\eta_s = 0, \eta_m = 1$, $\lambda = 1$); (2) Oldroyd-B ($\eta_s = 0.112$, $\eta_m = 0.888$, $\lambda = 1$); (3) PTT ($\varepsilon = 0.01$, $\zeta = 0.1$, $\eta_s = 0$, $\eta_m = 1$, $\lambda = 1$); (4) PTT ($\varepsilon = 0.01$, $\zeta = 0.1$, $\eta_s = 0.122$, $\eta_m = 0.888, \lambda = 1$); (5) MPTT ($n = 1, \varepsilon = 0.01, \zeta = 0, \eta_0 = 1, \eta_s = 0, \lambda = 1$); (6) MPTT ($n = 0.5$, $\varepsilon = 0.01$, $\zeta = 0$, $\eta_0 = 1$, $\eta_s = 0$, $\lambda = 1$); (7) Leonov ($\mu = 0.5, \eta_s = 0, \lambda = 1, \beta = 0$); (8) Leonov ($\mu = 0.5, \eta_s = 0, \lambda = 1, \beta = 9$); ----, planar elongation of Leonov fluid. The Trouton viscosity of the MPTT fluid approaches $2/\varepsilon$ at high strain rates.

where W is an 'elastic potential' function given by

$$W = \frac{1}{2}\mu\left(\frac{1}{2\mu}\operatorname{tr}(\tau) + 2\mu\operatorname{tr}(\tau^{-1}) - 6\right) \tag{4.32}$$

The significance of the function ϕ is discussed in detail by Larson.[16] If $\beta = 0$ we recover the original Leonov model. The effect of β on the properties of the model is discussed in the next section.

Another, similar model is that of Giesekus;[17] it will not be used here.

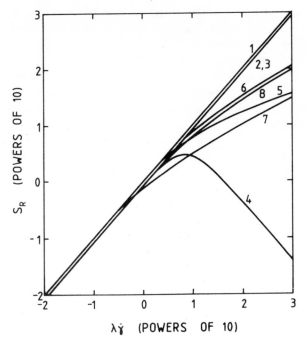

Fig. 4.4. Recoverable shear, S_R, as a function of the dimensionless shear rate, $\lambda\dot{\gamma}$. For legend, see caption to Fig. 4.3.

4.4.1. Steady Shear Behaviour

The rate-of-strain tensor in steady simple shear, with shear rate $\dot{\gamma}$, is given by

$$\mathbf{D} = 0.5\dot{\gamma}\begin{bmatrix} 0 & 1 & 0 \\ 1 & 0 & 0 \\ 0 & 0 & 0 \end{bmatrix} \tag{4.33}$$

The steady shear viscosity is simply $\eta_s + \tau_{12}/\dot{\gamma}$, where τ_{12} is the extra shear stress. A measure of the relative importance of the first normal stress difference, N_1, in shear flow is the recoverable shear, S_R, written as in eqn (4.1).

In some cases (Maxwell fluid, Oldroyd-B fluid and Leonov fluid with $\beta = 0$) it is possible to obtain analytical expressions for the steady shear viscosity and recoverable shear. In other cases it was necessary to solve the governing equations numerically. This was achieved by integrating eqn (4.24) through time, after the sudden application of the required steady shearing motion to a previously static body of fluid. A fourth-order Runge–Kutta algorithm was employed for this purpose. The integration was continued until steady state conditions were reached. The results are shown in Figs 4.3 and 4.4 where the steady shear viscosity and S_R are plotted against the dimensionless shear rate, $\lambda\dot{\gamma}$, which we shall call the Weissenberg number, W_e.

The viscosity in the Maxwell and Oldroyd-B models is independent of shear rate. A more realistic shear-thinning behaviour is exhibited by the MPTT, PTT and Leonov models. The parameter β has a negligible effect on the viscosity of the Leonov model. In contrast, a wide range of shear-thinning behaviour can be obtained using the PTT and MPTT models. Note that the steepest curve corresponds to the PTT model with $\eta_s = 0$. Indeed, the curve is so steep that the slope of the corresponding shear stress versus shear rate curve becomes zero at a finite shear rate, and becomes negative at higher shear rates. This is corrected by ensuring that $\eta_m/\eta_s \leqslant 8$; the case of $\eta_m/\eta_s = 8$ is illustrated in Fig. 4.3. However, this also imposes a lower limit on the viscosity at higher shear rates.

The behaviour of the recoverable shear (Fig. 4.4) is similar in all cases except for the PTT model with $\eta_s \neq 0$. In the case of the Maxwell model we find $S_R = \lambda\dot{\gamma}$, while $S_R = \eta_m\lambda\dot{\gamma}/(\eta_m + \eta_s)$ for the Oldroyd-B model. At low shear rates the recoverable shear corresponding to the PTT model ($\eta_s = 0$) is approximately $S_R = \lambda\dot{\gamma}$, and deviates only slightly from this at high shear rates. In the case of the Leonov model, it can be shown that S_R is proportional to $\sqrt{(\lambda\dot{\gamma})}$ at large values of the shear rate. An analytical expression for all $\lambda\dot{\gamma}$ can also be found for the case $\beta = 0$, by using the exact solution for steady shear flow.[13] The effect of β is clearly to increase S_R at a given shear rate. However, the effect is not particularly great; for large $\lambda\dot{\gamma}$ we find that S_R is increased by a factor of $\sqrt{(1 + \beta)}$. We will see later that β has a much greater effect on the elongational flow characteristics of the Leonov model.

In the case of the PTT model with $\eta_s \neq 0$, the relative importance of the first normal stress difference diminishes at high shear rates. Thus one might expect that any flow phenomenon attributable to the presence of first normal stress differences will diminish as some measure of the 'effective' shear rate (Weissenberg number) is increased. This was found to be so in the die-swell problem.

4.4.2. Steady Elongational Behaviour

The rate-of-strain-tensor in steady elongational flow, with strain rate $\dot{\varepsilon}$, can be written in the form

$$\mathbf{D} = \dot{\varepsilon} \begin{bmatrix} 1 & 0 & 0 \\ 0 & m & 0 \\ 0 & 0 & -(1+m) \end{bmatrix} \tag{4.34}$$

The direction of stretching (with principal rate of strain $\dot{\varepsilon}$) is the x_1 direction. The parameter m determines the type of elongational flow. The case $m = -1/2$ produces axisymmetric (uniaxial) elongation, while $m = 0$ corresponds to planar elongation.

The Trouton viscosity, η_E, is defined as (in uniaxial elongation)

$$\eta_E = (\tau_{11} - \tau_{33})/\dot{\varepsilon} \tag{4.35}$$

An analytical expression for η_E in both planar and uniaxial elongation of the Maxwell and Oldroyd-B fluids is well known.[1,3] It appears to be less well known that the Trouton viscosity corresponding to the planar elongation of the Leonov fluid ($\beta = 0$) can also be found explicitly. The surprising result is that

$$\eta_E = 8\lambda\mu \tag{4.36}$$

i.e. η_E is independent of the strain rate. Thus the Trouton viscosity of the Leonov fluid ($\beta = 0$) in steady planar elongation behaves exactly like that of a Newtonian fluid.

In all other cases is was necessary to evaluate the Trouton viscosity numerically. As before, eqn (4.24) was integrated through time, after the sudden application of the required elongational flow. Integration continued until steady state conditions were reached. The results are plotted in Fig. 4.3 as a function of the dimensionless strain rate $\lambda\dot{\varepsilon}$. To avoid cluttering the figure, only the case of uniaxial elongation is shown. These results are also characteristic of the planar case. For reference, however, the planar case for the Leonov fluid has been included.

The Maxwell and Oldroyd-B models show unsatisfactory behaviour in the sense that η_E is unbounded at $\lambda\dot{\varepsilon} = 1/2$. On the other hand, the Leonov model ($\beta = 0$) is unrealistic in that η_E varies only slightly (if at all) from the zero strain-rate value. The effect of β is significant and it can be shown that the high strain-rate asymptote is increased by a factor of $(1 + \beta)$. Recall that, in steady shear, β has very little effect on the steady shear viscosity and altered S_R at high shear rates by a factor of $\sqrt{(1 + \beta)}$. Thus the parameter β provides significant freedom to fit the Leonov model to elongational flow data, without greatly affecting the fit to shear data.[16]

On the basis of the foregoing discussion it can be concluded that several models represent promising fluids in the sense that they can potentially fit both steady shear and elongational data of real fluids successfully.

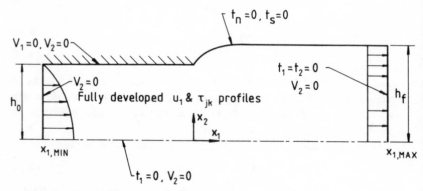

Fig. 4.5. Geometry and boundary conditions for (isothermal) extrusion of a plane sheet of material.

There are of course many other useful constitutive models[3] which do not follow the pattern of eqn (4.24). The main advantage of the Maxwell type models is that, when one is dealing with steady flows, and if the velocities are given, then the streamlines are the characteristic curves of the partial differential equations (4.24), and by integrating along the streamlines this part of the problem is reduced to solving three or four ordinary differential equations at each iteration step. This is straightforward and accurate in cases where no recirculating regions occur. Boundary conditions on the extra stresses τ_{ij} need to be supplied at inlet planes, in addition to the usual mechanical boundary conditions on traction and/or velocity. We thus have an iterative problem for solution,[3,13] and we now consider some results obtained using a boundary element scheme.[13]

4.4.3. Results for the Planar Swelling Problem

The geometry of the (isothermal) planar die swell problem is illustrated in Fig. 4.5. Also shown are the velocity and stress boundary conditions. In addition to these, suitable boundary conditions for the stream function were prescribed. The geometry was chosen such that $h_0 = 1$; $x_{1,\text{MIN}} = -2$ and $x_{1,\text{MAX}} = 3$, so that the channel half-width h_0 was used as a unit of length. The velocity and stress profiles imposed at the upstream boundary plane were the fully developed profiles for pressure-driven flow. In the case of the Maxwell and Oldroyd-B models, the velocity profile is the well known parabolic Newtonian profile. The corresponding stress field is easily evaluated. These results are also approximately true for the MPTT fluid, with $n = 1$, for $W_e < 1.5$ (in this range the shear viscosity is approximately constant). We also found that it is possible to solve exactly the equations for the Leonov model ($\beta = 0$, $\eta_s = 0$) to give

$$v_1 = \frac{-\mu}{P\lambda} \ln \left(\frac{4\mu^2 - P^2 x_2^2}{4\mu^2 - P^2 h_0^2} \right) \tag{4.37}$$

where P is the pressure gradient. Again the stress field is then easily evaluated. In other cases the velocity profile was obtained numerically. The governing equations were cast in a form that allowed the velocity gradient (shear rate) to be evaluated at any value of x_2. This was then integrated numerically, with the initial condition $v_1(h_0) = 0$, to yield the required velocity (and stress) profile.

Two measures of the importance of elastic effects can be used. The first, the Weissenberg number W_e, was defined as

$$W_e = \lambda \dot{\gamma}_w \tag{4.38}$$

where $\dot{\gamma}_w$ is the shear rate at the wall of the die far upstream. This definition can be applied to all elastic fluids, but it is often not a reliable measure of the true importance of elasticity. For example, W_e is not affected by the addition of more Newtonian solvent to an Oldroyd-B fluid, provided that the total viscosity is kept constant, despite the fact that the first normal stress difference has been reduced by this action. A more informative measure to use in these circumstances is the recoverable shear at the die wall, S_R (eqn (4.1)). Both of these measures were used by Crochet and Keunings[14] when studying the die swell of an Oldroyd-B fluid. The relationship between W_e and S_R for the various fluids is given in Fig. 4.4. Note that $S_R = W_e$ for the Maxwell fluid. Clearly, S_R is not a suitable measure to use with the PTT fluid ($\eta_s \neq 0$), and we must rely on W_e in this case.

The parameters of all models were chosen to give a zero-shear-rate viscosity of unity. For convenience, in the case of the Maxwell and Oldroyd-B models the upstream velocity profile was chosen to give a value of $v_1 = 1$ on the centreline, and the Weissenberg number was varied by altering λ. In other cases λ was set to 1 and W_e was adjusted by changing the flow rate.

All simulations were run on a Perkin-Elmer 3220 computer, in double precision. The Weissenberg number was increased in regular steps; the solution at the previous W_e was used to start the next series of iterations. The step used depended on the model. For example, W_e was increased in steps of 0·25 for the Oldroyd-B model, while steps of 0·5 were used for the PTT model and steps of 1·0 for the Leonov model. Generally, smaller steps were used at higher values of W_e if the numerical scheme showed

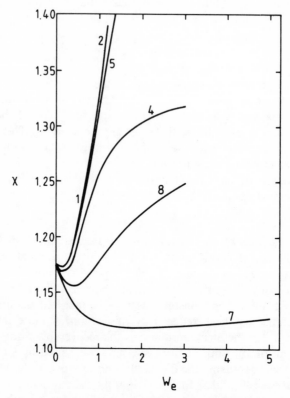

Fig. 4.6. Computed values of the swelling ratio χ as a function of the Weissenberg number, W_e. For legend, see caption to Fig. 4.3.

signs of instability. Each case was run for 20 iterations. In general, satisfactory convergence was obtained within 10–15 iterations. If significantly more than 20 iterations were required the Weissenberg number was not increased further. In the case of the Leonov and PTT models the process was stopped at Weissenberg numbers of 5 and 3 respectively, not because of poor convergence but because it was deemed that no further useful information could be gained by continuing the calculation.

The computed values of the swelling ratio $\chi = h_f/h_0$ are plotted in Figs. 4.6 and 4.7. There is clearly a wide range of behaviour exhibited by the models tested. The results corresponding to the Maxwell and Oldroyd-B models are identical when plotted against W_e. When increasing W_e in steps of 0·25 we were unable to achieve convergence with the Maxwell model

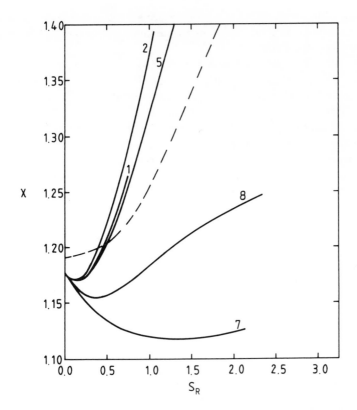

Fig. 4.7. Computed values of the swelling ratio as a function of the recoverable shear at the channel wall, S_R. For legend, see caption to Fig. 4.3. Dashed (———) curve is the elastic swelling formula (4·18) + 0·19. (The plane Newtonian swell is about 0·19.[3])

above W_e 0·75, as illustrated in Fig. 4.6. The Oldroyd-B model failed to converge above $W_e = 1\cdot2$ (with a step of 0·2). The reason for the failure in both cases was the emergence of numerical instability (due to the numerical formulation and, perhaps, inherent instability of the model) and, in particular, the occurrence of large spurious negative values of τ_{11}. This can be understood by reference to the Trouton viscosity shown in Fig. 4.3. It was noticed that the flow field near the lip became more like an elongational flow as W_e was increased. That is, the diagonal components of the rate-of-strain tensor increased in size, while the shear components diminished. By analogy with the pure elongational flow case illustrated in Fig. 4.3, the strain rate exceeded the critical value at which η_E is undefined. Beyond this point τ_{11} became negative, which is a physically unacceptable result.

The MPTT model (with $n = 1$) produced results very similar to those of the Oldroyd-B model in the range of W_e shown. Again this can be understood by reference to the steady shear and elongational behaviour of the model. Firstly, the steady shear behaviours of the MPTT ($n = 1$) and Maxwell/Oldroyd-B models are nearly identical in the range $\lambda\dot{\gamma} < 2$. Secondly, the behaviour of the elongational viscosity of the models is similar, in the sense that η_E rises sharply to a high value as the strain rate is increased for this choice of model parameters. The similarity between the performance of the MPTT model and Maxwell/Oldroyd-B model is therefore expected. It is important to note that numerical instability began to interfere with the solution for $W_e > 1.2$. However, with some perseverance, solutions up to $W_e = 10$ have been obtained. These are shown in Fig. 4.8. No problems associated with the appearance of non-physical solutions, as occurred with the Maxwell/Oldroyd-B models, were found.

The response of the PTT fluid is not unexpected. It has been demonstrated above that die swell can be predicted (semi-empirically) on the basis of the recoverable shear at the die wall. The recoverable shear is therefore important in die swell, as well as the elongational behaviour near the lip. By reference to Fig. 4.4 it can be seen that the rate of increase of S_R ($\eta_S \neq 0$) with shear rate begins to decrease significantly for $W_e > 1.5$. The slope of the swelling ratio curve is also seen to decrease steadily in this range. Although solutions for $W_e > 3$ could be obtained, this was not deemed productive. Notice that values of χ for the PTT model at a given value of W_e are consistently less than the corresponding χ for the Maxwell, Oldroyd-B and MPTT models. In a computer study of die swell of an inelastic power-law fluid[18] it has been demonstrated that shear-thinning effects tend to reduce the expansion ratio relative to the Newtonian case. In the case of the PTT fluid, the small reduction of χ relative to a similar fluid that does not exhibit shear-thinning is expected.

The behaviour of the Leonov fluid ($\beta = 0$) is less easily understood. The recoverable shear varies as $\sqrt{W_e}$ at large W_e, while for the other models it varies as W_e. However, in the range $W_e < 1$ the choice of model does not significantly affect S_R, whereas the expansion ratio for the Leonov model behaves very differently from that of other models. Note also that shear-thinning behaviour is not unusual in this range of W_e. Therefore the behaviour of the expansion ratio cannot be explained on the basis of S_R (evaluated at the wall) and shear-thinning alone. The explanation can be found by returning to the elongational behaviour. By considering the stiffness of elongated filaments on the outside of the extrudate, we have demonstrated above that die swell can also be predicted (semi-empirically) on the basis of elongational flow. Again this is not the whole explanation of swelling since shear effects are neglected. The important result is that, if the viscosity in elongation is independent of the strain rate (as is the case for the Leonov fluid with $\beta = 0$), then there is no swelling relative to the *base* flow. If the fluid is Newtonian, there is no swelling relative to the Newtonian base flow. In the case of the Leonov fluid, the theory states that there is no swelling relative to the equivalent shear-thinning base flow. At high shear rates the viscosity of the Leonov fluid follows the power-law behaviour, $m^{\dot{\gamma}-1}$. Thus the base flow at high shear rate is a plug flow; there is no expansion. At lower shear rates the shear-thinning behaviour is less severe, and the observed expansion of approximately 12% is not unexpected. In the range $W_e > 2$ the expansion ratio is observed to increase, indicating that other effects (such as the influence of S_R) are becoming important. It was not instructive to seek solutions for $W_e > 5$, although we believe they could be obtained without difficulty.

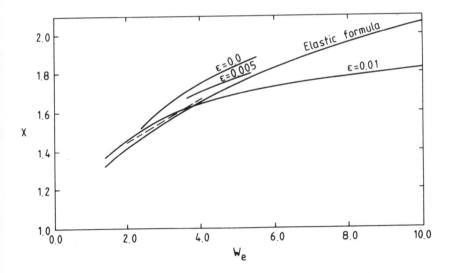

Fig. 4.8. Computed values of the swelling ratio for the MPTT model ($\xi = 0$, $n = 1$, $\eta_s = 0$, $\eta_o = 1$) for $\varepsilon = 0$, 0·005 and 0·01. Note that $\varepsilon = 0$ corresponds to the Maxwell model. Also shown is the elastic formula (4·18) + 0·19 and some results (––––) computed using a finite element programme with the PTT model ($\xi = 0$, $\eta_s = 0·112$, $\eta_m = 0·888$, $\varepsilon = 0·015$).

Further evidence of the importance of the elongational characteristics of a fluid in the swelling problem can be found by observing the case $\beta = 9$. The parameter β has a remarkable effect on the swelling ratio. Recall that β does not greatly affect the shear-thinning behaviour of the Leonov model, but it increases S_R at large W_e by a factor of $\sqrt{(1 + \beta)}$ and increases the maximum η_E by a factor of $(1 + \beta)$. The increase of S_R with β cannot wholly explain the large die swell. As seen in Fig. 4.6, at a given value of S_R at the channel wall, the die swell with $\beta = 9$ is still considerably greater than that for the case $\beta = 0$. Thus the changed elongational behaviour has a marked effect on the die swell. Again we have not proceeded beyond $W_e = 3$, although we believe solutions at higher values of W_e could easily have been obtained. We now have a great deal of freedom to fit the model to elongational and shear data, and to use the model to predict realistic swelling ratios.

The effect of the different models on the exit pressure loss has also been computed.[13]

TABLE 4.1
Swelling of MPTT Fluid

$W_e(= \lambda\dot{\gamma})$	0	0·25	0·5	0·75	1·0	2·0	3·0	4·0	5·0	7·0	10·0
S_R	0	0·25	0·5	0·75	1·0	1·9	2·7	3·3	3·9	4·8	5·9
$\lambda\bar{w}/h_0$	0	0·083	0·167	0·25	0·333	0·667	1·00	1·33	1·67	2·33	3·33
Swelling (%)	18	17	21	26	32	46	57	65	71	77	84

Parameters used here are $n = 1$, $\xi = 0·0$, $\varepsilon = 0·01$, $\eta_s = 0·0$, $\eta_0 = 1·0$. The value of the dimensionless number $\lambda\bar{w}/h_0$ is also given; here $\bar{w}$ is the mean speed in the duct.

Finally, in Fig. 4.8 and Table 4.1 we show results obtained using the MPTT model at higher $W_e < 10$. Note that the present numerical results confirm the trend predicted by elastic theory,[6] eqns (4.17) and (4.18). The boundary element results for the case $\varepsilon = 0$ (Maxwell model) at $W_e > 1$ were obtained by employing the solution for $\varepsilon = 0·005$ as a starting point. We believe these are the first reliable high Weissenberg number results for the Maxwell model (they do not agree with those of Crochet et al.[12,14]). Non-physical solutions did not arise at these values of W_e, indicating that solutions at higher W_e using the Maxwell (or Oldroyd-B) model can be obtained by employing very small increments in W_e. However it is much more practical to use a model that does not suffer from this limitation.

4.5 SUMMARY OF RELATION OF RHEOLOGY TO SWELLING

The following conclusions can now be drawn:

(i) The performance of a viscoelastic model on the numerical die swell problem can be related to the steady elongational and shear characteristics of the model. Both types of behaviour are important in the die swell problem. Swelling is clearly not a unique function of S_R (Fig. 4.7).

(ii) The Maxwell and Oldroyd-B models are capable of predicting significant die swell ($\sim 100\%$). However, experience gained indicates that with these models it is difficult or impossible to obtain convergent solutions at high Weissenberg numbers because of stability problems.

(iii) The MPTT and modified Leonov models show more realistic behaviour.

The prediction of swelling by eqns (4.17) and (4.18) has fitted some data[6-8] well but it does not always give a very accurate prediction. We may for example consider the results for extrusion of LDPE from long dies given by the IUPAC working party.[19] Table 4.2 shows the results at three nominal rates of shear $\dot{\gamma}_m$, where $\dot{\gamma}_m = 8\bar{w}/D$. In this table we have compared the experimental values of swelling with the value of χ given by eqn (4.17) (after adding 0·13 to account for the Newtonian swelling[3]) and with the results from eqn (4.19) (plus 0·13). In looking at the latter we note that we need to estimate R_i/R_o and η_i/η_o. We shall use the extensional viscosity η_E at the outer layer as being the most relevant quantity. Most of the expansion takes place within one tube radius (R) of the exit, and hence the material near the exit goes from zero speed to a speed of $\bar{w}/\chi^2$ in a distance of order R. Hence we will evaluate η_E at an average extensional rate of $\bar{w}/R\chi^2 = \dot{\gamma}_m/4\chi^2$. The inner viscosity η_i will be taken (somewhat arbitrarily) as three times the shear viscosity (3η) evaluated at a shear rate $\dot{\gamma}_m/4\chi^2$, equal to the mean extensional rate. The ratio R_i/R_o is taken to be 0·95 and is estimated empirically. Thus the form of eqn (4.19) used is

$$(\chi - 0.13)^2 = \left(\frac{R_i}{R_o}\right)^2 + \frac{\eta_E}{3\eta_s}\left[1 - \left(\frac{R_i}{R_o}\right)^2\right] \qquad (4.39)$$

TABLE 4.2
Swelling of Low-density Polyethylene[19] (Long Dies, 150 °C)

$\dot{\gamma}_m$	$\chi(exp.)$	$(N_1/\sigma)_w$	$\chi(eqn~(4.17)) + 0.13$	$\chi(eqn~(4.39))$	$\chi(numerical)$[20]
0·1	1·34	1·5	1·17	1·43	1·35
1·0	1·52	3·1	1·27	1·49	1·53
10	1·56	3·8	1·32	1·51	1·75

TABLE 4.3

Swelling Calculations for $S_R = 1·0$ for Various Constitutive Models (Plane Flow Case)

Model	Curve no. in Fig. 4.7	Numerical prediction of χ	W_e	Eqn (4.40)
Maxwell	1	1·35	1·00	1·31
Oldroyd-B	2	1·38	1·11	1·31
MPTT	5	1·33	1·00	1·27
Leonov	7	1·12	1·60	1·20
Modified Leonov	8	1·19	1·11	1·21
Eqn (4.18) + 0·19	–	1·265	–	–

The results, not surprisingly, show that eqn (4.39) is a better fit to the data than eqn (4.17), but neither formula is especially impressive. On the other hand, a full numerical simulation[20] (Table 4.2) of these experiments shows better agreement than either formula at low and medium rates of extrusion, without any empirical input. (The disagreement at higher extrusion rates may be due to wall slip, or deficiencies in the constitutive equations used, or other unknown factors; the matter is still under investigation. Shear heating is not the cause of this difference, as we have determined by simulation.)

We now consider the fit of the various theories to the calculated results given in the previous sections. From Fig. 4.8 we see that the elastic formula (4.18) for the plane case is a reasonable fit to the computed results for the Maxwell ($\varepsilon = 0·00$) and MPTT models up to Weissenberg numbers of order 10.

The results for several models can be examined in Table 4.3, computed for a recoverable shear (S_R) of 1·0. It is clear from previous discussion and Fig. 4.7 that S_R is not the only parameter in swelling. In these plane flows, the viscosities η_E and η are evaluated at the mean elongational rate of $\bar{w}/h\chi$, equal to $\dot{\gamma}_w/3\chi$. The formula used for χ is ($h_i/h_0 = 0·8$):

$$\chi = 1·19 + 0·2\left(\frac{\eta_E}{3\eta_s} - 1\right) \tag{4.40}$$

While the agreement shows correct trends at $S_R = 1$, at $S_R = 2$ the formula (4.40) overpredicts swelling for the modified Leonov model.

4.6. CONCLUSION AND NEED FOR FURTHER INVESTIGATIONS

It has been shown that the currently available theories predicting extrudate swell are only qualitative in character. Therefore it follows that it is generally not accurate to infer rheological properties from swelling experiments. By contrast, the complete numerical solution of the extrusion problem is potentially much more accurate. As a useful outcome it seems likely[20] that the sensitivity of χ to the elongational viscosity function is such that one can deduce a great deal about the η_E function from numerical simulation. With highly elastic (almost Maxwell) materials the elastic formulas (4.17) and (4.18) may sometimes be useful for deducing N_1/σ from results for χ; the inelastic results (4.19) and (4.20) may also be useful over limited ranges when a value of h_i/h_o (or R_i/R_o) can be estimated.

Further application to multi-phase materials is possible but is more complex. The author is unaware of any useful numerical solutions for multi-phase non-Newtonian extrusion. It is clear that further investigation needs to be done on the exact relation between rheological properties and swelling.

ACKNOWLEDGEMENTS

I thank Dr M. B. Bush and Dr N. Phan-Thien for their assistance with the material of this chapter.

REFERENCES

1. A. S. Lodge, *Elastic Liquids*, Academic Press, London, 1964.
2. J. J. Benbow and E. R. Howells, *Polymer*, 1961, **2**, 429.
3. R. I. Tanner, *Engineering Rheology*, Oxford University Press, 1985.
4. W. W. Graessley, S. D. Glasscock and R. L. Crawley, *Trans. Soc. Rheol.*, 1970, **14**, 519.
5. A. S. Lodge, D. J. Evans and D. B. Scully, *Rheol. Acta*, 1965, **4**, 140.
6. R. I. Tanner, *J. Polym. Sci. (A2)*, 1970, **8**, 2067.
7. L. A. Utracki, Z. Bakerdjian and M. R. Kamal, *J. Appl. Polym. Sci*, 1975, **19**, 481.
8. D. C. Huang and J. L. White, University of Tennessee, Polymer Science and Engineering Report No. 113, 1978.
9. J. R. A. Pearson and R. Trottnow, *J. Non-Newt. Fluid Mech.*, 1978, **4**, 195.
10. H. B. Phuoc and R. I. Tanner, *J. Fluid Mech.*, 1980, **98**, 253.
11. R. I. Tanner, *J. Non-Newt. Fluid Mech.*, 1980, **6**, 289.
12. M. J. Crochet, A. R. Davies and K. Walters, *Numerical Simulation of Non-Newtonian Flow*, Elsevier, Amsterdam, 1984.
13. M. B. Bush, R. I. Tanner and N. Phan-Thien, *J. Non-Newt. Fluid Mech.*, 1985, **18**, 143.
14. M. J. Crochet and R. Keunings, *J. Non-Newt. Fluid Mech.*, 1982, **10**, 85.
15. A. I. Leonov, *Rheol. Acta*, 1976, **15**, 85.

16. R. Larson, *Rheol. Acta*, 1983, **22**, 435.
17. H. Giesekus, *Proc. IX Int. Congr. Rheol.*, B. Mena *et al.* (Eds), Elsevier, Amsterdam, Vol. 1, 1985, p. 39.
18. R. I. Tanner, R. E. Nickell and R. W. Bilger, *Computer Meth. Appl. Mech. Eng.*, 1975, **6**, 155.
19. J. Meissner, *Pure Appl. Chem.*, 1975, **42**, 553.
20. R. I. Tanner, in *Numiform '86*, Proc. Second Int. Conf. on Numerical Methods in Industrial Forming Processes, Gothenburg, 1986, A. Samuelsson *et al.* (Eds), Balkema, Rotterdam, p. 59.

Chapter 5

Viscous Heating

R. C. WARREN

Weapons Systems Research Laboratory, Adelaide, South Australia,
Australia

NOTATION

A	pressure coefficient of viscosity
Bi	Biot number
Br	Brinkman number
C_p	heat capacity at constant pressure
C_v	heat capacity at constant volume
D	diameter of capillary
Gz	Graetz number
h	convective heat transfer coefficient inside die to die wall
h_0	convective heat transfer coefficient to die surroundings
k	thermal conductivity of fluid
K	coefficient in eqn (5.21)
k_w	thermal conductivity of die walls
L	length of capillary
m	power law consistency index
n	shear thinning index
Na	Nahme–Griffith number
Nu	Nusselt number
P	pressure
Pe	Peclet number
Δq	heat flux at die walls
Q	volume flow rate
r	radial variable
R	radius of capillary
T	temperature of fluid
T_0	initial temperature of flow and surroundings
T_w	temperature of die walls
ΔT_c	change in temperature at centre of flow from expansion cooling
v	average velocity
v_r	radial velocity
v_z	axial velocity
V	volume
w	mass flow rate
z	axial variable
α	thermal diffusivity
β	thermal coefficient of viscosity
$\dot{\gamma}$	shear rate
δ	die swell (%)

ε coefficient of volume thermal expansion
η shear viscosity
κ bulk compressibility
ρ density
σ_{ij} stress tensor
σ shear stress
σ_w shear stress at die wall

This chapter deals mainly with the effects of viscous heating and how to compensate for them. However, experimental conditions which cause problems with viscous heating often involve pressures sufficiently high for the pressure dependence of viscosity to be significant, so we will give a brief discussion of pressure effects before proceeding to viscous heating.

5.1. EFFECT OF PRESSURE ON VISCOSITY

The high pressures which occur in injection moulding and high rate extrusion can cause a considerable increase in viscosity. This increase in viscosity has been related to the decrease in free volume with increasing pressure, which restricts the mobility of the fluid molecules.[1] The pressure dependence of viscosity is usually assumed to be of the form

$$\eta = \eta_0 \exp (AP) \tag{5.1}$$

where η is the viscosity at pressure P, η_0 the viscosity at atmospheric pressure, and A the pressure coefficient. The value of A for polypropylene is of the order of $5 \times 10^{-9} \, \text{Pa}^{-1}$,[2] and this is typical of many polymers.[3]

The effect of pressure on viscosity is more easily handled than is the effect of temperature. For the case of a Newtonian fluid with a viscosity dependent only on pressure, Denn[4] solved the flow equations exactly to give the pressure drop along a capillary as a function of the exponent A. The solution indicated that choking would occur when the flow rate exceeded a finite value. However, Denn also showed that, if the viscosity was temperature dependent as well as pressure dependent, and the flow was totally adiabatic, then the decrease in viscosity due to viscous heating would be sufficient to prevent choking.

A pressure dependent viscosity can be fairly easily included in a numerical model of flow, and the boundary conditions are simpler than for thermal effects. However, data on the magnitude of the pressure dependence of viscosity are scarce, and the experimental procedures for measuring viscosity under a range of pressures are complicated. For example, Crowson *et al.* developed a rheometer for studying the effect of pressure at shear rates appropriate to injection moulding,[2] and they found that for polystyrene at pressures up to 140 MPa the effects of both pressure and viscous heating could not be ignored.

Many workers in this area make the assumption that at relatively low pressures the effect of pressure is secondary to the effect of viscous heating, and so can be neglected. However, this assumption should be checked for each particular case.

5.2. EQUATIONS OF FLOW IN CAPILLARIES

The general subject of viscous heating in materials processing and rheometry is very wide, and well beyond the scope of a single chapter. The following discussion will be confined to the situation of flow in capillaries in order to introduce the problems and the general methods of solution. It is relatively simple to generalise the discussion to extrusion through slits. For the effects of viscous heating in rotary rheometry the reader is referred to the excellent review by Winter.[5]

To introduce the nomenclature, we will start with the standard equations for viscous flow in capillaries. The shear stress at the die wall, σ_w, is given by

$$\sigma_w = \frac{PR}{2L} \qquad (5.2)$$

where R and L are the radius and length of the capillary, and P is the pressure drop along the capillary. The apparent shear rate at the capillary wall, $\dot{\gamma}_a$, is given by

$$\dot{\gamma}_a = \frac{4Q}{\pi R^3} \qquad (5.3)$$

where Q is the volumetric flow rate. The apparent shear rate equals the true shear rate, $\dot{\gamma}$, for Newtonian fluids, where the shear stress is given by

$$\sigma = \eta\dot{\gamma} \qquad (5.4)$$

where η is the Newtonian viscosity. For a fluid obeying the power law function of viscosity

$$\sigma = m\dot{\gamma}^n$$

where m is the consistency index and n is the shear thinning index. The effect of temperature on viscosity is assumed to be of the form

$$\eta = \eta_0 \exp [\beta(T_0 - T)] \qquad (5.5)$$

where η_0 is the viscosity at T_0, β is the thermal coefficient of viscosity, and T and T_0 are the local and reference temperatures respectively.

The flow will be considered to occur in a capillary with coordinates r and z in the radial and axial directions, with the relevant velocity components v_r and v_z. The fluid has density ρ, heat capacity at constant volume C_v, and thermal conductivity k. In order to reduce the problem of modelling the flow to practical proportions, the following assumptions are usually made:

(1) The fluid heat capacity and thermal conductivity are constant.
(2) Steady laminar flow prevails, and there is no slip at the die walls.
(3) The flow is axisymmetric.
(4) The radial velocity is sufficiently small to be neglected in the momentum and energy equations, and is included only in the continuity equation.
(5) The effects of inertia, gravity and normal stresses are negligible.
(6) Axial heat conduction is negligible compared to axial convection.

The general equations of continuity, momentum and energy, given for example in Bird *et al.*,[6] reduce, with the above assumptions, to

$$\frac{1}{r}\frac{\partial(\rho r v_r)}{\partial r} + \frac{\partial(\rho v_z)}{\partial z} = 0 \qquad (5.6)$$

$$\frac{\partial P}{\partial z} + \frac{1}{r}\frac{\partial}{\partial r}\left(r\frac{\partial \sigma_{rz}}{\partial r}\right) = 0 \qquad (5.7)$$

$$\rho C_v v_z \left(\frac{\partial T}{\partial z}\right) = \frac{k}{r}\frac{\partial}{\partial r}\left(r\frac{\partial T}{\partial r}\right) - \sigma_{rz}\left(\frac{\partial v_z}{\partial r}\right) - T\left(\frac{\partial P}{\partial T}\right)_\rho\left(\frac{\partial v_z}{\partial z}\right) \qquad (5.8)$$

Note the sign convention in eqn (5.7). The last term in eqn (5.8) allows for the effect of expansion cooling, and discussion of this effect will be given in Section 5.7. Initially the fluid will be considered to be incompressible, and hence the heat capacity will be the same when measured at either constant pressure or constant volume, so $C_v = C_p$. With these changes, eqn (5.8) becomes

$$\rho C_p v_z \left(\frac{\partial T}{\partial z}\right) = \frac{k}{r}\frac{\partial}{\partial r}\left(r\frac{\partial T}{\partial r}\right) - \sigma_{rz}\left(\frac{\partial v_z}{\partial r}\right) \qquad (5.9)$$

To make the solutions of the equations as widely applicable as possible, the equations are usually transformed to a non-dimensional form by making the following substitutions, where v is an average velocity and ρ_0 is the density at T_0:

$$r' = r/R \qquad\qquad z' = z/L$$
$$v'_r = v_r/v \qquad\qquad v'_z = v_z/v$$
$$\eta' = \eta/\eta_0 \qquad\qquad \rho' = \rho/\rho_0$$
$$P' = PR^2/\eta_0 vL \qquad\qquad \sigma'_{rz} = \sigma_{rz}R^2/\eta_0 vL$$
$$T' = (T - T_0)/T_0 \qquad\qquad \beta' = \beta T_0$$

The temperature can also be made non-dimensional by including the wall temperature and the temperature of the surroundings in the equation for T', but the above form has been chosen because the temperature environment for rheological characterisation should be uniform, with the inlet temperature, wall temperature and external temperature all equal to T_0.

5.3. DIMENSIONLESS NUMBERS DESCRIBING NON-ISOTHERMAL FLOW

When the non-dimensionalised variables are substituted into the flow equations, it is possible to write the coefficients in the equations in terms of dimensionless numbers. This procedure not only increases the generality of the equations, but the values of the resulting dimensionless numbers give an indication of the magnitude of the various factors affecting flow.[7] The appropriate numbers are defined and discussed below.

Brinkman Number
Newtonian fluid:

$$\mathrm{Br} = \frac{\eta_0 v^2}{kT_0} = \frac{\text{Rate of heat generated by viscous dissipation}}{\text{Rate of heat conduction to the walls}}$$

Power law fluid:

$$\mathrm{Br} = \frac{mv^{n+1}}{kT_0 R^{n-1}}$$

The Brinkman number compares the relative effect of temperature changes due to viscous heat generation to the absolute temperature of the capillary wall. The range of Br is $0 < \mathrm{Br} < \infty$.

Nahme–Griffith Number
Newtonian fluid:

$$\text{Na} = \frac{\beta v^2 \eta_0}{k} = \frac{\text{Heat generated by viscous dissipation}}{\text{Heat conduction in the radial direction}}$$

Power law fluid:

$$\text{Na} = \frac{\beta m v^{n+1}}{k T_0 R^{n-1}}$$

Na determines if viscous dissipation will lead to temperature changes sufficient to affect viscosity. The range of the Nahme–Griffith number is $0 < \text{Na} < 200$. For $\text{Na} < 0.1$ to 0.5 the viscosity is unaffected by temperature.[5]

Peclet Number

$$\text{Pe} = \frac{\rho_0 C_p v R}{k} = \frac{\text{Convected heat in the axial direction}}{\text{Conducted heat in the radial direction}}$$

Graetz Number

$$\text{Gz} = \frac{\rho_0 C_p v R^2}{kL} = \frac{\text{Heat convection in axial direction}}{\text{Heat conduction in radial direction}}$$

Gz is sometimes defined as $w C_p / kL$, where w is the mass flow rate. This version of Gz is π times the value of Gz used here. Gz can also be expressed as $\text{Pe} \cdot R/L$. The Graetz number compares the time required for heat to be conducted from the centre of the die to the wall with the residence time in the die. The range of Gz is $10^{-1} < \text{Gz} < 10^4$: $\text{Gz} < 1$, heat transfer is dominated by conduction; $\text{Gz} \gg 1$, convection is dominant, streamlines are isotherms; $\text{Gz} \simeq O(10)$, both conduction and convection are important.

Nusselt Number

$$\text{Nu} = \frac{hR}{k}$$

where h is the heat transfer coefficient from the fluid to the capillary.

Biot Number

$$\text{Bi} = \frac{h_0 R}{k}$$

where h_0 is the heat transfer coefficient from the capillary to the coolant.[8] Bi measures the ability of the walls to transmit heat to the cooling fluid. The equation for Bi can be rewritten as

$$\left(\frac{\partial T}{\partial r}\right)_w = \text{Bi}\left(\frac{T_w - T_0}{r}\right)$$

where T_0 is the temperature of the surroundings, and T_w is the temperature of the fluid at the die walls.

5.4. NON-DIMENSIONAL EQUATIONS OF FLOW

After substituting the non-dimensional variables into the flow equations, the dimensionless equations for continuity, momentum and energy reduce to

$$\frac{1}{r'}\frac{\partial}{\partial r'}(\rho' r' v'_r) + \frac{R\partial(\rho' v'_z)}{L\partial z'} = 0 \qquad (5.10)$$

$$\frac{\partial P'}{\partial z'} + \frac{L}{R}\frac{1}{r'}\frac{\partial}{\partial r'}\left(r'\frac{\partial \sigma'_{rz}}{\partial r'}\right) = 0 \qquad (5.11)$$

$$\text{Gz}\rho' v'_z\left(\frac{\partial T'}{\partial z'}\right) = \frac{1}{r'}\frac{\partial}{\partial r'}\left(r'\frac{\partial T'}{\partial r'}\right) - \frac{L}{R}\text{Br}\sigma'_{rz}\left(\frac{\partial v'_z}{\partial r'}\right) \qquad (5.12)$$

The following boundary conditions, in non-dimensional form, are usually used in solving the flow equations:

$$
\begin{array}{llll}
T' = 0 & z' = 0 & 0 < r' < 1 \\
v'_z = v'_z(r') & z' = 0 & 0 < r' < 1 \\
v'_r = 0 & z' = 0 & 0 < r' < 1 \\
P' = 0 & z' = 0 & 0 < r' < 1 \\
v'_r = 0 = v'_z & r' = 1 & 0 < z' < 1 \\
v'_r = 0 & r' = 0 & 0 < z' < 1 \\
\sigma'_{rz} = 0 & r' = 0 & 0 < z' < 1 \\
\partial T'/\partial r' = 0 & r' = 0 & 0 < z' < 1
\end{array}
$$

Extra thermal boundary conditions are required at the capillary wall, and these will be discussed in Section 5.6.

5.5. SOLUTION METHODS FOR THE EQUATIONS OF FLOW

5.5.1. Analytical Methods

The equations of energy and momentum are coupled through the temperature dependence of viscosity, and it is not possible to obtain an exact analytical solution to the equations in the general case. Analytical solutions obtained by decoupling the momentum and energy equations by assuming a temperature independent viscosity of a Newtonian fluid in a long pipe with isothermal walls have been obtained by a number of authors.[9,10]

Recently, Dinh and Armstrong[11] have obtained analytical expressions for the temperature distribution in flows where the viscosity is independent of temperature but can be an arbitrary function of shear rate. Both capillary and slit flow geometries were considered with an arbitrary heat transfer coefficient at the wall. This thermal boundary condition includes adiabatic and isothermal walls as extreme cases. While the results can only strictly be used where the viscosity is relatively insensitive to temperature, the procedure can be used as an adjunct to numerical solutions by providing a means for calculating the temperature from the calculated velocity distribution directly, and hence reducing the number of computations in numerical solutions.

Using the assumption of temperature independent viscosity, Ybarra and Eckert[12] converted the flow equations to an eigenvalue problem, and solved for the eigenfunctions numerically. The thermal boundary conditions were either adiabatic or isothermal walls, and for each case they presented functions defining the temperature distributions for the flow of power law fluids with values of n from 0 to 1. The results were illustrated by curves for various values of Br, n, and die length. The curves were mainly intended to be used for determining if the effect of viscous heating was likely to be significant in any particular case.

Perturbation methods can be used to obtain solutions where the viscosity is weakly dependent on temperature and pressure. Galili *et al.*[13,14] obtained solutions for Newtonian and power law fluids flowing in dies with adiabatic and isothermal die walls. However, the restriction to low Brinkman or Nahme–Griffith numbers limits the practical application of the results.

5.5.2. Empirical Methods

An empirical method of correcting measurements of pressure in a capillary rheometer for viscous heating effects has been developed by Kamal and Nyun[15] for the case of adiabatic walls. Starting from equations similar to (5.6), (5.7) and (5.9), with the assumptions considered above, they derived the following expression for the shear stress in a capillary of length L and radius R, with a pressure drop along the die of P at a volume flow rate Q:

$$\sigma_{rz} = -\frac{R}{2}\left(\frac{\partial P}{\partial L}\right)_{Q,R,T_0} \Bigg/ \left[1 + \frac{1}{rC_p}\left(\frac{\partial P}{\partial T_0}\right)_{Q,R,L}\right] \quad (5.13)$$

From measurements of the pressure drop in capillaries of various lengths, for a range of initial temperatures, the equivalent shear stress for isothermal flow at T_0 can be calculated. A flow curve of true shear stress versus true shear rate can be constructed by repeating the procedure at a range of flow rates and calculating the true shear rates by applying the Rabinowitsch correction in the standard manner.

A similar expression to eqn (5.13) was derived for the case of isothermal walls. However, to apply the expression, a knowledge of the heat flux through the die walls is required, and this involves a numerical solution of the flow equations. In these circumstances it is probably preferable to solve the flow equations directly.

5.5.3. Numerical Methods

Because of the coupling of the energy and momentum equations, the only way to calculate thermal effects in the general case is with the use of numerical methods. Finite difference methods are most commonly used for calculating the effects of heating for flow confined in dies,[16-21] but finite element methods are more suitable when free surfaces are involved.[22]

The following procedure is commonly used to calculate the temperature and velocity for all points in the die.[16,17,19] The temperature distribution is calculated from the energy equation (5.12), but since the velocities and stresses in the coefficients of the equation are not known *a priori* they must be calculated as part of the process for solving the energy equation. An iterative method of solving eqn (5.12) is used which involves rewriting the equation in terms of an iteration parameter, s:

$$\mathrm{Gz}(\rho' v_z')^s \left(\frac{\partial T'}{\partial z'}\right)^{s+1} = \frac{1}{r'}\frac{\partial}{\partial r'}\left(r'\frac{\partial T'}{\partial r'}\right)^{s+1} - \frac{L}{R}\,\mathrm{Br}\left(\sigma_{rz}'\frac{\partial v_z'}{\partial r'}\right)^s \quad (5.14)$$

where s denotes the values of the parameters calculated with the current estimate of temperatures, and $s + 1$ denotes the new values of temperature to be calculated. Equation (5.14) is solved by converting it to a difference equation, and calculating the differences on a grid filling the die, where the grid spacing is equal to the step size used to calculate the differences. New coefficients in eqn (5.14) are calculated for each step in the iterative process by the following procedure.

The definitions of viscosity and shear stress are combined to give

$$\sigma'_{rz} = -\frac{R}{L} \eta' \frac{\partial v'_z}{\partial r'} \tag{5.15}$$

Substituting into eqn (5.11),

$$\frac{\partial P'}{\partial z'} + \frac{L}{R} \frac{1}{r'} \frac{\partial}{\partial r'} \left(r' \frac{\partial \sigma'_{rz}}{\partial r'} \right) = 0 \tag{5.11}$$

and integrating gives

$$v'_z(r', z') = \frac{1}{2} \frac{\partial P'}{\partial z'} \int_1^{r'} \frac{\bar{r}}{\eta} \, \mathrm{d}\bar{r} \tag{5.16}$$

The mass flow rate through any section in the die must be constant, and this is expressed as

$$2\pi \int_0^1 r' v'_z r' \, \mathrm{d}r' = 1 \tag{5.17}$$

Combining eqns (5.16) and (5.17) gives an expression for the pressure gradient:

$$\frac{\mathrm{d}P'(z')}{\mathrm{d}z'} = \left(\int_0^1 \rho' \int_1^{r'} \frac{\bar{r}\mathrm{d}\bar{r}}{\eta'} r' \, \mathrm{d}r' \right)^{-1} \tag{5.18}$$

This value of $\mathrm{d}P'/\mathrm{d}z'$ is substituted into eqn (5.16) to give a new estimate of $v'_z(r', z')$. Integrating eqn (5.10),

$$\frac{1}{r'} \frac{\partial(\rho' r' v'_r)}{\partial r'} + \frac{R}{L} \frac{\partial(\rho' v'_z)}{\partial z'} = 0 \tag{5.10}$$

and substituting the new value of v_z gives

$$v'_r(r', z') = -\frac{R}{L} \frac{1}{\rho' r'} \int_1^{r'} \frac{\partial}{\partial z'} (\rho' v'_z) r \, \mathrm{d}r \tag{5.19}$$

The iterative process is started by assuming a constant temperature in the die and a velocity profile at the die inlet corresponding to isothermal flow. The integrals in eqns (5.16)–(5.18) are performed stepwise down the die to give the velocity distribution in the die. Equation (5.14) is then used to give the temperature distribution, which in turn is used to modify the viscosity. The new viscosity is substituted into the integrals and the process repeated until convergence is obtained.

Central differences are used in the radial direction, and backward differences are used in the axial direction. The reason for using backward differences is two-fold; the influence of downstream temperatures is eliminated, as required by the assumption that there is no axial thermal conduction, and also the difference equations are broken up into series of sets with one set for each slice in the axial direction. The equations for each axial slice can be solved separately, instead of one combined set of equations for all the points in the die which have to be solved simultaneously. For example, if there were 50 steps in the radial direction and 100 in the axial direction, then there would be 100 lots of equations in 50 unknowns, instead of 5000 equations in 5000 unknowns.

The accuracy of the procedure can be increased by using a finer grid where the flow variables change most rapidly near the wall and at the entrance.[16] However, rather than deal with the added complication of non-uniform grid spacings, the same effect can be achieved by transforming the spatial variables in the following manner:[17]

$$\phi = \exp(\xi r') \quad \text{and} \quad \psi = \exp[\zeta(1 - z')]$$

The resulting equations are solved in the same way as the untransformed equations.

5.6. THERMAL BOUNDARY CONDITIONS AT THE DIE WALLS

Even in numerical solutions, the thermal boundary conditions assumed at the die walls are only approximations, and the choice of wall thermal boundary condition can have considerable influence on the predicted flow behaviour. The general effects of applying the various boundary conditions are considered below, and they will be illustrated by a particular example of calculated behaviour of flow of a Newtonian fluid.

5.6.1. Adiabatic Walls
In this case the walls are assumed to be insulated, with no heat flow into the wall. Since the heat continues to be generated without any sink, the temperature continues to rise, and no steady state is achieved. However,

in sufficiently long dies the temperature profile attains a constant shape, with only the magnitude of the temperature continuing to grow.

The effect of viscous heating can be minimised in the adiabatic wall case by using the shortest practical dies with the largest diameter. These dies give higher shear rates and stresses for the same pressure drop, and hence temperature rise. This can be seen from eqn (5.2) which shows that pressure drop is proportional to the length and inversely proportional to the diameter of the capillary.

5.6.2. Isothermal Walls

In the isothermal wall case it is assumed that the cooling of the die walls is sufficiently effective for the walls to be maintained at a constant temperature. Near the die entrance the maximum temperature occurs adjacent to the wall where the rate of heat generation is greatest. However, heat will be conducted towards the cooler centre of the flow until the temperature at the centre is high enough for the thermal gradient from the wall to the centre to balance the rate of heat generated and the heat lost through the walls. This will be the steady state situation at long times. The flow can be considered to be fully developed when Gz is ~ 10 when approached from above.[23]

Shorter capillaries retain relatively more heat as there is less time for heat transfer to the walls, and thinner capillaries retain relatively less heat as there is a shorter distance for the heat to be conducted away.

5.6.3. Constant Heat Transfer Coefficient at the Die Walls

The true thermal boundary condition at the die walls is intermediate between the adiabatic and isothermal die wall cases, because there is a finite amount of heat lost through the die wall. Under these conditions a steady state flow is achieved in sufficiently long dies. The rate of heat loss depends on the temperature gradient at the wall, the die wall material, the efficiency of the cooling system and the distance along the capillary. An approximate method of setting a boundary condition is to specify a constant heat transfer coefficient at the walls. The heat flow at the wall, Δq, is assumed to be given by

$$\Delta q = h(T - T_0) = hT'T_0 \qquad (5.20)$$

There is no generally accepted way of specifying h. A method described by Cox and Macosko[16] uses the relationship

$$Nu = K \cdot Gz^{1/3} \qquad (5.21)$$

where Nu, Gz and K are given by

$$\mathrm{Nu} = \frac{hR}{k}, \mathrm{Gz} = \frac{\rho_0 C_p v^2 R}{kL}, K = 1.75$$

The relationship (5.21) was derived from a consideration of heat transfer from fluids in capillaries with a temperature difference between the fluid and the wall, and it strictly does not apply in the case of viscous heat generation. The use of the Nusselt number was questioned by Winter[5] because it relates the temperature gradient at the wall to the average temperature difference between the fluid and the wall. In the general case the wall temperature may be above the initial temperature of the fluid, giving a negative value of Nu. However, in the case of current interest where the wall and inlet temperatures are the same, the relation between Nu and Gz does provide a simple, objective method of specifying a more realistic boundary condition than either isothermal or adiabatic walls, and its use has some empirical justification from the work of Cox and Macosko[16] and Forrest and Wilkinson.[24]

An alternative method of specifying a thermal boundary condition at the wall, which mirrors the physical situation more exactly, involves the Biot number defined by $\mathrm{Bi} = h_0 R/k$ where h_0 is the heat transfer coefficient from the outside of the die wall to the coolant.[8] The heat flow through the walls is then given by

$$\Delta q = h_0(T_w - T_0) = \frac{\mathrm{Bi} \cdot k}{R}(T_w - T_0) \tag{5.22}$$

where T_w is the local temperature of the die walls and T_0 is the environment temperature.

There is a formal similarity between the Nusselt number and the Biot number. The main difference is that Nu involves a heat transfer coefficient from the fluid to the walls, whereas Bi involves a heat transfer coefficient from the walls to the surrounding coolant. This formal analogy may provide a reason for the apparent success obtained from the use of the Nu vs. Gz relationship (5.21) in specifying the boundary condition.[16]

A more satisfying method of specifying the heat transfer coefficient at the wall is given by Winter[5] who explicitly considers the total system of fluid, die wall and coolant. The thermal gradient in the fluid adjacent to the wall is taken to be proportional to the difference in temperature between the fluid at the die wall and the surroundings. The constant of proportionality is the Biot number. Equating the heat flux from the fluid to the heat flux to the coolant gives

$$k\left(\frac{\partial T}{\partial r}\right)_w = h_0(T_w - T_0) \tag{5.23}$$

Substituting for h_0 from the definition of Bi gives

$$\left(\frac{\partial T}{\partial r}\right)_w = \frac{Bi(T_0 - T_w)}{R} \tag{5.24}$$

If it assumed that the heat flux through the wall is governed by the thermal conductivity of the wall, and that the outer wall temperature is maintained at the initial temperature T_0, then the heat flux is given by

$$\Delta q = \frac{k_w}{R} \frac{(T_w - T_0)}{\ln(1 + S/R)} \tag{5.25}$$

where S is the wall thickness.[5]

Very large values of Bi (> 100) correspond to isothermal walls, and Bi $= 0$ corresponds to adiabatic walls. Winter also considered the case where the walls have thermal capacity and the thermal boundary is explicitly time dependent.[5]

5.6.4. An Example of the Effects of Different Thermal Boundary Conditions

To give an illustration of the effects of viscous heating, we will present the results of calculations of the flow of a Newtonian fluid with a moderate dependence of viscosity on temperature. The calculations were made using the finite element computer program THERMOVISC2 developed by Professor R. I. Tanner and co-workers at the University of Sydney, Australia.

The viscosity is given by $\eta = 1000 \exp[0{\cdot}05(300 - T)]$. The temperature at the die inlet is $300\,°C$, and the dimensions of the die are $R = 1\,mm$ and $L = 30\,mm$. The heat capacity and thermal conductivity of the fluid are $1000\,J\,kg^{-1}\,°C^{-1}$ and $0{\cdot}34\,J\,ms^{-1}\,°C^{-1}$ respectively. The corresponding flow parameters are:

Average velocity	$25\,mm\,s^{-1}$	$100\,mm\,s^{-1}$
Shear rate	$100\,s^{-1}$	$400\,s^{-1}$
Br	0.0061	0.098
Na	0.092	1.47
Pe	96	382
Gz	3.2	12.7

Three types of thermal boundary condition at the wall are considered: isothermal walls, adiabatic walls, and a constant heat transfer coefficient, h, at the walls. The value of h is arbitrarily chosen to be defined by eqn (5.21),

$$\text{Nu} = \frac{hR}{k} = 1.75\,\text{Gz}^{1/3}$$

Results for a temperature insensitive viscosity, $\beta = 0$, are also given for comparison. The axial profile of the relative pressure drop in the die at an average velocity of 100 mm s^{-1} is given in Fig. 5.1. For $\beta = 0$ the pressure gradient is constant, as expected. The adiabatic wall gives the greatest decrease in pressure compared with the $\beta = 0$ case, and there is considerable curvature in the pressure profile. The isothermal wall has the smallest effect on pressure.

The axial profiles of maximum temperature rise at a velocity of 100 mm s^{-1} are given in Fig. 5.2. In all cases the temperature increases rapidly at the start of the die, but the rate of increase progressively drops

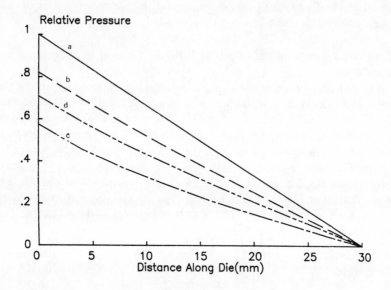

Fig. 5.1. Calculated axial pressure profile at an average velocity of 100 mm s^{-1}: a, $\beta = 0$; b, isothermal wall; c, adiabatic wall; d, constant heat transfer coefficient at the die wall.

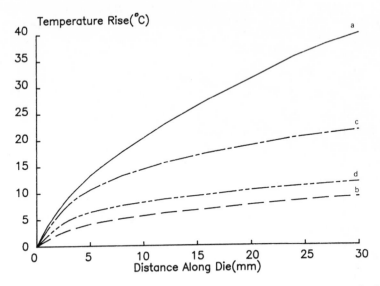

Fig. 5.2. Calculated axial profile of maximum temperature at an average velocity of $100\,\mathrm{mm\,s^{-1}}$: a, $\beta = 0$; b, isothermal wall; c, adiabatic wall; d, constant heat transfer coefficient at the die wall.

along the length of the die. At the exit of the die the temperature is almost constant in the cases where there is heat loss to the walls.

The radial profiles of temperature rise at the die exit for a velocity of $100\,\mathrm{mm\,s^{-1}}$ are given in Fig. 5.3. The most noticeable features are that the fluid has spent insufficient time in the die for heat to be conducted to the centre of the die, and also that the different thermal boundary conditions have no effect for half the radial distance in the die. The radial temperature profiles at the lower velocity of $25\,\mathrm{mm\,s^{-1}}$ are given in Fig. 5.4. The temperature rises are much lower, and the longer transit time in the die has allowed sufficient heat conduction towards the centre of the die for the profiles to have almost attained their equilibrium shapes.

5.7. EFFECT OF FLUID COMPRESSIBILITY AND EXPANSION COOLING

Equation (5.8) contains the heat capacity at constant volume, C_v, whereas the heat capacity is usually measured at constant pressure to give C_p. An

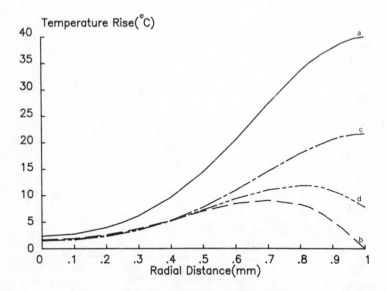

Fig. 5.3. Calculated radial temperature profile at an average velocity of $100\,\text{mm s}^{-1}$: a, $\beta = 0$; b, isothermal wall; c, adiabatic wall; d, constant heat transfer coefficient at the die wall.

equation in terms of C_p can be obtained by rewriting the expansion term:[21]

$$T\left(\frac{\partial P}{\partial T}\right)_\rho \left(\frac{\partial v_z}{\partial z}\right) = T\varepsilon v_z \left[\frac{\varepsilon}{\kappa}\left(\frac{\partial T}{\partial z}\right) - \frac{\partial P}{\partial z}\right] \tag{5.26}$$

where

$$\varepsilon = \frac{1}{V}\left(\frac{\partial V}{\partial T}\right)_P \quad \text{and} \quad \kappa = -\frac{1}{V}\left(\frac{\partial V}{\partial P}\right)_T$$

Combining eqns (5.8) and (5.26) and rearranging gives

$$\rho v_z \left(\frac{\partial T}{\partial z}\right)\left(C_v + \frac{T^2\varepsilon}{\kappa\rho}\right) = \rho v_z C_p \left(\frac{\partial T}{\partial z}\right) = \frac{k}{r}\frac{\partial}{\partial r}\left(r\frac{\partial T}{\partial r}\right)$$

$$- \sigma_{rz}\left(\frac{\partial v_z}{\partial r}\right) + T\varepsilon v_z \left(\frac{\partial P}{\partial z}\right) \tag{5.27}$$

The non-dimensional form of the equation is

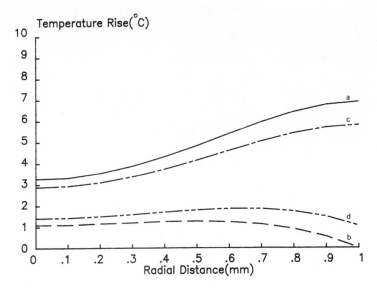

Fig. 5.4. Calculated radial temperature profile at an average velocity of 25 mm s^{-1}: a, $\beta = 0$; b, isothermal wall; c, adiabatic wall; d, constant heat transfer coefficient at the die wall.

$$\text{Gz}\rho'v'_z\left(\frac{\partial T'}{\partial z'}\right) = \frac{1}{r'}\frac{\partial}{\partial r'}\left(r'\frac{\partial T'}{\partial r'}\right) - \frac{L}{R}\text{Br}\sigma'_{rz}\left(\frac{\partial v'_z}{\partial r'}\right)$$

$$+ \text{Br}T\varepsilon v'_z\left(\frac{\partial P'}{\partial z'}\right) \tag{5.28}$$

The term $T\varepsilon$ is dimensionless, and hence it has not been necessary to rewrite it in dimensionless units. Since the effect of cooling is dependent on the product $T\varepsilon$, the effect can be large even though ε is usually small.

The consequences of expansion cooling were first emphasised by Toor[10] who calculated the temperature profile in long tubes where the profile was independent of distance along the tube. Additional assumptions were that the viscosity followed the power law and was independent of temperature, the pressure gradient was constant, and the heat transfer coefficient at the wall was constant.

The solutions of the equations for the temperature derived by Toor showed that the effect of expansion cooling was a maximum at the centre of the die and decreased to zero at the wall.[10] Hence the radial dependence of expansion cooling is opposite to the radial dependence of viscous heating which is a maximum near the wall. The change in temperature at the centre of the flow, ΔT_c, is given by

$$\Delta T_c = \frac{PvR^2}{kL} \frac{n}{6n + 2} \left[1 - T\varepsilon \left(\frac{5n + 1}{2n} \right) \right] \qquad (5.29)$$

The effect of expansion cooling alone is given by the ratio

$$\frac{\Delta T_c}{(\Delta T_c)_{T\varepsilon = 0}} = 1 - T\varepsilon \left(\frac{5n + 1}{2n} \right) \qquad (5.30)$$

Note that 'n' used by Toor is equal to $(1/n + 1)$ for n defined here. For a fluid with $n = 0.5$ the magnitude of the expansion cooling is sufficient to cancel the effect of viscous heating at the centre of the flow when $T\varepsilon \simeq 0.28$.

These equations can only be used to indicate the order of magnitude of the effect of expansion cooling, because of the restrictive assumptions made by Toor in deriving them. To determine the effect of expansion cooling in a particular case, the full set of equations including the expansion cooling term have to be solved. This has been done by Cox and Macosko[16] and also by Hulatt and Wilkinson.[21] They found that for moderate pressure drops the temperature change due to cooling was 2–5 °C.

In practice, the effect of cooling will be influenced by the measurement procedure. If the capillary is attached to a continuously operating extruder where the fluid entering the capillary is at thermal equilibrium, the effect of cooling will be a maximum. However, if a ram type capillary rheometer is used, the temperature of the fluid will be raised by compression heating when the pressure is applied to the ram. If the measurements are made before the heat can be conducted away, the cooling of the fluid as it expands in the capillary will tend to reverse the compression heating, and the overall effect will tend to zero.

5.8. MEASUREMENT OF TEMPERATURE RISE DUE TO VISCOUS HEATING

In principle, the bulk temperature rise of the material as it issues from the die can be readily determined by calorimetric means. However, there are usually difficulties in maintaining an adiabatic environment under experimental conditions. The wall temperature of the capillary can be measured with thermocouples soldered to the wall.[17] Alternatively, the surface temperature rise of the fluid issuing from the die can be determined with an infrared pyrometer.[16,25] While these techniques give limited information which is useful for fitting computer models of viscous heating, it is more desirable to obtain the full temperature profile in the fluid.

The most commonly used method of measuring temperature profiles in flowing polymeric fluids involves the use of thermocouple probes immersed in the flow. The probes have to satisfy three main requirements: (1) minimum disturbance to flow; (2) sufficient mechanical strength; (3) good accuracy. The performance of probes with various configurations was judged against these requirements by van Leeuwen who concluded that the most suitable configuration was a probe parallel to the flow and pointing upstream.[26]

Measurement accuracy is affected by a number of factors, including heat conduction along the probe and viscous heating in the layers of fluid adjacent to the probe. Conduction is important when the temperature of the fluid at the tip of the probe is different from the temperature at the root of the probe at the die wall. Van Leeuwen developed an expression for correcting for conduction[26] which was simplified by Hulatt and Wilkinson.[27] The temperature corrections calculated for conduction along the particular probe used were generally less than $0.1\,°C$, and hence were considered to be negligible.

Van Leeuwen also developed an expression for correcting for viscous heating of the probe,[26] but his expression overestimated the amount of heating when compared with experimental measurements. Hulatt and Wilkinson refined the viscous heating correction, and found that the values agreed well with experimental values.[27] In the particular case of LDPE flowing in a $12.9\,mm$ diameter tube at a velocity at the probe tip of approximately $50\,mm\,s^{-1}$, the magnitude of the correction was of the order of $2\,°C$.

Kim and Collins used upstream pointing probes which contained an additional thermocouple at the probe root to measure root temperature.[28] The probes also contained a small capillary to allow air to be blown into the probe root for cooling. The effect of conduction along the probe was calculated by a complicated procedure involving cooling the thermocouple root. The calculated errors were not listed explicitly, but from figures in the paper they appear to vary between 1 and $4\,°C$.

The effect of shear heating was determined by stopping the flow and monitoring the rate of decay of the temperature of the probe tip. The increase in tip temperature due to viscous heating was given by the product of the initial rate of temperature decay and the decay time constant. The values obtained were up to 8 °C, which indicates a significant disturbance to the flow by the probe.

5.9. COMPARISON OF CALCULATED AND EXPERIMENTALLY DETERMINED TEMPERATURE RISES

A comprehensive study of the effects of viscous heating was carried out by Gerrard *et al.*[17,18] They used a lubricating oil with viscosity 1·025 Pa s at 25 °C in capillaries with both adiabatic and isothermal wall conditions. A capillary 0·425 mm in diameter and 103·5 mm long was used for both adiabatic and isothermal walls, and longer and shorter capillaries were used for adiabatic walls. Wall temperatures were measured by thermocouples soldered to the walls, and the temperature profiles were measured in the flow as it emerged from the capillary with butt jointed thermocouples 0·076 mm diameter mounted across the flow. The flow was modelled using the usual assumptions, and an empirical relation was used for the combined temperature and pressure dependence of viscosity. Good agreement was reported between the calculated and experimental temperatures but, since no corrections were made to the thermocouple readings for conduction or viscous heating, the agreement may be partly fortuitous.

The different wall boundary conditions gave large differences in the measured temperature rises. For flow in the 0·425 × 103·5 mm die at a wall shear stress of 2·83 × 10⁴ Pa the maximum temperature rise in the isothermal wall case was 10·8 °C, while for the adiabatic wall case the maximum temperature rise was 33·3 °C. In the adiabatic case the calculated bulk temperature rise was 7·6 °C, so it can be seen that the bulk temperature rise considerably underestimates the maximum temperature rise seen by the fluid.

The axial wall temperature distribution in the adiabatic case showed an initial rapid rise in temperature, but the rise became more gradual as the exit was approached. For the longest die studied, 0·425 × 195 mm, at a shear stress of 1·5 × 10⁴ Pa the wall temperature rose by 200 °C and the measured viscosity decreased by 70%.

Another important finding was that it was impossible to achieve true isothermal wall conditions.[18] The heat transfer from the capillary to the coolant was improved by soldering a brass sleeve over the capillary and pumping the coolant at a rate of 12 litres min^{-1} over the sleeve. However, the wall temperature at the exit of the 0.425×103.5 mm die still rose by 2·8 °C at a pressure of 11·1 MPa. On the other hand, almost totally adiabatic walls were easily obtained.

Cox and Macosko calculated the effects of viscous heating on the flow of ABS and LDPE, and compared the results with experimental measurements of shear stress and surface temperature rise as measured by an infrared pyrometer.[16] The ABS was assumed to be incompressible, and the temperature dependence of the viscosity was fitted by a WLF equation. The temperature and pressure dependence of the viscosity of LDPE was given by an empirical relation. The thermal boundary coefficient at the die wall was specified by a constant heat transfer coefficient which had the value 0 for an adiabatic wall and ∞ for an isothermal wall. Intermediate values were determined by a relation between the Nusselt and Graetz numbers:

$$\text{Nu} = K \cdot \text{Gz}^{1/3} \tag{5.21}$$

The flow of ABS was studied in a slit die of section 0.457×4.03 mm and 26·83 mm long. At an initial temperature of 230 °C the surface temperature rose 23 °C at an apparent shear rate of 8200 s^{-1}. A plot of experimentally determined surface temperature rise versus apparent shear rate was well fitted by calculations assuming a thermal boundary at the walls given by eqn (5.21) with $K = 1$. The flow curve deviated from the calculated isothermal flow curve, but the deviation was not large enough to allow the fitting of any thermal boundary conditions.

For flow in a capillary die 3·18 mm in diameter and 95·3 mm long at 230 °C, the maximum surface temperature rise was 65 °C and the pressure was reduced by 30% at an apparent shear rate of 5730 s^{-1}. The plot of surface temperature rise versus shear rate was best fitted by assuming a thermal boundary condition based on a heat transfer coefficient given by eqn (5.21) with $K = 1.75$. The flow curves could not be fitted by assuming isothermal flow or isothermal walls. Calculated axial temperature profiles indicated that 50% of the maximum temperature rise was achieved in the first 20% of the length of the die.

An annular die with inner and outer radii of 5·08 mm and 10·2 mm and a length of 101·6 mm was used for LDPE. At an initial temperature of 199 °C a surface temperature rise of 25 °C was measured at an apparent shear rate of 235 s^{-1} (given by $4Q/\pi R^3$, where R is the outer diameter). The plot of temperature rise versus shear rate was well fitted by assuming a wall boundary condition given by eqn (5.21) with $K = 1.75$. Expansion cooling was calculated to give a temperature drop of the order of 2 °C in the centre of the flow.

Kim and Collins measured temperature profiles in a PVC blow moulding compound flowing in a 0·75 inch diameter die.[28] Temperature profiles were measured for die wall temperatures of 194·4 °C and 205·5 °C. The flow was modelled using the standard equations, with empirical values for the viscosity as a function of shear rate and temperature, and the calculation included the effect of expansion cooling. The measured upstream temperature profile and constant wall temperature were used as thermal boundary conditions. The agreement was very good at 194·4 °C but was less good at 205·5 °C. However, the distance for heating to occur was relatively small, and the temperature changes over the length were only of the order of a few degrees.

A more comprehensive study was conducted by Hulatt and Wilkinson.[21] Temperature and velocity profiles in the flow of a LDPE in a die of 12·9 mm diameter and 745 mm long were measured. Measurements were made of the inlet and downstream temperature profiles, the axial wall temperature distribution and the downstream velocity profile. The flow was modelled using the usual assumptions, with a temperature dependent power law viscosity, and the effect of expansion cooling was included. The inlet temperature profile and axial wall temperatures were used as thermal boundary conditions.

Good agreement was obtained between predicted and measured downstream temperature and velocity profiles for cases of wall heating and cooling, as well as when the wall temperature was near the average fluid temperature. Maximum temperature rises of the order of 10 °C were recorded, and expansion cooling at the centre of the die of up to 4 °C was measured. While this work gives some confidence in the accuracy of the calculations, it is not a strong test of the theory because of the relatively small size of the temperature changes.

The general conclusion from these studies is that the calculated effects of viscous heating, especially on viscosity, are in reasonable agreement with experimental results. However, a definitive comparison between theory and experiment still remains to be done.

5.10. EFFECTS OF VISCOUS HEATING ON DIE SWELL

The viscoelastic character of the material is often an important parameter in polymer processing. While quantification of the viscosity is a relatively well developed procedure, the quantification of elasticity is not. A commonly used measure of elasticity is die swell, and measurements of die swell and viscosity are often made simultaneously (see Chapter 6). It would be expected that in situations where viscous heating affected the measurement of viscosity there would also be an effect on die swell, but in general such an effect is poorly understood.

Numerical modelling of the extrusion of inelastic fluids has led to the discovery of a mechanism for the effect of viscous heating on die swell of these fluids. However, little success has been obtained so far in modelling the effects of viscous heating on elastic fluids. In this section we will discuss the inelastic theory of die swell, and also present some experimental results showing the effect of viscous heating on die swell of a viscoelastic fluid.

5.10.1. Inelastic Fluids
The effect on the die swell of inelastic fluids of a temperature gradient perpendicular to the flow direction was discovered by Phuoc and Tanner who used a finite element computer program to model non-isothermal flow effects.[22] They calculated the die swell of a Newtonian fluid emerging from a die with isothermal walls held at T_w into an environment at temperature T_∞, where convective cooling was assumed on the free surface. The non-dimensional temperature was chosen to be

$$T^* = \frac{T - T_w}{T_w - T_\infty}$$

The inlet velocity and temperature profiles were those given by Kearsley[9] for steady state flow in a long tube. In this case the dimensionless temperature is a maximum at the centre of the flow and is zero at the wall. Under these conditions viscous heating was found to increase die swell, and die swells of up to 70% were calculated. The swell was found to be a function of Nahme number only, and the following expression for die swell, $\delta = (D_e - D)/D$, where D_e is the diameter of the extrudate, was found to apply for Na up to 6:

$$\delta = 0.129 + 0.112\,\text{Na}$$

In the case considered above, the temperature profile was fully developed, with the maximum temperature at the centre of the flow. In most cases extrusion is carried out through short dies, and the maximum temperature is in the region of maximum rate of heat generation adjacent to the die walls. In these circumstances the temperature profile is the reverse of that considered by Phuoc and Tanner,[22] and die swell should be decreased from the isothermal value. This expectation was confirmed by finite element flow modelling by Huynh[29] who also calculated the effect of viscous heating on the die swell of power law fluids and found it to be qualitatively similar to the behaviour of Newtonian fluids.

A theory of die swell of inelastic fluids which explains the above results has been proposed by Tanner.[30] The theory considers the flow of an extrudate consisting of a thin outer layer with a viscosity different from that of the inner core. If the viscosity of the core is less than that of the surface layer then the extrudate is predicted to swell, whereas if the viscosity of the core is greater than the viscosity of the surface then the extrudate is predicted to shrink.

5.10.2. Elastic Fluids

While the inelastic mechanism of die swell undoubtedly applies to the extrusion of viscoelastic fluids, the die swell of these fluids is largely determined by their elastic memory (see Chapter 4). The effects of the memory can be approximately characterised by a time constant, and the time constant would normally decrease with increasing temperature. Hence viscous heating should decrease the die swell from the value obtained in isothermal extrusion by decreasing the fluid time constants. These effects are complex, and no satisfactory method of dealing with the problem has yet been developed.

In order to give an indication of the effect of viscous heating on die swell, some experimental results obtained by the author and R. E. Carter at Royal Ordnance (Waltham Abbey, UK) will be presented. The material is a particular double base propellant dough, consisting of 40 parts nitrocellulose, 60 parts nitroglycerine, plus processing solvents. A more detailed discussion of this type of material and its rheology is given in reference 25. Extrusion was made through capillary dies 2 mm in diameter and with lengths from 10 to 100 mm, at 20 °C, 35 °C and 50 °C.

Flow curves of true shear stress versus apparent shear rate are given in Fig. 5.5. At 20 °C the shear stress is decreased by viscous heating at high shear rates, and the effect increases with increasing die length. The magnitude of the viscous heating is indicated by the temperature rise of the surface of the fluid as it issues from the die, as illustrated in Fig. 5.6. The surface temperature was measured by an infrared pyrometer. For extrusion through the 100 mm long die at 20 °C the temperature rise at an apparent shear rate of $1200\,s^{-1}$ is 30 °C, with lower rises being recorded with shorter dies and at higher temperatures. Hence the viscous heating is

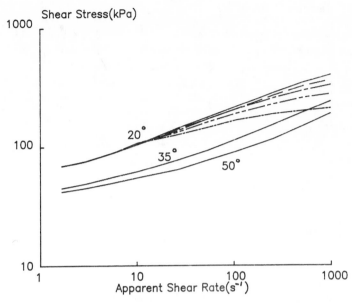

Fig. 5.5. True shear stress vs. apparent shear rate for a nitrocellulose propellant dough for various initial temperatures and die lengths. The 20 °C curves are, from top to bottom, for die lengths of 10 mm, 20 mm, 30 mm, 50 mm and 100 mm, respectively. The 35 °C and 50 °C curves are for 15 mm dies.

of considerable magnitude, and would be expected to have a large effect on die swell.

Plots of die swell from dies 10, 50 and 100 mm long at 20 °C and dies 15 mm long at 35 °C and 50 °C are given in Fig. 5.7. At 20 °C the die swell from each die initially increases with increasing shear rate, then it peaks and decreases with further increase in rate. The shear rate at which the die swell reaches a maximum decreases with increasing die length, and the shear rate corresponds to the shear rate at which viscous heating significantly affects viscosity. Hence it appears that the overall effect of viscous heating is to decrease die swell. We can see from Fig. 5.7 that as the extrusion temperature is increased from 20 °C to 50 °C the die swell decreases with increasing temperature, indicating that the time constant of the fluid decreases with increasing temperature. This decrease in time constant probably contributes in large measure to the decrease in die swell caused by viscous heating. With the advances in numerical modelling of

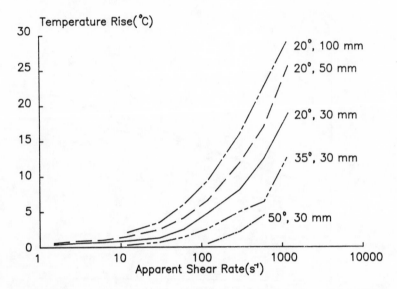

Fig. 5.6. Surface temperature rise vs. apparent shear rate for a nitrocellulose propellant dough for various initial temperatures and die lengths.

die swell which are currently occurring, it is expected that the effect of viscous heating on die swell will be well understood in the near future.

5.11. CONCLUDING REMARKS

Numerical methods have been developed to the point where realistic modelling of flow behaviour, including viscous heating, is a routine procedure. However, appropriate boundary conditions and accurate thermophysical properties of the fluid must be specified, and it is in the determination of these factors that the outstanding problems with viscous heating lie. An isothermal die wall is the preferred thermal boundary condition because it minimises the effects of viscous heating, but this boundary condition is the most difficult to realise in practice. Many commercial capillary rheometers are not designed to carry away the large amounts of heat which may be generated at high shear rates, and the assumption that the walls are isothermal may not be a sufficiently good approximation. In these circumstances a better way of determining the

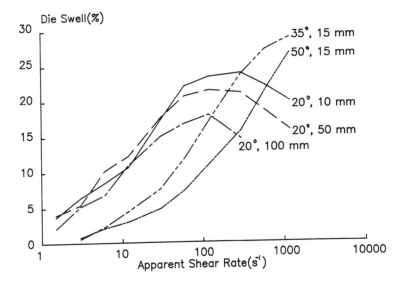

Fig. 5.7. Die swell vs. apparent shear rate for a nitrocellulose propellant dough for various initial temperatures and die lengths.

thermal boundary condition at the die wall is to mount thermocouples in the wall and measure the axial temperature profile directly.

Current methods of measurement of radial temperature profiles in the flow are not really satisfactory. Any probe immersed in the flow will cause a disturbance, although careful numerical modelling of the thermal environment of the probe may minimise errors in corrections for the effect of the probe. A non-intrusive method of measurement of temperature in the fluid is highly desirable but is only likely to be practical in special cases.

Further problems exist with the determination of physical properties of fluids, particularly polymers. Values have been obtained for thermal conductivity and heat capacity, and the variation of these properties with temperature has been determined at atmospheric pressure for many materials. However, there is less information on the effect of pressure on thermal properties. A complicating factor is that most thermophysical measurements are made on materials which are at rest, but flow at high shear rates can induce a large degree of molecular orientation which would lead to anisotropy in physical properties.

Because the effects of viscous heating are dependent on a wide range of factors, it has been possible only to give a general introduction to the subject. For a discussion of viscous heating in a range of geometries the reader is referred to the excellent review by Winter.[5] The effects of viscous heating in materials processing, particularly in polymer processing, are even more complex than in rheometry, as the thermal environment is poorly defined, and many processes occur under non-steady state conditions. For a discussion of some of the problems in polymer processing the reader is referred to the works of Pearson.[7,23,31]

REFERENCES

1. R. C. Penwell and R. S. Porter, *J. Polym. Sci. (A-2)*, 1971, **9**, 463.
2. R. J. Crowson, A. J. Scott and D. W. Saunders, *Polym. Eng. Sci.*, 1981, **21**, 748.
3. Z. Tadmor and C. G. Gogos, *Principles of Polymer Processing*, John Wiley, New York, 1979.
4. M. M. Denn, *Polym. Eng. Sci.*, 1981, **21**, 65.
5. H. H. Winter, *Advances in Heat Transfer*, 1977, **13**, 205.
6. R. B. Bird, W. E. Steward and E. N. Lightfoot, *Transport Phenomena*, John Wiley, New York, 1960.
7. J. R. A. Pearson, *Progress in Heat and Mass Transfer* (Monograph series of the *Int. J. Heat Mass Transfer*), W. R. Schowalter (Ed.), Vol. 5, Pergamon Press, Oxford, 1972, p. 73.
8. E. R. G. Eckert and R. M. Drake, *Analysis of Heat and Mass Transfer*, McGraw-Hill, New York, 1972.
9. E. A. Kearsley, *Trans. Soc. Rheol.*, 1962, **6**, 253.
10. H. L. Toor, *Ind. Eng. Chem.*, 1956, **48**, 922.
11. S. M. Dinh and R. C. Armstrong, *A.I.Ch.E.J.*, 1982, **28**, 294.
12. R. M. Ybarra and R. E. Eckert, *A.I.Ch.E.J.*, 1980, **26**, 751.
13. N. Galili, R. Takserman-Krozer and Z. Rigbi, *Rheol. Acta*, 1975, **14**, 550.
14. N. Galili, Z. Rigbi and R. Takserman-Krozer, *Rheol. Acta*, 1975, **14**, 816.
15. M. R. Kamal and H. Nyun, *Polym. Eng. Sci.*, 1980, **20**, 109.
16. H. W. Cox and C. W. Macosko, *A.I.Ch.E.J.*, 1974, **20**, 785.
17. J. E. Gerrard, F. E. Steidler and J. K. Appeldoorn, *Ind. Eng. Chem. Fund.*, 1965, **4**, 332.
18. J. E. Gerrard, F. E. Steidler and J. K. Appeldoorn, *Ind. Eng. Chem. Fund.*, 1966, **5**, 260.
19. R. A. Morrette and C. G. Gogos, *Polym. Eng. Sci.*, 1968, **8**, 272.
20. R. E. Gee and J. B. Lyon, *Ind. Eng. Chem.*, 1957, **49**, 956.
21. M. Hulatt and W. L. Wilkinson, *Polym. Eng. Sci.*, 1978, **18**, 1148.
22. H. B. Phuoc and R. I. Tanner, *J. Fluid Mech.*, 1980, **98**, 253.
23. J. R. A. Pearson, *Polym. Eng. Sci.*, 1978, **18**, 222.
24. G. Forrest and W. L. Wilkinson, *Trans. Inst. Chem. Engrs*, 1974, **52**, 10.
25. R. E. Carter and R. C. Warren, *J. Rheol.*, 1987, **31**, 151.
26. J. van Leeuwen, *Polym. Eng. Sci.*, 1967, **7**, 98.
27. M. Hulatt and W. L. Wilkinson, *Plast. Rubber Processing*, 1977, March, 15.

28. H. T. Kim and E. A. Collins, *Polym. Eng. Sci.,* 1971, **11,** 83.
29. B. P. Huynh, *J. Non-Newt. Fluid Mech.,* 1983, **13,** 1.
30. R. I. Tanner, *J. Non-Newt. Fluid Mech.,* 1980, **6,** 289.
31. J. R. A. Pearson, *Mechanics of Polymer Processing*, Elsevier Applied Science, London, 1985.

Chapter 6

Computer Control and Data Processing in Extrusion Rheometers

F. S. Baker, R. E. Carter and G. J. Privett

Royal Ordnance Explosives Division,* Waltham Abbey, Essex, UK

6.1. INTRODUCTION

In this chapter we shall not concern ourselves with the detailed architecture of microprocessor systems, but rather with the use of modern

---

* Now known as: Royal Ordnance plc, Research & Development Centre.

computer technology to enhance the efficiency and effectiveness of extrusion rheometers. We shall not deal in depth with those modern extrusion rheometers which are fully instrumented, since they are described elsewhere in this volume. However, users of these instruments may find our observations to be of value in sifting genuine material flow data from instrumental artifacts. We shall attempt to lead those unfamiliar with the field to apply modern instrumentation techniques to their extrusion rheometers. Throughout, an eye will be kept on cost, as the most expensive system is not necessarily the most cost-effective.

A glossary of terminology likely to be encountered is given, and we outline the principal types of instrumentation which could be used to automate extrusion rheometers. In addition, we present a buyer's guide in which we outline critical parameters which should be considered in selecting a microcomputer system. These will be illustrated with reference to equipment available at the time of writing. The authors are well aware, however, that developments in computing equipment are progressing at such a pace that the computing power of today's mainframe computers may be available more cheaply in tomorrow's microcomputers, and therefore the reader is urged to carry out his own market survey.

We list below the principal user-perceived benefits and disadvantages of computer-aided data acquisition and control of extrusion rheometers.

6.1.1. Potential Benefits

More efficient utilisation of staff
Allows unaided operation in some circumstances
Permits operation by less skilled operators
Faster results on test samples
Reproducible test conditions
Establishes a data-base of material performance
Sets limits of acceptance for quality control operations
Allows rapid analyses of data
More complex analyses can be performed quickly and efficiently
Allows on-line control of production processes

6.1.2. Potential Disadvantages

Initial capital outlay
Time needed for software development
Loss of data if system fails or storage media are damaged
Transient phenomena may be missed with multiplexed input systems
Undetected software bugs can give misleading results
Deters operators from thinking!

6.1.3. Types of Extrusion Rheometer[1]

Weight-driven piston type capillary rheometers (including melt flow indexers)

Gas pressure driven capillary rheometers

Capillary rheometers with hydraulic drive

Capillary rheometers with electromechanical drive

Continuous capillary rheometers

Slit die rheometers

The observations which follow are applicable to all these generic rheometer types to a greater or lesser degree. We shall use as examples a simple melt flow indexer and a driven-piston capillary extrusion rheometer.

6.1.4. Use of Computers with Extrusion Rheometers

There are three basic levels of using computers to aid the extrusion rheometer experiment:

Off-line data analysis

On-line data acquisition and analysis

On-line control, data acquisition and analysis

Before describing instrumentation techniques and the component parts of typical computer systems, we shall consider each of the above modes of operation in some detail.

6.2. OFF-LINE DATA ANALYSIS

Off-line data analysis is the simplest method of using a computer with a capillary rheometer experiment, and is often the most time-saving step. The experimental data are gathered manually, for example by taking equilibrium pressure readings from chart recorders or displays, at a series of known constant flow rates for a die of known geometry, and typing the data into a computer using a purpose-written program. The parameters of the particular rheometer used, such as piston diameter, are written into the software, as are any conversion factors needed to convert the measured and displayed units into consistent units. Constant calibration factors may be included in the software, and 'variable' calibration factors may be entered at the start of a day, together with such data as experiment number, date, operator's name, sample type, batch number, comments, etc. Most 'user-friendly' software uses a 'menu driven' program, in which the operator is presented with a list of options, from which the particular operating conditions may be indicated to the computer. A facility to correct typing errors at this stage is invaluable. At the completion of the experiment, the data, together with the headings described above, can be printed out as a hard copy to any format the user wishes.

This hardly taxes the power of even the cheapest microcomputer, and suitable 'purpose built' software may be written easily, even by absolute beginners. Indeed, wherever possible, it is recommended that the user writes his own software in order that he knows exactly what is happening to his data. The cost of programming in manpower terms will seem high, but the user will know that the resulting software will exactly fulfil his needs. Beware of using programmers not conversant with the field of application, since many mathematical manipulations may be carried out on a given set of data, yet the results may have little physical relevance. Cruel experience also leads us to suggest that *all* software (whether commercial or home-written) be thoroughly checked for errors using a set of test data for which the results have been evaluated by other means. The old adage 'rubbish in = rubbish out' can (and will!) manifest itself in many irritating and misleading ways.

The raw data can be converted easily into apparent shear rate and apparent shear stress. These calculated quantities are stored in the computer memory as arrays. The calculated data may be plotted on the screen, provided that graphics are available on the specific system used, so that the experimenter can see within seconds the flow characteristics of the material. The data can be analysed to give the viscosity, if the material is Newtonian, or the apparent consistency index and flow behaviour index for a power-law material. Should the material exhibit Bingham or Herschel–Bulkley behaviour, the curve can be analysed to estimate yield stress, the apparent consistency index and flow behaviour index. By examination of the flow curves the presence of such phenomena as wall-slip and shear heating can be deduced.

Having entered the data into the computer and performed the necessary calculations, the data and results must be stored in some 'non-volatile' device. Experience suggests that the raw data should be stored at the earliest opportunity, since losses and corruption of data in 'virtual' memory can occur, due usually to voltage spikes carried on the mains power supply caused by switching inadequately protected high power equipment (such as air compressors). Thunderstorms can also be a source of spikes which can corrupt software and damage hardware. A mains filter specially designed for computer systems should be used, and *all* the components of the computer system powered through this filter.

Typical mass storage devices used in microcomputer systems are floppy disc units and hard disc units (Winchesters). In these devices, described in the glossary, the data are stored on a magnetic medium, very much like music on a tape recorder. However, tape cassette players such as those provided with many home computer systems are not recommended for technical work as they are not very reliable and are often slow. Floppy disc units are cheaper than hard disc units, and have the advantage of added security, since the floppy discs can be removed from the drive unit in order to avoid inadvertent corruption or erasure of the data and unauthorised access. Hard disc units have the advantage of higher capacity and speed of access, but are more expensive and generally reside with the computer system. Whichever storage system is used, it is recommended that 'back-up' copies of programs and crucial data be made regularly, and that these be kept separate from the working copies. (The authors are aware of a case in which the back-up copies were kept in the same disc box as the working copies. All was well until a water pipe burst directly above the box!)

6.3. ON-LINE DATA ACQUISITION AND ANALYSIS

6.3.1. Example 1: Simple Melt Flow Indexer

To illustrate how one would go about upgrading a purely mechanical machine to a computer-based system, we shall consider a simple melt flow index machine possessing no instrumentation other than temperature control. The operation of a such a machine is broadly as follows.[2]

The sample to be tested is loaded into the machine, which has been heated to the correct temperature for the measurement. A piston (of known weight and geometry) is lowered on to the sample. When the fluid has equilibrated to the temperature of the barrel, a standard load is applied to the piston. This load, usually in the form of weights, causes the material to extrude through a capillary die of standard size. The extrudate is caught in a receptacle, and the mass of material extruded in a given time within a specified range of the piston stroke is measured. From this is calculated the mass flow rate which, expressed in grams extruded per 10 min, is known as the melt flow index (MFI).

Clearly, this operation is subject to operator skill and judgement. The operation can be made more accurate and reproducible by using the computer to monitor and control the experiment. One microswitch and a solenoid operated cutter are required. As can be seen in Fig. 6.1, the microswitch is placed such that it will be activated as soon as the tray carrying the weight starts to fall and starts extruding the sample. The

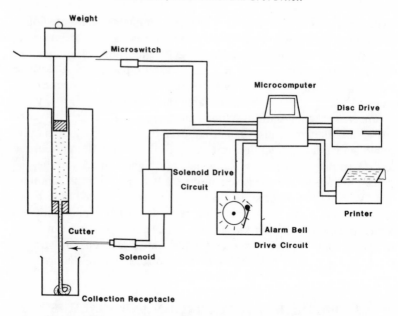

Fig. 1. A schematic diagram of instrumentation for a simple melt flow indexer.

switch then makes the circuit which will supply 5 volts (TTL logic level) to the user port of a microcomputer. This voltage pulse is sensed via the program and resets either an internal or an external clock. When the specified time has elapsed, the clock sends either a signal from the computer via the user port to a relay, or simply in the case of the external clock closes a switch. In any event, a circuit is triggered which will allow a solenoid to be operated. The solenoid interrupts the flow of the sample into the receptacle. At the same time an audible signal is activated, whereupon the operator, now alerted, can take the receptacle away for weighing.

One can reduce operator time even further, particularly if many tests are required for quality control. There are on the market now balances which have either RS-232C or IEEE circuits which will interface directly with many microcomputers. Thus the computer can record the weight of the empty receptacle. As the material fills the container the balance weighs the sample and a few seconds after the extrudate has been cut the computer is instructed to store the information given by the balance. A very simple computer program then subtracts the two masses and can display on the VDU or on a printer the sample name, the date of the test, any other comments, and the melt index, in a neat easily legible format. All the operator has to do is load the sample, write the details of the sample into the computer, set the machine going, and clean up afterwards.

6.3.2. Example 2: Driven-Piston Capillary Extrusion Rheometer

Consider now the method of abstracting data from a typical capillary extrusion experiment using a constant-rate driven piston rheometer. The rate of descent of the ram is set manually and the pressure required to extrude the material is measured when the flow through the die is constant. The ram rate is changed again and the pressure reading taken when it reaches a constant value. This is repeated time and again until all of the sample in the barrel of the rheometer has been discharged—a simple operation but, as those who carry out these experiments will vouch, taking measurements at high extrusion speeds can be quite exhausting! Additionally, cleaning, loading and temperature equilibration occupy a significant part of the test cycle. The more data per cycle that can be gleaned, the more cost-effective is the use of equipment and staff.

It is in just such a situation that data acquisition by a computer becomes such a boon. The analogue voltage signals from the pressure-measuring electronics and from the motor speed sensor are passed through an analogue-to-digital converter. As its name implies, this device converts the d.c. voltage signal to a sequence of digital pulses which the computer can process. The computer now knows the magnitude of the voltages being fed into it. By writing a program, the computer can be instructed to calculate the apparent shear stress and the apparent shear rate, and to print the resultant flow curve on the visual display unit (VDU), or on a digital plotter or printer/ plotter. Of course, one need not stop there; the curve can be analysed, and the resultant rheological parameters calculated. If a series of dies with different length-to-diameter ratios are used, the experimental results from the batch of experiments can be logged either in the computer memory or on a storage medium such as a floppy disc. These data can be called up by the user's own program to calculate automatically entrance pressure effects and to correct the curves to give the true shear stress against true shear rate. The time saving in this operation alone is worth the time spent programming and the cost of setting up the system.

6.4. ANALYSIS OF DATA[3-5]

The major advantage of a computer in the study of rheology is in its ability to make mathematical calculations at a very high speed. A cheap home microcomputer can perform complex calculations and manipulations thousands of times faster than the most skilled calculator-user. Even a very simple program can save hours of tedious manual computation, freeing skilled manpower to undertake more profitable work.

Before buying a particular computer, it is worth checking that it will support all the mathematical functions which are likely to be required, and their inverse forms. For instance, some very cheap microcomputers do not have all the inverse trigonometric functions.

The most common application of the computer to rheological experiments is in the calculation of the flow curve from raw data. To do this, the program must contain physical information on the rheometer, such as the ram diameter and die dimensions. This sort of data can be entered as part of a 'start of day' routine at the beginning of the program or, if the equipment is seldom varied, may be written in the program as constant values. The latter approach is more suited to routine quality control testing, whereas the former is more appropriate to a research environment. Additionally, if the Bagley end correction is known, then end effects may easily be estimated to deduce a machine-independent flow curve.

Having derived shear rate/shear stress values from the raw data, it can be very helpful to display the information in graphical form, possibly as a log–log plot. Such a plot facilitates detection of such phenomena as wall slip, yield stress and viscous heating. Sudden transitions in flow properties and long-term relaxation processes also may be highlighted. Once the data have been plotted, using a medium-to-high resolution display, other experimental data or comparison standards may be superimposed to allow trends or differences to be identified. A simple addition to the plotting routine might colour-code the data points to aid, for example, the identification of the shear rate at which viscous heating becomes significant.

Another possibility is to plot both a theoretical flow curve and the experimental data. By adjusting the rheological parameters of the theoretical curve in such a way as to minimise the differences between the curves, the rheological parameters equivalent to the experimental data may be approximated iteratively. The same result can be obtained easily using a linear regression for materials with 'simple' flow behaviour, e.g. power–law flow. The calculations required for a material with a yield stress are more elaborate but may take the computer only 30–40 s to perform. It must be stressed that this sort of analysis is very sensitive to the accuracy of the raw data, particularly with regard to yield stress. Scattered data will certainly lead to unreliable and misleading results. In short, the more data points the better, especially at low shear rates if viscous heating or wall slip effects are likely.

It should be emphasised that, no matter what analysis routine is adopted, the data points should always be visually scrutinised so that dubious points will not be included in the analysis. Where any doubt exists as to whether a data point is spurious or reflects the true flow behaviour of the material, the experiment should be repeated until consistent results are obtained. For example, atypical data may be obtained if the extrusion pressure had not stabilised at the time the reading was taken. It is sensible therefore to display the extrusion pressure continuously, either on a chart recorder or on the VDU. Such a record has the additional advantage of allowing stick–slip phenomena to be readily observed (provided that the frequency of oscillation is within the band-width of the recorder). Without a continuous display it is difficult to deduce the existence and nature of anomalous flow behaviour.

It must be remembered always that the computer is without intelligence. It can analyse the data swiftly and can draw graphs, but it will not (without extensive programming) pick and choose the points which may be in error in the manner of a human operator. With the exception of the simple tasks, the operator must still play a vital role in the interpretation of the results.

One possible approach to analysing a flow curve, using a Herschel–Bulkley fluid as an example, is outlined below.

Examination of the Herschel–Bulkley formalism shows that logarithmic plots of shear stress versus shear rate can be straight lines only if the material does not possess a yield stress. It is clear that, if the correct yield stress value is subtracted from the shear stress values, a straight line plot will result. The problem therefore is to deduce the correct yield stress value, after which the consistency index and flow behaviour index may be calculated, using iterative techniques.

There are two inherent limits to the range of possible yield stress values, since the yield stress cannot physically be lower than zero and cannot be greater than the shear stress measured at the lowest shear rate. It is a simple matter to choose as a 'first guess' a random value between these two limits, subtract this value from the calculated shear stress values, and perform a linear regression for the logarithmic corrected shear stress/shear rate data. This process is repeated for a number of yield stress guesses (taking care not to erase or overwrite the original data), and a plot is made showing the linear regression coefficient (R^2) against the yield stress guesses. This plot will usually be a parabola with the maximum at the correct yield stress value. Alternatively, it is possible to take regressions at three yield stress values (upper limit, lower limit and midpoint) and use the regression coefficient to indicate which of the three potential yield stress values is furthest from the 'best fit' value. It is then possible to narrow the range by changing the value of the appropriate limit (up or down) and re-calculating the midpoint. The process may then be repeated until the values of the upper and lower limit are very close together or the regression coefficients differ by some small, predetermined amount. This often occurs within 20 iterations.

Both of these approaches will give sensible results for good data, and with some modification they can even tolerate quite noisy data. The choice of technique is very much a matter of personal preference and experimentation on the part of the user. These are by no means the only methods that might be used to deduce rheological parameters, but they do represent examples which are easy both to understand and to program.

6.4.1. Schematic Flow Diagram

Initially the task of programming a microcomputer to control and/or monitor a rheometer may seem a little daunting. However, if the task is broken down into smaller parts (modules) it becomes much simpler to understand and to achieve. The module numbers in the following description refer to the numbers alongside the various sections of the schematic flow diagram in Fig 6.2.

It is essential to avoid situations where the operator could be injured or the equipment damaged. To that end, all primary safety systems, such as over-pressure detection and end-of-travel limit switches, should be hard-wired and connected by high-speed circuitry such that the drive can be stopped immediately. It is most unwise to rely on a microcomputer for such basic safety measures, as the time taken for the computer to detect the problem and react to it can be significant. The computer can, however, be used to control the instrument within the hard-wired safety limits.

Module 1

The first task of the program must be to create the variables and to reserve space for arrays in which to store the data. Where possible, it is useful to use variable names which reflect the nature of the variable, e.g. Ram speed or Swell. This can save a lot of time and mental effort in later programming stages. It is sensible to keep a list of variables as they are used, so that duplication can be avoided in later modules and to aid program debugging.

Fig. 6.2. A flow diagram showing the program control structures and some of the modules that will be needed. Some modules will themselves be made up of simpler units.

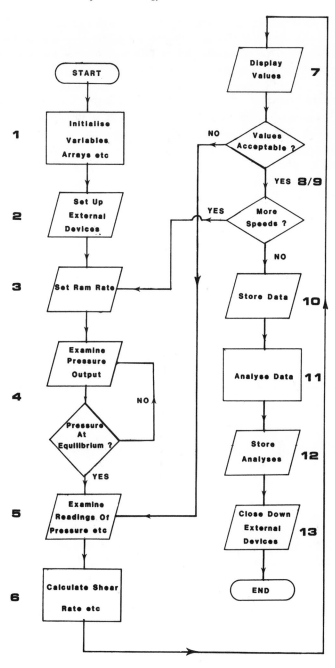

Module 2

It is essential that all peripheral devices be properly set up ('initialised') before any readings are taken. Wherever possible, assume that the user is not familiar with the equipment. For example, if the 0 to 1 V scale on a voltmeter should be used, either set this directly from the software or tell the operator to set the switch manually. It is highly frustrating to spend all day taking readings, only to discover that resistance or current rather than voltage has been recorded!

Module 3

Setting the ram speed may be done by hand (e.g. by a multi-turn potentiometer), or possibly by computer. This is usually quicker and less prone to error if it is done by the software, but some operational flexibility may then be sacrificed. Computer control is very good for routine work, but careful programming is required to allow sufficient versatility.

Module 4

Judging whether the extrusion pressure has reached equilibrium can be a very difficult task. For rheologically simple materials, this may involve taking several readings and looking for a trend, using e.g. a linear regression or a skewness/kurtosis study. More complex materials, exhibiting such effects as viscous heating or stick-slip, are not so easy to work with since the trend may vary from moment to moment. If possible, the pressure readings should be displayed as a function of time, using a chart recorder or the VDU, so that important material properties are not overlooked.

Module 5

When the pressure has become stable, readings may be taken from each input. This may be accomplished using a computer-activated relay bank to select a chosen input and then taking a reading using a digital voltmeter. Electromechanical relays must be allowed to settle for a few tens of milliseconds, to allow for contact 'bounce', before the reading is taken. Generally, it is better to take several readings from each input and average them. Of course, when the ram is moving very slowly, the number of readings may be quite large, perhaps several hundred, because only a small amount of the test material will have been extruded. However, at higher ram rates the number of readings will need to be reduced in order to avoid wasting material. It is often best to measure the ram speed first, and then decide via a suitable algorithm the number of data readings which should be taken at that rate.

Modules 6 and 7

Calculating the apparent shear stress, apparent shear rate and other derived quantities is simply a matter of converting the measured voltage to the proper units. If possible, the result should be displayed with the previous results of the experiment in order that the operator might compare results and decide whether to check apparently anomalous points. A buffered printer would be ideal to display this information, especially if the VDU is used to display the data graphically. Use of a printer in this 'on-line' mode has the added advantage of giving a record of the experiment should, for example, a power failure occur.

Modules 8 and 9

These decisions are very much a matter of personal preference. One may choose to keep all data, good or bad, and edit later, or one may wish to repeat a reading which appears anomalous due, for example, to an unstable pressure signal.

Module 10

When an experimental run has finished, the data should be saved to disc as soon as possible, preferably automatically to preclude operator forgetfulness. The first part of the information saved should be a code defining what data, and how many data points, have been saved. This is done because, at a later date, the number of data channels may be changed, and a program loading data back from storage will need to be told what the stored values represent.

Module 11

As a general rule, it is good practice to display the data graphically as a function of, for example, shear rate. This will aid in identifying phenomena such as wall slip, and will allow the occasional bad data point to be edited out. This is discussed more fully elsewhere.

Module 12

Having taken the trouble to analyse the data, often a lengthy process, it is useful to save the results of the analysis together with any user comments in a separate disc file. This may then be accessed at a later date, or may be used with other software.

Module 13

It is worthwhile ensuring that, when the equipment is not in use, the relay box is configured in such a manner that the digital voltmeter is disconnected from the rheometer. This will reduce the possibility of damaging the voltmeter during repairs or wiring modification.

6.5. ON-LINE DATA ACQUISITION AND INSTRUMENTATION

Let us now return to the problem of how to improve the use of a capillary extrusion rheometer. In order to remove errors due to operator variability and to increase the effectiveness of the machine (i.e. more useful data per man-hour), one must first consider how information concerning the experiment is to be measured and collected by the computer system. In order for a computer to sense the operational parameters of the extrusion experiment, there must be a means of converting information about the experiment into electrical signals which can be read by the computer. In other words, it is necessary to fit transducers to the equipment. Apparatus will be needed which, for example, generates analogue signals representing pressure, load, temperature or piston speed. The following (not exhaustive) list is intended to give the user sufficient information from which he may decide to what level and by what means he wishes to fit instrumentation to his equipment.

6.5.1. Temperature Measurement and Control
All commercially available extrusion rheometers have fitted some form of temperature control. Accurate temperature control is essential, since the temperature coefficient of viscosity can be very large indeed. For operation at temperatures predominantly below about 70 °C, control may be achieved by a fluid circulation heat-exchange system. For operation at and above 70 °C, most systems use electrical heating whereby electrical power is applied to resistive elements. Some older instruments use variable voltage transformers to set the temperature, the temperature being measured by an independent mercury-in-glass thermometer or, latterly, an electronic thermometer. Such systems are acceptable where the instrument will be used at only one test temperature. However, where data are required over a range of temperatures, it is more sensible, in order to achieve rapid thermal stabilisation, to fit a temperature control system using a negative feedback loop. In such a system, a temperature-sensing element is sited in the barrel wall, and the electrical signal from this device is used to regulate the amount of power being applied to the heating elements.

Many modern controllers are available at reasonable price (about £500 for a system), and these will effect three-term, or PID (proportional integral and differential), control.[6] Such instruments allow the heating system to be matched to the thermal losses and thermal lags present in the system to be controlled. Many controllers may now have computer interfaces fitted, and the latest of these instruments have an 'auto-tuning' facility which, by measuring the response times of the system being controlled during a test heating cycle, will calculate the three PID terms for that temperature and for those conditions. If these terms are entered into the controller, the next time that the equipment is used under those conditions the controller will bring the temperature to the set temperature with maximum speed and minimal overshoot. When using such a system, it must be remembered that the tuning conditions *must* be the same as the experimental conditions. For example, if the tuning run is carried out without the die in the barrel, convection currents will give higher losses, and erroneous control parameters will be obtained. This will, of course, be more noticeable at higher temperatures.

As an aside, some modern materials demand high test temperatures (over 400 °C), and rheometers are therefore being used at their higher temperature limits. Without a well defined control system there is a very real danger that, if the high temperature is called from a much lower temperature, the temperature of the barrel will overshoot the set value by a considerable amount. This could damage pressure transducers, and might reduce the temper of the steel used for the barrel. When working at these high temperatures it is prudent to set the temperature about 100 °C lower than the desired temperature, and allow the system to equilibrate before cautiously approaching the set temperature.

Most controllers are available with user-settable relay limits which may be programmed to switch at a predetermined temperature, and (if so wired) can sound alarms and switch off the power supply.

Regarding temperature sensors, cheap thermocouples should be avoided, as these can be in error by several degrees. Although there are some other temperature transducers on the market, such as thermistors, platinum resistance thermometers (PRTs) provide accurate, stable and reasonably priced sensors. These may be supplied in a range of geometries, often within a stainless steel sheath. Grade 1 probes should be specified, and three- or four-wire probes used in preference to two-wire probes as, with a matched controller, the former allow for compensation for lead resistance, etc. Calibration certificates can be supplied by most manufacturers for controllers and probes. The accuracy of temperature sensors can drift with time, and thus, if only for peace of mind, they should be calibrated against a known standard at least once a year.

Control of the power to the resistive elements is achieved via a solid-state switch which is activated by a low-level signal from the controller. A schematic diagram of a typical heater control circuit is shown in Fig. 6.3.

6.5.2. Pressure Measurement

It is highly desirable, in order to minimise frictional errors, that the pressure in the material directly above the die entrance be measured, and not merely the load on the ram. In order to achieve this, the rheometer design must allow for the use of such a sensor by having a machined port and fixing device to allow the tip of the probe to protrude through the barrel wall. Probes used generally for pressure measurements at elevated temperatures were developed for the plastics industry and are generically known as 'melt pressure transducers'. Several makes of melt pressure transducer are available on the market, and generally have similar external geometries to enable mounting in a 'standard' pocket. Typically these instruments are priced at £450 to £650, depending on pressure range, accuracy, the need for abrasion-resistant tips, etc. Some instruments are available with built-in thermocouple sensors which, although useful, will not give a rapid response to changes in material temperature since, of necessity, the temperature sensing element is inside the body of the transducer.

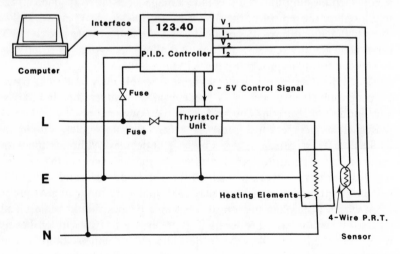

Fig. 6.3. A typical circiut layout for temperature control.

The pressure exerted by the material is experienced by a thin diaphragm rigidly fixed to the body of the probe. The diaphragm is elastically deformed by the pressure and this displacement of the diaphragm is transmitted to another diaphragm remote from the sensing head. The movement in this sensing diaphragm is monitored by a strain gauge, and the output from the strain gauge is thus a measure of the pressure exerted on the front diaphragm of the probe. In good melt pressure transducers, the output is almost linearly proportional to the pressure, and shows little hysteresis (typically less than 0·5% of full scale output).

A major problem with many pressure transducers is that they respond not only to pressure but to fixing torque and to temperature. Although impressive temperature sensitivities are often quoted, the response time to a change in temperature is often not quoted, and with good reason! These devices can exhibit dramatic changes in zero point and sensitivity with temperature, a useful experiment being to record the transducer zero output and span (by a built-in calibration resistor if possible), as the rheometer barrel warms up. Transducers which use a simple mechanical force-rod to transmit the deflection from the pressure-sensing end of the transducer to the strain gauge assembly are particularly prone to these zero point shifts.

Transducers have been developed[6] which use a flexible liquid column to transmit the deflection to the strain gauge, and a novel transducer just on the market uses a refined mechanical system to achieve improved temperature insensitivity. One cause for concern with all pressure transducers is in accurate calibration at the working temperature, a feat which is rarely accomplished.

The transducer must be supplied with a voltage to excite the strain gauge bridge (Fig. 6.4). The imbalance due to applied load of the Wheatstone bridge arrangement of strain gauges is a small signal, typically 2–3 mV/V of bridge supply voltage, although some higher-response transducers are available. Thus an amplifier is required to sense the out-of-balance voltage linearly and accurately. The strain gauge element on pressure transducers must be supplied with an excitation voltage (5–20 V a.c. or d.c., depending upon the instrument), and a linear amplifier circuit is required to amplify and normalise the signal resulting from an applied pressure. Many such amplifiers are available on the market, ranging from do-it-yourself modules at around £60 to ready-built devices with high and low presettable alarms, isolated analogue signals and computer interfaces, costing up to £500.

With better transducers, calibration of pressure transducers may be

Typical Strain Gauge Bridge

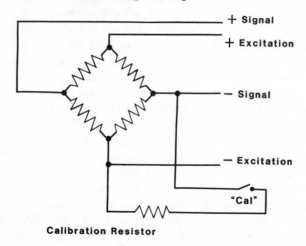

Fig. 6.4. A Wheatstone bridge circuit similar to those used for strain gauge measurements.

checked *in situ* by shorting-out a precision-resistor built into the transducer to simulate a specified deflection. By placing a prompt into the program for running the data acquisition system, the operator is automatically given an *aide-mémoire* for ensuring that he carries out not only this operation but also any other details of the experiment that have to be logged, or carried out before measurements are actually taken. Routine calibration with a dead-load tester is essential, in order that any long-term drift may be detected. However, the comments above regarding calibration at working temperatures should be borne in mind.

6.5.3. Load Measurement

Piston load measurement is often effected on driven-piston rheometers by placing a load cell between the piston and the drive mechanism. Where such a device is fitted to the rheometer as standard, care must be exercised to ensure that no overload protection circuits are disrupted when seeking to extract a load signal. Load cells, like pressure transducers, are generally based upon a strain-gauge element bonded to a calibrated spring component which is linearly deformed by the applied load. The piston load must be applied axially to the load cell; otherwise erroneously low readings will result. Calibration may be made by shunting a precision resistor across one arm of the strain-gauge. Periodic testing with a comparator is essential. Some small strain-gauge devices are now available which may be useful for specialist applications such as measuring the load directly under the piston. As with pressure transducers, load cells are in the main temperature-dependent.

6.5.4. Piston Displacement and Speed Measurement

Another important parameter to measure in the capillary extrusion experiment is the rate of descent of the ram, so that volume throughput per unit time can be calculated.

Electromechanically driven rheometers usually have a tachogenerator coupled to the motor. The tachogenerator is a dynamo which provides a voltage which is proportional to the speed of the rotating shaft of the motor, or some other rotating shaft which is directly linked to the drive system of the rheometer. This voltage provides the signal for a negative feedback loop to the drive circuit to ensure that the motor speed, and hence the rate of descent of the ram, is kept constant at the selected speed. This same signal could of course be used to give the computer a voltage which determines the rate of descent of the ram, provided the gearing ratios between the motor and the ram are known. Since the ram rate is known it is an easy matter, assuming minimal 'flash' past the piston, to compute the volume throughput and hence the apparent shear rate at the wall of the capillary. Note that, if the tachogenerator signal is used, then it must be fed to the computer via a high impedance circuit to ensure that the current drain on the tachogenerator does not corrupt the voltage output to an extent that proper feedback signals are not fed to the motor speed control circuitry. For safety and to minimise electrical noise, the signal from the drive system should be electrically isolated (preferably optically) from the computer. This may be achieved by ensuring that the A/D converter is equipped with an isolating circuit.

Piston displacement may be measured directly by several means. With the exception of optical-based metrication systems, one of the most accurate means is to attach a linear variable differential transformer (LVDT) transducer to move in parallel with the piston. These devices and the associated conditioning amplifiers are readily available from a number of suppliers, although the price for a system approaches £1000. Similarly, linear potentiometers are available (at around £250 for the lengths commonly required), which may be simply powered and provide a voltage signal proportional to ram stroke. For the shoestring budget, a solution is to use a multi-turn potentiometer attached to a drum of known diameter, driven by an inelastic cord attached to the piston drive mechanism. Return and tensioning can be achieved by a simple counter-weight. Care must be taken with 'constant load' rheometers such as melt flow indexers to ensure that the piston load is not affected by such a sensing mechanism.

6.5.5. Piston Speed Control

A modification which can prove worthwhile is to substitute for the manual speed adjustment potentiometer a series of presettable potentiometers which may be selected by push-buttons (or by a computer control system) in order to allow essentially the same speeds to be selected for each test run. Such a facility saves on operator time and fatigue, ensures reproducibility between runs and comparability of data, and, by removing the trial-and-error element in speed selection, allows more data points per rheometer loading. Wherever possible, the advice of the manufacturer should be sought before attempting such a modification. A typical circuit is shown in Fig. 6.5. Due attention must be paid to safety considerations, especially whether the voltages on the speed control potentiometer are referred to earth or whether they are floating at mains voltage. In any case, where an option to allow the preset speeds to be selected by a computer is desired, the computing equipment should be electrically isolated from the drive system. If in doubt, seek professional advice, as mistakes can be expensive and could injure someone. Care should be taken to ensure that the total current drain through the new potentiometer network is no more

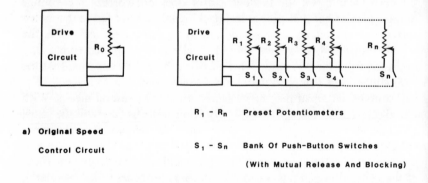

R₁ - Rₙ   Preset Potentiometers

a) Original Speed

Control Circuit

S₁ - Sₙ   Bank Of Push-Button Switches

(With Mutual Release And Blocking)

b) Modified Speed Control Circuit

Fig. 6.5. Two possible methods for establishing motor speed control.

than the drain through the original single potentiometer. In other words, the total resistance of the new potentiometer network must equal the resistance of the original potentiometer: $R_n = nR_o$, where R_o is the resistance in ohms of the original potentiometer, n is the number of potentiometers in the new potentiometer network, and R_n is the resistance of each new potentiometer. Also, test briefly what happens to the drive system if the switched potentiometer wiper goes 'open circuit', as can happen if, for example, a speed selector button fails to operate correctly. If the drive system does not move, then all is well. If the drive defaults to full speed, then it is recommended that an independent safety cut-out be fitted. This could be in the form of a 'voltage sensing relay' wired to trip a contactor in the mains supply if the motor speed exceeds a preset maximum.

6.5.6. Extrudate Speed Measurement

The technique selected to measure the linear extrudate speed depends greatly on the physical nature of the extruding material. Non-sticky materials may be measured by allowing the extrudate to pass over a light, rotating drum of known circumference and to which is attached a speed detector such as a rotary optical encoder. Laser-Doppler instruments are available which may be used for speed measurement, although these are very expensive. More simply, the time taken may easily be measured for the cut end of the extrudate to pass between two sensors (such as light beams, fluidic sensors, or mechanical probes) spaced a known distance apart, to give an average speed of extrusion. Allowance must be made for any post-extrusion relaxation effects.

6.5.7. Extrudate Swell Measurement

The measurement of extrudate swell as part of an extrusion rheometer experiment can give an estimate of the elasticity of the sample, and can be very useful for comparative purposes. The results should be treated with caution, as the observed results will be specific to the conditions of the experiment, in that the observed swell is a function of the experimental time-scale and of the heat-transfer characteristics of the rheometer (especially if the material is subject to viscous heating). Wall slip phenomena can affect extrudate swell results. Additionally, the extruding material may 'draw down' and neck under its own weight, and give a misleading low extrudate swell value. Some materials may continue to recover for some time after extrusion, so a 'one off' measurement of size at a fixed distance from the die may not convey the whole picture.

Since the extruding material will in the main have little mechanical strength, it is expedient to select a non-contacting measurement system. Several optical devices are available whereby the extrudate is imaged on to an integrated circuit chip containing a line of accurately spaced light-sensitive elements. These elements may be electronically scanned (at, typically, 2–6 MHz) to determine which elements are illuminated and which are eclipsed. By prior calibration, the size of the extruding material may be speedily and precisely determined. Other devices available on the market include those which measure the reduction in output from a light-sensitive cell when the extrudate is interposed between the cell and a light source. A careful check of the linearity of the output signal with extrudate diameter is advised here. Also, misleading results may be obtained when measuring transparent samples.

6.5.8. Extrudate Temperature Measurement

It is useful to measure the surface temperature of the extrudate issuing from an extrusion rheometer in order to estimate the effects of frictional heating as a function of, for example, shear rate and stock temperature. Modelling work[7] has shown that the highest temperature rise (for capillary flow) occurs close to the die wall. Measurement of the extrudate temperature is usually best achieved using an infrared pyrometer system, since this is a non-contacting means of measurement. It is necessary to specify the emissivity of the material and the operational temperature range in order that an instrument with the correct characteristics may be supplied. Although there are on the market several infrared pyrometer systems for measuring, for example, the temperature in internal mixers, there are few which will deal with the necessary small target size of around 1 mm diameter, and these are quite expensive, costing around £5000. Instruments which work with this target size often have lens-to-target distances of 100–150 mm and, since the detector units have a diameter of around 100 mm, care must be exercised to ensure that the proposed instrument can be positioned correctly in relation to the target. A standard photographic tripod will usually suffice to support the detector units, and the signal conditioning equipment may be built into a control console. To avoid false readings, it may be necessary to restrict oscillation of the extrudate in order to keep the extrudate within the field of view of the pyrometer.

The principle of operation of these instruments is to detect over a fixed bandwidth the amplitude of infrared radiation emitted by the sample. This amplitude will depend upon the temperature of the sample, upon the emissivity of the sample, and to a lesser extent upon the quality of the sample surface. In order to obtain accurate temperature readings, it is therefore, necessary to calibrate the instrument for the sample emissivity, and this is best done by using a sample of the test material held at a known temperature, as determined by, for example, a thermocouple embedded in it. Black materials, such as many rubber compositions, may be assumed to have an emissivity of unity for all practical purposes. Blackbody calibration devices are available for use with infrared pyrometers, but these are considered to be an expensive luxury when emissivity still has to be accounted for.

The signal conditioning units supplied with infrared pyrometer systems can be supplied with an analogue output signal, which may be logged by the computer data-acquisition system via an A/D converter.

6.5.9. Interfacing to the Computer

Analogue signals may be converted to a digital representation and passed to a computer by use of an analogue-to-digital converter. Such devices form part of digital voltmeters. The accuracy of the resulting measurements is determined in a manner described in the glossary. Care must be taken to ensure that the resolution of the converter is sufficient to reflect accurately the quality of the input signals.

Additionally, consideration must be given to the speed of data access by the computer system. Generally, the higher the resolution the slower the conversion time from analogue to digital form; also, for a given resolution, faster conversion time instruments cost more money. In the case of the capillary extrusion rheometer, it may be that, once the operator has decided that the pressure has reached equilibrium, a series of readings should be taken in bursts of maybe five readings per second at 1 s intervals for 7 s. These readings are stored in the computer and can be presented as either raw data or the apparent shear rate, and apparent shear stress can be calculated. As described earlier, the data can be displayed as a flow curve; from the flow curve an analysis can be made to ascertain the flow curve law, and hence the underlying constitutive equation.

6.6. COMPUTER CONTROL WITH ON-LINE DATA ACQUISITION

So far, we have considered the use of computers only for data acquisition. With microcomputers though, a new vista is revealed, particularly where

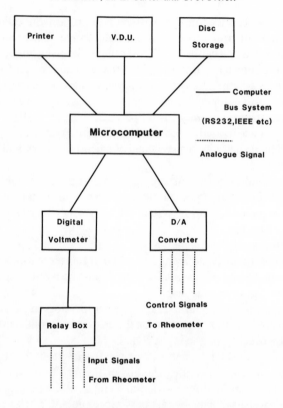

Fig. 6.6. A schematic diagram of a microcomputer system capable of monitoring and controlling a rheometer.

quality control is of the essence. Provided enough basic rheological work has been carried out on a product, it is possible to generate a flow curve for the material which represents the mean performance of that material over a given shear rate and temperature regime. Thus it becomes a relatively easy matter to measure a batch of material in the capillary rheometer, calculate the parameters for the flow curve and either compare analytically against the constants for the 'standard material', or simply to superimpose the two flow curves and compare visually whether the sample falls within acceptable limits against the 'standard'. This technique equates to overlaying standard templates on the curve of the test results.

As suggested in modules 3 and 4 (Section 6.4), the microcomputer can be made to control the rheometer drive provided that the pressure equilibrates quickly and smoothly with increasing ram rates. This may be achieved in a number of ways; all involve supplying an analogue voltage to the motor speed control unit, for example, by causing the computer to operate a relay in order to select a preset potentiometer, or by controlling a stepper-motor which in turn drives a speed-control potentiometer, or by using a digital-to-analogue converter to provide a reference signal to the speed control electronics directly. The equilibrium pressure is recorded, together with the ram rate, the next speed is selected, and so on until the sample is fully discharged. The motor is automatically reversed to bring the ram back to its start position in readiness for the next sample, and the operator's attention is gained by sounding an audible warning. The results from the experiment are then analysed as described. It should be noted that, where an equilibrium pressure is not achieved, for example because of 'stick-slip' flow behaviour, some degree of 'intelligence' must be written into the software, e.g. to summon the operator if equilibrium pressure within a defined tolerance band is not attained within a specified time-scale. A system configuration that would allow this to be done is shown in Fig. 6.6.

Thus the rheometer may be used as a quality control check, for the raw ingredients before processing and/or as an instrument to check the quality of the material being produced.

ACKNOWLEDGEMENTS

The authors wholeheartedly thank Mr Paul Weaver and Mr Peter Robson for their help in the preparation of this chapter. Miss Kate Turner is to be commended for her delightful figure work.

REFERENCES

1. J. M. Dealy, *Rheometers for Molten Plastics*, Van Nostrand/Reinhold, The Hague, 1982.
2. British Standard 2782, Part 7, Method 720A, 1979.
3. R. W. Whorlow, *Rheological Techniques*, Ellis Horwood, Chichester, 1980.
4. K. Walters, *Rheometry*, Chapman and Hall, London, 1975.
5. J. A. Brydson, *Flow Properties of Polymer Melts*, 2nd edn, George Godwin Ltd/Plastics and Rubber Institute, 1981.
6. C. Rauwendaal, *Polymer Extrusion*, Carl Hanser, Verlag, Munich, 1986.
7. R. E. Carter and R. C. Warren, *J. Rheol.*, 1987, **31**(2), 151–73.
8. G. Loveday, *Practical Interface Circuits For Micros*, Pitman, London, 1984.
9. R. A. Penfold, *Micro Interfacing Circuits*, Books 1 and 2, Bernard Babani, London, 1984.

APPENDIX 6.1: GLOSSARY

A/D converter. This is a device which converts an analogue signal into a digital form to a degree of approximation defined by the number of bits specified. An 8 bit device is accurate to 1 part in 256 (1 part in 2^8), 12 bits to 1 part in 4096 (2^{12}), and so on. The conversion time usually increases as the resolution increases, thereby giving a slower response (there are, however, some high speed, high accuracy—and high price! —transient recorders for the study of fast events). When choosing a converter it should be remembered that many transducers are only accurate to less than 1 part in 200, so accuracies greater than 12 bits are not usually justified. Some digital panel meters are equipped with suitable interfaces, and can make very cost-effective A/D converters.

ADA. A language originally based on the highly structured language PASCAL. Its advantage is that it was designed specifically for real-time control applications. It is therefore ideally suited to plant applications, hazardous environments and any application where monitoring of a large number of inputs may be necessary. Unfortunately it is not yet widely available for microcomputers, but it should become increasingly common in the future. It is not a language for the beginner.

ASCII. American Standard Code for Information Interchange. Each character which the computer can generate has its own ASCII code. This generally holds true for alphanumeric and some control characters such as 'carriage return', 'line feed', 'bell' etc. However, each system tends to have its own peculiarities, especially where graphics fonts are available. Also, some peripheral devices use some control characters for specific tasks. It may be necessary to write a simple translation program to convert from one machine to another.

Assembler level languages. These are languages that operate according to rules defined by the microprocessor chip running the computer. All data manipulation is done at a very low language level, many assembler language instructions being required to fulfil tasks called for in high level languages. Programs written in such languages are very fast but they are much more difficult to write, take longer to correct, and are a lot more difficult to modify. They are only really worth the effort for routines that must be very fast.

BASIC. Probably the best-known programming language in the world. This language is extremely easy to use, allowing the user to produce working programs quickly and simply. It is generally loathed and despised by professionals owing to its lack of structure (see Structured programming). Despite that, BASIC is often used to very good effect. Most implementations allow a wide range of mathematical functions support arrays and graphics displays. It is a good choice for all but the most experienced buyer or professional programmer.

Baud rate. This is closely related to the rate at which data may be transmitted between the computer and peripheral devices. For communication between devices to be possible they should be capable of transmitting/receiving at the same rate (many devices are capable of communicating at more than one rate). The rate of data transfer may be found approximately by dividing the baud rate by the number of bits in the data bus added to the number of parity and start/stop bits employed.

Benchmarks. These are short high level language routines that repeatedly use some aspect of a machine's capabilities. They might, for example, calculate the logarithm of a number several thousand times or write text to the screen repeatedly. By comparing timings for the same routine run on different machines, it is possible to judge which machine is fastest in a given field of operation. Several of the more serious computing magazines regularly publish lists of timings for machines they have reviewed. An example is included in this Appendix.

Bit. Within computers numbers are stored as series of electrical yes/no statements which are termed bits. A series of such bits make up a word and define a binary representation of a number or some other formalised representation of data. Each bit represents one binary digit of the number.

Buffer. Owing to the difference in speed between peripherals and the computer it is often the case that the computer may try and send data to peripherals faster than they can deal with it. Whilst none will be lost due to the use of sophisticated handshaking routines, the computer will spend time waiting for the peripheral to respond when it could be doing something more useful. To avoid this, many peripherals have an area of RAM used for temporary storage of incoming data. This allows the peripheral to take in a lot of data at the rate the computer operates and deal with it at its leisure. This can be extremely useful particularly if results are being outputted to a printer. Additionally, stand-alone inline buffers are available for the common interface configurations, and are very effective in freeing the computer for the next set of data while, for example, the results of the previous experiment are being printed.

Bug. No matter how experienced one is, it is likely that the first time one runs a new program an error will be found, either syntactic or semantic. These are generally termed bugs (a sort of mid-Atlantic gremlin) and are a fact of life. They usually turn up at the worst possible moment. Some of the structured languages tend by their very nature to produce less errors and make them easier to locate.

Bus. Information is transferred between the component parts of a computer and/or the outside world (peripherals) via a series of electrical pathways known as the bus. This is made up of three major parts: the data, address, and control buses. Generally, computers with data buses of 8 bits are slower than those with 16 bits when it comes to number manipulation and input/output operations.

Byte. An 8-bit number, i.e. a number within the range 0–255.

Centronics parallel interface. A standard type of connection between a printer and a computer. It is extremely popular and strongly supported by a wide range of manufacturers.

Clock speed. The operation of all computers is carefully coordinated by a timing pulse generated by an oscillating quartz crystal. It is common for manufacturers to quote the clock speed of the microprocessor at the heart of any computer. A typical value might by 2 MHz. One should not be misled—a machine operating at 8 MHz is not twice as fast as a different kind of machine operating at 4 MHz. This is governed by a wide range of factors such as the internal architecture of the computer. See Benchmark.

COBOL. A language extensively used for accounting and administrative purposes, but of little use in the laboratory or for process control.

Compilers. There are two principal ways in which a computer program may be executed. These are via interpreters or by use of a compiler. The former works through a program line-by-line converting each part to a form the computer understands (assembly language level) as and when that line is about to be used. The latter operates by converting the whole program into a form the computer understands prior to its being used. Both lead to the same ultimate result but there are two major differences: the interpreted language is easier and simpler to use but compiled languages perform an equivalent task considerably faster. Unless speed is extremely important, the difference is probably not terribly important. It is not uncommon within a high-level language program to use a compiled sub-routine to achieve adequate speed for some data input and control operations, and for some data manipulations.

CP/M. When first switched on, some machines are essentially empty of either a programming language or a working environment, rather like a blank sheet of paper. CP/M is a system wherein, upon 'power-up', programs are loaded from disc into the empty RAM. They are then available for use, allowing languages or other utilities to be loaded and run, or allowing manipulation of disc files. There is a very wide range of software available for the CP/M type systems which thus can make them a very attractive purchase.

D/A converter. Digital to analogue converter. A device which converts a digital number into an analogue output signal, usually a voltage. See A/D converter.

Editor. A piece of software/hardware used in conjunction with a compiled language.

Floating point numbers. Very large or very small real numbers may be stored and manipulated by computers despite the fact that data are stored as integer values. Generally, real numbers are stored as several words/bytes (often 5) which the computer interprets. Some bits represent sign, others the exponent, and the remainder an approximation to the value. The greater the number of bits used to define a real number, and consequently the more memory used, the more accurate the approximation and the greater the permissible range of values.

Floppy disc. A thin plastic disc coated with a magnetic material and kept within a protective cover. It may be used with a disc drive to store data in a reusable form. The devices store data quite quickly, typically taking only a few seconds to store a thousand data points. Three disc sizes are commonly available 8, 5·25 and 3·5 inches in diameter. It is often the case that discs used with one make of computer cannot be read using a different type, though some manufacturers may be able to assist in some cases. This is not because the discs are different but is due to differences in how data are arranged on the disc. Discs are usually capable of holding between 150 and 1000 kilobytes of information.

FORTRAN. This is a high level language specifically designed with the scientist/engineer/mathematician in mind. As such it has good facilities for doing high precision calculations rapidly and can even perform operations on complex numbers. A wide range of mathematical software has been published in professional journals, and some of this might be used to help reduce software development time/cost.

Handshaking. To ensure that data are successfully transferred between computers and peripherals, a complex system of signals passes between the two devices. These serve the purpose of coordinating actions, ensuring that both parties know what is going on and who should do what next.

Hard disc. A reusable storage medium working on the same principles as the floppy disc (and to some extent a tape recorder) but much more quickly and with a far greater capacity, typically 10–60 Mbytes. They are, however, more expensive and are fixed units, since the discs are sealed within an air-tight precision enclosure. When a hard disc is full, older data/programs may be 'downloaded' on to floppy discs using a floppy disc or tape drive (often supplied as part of the hard disc unit) for long-term storage in order to create space for new information.

Hardware. Basically these are the substantial items that make up the computer and peripherals, i.e. chips, wire, metal etc. The hardware is controlled by software which is stored either in RAM (after loading) or in ROM form.

High level languages. These are environments provided by software or hardware which allow complex operations to be performed in a sequence (program) defined by the user. Their greatest virtues are that the user needs no chip level understanding of the computer, the tasks performed are easily corrected (debugged) if in error, and it is possible to produce programs that are easily read and understood by other people.

IEEE parallel interface. This is a device which allows a computer to communicate with a similarly equipped peripheral. This system is commonly found on scientifically orientated equipment. It is faster than the RS-232C serial interfaces since several bits of information are sent simultaneously. It is however more expensive to send signals over distances greater than 5 m. HPIB and GPIB are embodiments of this standard interface. Always check with the manufacturers before mixing the systems, as each system has its own idiosyncrasies.

I/O. The operations which allow communication between a computer and a peripheral, whether sending data (writing) or receiving data (reading), are generally termed I/O operations, i.e. input/output.

Kilo. The value 1024 (2 raised to the power of 10) is often used to denote RAM or ROM memory size. The difference between this kilo and the normal metric 1000 stems from the binary origins of computer memory. As an example, a 48 kilobyte memory contains 49 152 byte locations.

Memory. This denotes the amount of space available for storage of data, programs and display data for example. It is measured in kilobytes or kilowords and comes in two forms: RAM or ROM. The former is of most interest to the user. Obviously, the more one can get the better, particularly if one wishes to apply techniques like FFTs (fast Fourier transforms) to the data. As an example, 1000 pairs of data points stored in a floating point array require about 10 kilobytes of memory. By comparison, if saved as an integer within the range $-32\,000$ to $+32\,000$, the memory used would be 4 kilobytes (using an 8-bit machine).

MS-DOS. An operating system found on a large number of microcomputers.

Multiplexer. In computer terms, a multiplexer (MUX) is a switching device which will allow, for example, one A/D converter to be used to read more than one analogue input channel into the computer. Naturally, this is slower than using an individual A/D per channel, but considerably cheaper. Note that, when employing multiplexers which use relays, a delay must be allowed between channel selection (i.e. energising the relay) and taking a reading from the A/D converter. This is to allow for contact bounce, and typical delay times are of the order of 20–50 ms. Multiplexers using solid-state switches do not have the contact bounce problem, but the authors have had problems with long-term stability on some of these devices.

Parity bits. To avoid the danger of data transmission between devices being corrupted by a noisy signal pathway, it is common to send both data, stop/start timing bits and some parity bits. The parity bits are related to the data in a way related to the number of bits set to 1 in the data sent. This makes it possible to detect if any of the bits transmitted have been corrupted. Many systems automatically re-request a previous transmission if a signal appears to have been corrupted.

PASCAL. A highly structured high level language. Though initially a rather pedantic and intolerant language, PASCAL has many virtues for the experienced user. It supports a wide range of data structures and allows programs to be written systematically in a clear and concise form. Some versions may have only a limited ability to communicate with peripherals. It is worth checking this aspect prior to purchase.

Peripheral. These are essentially anything that can be coaxed into swapping information or be controlled by a computer. Generally they are storage devices, data display units, control systems or input/output devices.

Pixel. Graphical displays on VDUs have a resolution defined in terms of pixels. A pixel is the smallest picture element that can be individually displayed. For comparison purposes a television screen is about 625 (in the UK) pixels high from top to bottom. Display potential is often described as high, low or medium resolution. There are no formal definitions, but a low resolution display will be less than 80 pixels by 80 pixels (80 × 80), medium resolution around 320 × 200, and high resolution anything greater than 400 × 300. One may be offered displays with much higher resolution but these are only really an advantage for CAD work or molecular modelling. In addition, a high resolution screen display may use up a lot of the RAM. Do not forget that the number of colours that may be displayed simultaneously is often more limited with higher resolution displays. Medium resolution displays are often a good compromise between cost and effectiveness.

Program. A sequence of instructions which, when converted to a form that the computer can act upon via compilers or interpreters, performs a given task.

RAM. Random access memory chips. These are memory devices that may be used as temporary storage for programs data or screen information. Information is stored as words that are interpreted by the language or environment in use. It is best to purchase machines with at least 64 kilobytes of RAM available to the users, and preferably in excess of 128 kilobytes. Though this may seem a lot, it makes life easier for comparing data from different experimental runs. It is worth bearing in mind that many computers, in particular those operating CP/M, may use some of the RAM for its own purposes, such as storing a high level language or providing memory for a screen display. A good example was the original BBC microcomputer, which used over 20 kilobytes of its RAM to provide a high-resolution screen, leaving a paltry 12 kilobytes for programs and data. This is not the case for the later BBC micros such as the Master series, where more RAM is available. The rule should be to ask how much memory one will have when the chosen language and the screen resolution have been defined.

ROM. Read only memory chips, in which instructions are stored in a manner that cannot be changed, short of by physical damage. They are often used to store languages operating systems or other information essential to the computer. It is usually possible to read what they contain or use some of them via assembler level languages.

RS-232C/422/423 serial interfaces. These are devices allowing a computer to talk to a similarly equipped peripheral. The exchange of information is slower than for an IEEE interface but may be transmitted over far greater distances at lower cost. The different numbers signify slightly different handshaking arrangements and different voltage levels. Converters between the types are available.

Software. This consists of a program and/or data which, when run, allows some complex operation(s) to be carried out. It is worth remembering, when writing a program, that the movement of the cursor, keyboard interpretation and conversion of the program into the machine level instructions are all performed by a program. Often software is provided for different tasks such as helping to debug programs (a 'toolkit'), or word processing.

Structured programming. This is an approach to programming wherein an attempt is made to ensure that the programs are easy to debug, read and modify. Structured languages impose constraints on the programmer which help to stop programs from becoming unreadable networks of interdependent clauses. This may not seem of great importance for small programs (less than 30 kilobytes of program) but, as the level of complexity grows, it becomes invaluable, particularly if a program is being developed by a team or is likely to be modified at some future date.

VDU. Visual display unit; a television or monitor display. Monitors give a sharper and more stable picture, but for some purposes televisions may be acceptable and are also considerably cheaper. Some domestic TV sets are now equipped with a 'monitor' socket for use with computers.

Winchester. See Hard disc.

APPENDIX 6.2: BUYING GUIDE

Buying a computer system is never easy, even for experienced hands. There are a large number of factors that need to be considered; however, since the market is changing extremely rapidly, it is futile to consider specific computer systems in depth. Rather, general principles will be dealt with. Bear in mind that an older model may meet your particular demands more cheaply than the more recent (and expensive) types, and may have much software and many technical books available. Check before purchase that there is a local service agent for the instrument under consideration.

The following points are worth considering before committing oneself to a specific system:

1. How much money is available for purchasing the computer?
2. What *exactly* is the computer to do?
3. What peripherals will be needed?
4. Will the computer be used for other purposes such as word processing?
5. So that the capital investment may be shared, is a multi-user system a practical proposition for the application?
6. How are the most promising candidates to be evaluated?

One thing worth remembering is that, in all probability, other people have already done what you are attempting. You are in a position to profit from their mistakes, as many problems which you might encounter have already been solved. It can be very helpful to talk to people who already use computers for scientific work (whatever the field) and ask them to show you what their equipment does and—of equal importance—what it does not do. Obviously, a wide range of opinions and the occasional case of obsession will be encountered, but often more can be learnt over a cup of coffee than from a week of examining technical specifications.

In common with all other equipment, your computer may break down out of warranty. Cheaper machines (such as some home computers and low-priced business machines) may have to be sent back to the service agent's premises for repair, which can put you out of action for several weeks. For this reason you may wish to put some of your budget aside for a service contract, where you may call the service engineer to your laboratory. In addition, it is worth remembering that during the year you will use some discs and a quantity of printer paper and ribbons or ink, particularly if you use the system for word processing. A dust cover is a worthwhile investment if the equipment is not going to be used for protracted periods of time. Purchase of a robust storage container for floppy discs etc. is advised. It can be profitable to shop around for these consumable items. Consult the popular computing magazines, and specialists in computer stationery.

It is worth defining exactly what you intend to do with your computer. If you intend doing only a small part of those tasks outlined here, then your requirements will not be very high (unless you envisage extending your system at some later date). There is little point in buying the latest megabyte memory microcomputer if what it does could be equally well done by a simple home computer.

Peripherals such as A/D converters are often the limiting factor when selecting a new computer. Most will contain RS-232C or IEEE interfaces as part of their design or optional extras. This can make life very easy since most of the computers available today also conform to one of these standards. When purchasing, it is worth making the successful interfacing of the computer with peripherals a condition of the sale. Most reputable companies will agree to this, so ask for a copy of the demonstration program, so that you can build it into your own program as a subroutine (having checked with the supplier that the copyright holder permits this).

When deciding which computer to buy, it is worth remembering that, in addition to controlling and monitoring equipment, it can be invaluable as a word processor, data base, or for carrying out intensive mathematical calculations. Though a secondary consideration, these can be of great additional value to a development section or a research team.

Most of the popular makes of microcomputer have word processing and similar software available. This is particularly true for CP/M and IBM machines, for which a phenomenal amount of software has been written ranging from simple word processors to complex three-dimensional molecular modelling packages. It has recently become increasingly common for manufacturers and retailers to provide 'bundled software' with a given computer. This usually comprises a word processor, data base and spreadsheet. Though they are not always the best available they often can be of use.

Special mention should perhaps be given to the IBM–PC microcomputer, since worldwide, it is one of the most popular machines. Whilst a trifle sluggish and primitive by today's (1988) standards the machines are well catered for in terms of add-on boards such as I/O interfaces or A/D converters, and it should be remembered that not all experiments need state-of-the-art technology. In particular, there are now a number of IBM compatible 'clones' available that are considerably cheaper and faster than the original.

Multi-user systems allow a number of users simultaneously to make use of a computer and its peripherals using separate terminals. This is often done via a sophisticated software environment such as UNIX. This can be a very cost effective way of running more than one experiment at a time. On the whole, however, such a system may impose restraints on data acquisition rates and program structure, especially when devices such as printers are shared. Whilst they may not cause serious problems for the user experienced in juggling priorities, they may not initially be worth the extra expenditure. On a reduced level, it is possible to link several micro-computer systems to form a 'local area net' (LAN), to achieve data transfer between systems and for distributed control applications. Simpler yet, a device known as a T-switch, costing about £100, will allow, for example, several computers to share one printer.

It is not a practical proposition to evaluate each and every computer within a price range with each and every peripheral. In order to draw up a ranked short-list of the available systems it is advisable to have a test program which will check independently each computer system. As an example, the authors wished to select a computer system for a process control application, for which speed of operation was important. In addition to comparing the technical specifications, prices and available discounts, we devised a simple benchmark program which could be quickly entered into a computer. We stress that this is by no means an exhaustive test, but does give a ranking of the speed of operation, from which systems may be selected for more exhaustive tests:

The test program (in BASIC) was as follows

```
10 FOR I = 1 TO 1000
20 A = I * COS(I) * TAN(I) + 10^ABS(LOG(I))
30 NEXT I
```

The time for each computer system to complete this loop was recorded with a stop-watch, and the results obtained, in seconds, are listed below. To give some perspective, the same program was also run on some main-frame systems, desk-top computers and microcomputers.

Commodore 4032	160 s	~ £600
Amstrad/Schneider CPC464	87 s	~ £550
IBM-AT	35 s	~ £1000
Hewlett-Packard 310 (desktop)	6 s	~ £6000
Hewlett-Packard A600 (mainframe)	1·7 s	~ £50 000

Summary. Check that your computer is capable of doing *your* job, that it is compatible with your peripherals, and will run all additional software you may want to purchase. Finally, ensure that you will still be able to afford consumable items such as printer paper during the year. In addition, always get demonstrations of compatibility before purchase.

Other Possible Systems

The method of data acquisition described is both easy to use and easy to understand. It is not, however, the only way such readings may be taken, and by no means the cheapest. Many people find it easier to use 19-inch modular rack instruments such as that produced by Mowlem Microsystems or Biodata. In such a system, the user initially buys a controlling module which interfaces to the computer, then selects a number of other modules from a wide range which can perform tasks such as relay control or D/A conversions. This allows a user to choose a configuration that perfectly fits the task requirement with little or no excessive capacity. Such instruments are again easy to use and very popular. Unfortunately, in common with the system described previously, this is not a particularly cheap way of doing things (£700–£8000, depending upon complexity).

The user with less money available may find it necessary to use a home microcomputer. Several types of approach are then possible. Although some of the cheaper microcomputers do have interfaces available, normally RS-232C rather than IEEE, they should be very thoroughly tested before acceptance. Others may find they are forced to provide their own control or signal monitoring. Such a task can be difficult and slow but very rewarding. In such a case it is essential that the computer is very carefully chosen. In particular it is worth looking for microcomputers with

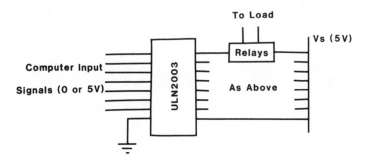

Fig. 6.7. An outline circuit showing how a Darlington driver circuit might be used to activate a bank of relays.

an easily available I/O user port (often based on a VIA 6522 IC), a parallel printer port and joystick socket(s). If these are available it is usually possible to switch relays successfully, operate simple A/D converter circuits, and control D/A converters via a small amount of digital circuitry.

For example, a simple circuit, such as that shown in Fig. 6.7, can be used to control up to 8 relays and is very simply driven via a programmable I/O port. If this approach is to be taken, special consideration should be given to the Acorn BBC series computers which fulfil the requirements, and in addition contain four 12-bit A/D converters, making life very easy indeed! If no advice is available, some dedicated books[8,9] may be of assistance in providing a gentle introduction.

Alternatively the user might purchase one of the S-100 or VME bus type microcomputers. These consist of plug-in boards that share a common bus system. There are a large number of board types available, such as A/D converters, printer interfaces and stepper motor controllers. This system has proved extremely popular over the years, particularly in the USA, and has been used very successfully for a wide range of applications. These systems, although ideal for industrial environments, tend to be quite expensive.

Chapter 7

Commercial Instruments

G. H. FRANCE

Department of Applied Physics, Sheffield City Polytechnic, Sheffield, UK

7.1. INTRODUCTION

The aim of this chapter is to describe the main features of a selection of commercially available extrusion rheometers, together with any accessories which may be obtained as optional extras. The instruments have been divided into two categories, extrusion plastometers and capillary rheometers. All technical information has been supplied by the manufacturers

189

together with any photographs used. However, care must be exercised since most manufacturers, in order to maintain a technological gain, are continually improving their products, and thus this chapter must be used only as a guide.

7.2. EXTRUSION PLASTOMETERS/MELT FLOW INDEXERS

Traditionally, extrusion plastometers, commonly known as melt flow indexers, provided the cheapest and most widely used method for obtaining rheological data from a capillary system. Although they are still widely used, the cost of some of the computerised instruments is approaching that of some manually operated extrusion rheometers.

However, these instruments are ideally suited for routine quality control, being robust, simple to use, and giving accurate data, so that the melt flow index (MFI) and melt volume index (MVI) can be calculated, these being an indication of the mass and volume of specimen flowing in a given time. By comparing the flow rates at two different loads, an indication of the pseudoplasticity can be obtained, i.e. the flow rate ratio (FRR).

All the melt flow indexers described can be used for tests which comply with a variety of international standards, but care should be taken to select the correct model since each model may only be suitable for a few selected tests. Also, the cost of the instrument in some cases can be reduced. In particular, if the user does not need to test to ASTM D.2116-83 and D.3159-81 standards, then a cheaper barrel and piston can usually be fitted since these tests are for corrosive materials.

In the standard ASTM D-1238 test, two methods are described, procedures A and B. For non-automated instruments procedure A is followed. This involves simply weighing the amount of material that is extruded in a 10 min period. Procedure B requires a precision timer to provide the time taken for the piston to fall through a precise distance.

$$ \text{MFI} = (Al\rho/T) \times 600 $$

where A is the average cross-sectional area between piston surface and extrusion channel, a constant for a particular instrument (cm^2), l is the length of the extrusion channel (cm), ρ is the density of the material (g cm^{-3}), T is the time taken for the piston to fall a known distance, and 600 is the conversion factor since the MFI is expressed in g/10 min.

Similarly

$$MVI = (Al/T) \times 600$$

Some of the major manufacturers of melt flow indexers attempt to make their instruments in a modular fashion, so that the user, if he so wishes, can start with a basic instrument and, as his needs develop, can add on with minimum amount of time and redundant modules.

7.2.1. CEAST Modular Flow Indexer

Figure 7.1 shows the CEAST modular flow indexer 6542/000. The basic instrument comes complete with all ancillary parts required for basic

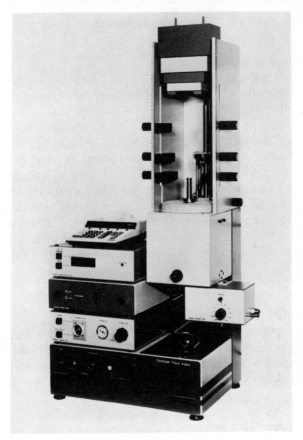

Fig. 7.1. CEAST modular flow indexer 6542/000. (By courtesy of the manufacturer.)

manual operation. Temperature regulation is by two CEAST regulators with a single control giving a working temperature range of 100–400 °C. The extrusion cylinder, piston and nozzle on the basic instrument are manufactured from deformation-free steel but tungsten carbide or hast-alloy versions are available. By the combination of different modules, varying degrees of sophistication can be obtained. A typical manual instrument could consist of the basic unit together with a pneumatic weight lifter and digital read-out of time. A dedicated calculator is available from CEAST which calculates the MFI. At the top of the range the instrument can be made fully automatic with the addition of an interface and a HP41 CV and an automatic weight lifter.

Price range £3000–£6000.

7.2.2. Davenport Melt Indexer

Daventest manufacture a complete range of melt flow indexers, starting with a utility model which consists of a temperature controlled barrel and stand together with all ancillary parts. Daventest also manufacture two other manually operated instruments giving improved performance. At the top of Davantest's range is the model 5 (Fig. 7.2) which can be purchased with a manual control rack or a computer interface for use with a Commodore 64 microcomputer. The software is supplied with the interface so that the computer may be purchased separately. However, the software is on cassette, giving rise to all the problems associated with this form of data storage medium. There is no automatic extrudate cutter or weight lifter available, therefore limiting the degree of automation, and requiring more of the operator's attention.

Price range £1100–£5300.

7.2.3. Göttfert Melt Indexer

Göttfert manufacture a range of melt flow indexers. The microprocessor models are programmed by a six digit code, and an IEEE-488 interface is provided which will allow the user to connect several instruments together to be controlled by the interface or by a host computer that has a similar interface.

7.2.4. Kayeness Melt Indexer

Kayeness supply a range of melt flow indexers. At the bottom of the range is the economy model which is completely manual in operation and has

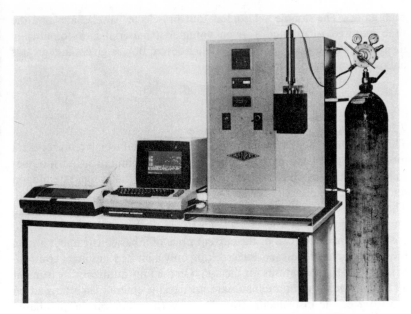

Fig. 7.2. Davenport melt indexer. (By courtesy of the manufacturer.)

none of the sophistication of the other models in the range. The temperature must be checked against a thermometer but it has the same temperature controller as the others. The other two models are similar, differing only in that the top of the range model has computer control. These instruments have digitally displayed temperature as standard, and a pneumatic weight lifter can be added as an option. The non-computerised model can be upgraded with the computer at a later date. With the computerised version a variety of programs may be selected and the computer will print all data collected.

7.2.5. Monsanto Automatic Capillary Rheometer

Monsanto manufacture two versions of melt flow indexer. The basic model is very standard, being totally manual in operation. The second version, known by Monsanto as an automatic capillary rheometer, can be obtained either as a single-pressure instrument or equipped with a pressure switching unit allowing for four different pressures in a single run. In this model the driving force for the piston is a 160 psig regulated nitrogen supply. Two pressure gauges are mounted on the top of the stand; the use of two gauges allows precise pressure measurements within the range of each gauge. The sample is tested at four preselected dwell times and the time required to extrude a given volume of material is automatically measured. A die swell tester (a detailed description is given later in this chapter) can also be fitted.

Price range £6500–£17000.

7.2.6. Zwick 4105 Extrusion Plastometer

This instrument (Fig. 7.3) is purchased as a base unit which requires extra modules to give basic manual operation; by combining various modules full automation can be obtained. It must be noted that a separate plug-in temperature programmer is necessary for every test temperature required. There are eleven temperature programmers available, giving a working temperature range of 150–373 °C. To stock all the programmers would cost approximately 10% of the current price of a basic instrument and in most cases is not necessary, but stocking only a limited supply of controller must lead to frustrations for the user. On the fully automatic instrument all the information on the material under test is entered via a keypad on the front of the instrument. However, a card reader can be purchased which allows the user to program the microprocessor by means of a plastic program card. The program required can be marked on the card by the user. Standard with the microprocessor is an 8-bit parallel or RS-232-C-/20mA interface for the transmission of either individual or statistical data. Software is available for an IBM personal computer which will collect and store the data which may then be plotted (i.e. mean MFI over a period of time).

Price range £3800–£10500.

7.3. CAPILLARY EXTRUSION RHEOMETERS

Most of the commercially manufactured extrusion rheometers commonly available may be purchased in an automated form. The software packages provided can usually be considered in three sections: control, data acquisition, and data storage and display. When an extrusion rheometer is used in a manual mode the decision as to when steady state conditions are achieved is the responsibility of the operator. Similarly the data taken are processed by equations known to the operator. When the rheometer is used in an automatic mode these decisions are taken away from the

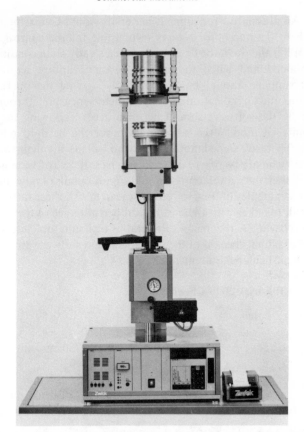

Fig. 7.3. Zwick 4105 extrusion plastometer. (By courtesy of the manufacturer.)

operator; therefore, when considering a rheometer, an appreciation of how the software collects the data and applies the equations and corrections used in the subsequent data processing should be known. Although most polymers will process with the rheometer driven automatically, there will inevitably be some which fail for a variety of reasons. The controlling software may assume that steady state conditions have been achieved when in reality the pressure is fluctuating rapidly. Since one of the main benefits of automation is that of freeing the operator to perform other tasks, this effect can go unnoticed. Some manufacturers attempt to accommodate this by limiting the number of readings of pressure at each piston speed. If the maximum value is reached, that particular data point is flagged. An alternative for difficult materials would be a semi-automatic mode where the microprocessor is responsible for the control and data collection but the operator determines when steady state conditions have been obtained and when to initiate the data capture sequence. The software supplied should be 'user friendly', giving the operator clear instructions and an indication of the parameters measured throughout the test. Ideally the software should be open access, allowing the user the opportunity to modify the software without the need to refer to the suppliers. There are some maufacturers who will modify their software for those users who are unable to do so themselves. If the software is supplied protected, then the manufacturer should supply details of how the data are stored and examples of how to retrieve the data. All these facts should be considered, together with the mechanical performance of the instrument, when purchasing a rheometer. Preferably a 'hands on' test should be arranged as a final check that the instrument and software are suitable for the user's particular requirements.

7.3.1. ACER Series 2000 Rheometer

Temperature range	Range 1: -20 to $+80\,°C$
	Range 2: $+80$ to $+450\,°C$
Piston speed range	0·5 or 0·05 to 750 mm min^{-1}
Dynamic range	1500:1 or 15 000:1
Shear rate range	Min. 0·3 s^{-1} (2·5 mm die)
	Max. 62 500 s^{-1} (1·0 mm die)
Pressure range	Max. working pressure 200 MPa

Figure 7.4 shows the ACER series 2000 capillary extrusion rheometer manufactured by Carter Baker Enterprises (CBE). This instrument is available with a choice of temperature range, piston speed range, and barrel size. Both the force on the ram and the entrance pressure are measured using a load cell on the piston and a pressure transducer sited in the cylinder wall above the die entrance. The piston speed range is achieved by the use of a reduction gearbox. This presents no problem for the automation sequence since the gearbox is electrically operated. The volume of polymer remaining in the barrel may be calculated, since a transducer may be used to monitor the position of the piston, which may be displayed on the control panel. Compressed air can be used to cool the barrel and die rapidly. On the manual versions all control is via the control module. All the signals measured by the rheometer are readily available, therefore the user who wishes to interface his own computer to the

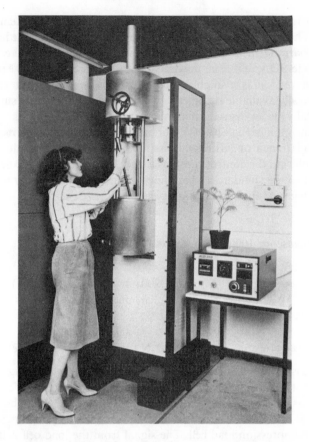

Fig. 7.4. ACER series 2000 rheometer. (By courtesy of the manufacturer.)

rheometer will have very few problems. The signals from the control module are in the range 0–10 volts. However, CBE can supply a desk-top computer, control console, and software.

CBE also manufacture a range of accessories for their own and other manufacturers' rheometers. These include a non-contacting optical system which measures the extrudate diameter. An optical pyrometer known as an extrudate temperature accessory (ETA) is available and consists of a measuring head and control console. The standard ETA unit will measure a target size of nominally 1 mm diameter, with a lens to target distance of 107 mm. The unit is offered as standard with a choice of two temperature ranges 0–150 and 150–500 °C. The slit die accessory (SDA) for rheometers and extruders has four pressure ports and a choice of two temperature ranges. The four pressure transducers are flush mounted on one half of the die. This arrangement allows for different size slits to be fitted economically to one SDA unit. The maximum standard pressure is 70 MPa but a 200 MPa version is available. The SDA can be fitted to a variety of commercially available rheometers with the use of an adapter supplied by CBE. All the accessories manufactured by CBE have, as standard, analogue output signals (0–10 V) for all test parameters so that incorporating them into new or existing automated systems has been made as simply as possible. All the control consoles for the rheometer and accessories are designed to the standard 19 inch format, and thus may easily be built in to an integrated instrumentation system.

7.3.2. Rheoscope 1000

Temperature range	100–400 °C
Piston speed range	0·5–200 mm min^{-1} (preselected)
	0·3–300 mm min^{-1} (continuous)
Shear rate range	Min. 1 s^{-1} (2·1 mm die)
	Max. 40 000 s^{-1} (0·5 mm die)
Pressure range	0–10^4 N (other ranges available)

The Rheoscope 1000 manufactured by CEAST is shown in Fig. 7.5. This instrument may be purchased as an extrusion instrument only, or together with a tensile testing module. In either case the rheometer can be obtained in manual or automated form. The total force on the piston is measured using a compression load cell. The signal from the load cell is displayed digitally and an analogue output allows for a continuous recording on a chart recorder. The maximum load allowed is 10^4 N. The required piston speed is preselected by nine push-buttons, or alternatively continuously variable speeds are obtained by hand operated control. The selected speed is displayed digitally. When tensile measurements are required the extrudate from the rheometer is passed through a pulley system and then pulled by two counter-rotating rollers, the velocity of which can be varied by hand operation in the range 1–1000 rpm. The velocity of the rollers can also be varied from a preset value to 1000 rpm with three constant accelerations. The force detector used is connected to the first pulley. The rotational speeds and the tensile forces are displayed digitally and these can be recorded. The rotational speed of the roller at the breaking point of the filament is retained on the display. For constant temperature tests

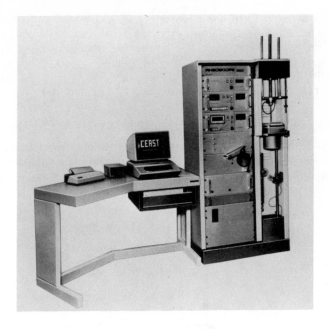

Fig. 7.5. CEAST Rheoscope 1000. (By courtesy of the manufacturer.)

a thermostatic window chamber is available. The Rheoscope 1000 has a microprocessor option consisting of an interface for the rheometer and an Apple microcomputer equipped with several interface cards. The software is supplied on disc and is divided into two sections: data acquisition and data elaboration. The data acquisition software allows the user to select up to a maximum of 32 piston speeds with a minimum step increase of $0.6\,\text{mm}\,\text{min}^{-1}$ and the time at each piston speed. The operator is also allowed to define an instability condition for the extrudate flow, at which point the test is automatically aborted and all data collected to that point are transferred to the computer which indicates that an instability condition has occurred. Once all the initial parameters have been entered and the barrel filled, the test will then be carried out automatically. The data elaboration software displays and prints out the rheological curves from the data obtained. The curves displayed are shear stress and viscosity versus shear rate. The software will also calculate and display the Bagley correction and a 'graphical' scanning of each curve, the relevant typical points being stored.

7.3.3. Davenport Extrusion Rheometer

Temperature range	100–300 °C
Piston speed range	0·125–25 cm min^{-1}
Dynamic range	10 000:1
Shear rate range	Min. 62·5 s^{-1} (1·0 mm die)
	Max. 12 500 s^{-1} (1·0 mm die)
Pressure range	Max. working pressure 1400 kg cm^{-1}

Figure 7.6 shows a typical Davenport extrusion rheometer. The only rheometer available at present from Daventest is their manual version, but they have indicated to the author that a completely new automated model

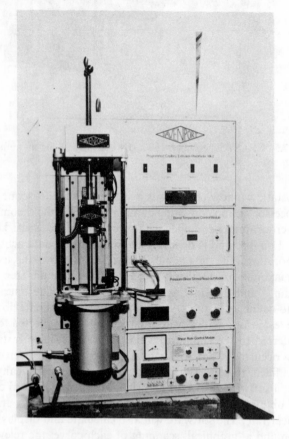

Fig. 7.6. Davenport extrusion rheometer. (By courtesy of the manufacturer.)

is under development and should be available in the near future. It should be noted that manual versions can be automated as mentioned in Section 7.4. The rheometer supplied at present is driven by a thyristor controlled d.c. shunt motor via a manually operated two-speed gearbox. The speed of the piston is indicated by means of an electric tachometer, the speed being maintained to a high degree of accuracy using the tachometer signal to monitor and control the thyristor unit. The speed of the piston is continuous throughout the range and displayed on the control panel. The entrance pressure is measured by a transducer sited above the entrance to the die. The total force on the piston can be measured by fitting a compression load cell on top of the piston, but usually a load ring is fitted which simply acts as a safety switch. The pressures developed are displayed on the control panel and the facility for a chart recorder is provided. Any chart recorder can be employed to record the pressures, provided they can give full scale deflection at 10 mV signal input. A comparator is supplied with the rheometer to enable the user to calibrate the meter, or chart recorder, periodically.

7.3.4. Göttfert Rheograph 2001

Göttfert manufacture a complete range of test instruments for rheological measurements. The Rheograph 2001 (Fig. 7.7) is a high pressure capillary rheometer with microprocessor. The piston on the rheometer is driven by a hydraulic system consisting of an oil tank with a high pressure internal gear wheel pump dipping into the tank. An electro-hydraulic linear amplifier converts the rotation of a stepper motor into a linear movement of the piston. The barrel temperature is controlled by three electronic temperature controllers with structure switch-over PD-PID behaviour. Also the melt temperature is determined by two iron–constantan thermocouples positioned at the entrance and exit of the die. The entrance pressure is measured using a transducer sited in the barrel above the entrance to the die. As software for the instrument is supplied on ROM, the rheometer is ready to operate immediately the unit is switched on. There is a maximum of 18 different preset piston speeds or test pressures since the machine can be operated in two modes: constant piston speed or constant pressure. An interface may be obtained which allows the rheometer to be connected to a host computer or plotter. The software to supplement these options is also available and is supplied on ROM. All the ROMs available are fitted into the host computer interface. The software for the host computer application gives the user the facility for the bi-directional transfer of data. Included in the host computer ROM package

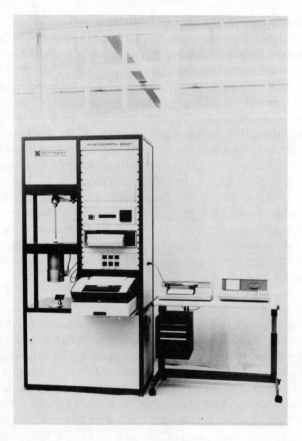

Fig. 7.7. Göttfert Rheograph 2001. (By courtesy of the manufacturer.)

is a program cassette and listing, together with an example program for an HP-85 desk-top computer. A manually operated rheometer is also available from Göttfert and is similar to the Rheograph 2001. The dual mode operation is maintained, and all the test parameters are displayed on the control panel.

Göttfert manufacture round hole dies, annular dies and slit dies. All these dies can be fitted to the standard barrel of either rheometer. The slit die can be obtained in a variety of sizes and in each case has three pressure ports, but by using the slit die in conjunction with a measuring ring a further pressure port, which measures the inlet pressure loss, and an extra temperature port may be gained. The rheometers may be fitted with a die swell tester; this measures the extrudate diameter and comes complete with a manually operated extrudate cutter. This unit generates a signal which is fed into the rheometer interface and is processed by the on-board microprocessor. The die swell is measured statistically and dynamically during the test, the average value and standard deviation being calculated and stored.

A tensile tester (Rheotens) is available, having haul-off speeds in the range 0–1200 mm s^{-1}. This unit will measure the tensile force and the rotational speed of the drum at the breaking point of the extrudate. Both signals from the unit can be permanently recorded on an X–Y chart recorder. The Rheotens can be fitted to a variety of instruments, and deflectors can be obtained. One of these is a continuous capillary rheometer (Minex-rheometer). This employs a small extruder both to melt the polymer and to pump it through the capillary. The extrudate is then fed into the tensile tester. For those who wish to take continuous on-line measurements of viscosity, Göttfert manufacture a bypass-flow-capillary rheometer, which is capable of testing both low and high viscosity materials, and the facility for both data acquisition and processing.

7.3.5. Instron Rheometers

Instron manufacture a high pressure capillary rheometer model 3211. This system is totally self-contained in a table-top cabinet including control and

Temperature range	40–350 °C
Dynamic range	333:1
Piston speed range	0·6–200 mm min^{-1}
Shear rate range	Min. 0·12 mm s^{-1} (1·524 mm die)
	Max. 400 mm s^{-1} (0·762 mm die)
Pressure range	Max. working pressure 20 kN

drive mechanisms. The piston speed is selected via a series of six push-buttons. Range extensions are available through special gear ratios. The pressure is measured using a load cell and displayed on a vane meter as standard, but a digital meter or recorder is available on request. This instrument may also be used to perform melt index testing through the use of a capillary meeting ASTM specification D-1238.

Instron also manufacture a high pressure capillary rheometer as an accessory model 3210 for their universal testing machines 1193 and 1195. Special adapters are available for other Instron machines on request. This rheometer consists of an extrusion assembly mounted on the base of a standard Instron testing machine. The temperature controls for the

Temperature range	40–350 °C
Piston speed range	0·5–500 mm min^{-1}
Shear rate range	Min. 0·005 s^{-1} (1·524 mm die)
	Max. 1000 s^{-1} (0·762 mm die)
Pressure	Max. working pressure 13 kN

heating system are contained in a separate console. The force is measured using a load cell and is plotted on a chart recorder. This rheometer has a wide range of piston speeds as standard, but special speeds are available on request. The instrument can be operated in either constant shear rate or constant stress mode.

7.3.6. Kayeness Rheometer 2052

Temperature range	Range 1: 26–300 °C
	Range 2: 26–375 °C
Piston speed range	0·04–24 in min^{-1}
Pressure range	Max. working pressure 1000 lb

Figure 7.8 shows the Kayeness microcomputer controlled rheometer model 2052. Three versions of this model are currently available. Model 2052A known as a rubber scorch rheometer (ram speed 0·05–5 in min^{-1}), Model 2052B a constant shear rate (0·04–20 in min^{-1}) and Model 2052C a constant shear rate of constant shear stress (ram speed 0·04 in min^{-1}) or (load 0–600 or 0–1000 lb). The servomotor which determines the ram speed on all models is digitally controlled by the computer. A force transducer (accuracy 0·02%) sited on top of the piston feeds data to the computer for preload control and stress calculations. Using the computer, five increments can be programmed for one constant shear rate, with the option of a dwell time between the increments, or up to a maximum of five different shear rates in one test. Preload and preheat times are programmable. The microcomputer control panel has indicator lights to assist the operator in entering the program; thus the minimum of training is required. On completion of the test, the data are printed on any Epson compatible printer, in metric or English form. A data processing option is available and consists of an IBM computer system model 256K IBM-XT with dual disc drives and an RS232 interface together with some basic software. The software package allows for data storage and retrieval, straight line curve fits of viscosity vs. shear rate, calculation of the slope of the curve and the sequence control of a Bausch and Lomb plotter, plus the program to plot viscosity vs. shear rate.

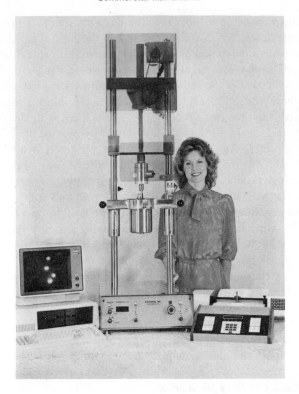

Fig. 7.8. Kayeness rheometer 2052. (By courtesy of the manufacturer.)

7.3.7. Monsanto Processability Tester

Temperature range	70–287 °C
Piston speed range	$0 \cdot 25$–$250 \, \text{mm} \, \text{min}^{-1}$
Shear rate range	Min. $1 \cdot 5 \, \text{s}^{-1}$ ($2 \cdot 0 \, \text{mm}$ die)
	Max. $25 \, 500 \, \text{s}^{-1}$ ($0 \cdot 03 \, \text{mm}$ die)
Pressure range	Max. working pressure $15 \, 000 \, \text{psi}$

Monsanto Instruments manufacture this capillary rheometer (the MPT) which is driven hydraulically and features a temperature controlled piston and barrel. The pressure, measured by a transducer sited in the barrel above the entrance to the die, is displayed both digitally and for a permanent record on a chart recorder. The barrel assembly has been designed to pull forward to give easy access when loading a sample. Once the barrel is loaded with the sample under test, there is a choice of six principal test sequences, each selected by a code entered on the control panel. A typical test run involves a maximum of four programmed shear rates, the pressure and die swell being measured at each state. However, a pause or dwell time can be introduced after the end of each of the four tests. Also, after the last test a stress relaxation measurement can be taken. Manual operation is also allowed, the operator selecting the piston speed with the rheometer collecting the data. In all the tests the data are presented digitally and as a continuous plot. As an optional extra, a printer is available which connects to the rheometer and gives the user a hard copy of the averaged data, the raw data collected can then be processed by the operator. A main feature of the MPT is the built-in die swell tester and controlled heated environment chamber. This unit can also be fitted to the melt flow indexer supplied by Monsanto and to any other manufacturer's rheometer. A collimated laser beam is used, projected through a rotating prism to produce a translating scan which sweeps across the extrudate. The shadow cast by the extrudate falls upon a receiver and is directly proportional to the diameter of the extrudate. The receiver converts the image into equivalent electrical signals which are then processed. The extrudate diameter or percentage swell is then displayed digitally on the rheometer, and on the chart recorder. A useful feature is the vertical laser scanning mechanism which allows the unit to define the extrusion profile.

7.3.8. Rosand Capillary Rheometer

Temperature range	45–400 °C
Piston speed range	$0 \cdot 012$–500 mm min^{-1}
Dynamic range	50 000:1
Shear rate range	Min. $0 \cdot 1$ s^{-1}
	Max. 192 000 s^{-1}
Pressure range	Max. working pressure > 10 t

Rosand Precision seem unique in that they manufacture multi-barrel capillary rheometers. These are available in single bore single barrel format, but twin bore single barrel and twin double barrel systems are available. There is a choice of three bore diameters: 12, 15 and 19 mm. The frame of the rheometer is rated in excess of 10 tonnes; the drive is of 5 t as standard, but a 10 t drive is available. In all the formats the pressure transducers are sited above the entrance to the die. A Rosand stainless steel force transducer is used to measure the total force on the piston. All the rheometers are floor standing and incorporate a forced air fume extracter for the operators' safety. The single bore single barrel version can be supplied with an 'intelligent' control panel as an alternative to full computerisation, yet this model can be easily converted to full computer operation. Using a multi-bore rheometer allows for the simultaneous determination of pressure drop across a long and a short die. Either a zero length die can be used or a short die, in which case a full Bagley correction is automatically applied. This facility of twin bore double barrelled rheometers enables a single technician to obtain all the information needed from a test in a fraction of the time required using a conventional rheometer. The computer system supplied by Rosand with the rheometer has a twin screen facility. One of the screens acts as a console showing all the experimental parameters while the second screen displays all the data collected or the derived curves. The software performs all the computations on the data, including Bagley and Rabinowitsch correction when required. Presentation of the results is up to report standard and consists of tabulated data and a selection of graphs. Several other features offered by the automation during a test include ramped or other preselected speed inputs, and constant shear stress as opposed to constant shear rate, set shear rates or relaxation experiments.

Rosand also manufacture a melt tension tester. This may be fitted into a glass-fronted temperature controlled environment chamber allowing controlled temperatures in the range 40–199 °C. Two types of haul-off are currently available: one with a standard drum speed of $0·01–10 \text{ m min}^{-1}$ and a high speed version with drum speeds of $0·3–300 \text{ m min}^{-1}$. Tensions from $0·5$ to 50 N fsd can be measured as standard but a special high load device (2 kN) is available. There is a choice of capillary sizes and entry angles of the supplied dies. Other die geometries manufactured by Rosand include slit dies and annular dies; both types can be obtained in a variety of sizes with single or multi-point pressure ports if required, but Rosand will manufacture one-off specials to suit individual requirements.

7.4. CONCLUSION

All the capillary extrusion rheometers described in this chapter are in the price range of £12 000 to £55 000. For an automated capillary rheometer the prices start at approximately £20 000. For establishments that already possess an old non-automatic rheometer, the high cost of purchasing a new computerised model may be prohibitive. There are always alternatives, one being to convert the instrument to accept computer control 'in house'. The time and skills necessary to undertake this upgrade are quite considerable and the end result may not perform as originally intended. There are companies who specialise in converting manually operated instruments to full computer control at a fraction of the cost of a new machine. One such company is CFM Electronics who offer a conversion package for the Davenport extrusion rheometer. These companies offer a package which usually refurbishes the rheometer, and they provide a suitable interface to connect to a computer which controls and collects the data. In some cases a choice of computer is allowed. The instrument can still be used in a manual mode but fully and semi-automatic modes are provided. The software will allow long and zero length die tests or tests using dies having different L/R ratios to give a Bagley plot. Software to perform all computations, data presentation and a graph plotting routine can be supplied. This type of conversion is useful since it gives a new lease of life to an old instrument and is flexible enough to allow for any unique alterations that a particular user needs.

The choice of capillary rheometers (automated or manual) on the market at present is limited but, knowing one's own particular requirements, a suitable machine can be obtained. When the final choice has been made (either a new instrument or an upgrade) a 'hands on' test should still be arranged.

APPENDIX 7.1. MANUFACTURERS AND THEIR AGENTS' ADDRESSES

Manufacturer	Agent
Carter Baker Enterprises, 83 Cherry Garden Lane, Newport, Essex CB11 3QB, UK	
CEAST SpA, Via Asinari di Bernezzo 70, Torino 10146, Italy	Engelman & Buckham, Willian Curtis House, Alton, Hants GU34 1HH, UK

Daventest Ltd,
Tewin Road,
Welwyn Garden City,
Herts
AL7 1AQ,
UK

Göttfert Werkstoff-Prüfmaschinen GmbH,
D-6967 Buchen/Odenwald,
Siemensstr. 2,
Postfach 1220,
Federal Republic of Germany

Instron Limited,
Coronation Road,
High Wycombe,
Bucks HP12 3SY,
UK

Kayeness Inc.,
RD 3,
Box 30,
Honeybrook,
Pennsylvania 19344,
USA

Monsanto Company,
2689 Wingate Avenue,
Akron,
Ohio 44313,
USA

Monsanto Limited,
Edison Road,
Dorcan,
Swindon,
Wiltshire
SN3 5HN,
UK

Rosand Precision,
11 Little Ridge,
Welwyn Garden City,
Herts
AL7 2BH,
UK

Zwick Testing Machines Ltd,
Southern Avenue,
Leominster,
Herefordshire
HR6 0QH,
UK

CFM Electronics Ltd,
PO Box 297,
Sheffield
S1 1UZ,
UK

Chapter 8

Elongational Rheometers

R. K. GUPTA

Department of Chemical Engineering, State University of New York at Buffalo, Buffalo, New York, USA

and

T. SRIDHAR

Department of Chemical Engineering, Monash University, Clayton, Victoria, Australia

NOTATION

A_0	cross-sectional area of nozzle exit in eqns (8.18) and (8.19)
a_1 to a_5	constants in eqn (8.17)
D	diameter
F	force (used with various subscripts)

g	acceleration due to gravity
l	sample length
L	capillary length
L_0	initial length in eqn (8.7)
l, l_0	sample length at time t and $t = 0$
n	power law index
P_{Ent}	entrance pressure drop
P_0, P_1	pressures in viscometer before and after stretching in eqns (8.20) and (8.21)
Q	volumetric flow rate
Q_0, Q_1	volumetric flow rate without stretching and with stretching in eqns (8.20) and (8.21)
r	radius
R	capillary radius
T_r	Trouton ratio
v_1, v_2, v_3	flow velocity components
V_0	average flow velocity at nozzle exit in eqn (8.19)
x_1, x_2, x_3	coordinate directions, with flow in x_1 direction
γ	surface tension
$\dot{\gamma}_A$	apparent shear rate
$\dot{\varepsilon}$	tensile strain rate
$\dot{\varepsilon}_E$	net average extension rate
η_E	tensile viscosity
η_E^+	tensile stress growth coefficient
η	shear viscosity
ρ	polymer density
$\boldsymbol{\sigma}$	total stress tensor
σ_{11}	total stress at x
σ_E	net average extensional stress
$\boldsymbol{\tau}$	extra stress tensor
$\tau_{11} - \tau_{22}$	first normal stress difference

8.1. INTRODUCTION

The study of the elongational or extensional flow of polymeric fluids has been the subject of intense research for most of the last two decades. Continuing interest in this area stems from the fact that several industrially important polymer processing operations such as fibre spinning, blow moulding, flat film extrusion and film blowing involve a predominantly extensional mode of deformation. This flow field is also highly effective in orienting polymer molecules in the flow direction, and the high deformation rates which typically occur in industrial operations, albeit for a short duration, result in the presence of unusually large fluid stresses; the theoretical prediction of these stresses is an unsolved issue which represents an intellectual challenge to every rheologist.

Although most of the literature on extensional flows is devoted to work on polymer melts, an increasing amount of effort is now being directed at polymer solutions as well. The stretching flow of polymer solutions is encountered, for instance, in applications like coatings, enhanced oil recovery, lubrication, turbulent drag reduction, and the break-up of jets into droplets. In addition, extensional flow data, where available, are useful for polymer characterization and quality control purposes since these are often sensitive to subtle changes in the polymer structure.

In order to understand and interpret rheological measurements properly it is necessary that the results depend neither on the technique of measurement nor on any assumptions regarding the constitutive behaviour of the material. It is for this reason that one usually defines material functions which characterize the fluid response in simple flow situations. For extensional flows, this requires that data be obtained under conditions of constant stress or constant rate of strain. Unfortunately this is an extremely daunting task which has been accomplished only for highly viscous materials, and that too for low values of the rate of strain and the strain itself. The difficulty arises from the mobile nature of liquids and the impossibility of gripping them and making them stretch in a prescribed manner. As a consequence, several ingenious techniques have been devised to create stretching flows and also to measure the fluid stresses and the attendant rates of strain. These latter techniques, however, yield transient data since a constant stretch history is not involved. Nonetheless, these data can be extremely useful for the purpose of developing and testing rheological constitutive equations provided that the kinematics are well defined and known.

Different aspects of extensional flows have been reviewed in the past. Table 8.1 presents a sample of recent reviews; it appears that the emphasis has been on polymer melts, but most of the recent progress has taken place in the area of polymer solutions and it is to this topic that we primarily address ourselves.

TABLE 8.1
Recent Reviews on Elongational Rheometers

Authors	Year	Title
Hill and Cuculo[1]	1976	Elongational flow behaviour of polymeric fluids
Petrie[2]	1979	Elongational flows
Bogue[3]	1978	Tensile viscosity: a review
Dealy[4]	1978	Extensional rheometers for molten polymers
White[5]	1978	Experimental studies of elongational flows of polymer melts
Cogswell[6]	1978	Converging flow and stretching flow
White[7]	1981	Dynamics, heat transfer and rheological aspects of melt spinning
Dealy[8]	1982	Rheometers for molten plastics
Meissner[9]	1985	Experimental aspects in polymer melt elongational rheometry

8.2. EXTENSIONAL FLOW KINEMATICS

Most elongational rheometers measure the fluid response in uniaxial extensional flow. In a rectangular cartesian coordinate system, this flow can be described by expressing the three velocity components as

$$v_1 = \dot{\varepsilon}x_1 \tag{8.1}$$

$$v_2 = -\dot{\varepsilon}x_2/2 \tag{8.2}$$

$$v_3 = -\dot{\varepsilon}x_3/2 \tag{8.3}$$

where the stretch rate, $\dot{\varepsilon}$, may depend on both time and position. Here x_1, x_2 and x_3 are the coordinate directions, and flow is assumed to take place in the x_1 direction; also it is understood that the material is incompressible.

If a specimen, initially of length l_0, is stretched at constant stretch rate for time t, integration of eqn (8.1) yields

$$\ln (l/l_0) = \dot{\varepsilon}t \tag{8.4}$$

where l is the sample length at time t and the right-hand side of eqn (8.4) is the elongational strain, often called the Hencky strain. Clearly the sample length increases exponentially with time.

Although other kinds of extensional flow such as biaxial extension and planar extension can be defined,[8] we shall not be concerned with these in this chapter.

8.2.1. Elongational Viscosity

In uniaxial extension both the extra stress tensor, τ, and the total stress tensor, σ, are diagonal and the stress components in directions normal to the flow direction are equal to each other. As a consequence, the only non-zero material function is the stress difference $(\sigma_{11} - \sigma_{22})$ and this also equals $(\tau_{11} - \tau_{22})$.

For constant stretch rate homogeneous deformation which begins from rest, one can define a tensile stress growth coefficient.

$$\eta_E^+ = (\tau_{11} - \tau_{22})/\dot{\varepsilon} \tag{8.5}$$

which has the dimensions of viscosity. The limiting value of this quantity as time tends to infinity is termed the elongational or tensile viscosity, η_E. In general η_E can be expected to be a function of the stretch rate $\dot{\varepsilon}$, although for Newtonian liquids the extensional viscosity is independent of $\dot{\varepsilon}$ and is exactly three times the shear viscosity; this result is called Trouton's law.[10] For polymeric liquids, the Trouton result is expected to hold only in the limit of vanishing low deformation rates,[11] i.e.

$$\lim_{\dot{\varepsilon} \to 0} (\eta_E/\eta_0) = \lim_{\dot{\varepsilon} \to 0} T_r = 3 \tag{8.6}$$

where η_0 is the zero shear viscosity.

As opposed to a constant stretch rate experiment, one may carry out a creep test and impose a constant stress and measure the strain as a function of time. The extensional viscosity is then obtained as the large strain asymptote.

In closing this section, we emphasize that steady state stress levels are obtained only at low deformation rates and at long times of deformation provided of course that a constant stretch rate extensional flow field can be generated at all in the first place. The stretch rates encountered in industrial practice are normally orders of magnitude greater than those for which eqn (8.6) applies or for which a Lagrangian steady state can be achieved. It is therefore not surprising that it has become common practice to compute the ratio of the instantaneous stress to the instantaneous stretch rate, even in a spatially non-homogeneous flow field, and to call the result an apparent extensional viscosity. While this may be a useful comparative parameter, it is not a quantity of fundamental interest or significance.

8.3. HOMOGENEOUS STRETCHING OF POLYMER MELTS

The uniform uniaxial stretching of a polymer sample is the preferred testing method from the viewpoint of obtaining fundamental rheological information. The technique, however, is limited to very viscous polymer melts and to low rates of strain. Tests can be conducted at constant stretch rate, constant stress, constant velocity or constant force. Only the first two conditions, though, allow for the determination of the extensional viscosity. Experimentally, most published reports utilize one of the two basic designs, one involving a constant sample length and the other a variable sample length.[3,4,12] Often the test is terminated before a Lagrangian steady state is reached. The major difficulties encountered are related to temperature and stretch rate uniformity and the need to prevent gravity from contributing to the deformation. Despite these problems, enough reliable data are now available on several polymers that some general comments can be made regarding the nature of the extensional viscosity. Also, at least two extensional rheometers are now available commercially.[8]

8.3.1. Constant Stretch Rate Experiments
In this technique, a cylindrical sample, typically in the shape of a dumbbell, is attached at one end to a force transducer while the other end is moved outwards so that the sample length increases as described by eqn (8.4). The sample is generally moulded under vacuum to eliminate air bubbles and it is annealed at the test temperature for some time before being stretched. Ballman[13] used a standard tensile tester and an isothermal oven to extend a vertical polystyrene filament at different deformation rates up to $0.022\,s^{-1}$. At these low stretch rates, he obtained a steady state in each instance and found that the extensional viscosity was essentially constant but about two orders of magnitude greater than the shear viscosity. Stevenson[14] used a similar set-up and verified the validity of eqn (8.6) for an isobutylene–isoprene copolymer at $100\,°C$. For *cis*-1,4-polyisoprene, however, he could not get a steady state at any of the stretch rates studied. In order to eliminate the influence of gravity, Vinogradov *et al.*[15] used a horizontal device with the polymer specimen kept floating on the surface of an inert liquid; Trouton's rule was found to hold for polyisobutylene. Horizontal extensiometers have also been described by Rhi-Sausi and Dealy[16] and Agrawal *et al.*[17] The former authors used polyethylene at stretch rates up to $0.1\,s^{-1}$ and found that the extensional viscosity was an increasing function of the extension rate. The latter set of authors, using the apparatus sketched in Fig. 8.1, obtained similar results for

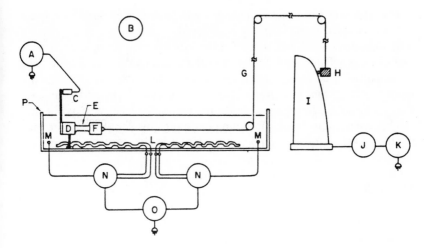

Fig. 8.1. The apparatus of Agrawal *et al.*[17] (Reproduced with permission of John
Wiley & Sons, Inc. Copyright © 1977, John Wiley & Sons, Inc.)

polystyrene although a steady state could not be attained in several of their
runs. It should be noted that the duration of the experiment is limited to
the time taken for the moving end of the sample to traverse the length of
the constant temperature bath. Errors arise if the sample temperature rises
or if the sample does not deform uniformly. Also, it is necessary for the
end of the sample to go instantly from rest to a finite predetermined
velocity at the inception of stretching. Finally, the method is suitable only
for polymers having a shear viscosity in excess of about $10^4 \, \text{N s m}^{-2}$ at the
temperature of interest.

8.3.2. Constant Stress Experiments
Constant stress rheometers are fairly similar to the constant strain rate
rheometers described in the previous section except that the pulling force
varies in order to provide a constant stress. Cogswell[18] used a spiral shaped
cam as a pulley together with weights to achieve this purpose (the design
equations are given by Dealy *et al.*[19]). Since the sample cross-sectional area
decreases continuously, the force must also decrease so that (assuming
incompressibility)

$$F = F_0 L_0 / L \qquad (8.7)$$

where the subscript zero denotes initial conditions. The strain is monitored as the experiment proceeds, and if it begins to increase linearly with time a constant extensional viscosity is achieved.

Vinogradov *et al.*[20] used a much more sophisticated set-up compared to that of Cogswell and showed the equivalence of extensional viscosity data obtained using constant stretch rate and constant stress instruments for molten polystyrene. The unusual feature of the constant stress results was that the strain rate was found to decrease initially, as expected, but then exhibit a minimum before becoming constant; this suggests the presence of stress overshoots and implies a maximum in the transient extensional viscosity.

Other constant stress extensiometers have been developed by Munstedt;[21,22] a sketch of his 'creepmeter' is shown in Fig. 8.2. Here the sample is extended vertically and a tenfold increase in length is possible. The later version has the flexibility of being used in the constant stretch rate or the constant stress mode, and it is also the basis of commercial instruments marketed by the Rheometrics and the Göttfert companies.[8]

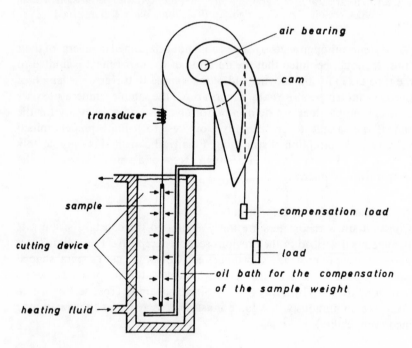

Fig. 8.2. The Munstedt Creepmeter.[21] (Reproduced with permission of Steinkopff-Verlag Darmstadt.)

The Munstedt[22] design employs electronic feedback control and uses small samples (3–10 mm diameter, 10–50 mm long) fixed to a load cell located in the oil bath itself. The maximum Hencky strain that can be achieved is 3·9 and strain rates up to $0·5 s^{-1}$ are possible.

The major advantage of the constant stress rheometers over the constant strain rate ones appears to be that a Lagrangian steady state is achieved at a significantly lower value of the total strain. This extends the range of strain rates at which the extensional viscosity can be determined for an apparatus of a given size.

8.3.3. Constant Sample Length Experiments

The maximum strain limitation imposed by the size of the apparatus can be removed if one stretches a sample at constant length. For a constant stretch rate experiment this necessitates maintaining the velocity of the sample ends constant. This was done by Meissner[23] with the use of rotary clamps—two pairs of gears which grip a specimen and provide stretching by rotating in opposite directions. A version of Meissner's extensional rheometer, together with the rotary clamps, is shown in Fig. 8.3. The

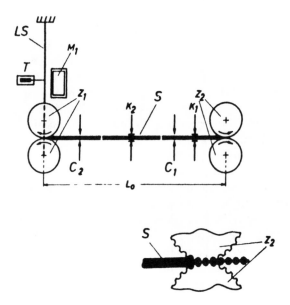

Fig. 8.3. Meissner's rheometer and rotary clamps.[24] (Reproduced with permission of John Wiley & Sons, Inc. Copyright © 1981, John Wiley & Sons, Inc.)

major advantage of the rotary clamps is that they continuously transport material from within the clamps to the outside so that necking does not occur and Hencky strains as large as 7 are possible.[24] The limiting factor for still larger extensions seems to be the homogeneity of the initial cross-sectional area along the sample. In this regard, note that samples as long as 75 cm are needed in this instrument.

The development of the rotary clamp extensional rheometer has been described by Meissner[25] and further progress has been reviewed more recently.[9,26] The polymer sample is immersed in an oil bath and the stretching force is determined by mounting one set of gears on a vertical leaf spring; the deflection of the spring is noted by a displacement transducer which is calibrated to yield the force. The stretch rate is related in a simple way to the velocities v_1 and v_2 in opposite directions of the two sets of clamps:

$$\dot{\varepsilon} = (v_1 + v_2)/L \tag{8.8}$$

where L is the sample length between the clamps. Recent modifications to the rheometer design allow it to be run under constant stress conditions. A less complicated but similar set-up has been used by Ishizuka and Koyama.[27]

A simple apparatus which also uses a constant sample length and yields a constant stretch rate has been developed by Ide and White.[28] It consists of a constant temperature silicone oil bath, an Instron load cell to which is fastened one end of the polymer sample, and a rotating roll attached to a motor with a speed controller. The polymer filament is stretched by the roll and wraps around it. The stress is determined with the help of the load cell while the stretch rate is given by the ratio of the linear roll velocity to the filament length.

Rotational viscometers are also sometimes adapted to act as stretching devices with the rotor of the apparatus serving as a roll on to which one end of the specimen being stretched is wound. The other end of the sample is attached to a slotted vertical spindle and the force exerted by the polymer on this spindle is measured. The winder is usually raised during the course of the experiment to ensure that the filament does not wrap on itself. This technique has been used by Macosko and Lorntson,[29] Everage and Ballman[30] and Connelly et al.[31] among others.

Although almost all the studies mentioned so far were conducted under isothermal conditions, Matsumoto and Bogue[32] have constructed a device which allows different cooling rates to be imposed during elongation at constant stretch rate.

8.3.4. Experimental Results

In the previous sections, mention has been made of the different observations concerning the extensional viscosity. Its value was found, by different investigators, to be constant and equal to three times the zero shear viscosity, constant but greater than three times the zero shear viscosity, an increasing function of the stretch rate, a decreasing function of the stretch rate, a function of the stretch rate which exhibited a maximum, and so on. A reason for this diversity of results was that data had been obtained over narrow ranges of experimental conditions and on very different materials, with few efforts made to compare results using different techniques in different laboratories. The first major attempt to generate consistent data on a single polymer was made by the IUPAC working party on structure and properties of commercial polymers which reported work done on three low density polyethylene samples.[33] One of these well characterized samples was subjected to extensive elongational testing by Laun and Munstedt[34] who showed that identical results were obtained irrespective of whether the Meissner[25] or the Munstedt[21] instrument was used. Laun and Munstedt[35] found that for constant stretch rate stretching the stress increased monotonically and ultimately became constant. This was found to be the case for stretch rates as high as $10 \, s^{-1}$, and their results for the elongational viscosity are shown in Fig. 8.4. The results span six decades of stretch rate and display every kind of behaviour mentioned at the beginning of this section; at low deformation rates, Trouton's rule is obeyed and then one witnesses elongation strengthening but this gives way to a maximum and then the extensional viscosity decreases to a level even below that of the zero shear viscosity. The shape of the extensional viscosity versus extension rate curve was found to be similar at different temperatures, and data could be made to overlap using time–temperature superposition;[36] the temperature shift factors were the same as those obtained from shear data. Other variables which influence the extensional viscosity are the polymer molecular weight, molecular weight distribution and chain branching. Data on several polystyrenes[37] seem to suggest that at low deformation rates the extensional viscosity depends only on the molecular weight and is proportional to the 3·5 power of the weight average molecular weight. In the non-linear region, though, the extensional viscosity increases with broadening of the molecular weight distribution, a result which is also found to hold for low density polyethylene.[38] Generalizations, however, become difficult to make since the behaviour of high density polyethylene is found to be different from that of low density polyethylene.[38] A separate point of concern is that there is dispute between

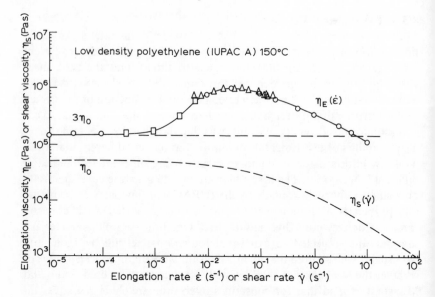

Fig. 8.4. Extensional viscosity of LDPE.[35] (Reproduced with permission of Stein-kopff-Verlag Darmstadt.)

different researchers as to whether a steady state is actually reached or not in the constant stretch rate experiments.[39]

Extensional flow data on different polymer melts have been summarized by White,[5] Ide and White[28] and Petrie.[2] The theoretical prediction and explanation of these results is a central problem in polymer melt rheology. We merely refer the reader to standard books[2,40–42] on the topic of rheological constitutive equations. The review of Bird[43] is also relevant to the problem at hand.

8.4. NON-UNIFORM STRETCHING OF POLYMER MELTS

The uniaxial extensiometers described so far are suitable for use with very viscous materials only. They cannot, for example, be used to measure the properties of such commercially important polymers as nylons and polyesters which may have shear viscosities as low as $100\,\mathrm{N\,s\,m^{-2}}$ at processing temperatures. Consequently other techniques are needed, but these invariably involve non-uniform stretching. Here one cannot require that the stress or the stretch rate be constant. Also the material is usually not in a virgin stress-free state to begin with. Therefore one cannot obtain the extensional viscosity from these measurements. Nonetheless, data from properly designed non-uniform stretching experiments can be profitably analysed with the help of rheological equations of state. In addition, such data provide a simple measure of resistance that polymeric fluids offer to extensional deformations.

8.4.1. Melt Spinning of Fibres

Polymer melt spinning is one of the major processes for the manufacture of synthetic fibres. Typically a polymer melt is extruded vertically downwards through a spinneret or die which could have hundreds of openings. The resulting filaments are simultaneously cooled by cross-flow air and stretched by the action of rollers. On solidification, the yarn is wound on to a bobbin. Different aspects of this operation have been described by Hill and Cuculo,[1] Ziabicki,[44] Walczak,[45] Petrie,[2] Denn,[46] White[7] and Ziabicki and Kawai[47] among others. When the fibre spinning process is used as an extensional viscometer, the set-up is simplified and only a single filament of circular cross-section is employed. This is shown schematically in Fig. 8.5. The flow under consideration is a circular filament whose cross-section varies along the flow direction (see figure). The assumptions normally made are that the liquid is incompressible, the flow is steady and axisymmetric, and the velocity is uniform across the cross-section. Under these conditions

$$V = V(x_1) \tag{8.9}$$

$$A = A(x_1) \tag{8.10}$$

Flow visualization studies on liquid jets have been carried out by Matthys and Khatami.[48] These investigators used a photochromic dye which becomes dark when activated by ultraviolet laser light. Use of laser pulses along with high speed photography allows the computation of velocity profiles. Results on a tubeless siphon (see Section 8.5.2) show a large variation of axial velocity with radial distance. For fibre spinning, however, the assumption of a flat velocity profile may not be too unreasonable. The force F_L needed to draw the fibre is usually measured at some distance L away from the spinneret at a position where the melt has solidified. This is generally done using a tensiometer although Spearot and Metzner[49] have used a novel technique to achieve the same purpose. Spearot and Metzner extruded a horizontal fibre into an isothermal oven.

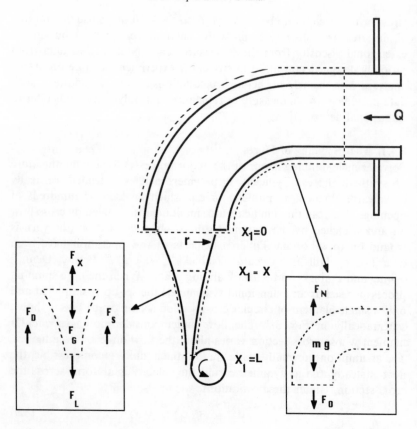

Fig. 8.5. Schematic diagram of a fibre spinning device showing force balances.

The filament leaving the oven passed over a frictionless pulley attached to the end of a leaf spring. The vertical deflection of the spring was used to obtain the tension in the threadline. The stress in the filament at any position x_1 between zero and L is obtained by carrying out a momentum balance with the assumption of a flat velocity profile. The validity of this assumption has been examined by Matovich and Pearson[50] and Phan-Thien and Caswell.[51] With reference to Fig. 8.5, the force balance becomes

$$\rho Q[v_L - v(x_1)] = F_L + \int_{x_1}^{L} \rho g \pi r^2(\xi) d\xi - \sigma_{11} \pi r^2(x_1) - 2\pi\gamma$$

$$\times [r(x_1) - r(L)] - F_d \qquad (8.11)$$

where ρ is the polymer density, Q the volumetric flow rate, g the acceleration due to gravity and γ the coefficient of surface tension. The second term on the right-hand side of eqn (8.11) represents the influence of gravity, the third term the viscoelastic stress, the fourth term surface tension and the last term is the air drag. The radius $r(x_1)$ is determined experimentally and this, together with the measured value of F_L, yields the total stress σ_{11} as a function of position x_1. Since the stretch rate is simply dv/dx_1, the apparent extensional viscosity can also be calculated with ease.

Data on extensional stresses in fibre melt spinnng and their constitutive modelling for both isothermal and non-isothermal situations can be found in the several books referred to earlier. Further modelling efforts are described in Denn.[52] In closing this section, we mention that fibre spinning data are available for polymer blends and filled polymers as well. Good summaries have been provided by White[7] and Han.[53,54] We return to the topic of fibre spinning (but for polymer solutions) in Section 8.5.1.

8.4.2. Converging Flows

If fluid is made to flow through a conical channel as discussed in Chapter 3, the average velocity increases monotonically as fluid elements move towards the apex. Clearly then, one has an extensional flow field. The presence of walls and the no-slip boundary condition, though, introduce a shearing component into the deformation rate tensor. The relative amount of shear and extension will obviously depend on the channel geometry, the volumetric flow rate and the fluid properties. A similar flow field arises in the entrance region leading from a reservoir to a capillary, and according to Cogswell[6,55,56] the situation can be exploited for the purpose of determining an apparent extensional viscosity, as has been discussed in Chapter 3.

The essential difficulty associated with this flow situation is that neither the stress nor the rate of strain can be calculated as a function of position from pressure drop–flow rate data which are the only measurements that can be made. As a consequence only average quantities can be computed. Even so, some rather drastic assumptions have to be made. Cogswell assumes that the entrance pressure drop, P_{Ent} can be separated into a shear contribution and an extensional contribution. He derives expressions for the average net extensional stress, σ_E, and the average extension rate $\dot{\varepsilon}_E$ as

$$\sigma_E = (3/8)(n + 1)P_{Ent} \tag{8.12}$$

$$\dot{\varepsilon}_E = \frac{4\eta\dot{\gamma}_A^2}{3(n + 1)P_{Ent}} \tag{8.13}$$

where η is the shear (thinning) viscosity, n the power law index and $\dot{\gamma}_A$ the apparent shear rate in the capillary whose radius is R such that

$$\dot{\gamma}_A = 4Q/\pi R^3 \qquad (8.14)$$

Knowing σ_E and $\dot{\varepsilon}_E$, one can calculate the apparent extensional viscosity as the ratio $\sigma_E/\dot{\varepsilon}_E$. The main virtue of this technique appears to be the ease of measurement.

8.4.3. Miscellaneous Methods

The presence of the shearing deformation in the converging flow into a capillary can be minimized by introducing a low viscosity liquid in the wall region. This technique was used by Everage and Ballman[57] in their extensional flow capillary. Good agreement was found with polystyrene data obtained earlier using a Meissner type set-up.

Johnson and Middleman[58] have proposed a bubble collapse method for measuring the extensional viscosity of low viscosity polymer melts. By measuring the pressure of gas in a bubble and the volume of the bubble collapsing in a body of still liquid they calculated an apparent extensional viscosity. When compared to measurements made using the Munstedt viscometer, good agreement was found for mildly elastic melts but not for highly elastic ones.[59]

Other techniques for determining the extensional properties of polymer melts include the weight dropping extensiometer of Takaki and Bogue[60] wherein sample rods are extended isothermally at constant force. The major advantage here is that large extensions can be obtained and the mode of sample failure can be studied.

8.5. EXTENSIONAL RHEOMETERS FOR SOLUTIONS

While rapid advances have been made in the development of extensional viscometers for polymer melts, progress for solutions has been relatively slow. Recently some new designs have been proposed and these may rectify the problem. In any case, imposing a constant stretch rate on these fluids is a task that still defies solution. Consequently, there are few or no data on the steady extensional viscosity. This is related to the fact that in every apparatus the flow field is unsteady in the Lagrangian sense.

As mentioned in the introduction, the impetus for the study of the extensional deformation of solutions comes from its importance in a variety of applications. It is to be noted that on the theoretical side our ability to model the constitutive behaviour of polymer solutions is largely restricted to dilute solutions. In this regard, simple mechanical models have led to a whole host of constitutive equations whose predictions in extensional deformation are only now being put to the test. In order to be useful for this purpose one needs to subject the polymer solution to a well defined deformation field and measure the resulting tensile stresses developed. The deformation field described by the stretch rate, while not necessarily constant in time or position, should at least be measurable. The concept of a constant stress experiment introduced earlier for melts has not yet found its counterpart in the study of solutions. While a number of extensional viscometers have been proposed for solutons, most of these are variations (sometimes significant) on a central theme of stretching a fluid jet emerging from a nozzle and in some manner measuring the resultant tensile force or stress. This category includes the viscometers developed by Nitschmann and Schrade[61] and Zidan[62] and the improved versions of Weinberger and Goddard,[63] Baid and Metzner,[64] Ferguson and coworkers[65,66] and Khagram *et al.*[67] (all under the generic title of fibre spinning devices). Although slightly different, the triple jet instrument,[68,69] the Fano flow apparatus[70] and the recent pressure drop technique of Sridhar and Gupta[71] are also included in this list. Table 8.2 lists these devices and their differences. Typically the description of these instruments can be divided into the nature of the flow field (which is common to all; see Section 8.4.1), the method of achieving the stretching, and finally the techniques used in measuring the tensile stresses. We discuss these

TABLE 8.2
Classification of Spinline Rheometers

Generic name	Flow direction	Stretching technique	Force measurement	Ref.
Fibre spinning	Down	Take-up wheel	Transducer	63, 64, 72–78
Fibre spinning	Down	Suction device	Microbalance	67
Fibre spinning	Down	Suction or take-up wheel	Pressure drop	71, 79
Triple jet	Horizontal	Impinging jets	Transducer	68, 69, 80, 81
Fano flow	Up	Suction	Weighing	70
Fano flow	Up	Suction	Transducer	82–88

below. Viscometers which are radically different from these are examined later.

8.5.1. Stretching Techniques

The original viscometer designed by Nitschmann and Schrade[61] utilized a rotating drum to elongate a liquid filament, and this has been the most common method of producing extensional flow in fibre spinning devices. The fluid sticking to the drum is removed continuously using a doctor blade. The method is easy to use and variation in stretching rates is achieved by controlling the rotational speed. There is obviously some velocity rearrangement that takes place as the liquid approaches the drum, and it is common to ignore data obtained from the region near the drum. One disadvantage of the rotating drum technique is that the range of stretch rates obtained is less than $10\,s^{-1}$ and the method seems to work best with high viscosity liquids. Liquids with viscosities less than $10\,N\,s\,m^{-2}$ often do not adhere to the drum. Khagram et al.[67] overcame this problem by using a suction device wherein the liquid emerging from a capillary is sucked into another capillary of still smaller diameter, producing a stretched jet in the air gap between the capillaries. This device is especially suitable for liquids with viscosity less than $1\,N\,s\,m^{-2}$ and the stretch rates produced can be as large as $1000\,s^{-1}$. Note that stretching for the Fano flow is also normally produced by using vacuum, but the stretch rates obtained are quite small. The triple jet system uses auxiliary jets which impinge on the main jet and thereby stretch it. In such cases, the jet lengths that can be obtained are small and, while high stretch rates $(100-800\,s^{-1})$ can be obtained,[68,69] the procedure is not simple.

In the spinline viscometer, the stretch rate can vary from nozzle to take-up depending on the fluid used. Local stretch rates are calculated by measuring the diameter profile of the jet. For a constant flow rate Q, assuming no radial variation in the velocity, the local velocity and stretch rates are given by

$$V = Q/\pi r^2 \qquad (8.15)$$

$$\dot{\varepsilon} = dV/dx_1 = -\frac{2Q}{\pi r^3}\frac{dr}{dx_1} \qquad (8.16)$$

The diameter profile is usually measured by photographing the filament, but there is some concern about the accuracy of this technique. A more convenient and accurate method is to use a light source–lens arrangement and cast a shadow of the filament on a screen. Using this method magnifications of up to 17 were obtained by Sridhar *et al.*[79] Commercial instruments which measure diameters by light attenuation techniques are available and these offer high accuracy and are particularly useful for dynamic studies.[89] In order to obtain stretch rates, these diameter profiles have to be numerically differentiated. This procedure can introduce large errors. To minimize this problem, it is common to fit the diameter–distance data to an equation and differentiate the equation. A variety of equations are available and one such is the equation suggested by Mewis and De Cleyn:[90]

$$D(x_1) = a_1(x_1 + a_2)^{-a_3} \exp\left(\frac{a_4}{x_1 + a_5}\right) \qquad (8.17)$$

where a_1 to a_5 are constants.

8.5.2. Force Measurements

The force exerted on the nozzle due to the stretching can be measured using a variety of techniques. The most common force measuring technique is to use a torsion bar which allows deflection of the nozzle and a displacement transducer which measures the deflection. Figure 8.6 shows the prototype fibre spinning device developed by Weinberger.[63] Subsequent investigators[64–66,77,78] have modified this design to increase its sensitivity. The modification by Metzner and Prilutski[77] represents the state of the art in this measurement. Here torsion was provided by a thin walled brass tube forming the delivery line, and the entire assembly was mounted on a knife edge. A slightly better sensitivity was achieved by Khagram *et al.*[67] by mounting the nozzle on a micro-balance. This allowed forces as low as 8×10^{-5} N (corresponding to a tensile stress of approximately $25 \, \text{N m}^{-2}$) to be measured. It should be appreciated that the actual deflections that need to be measured are very small. In the apparatus used by Weinberger a force of 10^{-4} N corresponds to a deflection of $0.1 \, \mu\text{m}$. In the more recent version of Metzner and Prilutski such a force would yield a deflection of $1 \, \mu\text{m}$. The increase in instrument sensitivity leads to operational problems, with instrument alignment becoming critical. As Becraft and Metzner[78] warn, simply walking around the instrument causes large deflections not just due to air currents but due to movement of the floor. The above paper highlights another problem with this scheme of force measurement that seems to have been ignored by many previous investigators. This concerns the distortion of the tube due to Bourdon pressure effects, with the degree of distortion increasing with flow rate and fluid viscosity. The zero offset due to these effects is large even at low pressures

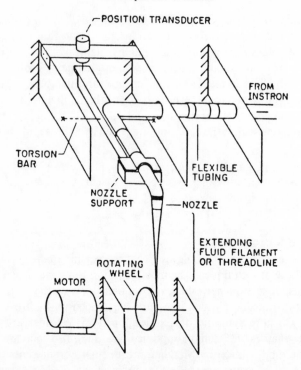

Fig. 8.6. Schematic diagram of the device developed by Weinberger.[63]

(< 50 psig), causing the computed axial stress to be meaningless. The paper of Becraft and Metzner provides ample details of how this problem could be reduced through careful design and pressure testing. The above problems are magnified when operation at higher temperatures is desired due to expansion of the various members.

Another source of error concerns the method of calibrating the force transducer (see Fig. 8.5). This effectively designates the reference condition for zero force on the nozzle and allows the fluid tensile force at the nozzle, F_0, to be determined from the measured force, F_N. An analysis of the literature indicates that very few papers give explicit details of the calibration. In what follows we shall consider different reference conditions and derive a relationship between F_0 and F_N.

Suppose the reference condition for zero force is specified as that when there is no liquid flow in the apparatus. After inception of flow the fluid emerging from the nozzle is stretched and the resulting force on the nozzle,

F_N, is measured. The forces on the nozzle assembly are detailed in Fig. 8.5. The mass of liquid (m) contained in the tube connected to the nozzle will exert a distributed load downwards, but for the present purpose this is shown as a force mg on the nozzle. The actual value can be established only by a moment balance about the support and hence will depend on system dimensions. A momentum balance on the control volume shown in Fig. 8.5 yields

$$F_0 = F_N + \rho V_0^2 A_0 - mg \qquad (8.18)$$

which allows calculation of the force F_0 on the fluid at the exit of the nozzle. The force at any other position can be calculated using F_0 and an appropriately modified version of eqn (8.11).

In eqn (8.18) the jet thrust is usually negligible at the low velocities commonly utilized. However, the force measured and the gravitational correction can easily be of the same order of magnitude and hence F_0 is not precisely estimated. This is because the magnitude of the measured force in polymer solutions is typically in the range 10^{-2}–100^{-3} N only. In addition, even a few drops of liquid sticking to the nozzle can also lead to large errors. The force due to stretching will be overestimated if the correction in eqn (8.18) is ignored. In many cases the resulting errors can be as high as 200–300%. Such a reference condition is clearly to be avoided.

If, alternatively, the nozzle assembly is filled with liquid (no flow) and the force transducer is zeroed, flow is initiated and the inception of stretching causes a force F_N to be measured which will be less than that encountered using the previous reference condition. Under such conditions it is obvious that

$$F_0 = F_N + \rho V_0^2 A_0 \qquad (8.19)$$

Since the jet thrust is again negligible compared to F_N, the force on the nozzle is nearly equal to the extensional force on the liquid. The correction in such a case is small and known. Hence this is the recommended procedure.

Measurement of forces in the Fano flow apparatus has been configured similar to spinning but is possible for few liquids and this depends on a combination of factors which are lumped into the, as yet, imprecisely defined term 'spinnability'. The influence on the stress of the prior history of deformation is possibly not as great as in fibre spinning and the measurement technique has been described by Astarita and Nicodemo.[70] A better procedure was used by Acierno *et al.*[82] and Nicodemo *et al.*[84] who suspended the nozzle on a scale system or load cell. See also the more recent designs of Peng and Landel,[85] Balmer and Hochschild[86] and Mac-Sporran.[87] In these cases, while the sensitivity is not different from that in the traditional fibre spinning devices, the filament length may be only 2 mm and end effects can be severe.

The problems of sensitivity in force measurement can be overcome in the apparatus proposed by Sridhar and Gupta.[71] Instead of measuring forces, this instrument measures the tensile stress at the nozzle. The technique is best understood by referring to Fig. 8.7. Under steady state conditions the fluid is pumped into the viscometer and exits through a capillary. If one lets subscripts 0 and 1 refer to the case without and with stretching, an overall momentum balance around the upper capillary yields (for a Newtonian liquid)

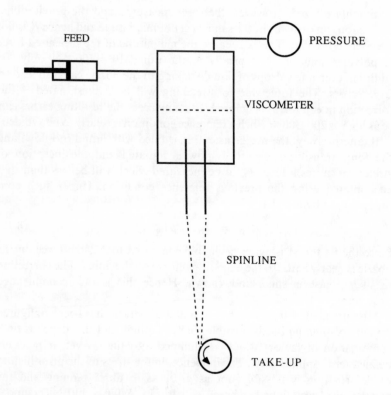

Fig. 8.7. Schematic diagram of the rheometer developed by Sridhar and Gupta.[71] (Reproduced with permission of Steinkopff-Verlag Darmstadt.)

$$Q_0 = \frac{\pi d^4}{128 \eta L} (P_0 + \rho g L) \qquad (8.20)$$

$$Q_1 = \frac{\pi d^4}{128 \eta L} (P_1 + \sigma_E + \rho g L) \qquad (8.21)$$

where σ_E is the net tensile stress due to the stretching encountered at the capillary exit, P_0 and P_1 are the pressures in the viscometer before and after the stretching, d is the capillary diameter, L is the capillary length, η is the shear viscosity, and ρ is the solution density. Since Q_0 equals Q_1, the above equations yield

$$\sigma_E = P_0 - P_1 \qquad (8.22)$$

and the result can be shown to be valid even for non-Newtonian liquids if one uses the power law equation to describe the shear flow of dilute polymer solutions or if one simply uses dimensional arguments.

The assumptions embodied in the above analysis are that the exit and entrance losses in the capillary do not change significantly when the fluid is stretched. Chan[91] examined entry flow patterns in the viscometer and found that these were unaffected by the stretching imposed downstream. Regarding exit losses, these are in general much smaller than entrance losses.[92] In addition, data on Newtonian fluids have been used to verify the technique. The advantages of this instrument are many. The instrument is rigid and suffers none of the problems associated with the original fibre spinning device. Pressure drop measurements can be made with great accuracy. For example, the lowest tensile stress obtained in the Metzner and Prilutski[77] device would correspond to a pressure reduction of 4 mm of water, which is well above the capabilities of currently available pressure transducers. The rigidity of the instrument also means that operation at higher temperatures is possibly easier than with traditional methods of measuring force.

8.5.3. Miscellaneous Techniques
In this section we describe some devices which use a variety of flow configurations to impose an extensional deformation. The one common feature of these instruments is that the magnitude and history of prior deformation is uncertain; however, approximate stretch rates can be calculated. These devices are convenient for studying auxiliary phenomena which depend on the stretching of macromolecules. Some of them have been used for polymer melts and have been described earlier. For

example, Cogswell[6] has presented a review of viscometers based on converging flows.

The earliest of these devices was based on the observation of a wine glass profile in converging flows.[93] Metzner and Metzner[94] interpreted such flows as being, primarily, extensional in character and developed a method of measuring extensional properties using flow through a sharp edged orifice. In this study, the jet thrust exerted by the fluid on the orifice was measured using leaf springs and a displacement transducer while the stretch rate was calculated from the angle of convergence. Similar studies were also carried out by many subsequent investigators.[95,96] In some of these latter studies the tensile stress was calculated from the measured pressure drop.[96] However, both the stretch rate and the tensile stress in an overall sense can only be calculated approximately. Each of these authors has proposed different equations for the stretch rate, although for angles of convergence less than 25 ° they yield the same numerical value.[6] Estimates of the tensile stress vary from $0.5 P$ to P, where P is the excess pressure drop. There are nonetheless certain advantages in this technique. Large stretch rates ($\sim 1000 \, s^{-1}$) can be achieved and the liquids need not be spinnable. Cogswell's[55] analysis of entry flow patterns has been detailed earlier and this analysis suggests a unique relationship between excess pressure drop and the angle of convergence in entry flows. Nguyen[97] has used the entry profile and pressure drop measurements to test the Cogswell analysis and has concluded that it is only qualitatively correct. Cogswell[6] himself says, in his review of such instruments, that these instruments give qualitative and comparative rather than definitive data.

Hsu and Flummerfelt[98] introduced the spinning drop technique in which a drop of fluid is placed in a rotating field of a fluid of higher density, where it experiences axisymmetrical extension. The shape of the drop as it elongates is measured and this allows the stretch rate and tensile stress to be calculated. The technique is restricted to stretch rates less than $0.3 \, s^{-1}$. For high accuracy, the viscosity of the fluid drop should be at least two orders of magnitude larger than that of the surrounding fluid and hence the technique may not be useful for dilute polymer solutions.

Pearson and Middleman[99] proposed the bubble collapse method for measuring apparent extensional viscosities. However, in this method a direct determination of the stresses is not possible unless a constitutive equation for the fluid is postulated. This is a serious disadvantage and could account for the authors not obtaining good agreement with the Munstedt viscometer for elastic melts (see Section 8.4.3).

Fuller *et al.*[100] have recently described a viscometer which uses opposing nozzles immersed in the test fluid. Sucking fluid into these nozzles, using vacuum, creates an approximate extensional flow in the small gap between the nozzles. One of these nozzles is fixed, while the other is mounted on a knife edge. The tensile stress causes the nozzles to approach each other and the resultant force is measured by a force transducer. Very large stretch rates $(400–4000 \, s^{-1})$ can be generated even for liquids that are not spinnable. In addition, a closed system, using this concept, can be arranged so that toxic fluids can be used. The residence time for various fluid elements in the flow field is not uniform and the stretch rate evaluated is an average value. The small gap between the nozzle also means that end effects will be prevalent.

Schummer and Tebel[101] have used a free jet rheometer based on liquid jets issuing from a harmonically vibrating nozzle. This produces a jet consisting of drops connected by filaments between them. The extensional viscosity can be calculated from the filament profile provided the filaments remain cylindrical. James[102] has used flow in a conical channel to measure extensional viscosities, with the tensile stress being inferred from the measured pressure drop.

8.5.4. Experimental Results and Modelling Aspects

Available experimental data on polymer solutions have been mainly accumulated in the past two decades. Early data were essentially of a qualitative nature, but recently the data are being subjected to more rigorous analysis. The need for modelling arises due to two reasons. The first is our interest in developing and testing constitutive equations. The second reason has to do with the fact that data available, except for Newtonian liquids and some solutions, using the instruments described earlier are in the form of an apparent extensional viscosity. Such a quantity has very little fundamental significance, since it is an unknown function not only of the local stretch rate but also of the deformation history. There is no technique, currently available, which allows one to measure the steady state extensional viscosity. Hence, at the present time, it is imperative that the data be examined in the context of a particular constitutive equation whose parameters have, preferably, been evaluated earlier using steady shear and dynamic data. This section compiles the data reported in the literature and shows how, in some cases, such data can be accurately modelled.

It is not our intention to review the constitutive equations that have been used for modelling polymer solutions except to point out that no particular equation has yet been totally successful and new equations are

constantly being formulated. Reviews on this aspect are available[40,43] and
it is dealt with in Chapter 15.

For Newtonian liquids, the ratio of extensional to shear viscosity
(Trouton's ratio) is equal to 3. This has provided a convenient way of
verifying the operation of any extensional viscometer. Figure 8.8 shows
the data obtained by Sridhar and Gupta[71] using the pressure drop technique. Such a measurement incorporates errors from both the force measurement and the diameter measurement and is therefore a good indication
of instrument accuracy and sensitivity. Results of other investigators are
presented in Table 8.3. The early instruments were tested using high
viscosity oils, while the more recent ones show their improved sensitivity
in handling lower viscosity liquids.

Solutions of polyacrylamide (PAA) and polyethylene oxide (PEO) in
glycerol–water mixtures have been widely used as test fluids. Table 8.4
shows the range of operating parameters and the apparent extensional

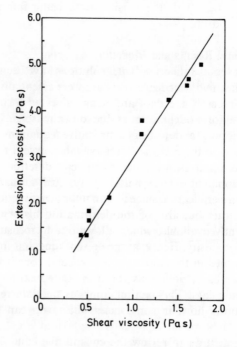

Fig. 8.8. Extensional viscosity of Newtonian liquid.[71] (Reproduced with permission of Steinkopff-Verlag Darmstadt.)

TABLE 8.3
Extensional Viscosity of Newtonian Liquids

Authors	Liquid	Viscosity (Nsm^{-2})	Stretch rate (s^{-1})	Trouton's ratio
Weinberger and Goddard[63]	Silicone oil	102·5	0·5–10	2·4–3·6
Mewis and Metzner[72]	Polybutene	24	1·6–5	2·7–3·3
Baid and Metzner[64]	Polybutene	23	2–10	2·6–3·8
Chang and Denn[74]	Corn syrup	25	–	~4
Hsu and Flummer-felt[98]	Oil	750	0·08–0·14	3·1–3·5
Jackson et al.[103]	Maltose syrup	104	2–5	5
Balmer and Hochschild[86]	Glycerol–water	0·357	4000–9000	1·7–3·36
Sridhar and Gupta[71]	Glycerol–water	0·4–1·7	40–180	2·7–3·3
Fuller et al.[100]	Glycerol–water	0·12–0·25	200–4000	2·4–3·9
Becraft and Metzner[78]	Viscasil	30	1–30	2·4–3·9

viscosity values obtained. Stretch rates range from as low as $0·1\,s^{-1}$ in Fano flow devices to as high as $19\,000\,s^{-1}$ in converging flow devices. The reported values of the Trouton ratio (T_r) or apparent extensional viscosity also vary considerably. Some of the discrepancy is no doubt due to experimental errors. However, comparing data from different experiments is complicated by the fact that the deformation history is different; indeed there is no reason to expect quantitative agreement. The behaviour of polymer solutions is also strongly dependent on the method of preparation since dilute polymer solutions are particularly prone to degradation due to scission of polymer chains or other changes in conformation. Nonetheless, these data serve to emphasize the considerable effect that small amounts of polymer can have in flow fields with significant extensional deformation. There have been some efforts[65,66,75,76,104] devoted to discovering specific relationships between the apparent extensional viscosity, the stretch rate, strain or other similar variables. However, the fundamental basis for the existence of any such relationship has never been provided. Petrie[2] rightly points out that many such relationships are fortuitous and do not shed any light on the constitutive behaviour.

Recognizing the need for rigorous modelling, Baid and Metzner[64] used Maxwell and Oldroyd models to predict extensional stresses along a spinline for solutions of polyacrylamide. It was found that different par-

TABLE 8.4

Solute[a]	Solvent	Concn. (%)	$\dot{\varepsilon}$ (s^{-1})	η_E^+ (N s m^{-2})	T_r	Ref.
PAA	Glycerol	1·5	0·1–10	2–8×10^3	–	63
PAA	Water	1·0	8–230	2·4–250	–	87
PAA	Glycerol	1·0	1–10	–	0·1–6·0	99
PAA	Glycerol	0·175–0·5	0·17–1·4	–	20–1000	82, 83
PAA	Glycerol	0·5	0·1–0·2	1–5×10^4	–	70
PAA	Maltose	0·1	0·5–5·0	–	~70	103
PAA	Water	0·1	100–750	–	3000	69, 80
PAA	Water	0·1	40–80	–	250–400	81
PAA	Water	0·01–0·5	33–19 000	–	500–29 000	94
PAA	Corn syrup	0·05	–	–	~300	74
PAA	Glycerol	0·01–0·03	4–17	30–100	–	64
PAA	Glycerol	0·005–0·05	50–1400	1–100	–	100
PAA	Water	0·0051	50–800	0·5–25	–	91
PEO	Sucrose	3·0	1–20	20–500	–	104
PEO	Glycerol	3·0	0·4–2·0	0·4–7·0×10^6	–	63
PEO	Water	0·1	100–750	8–11·4	–	69, 80
PEO	Water	0·1	40–80	–	1500–2400	81
PIB	Decalin	6·4–11.6	2–100	0·5–7	–	65, 66
PIB	Kerosene	3·0–4·0	3–100	–	1·2–40	85
PIB	Polybutene	0·18	0·4–3·0	–	3–30	79
XG	Glycerol	0·03–0·05	20–40	1–10	–	67
XG	Glycerol	0·005–0·01	50–1400	1–8	–	100
HPC	Water	2·0	0·1–1·0	–	2·0–5·0	99
HPC	Acetic acid	40·0	0·01–10·0	–	~10	77
HC	Jet fuel	0·4–1·0	3–40	–	80–2000	85
PU	DMF[b]	18–30	–	8–30	–	76

[a] PAA, polyacrylamide; PEO, polyethylene oxide; PIB, poly-isobutylene; XG, xanthan gum; HPC, hydroxy-propylcellulose; HC, hydrocarbon; PU, polyurethane.
[b] DMF, dimethylformamide.

ameter values were required to describe data in steady shear and extensional deformation. Khagram *et al.*[67] obtained a constant viscosity for solutions of xanthan gum, a semi-rigid polymer. The magnitude of these viscosities seemed to be in reasonable agreement with the theory for suspensions of rigid rods developed by Batchelor.[105]

A part of the problem in understanding the behaviour of polymer solutions is the presence of both shear thinning and elasticity. At present, no simple constitutive equation adequately models these characteristics. An experimental approach to overcome this problem was proposed by Boger[106] who developed a new solution which exhibited constant viscosity and yet high elasticity. Chang and Denn[74] examined the spinning behaviour of such fluids and concluded that the spinline forces were underestimated by a Maxwell type constitutive equation unless the relaxation time was taken to be larger than that measured in steady shear experiments. The Maxwell model also fails to describe the behaviour of these fluids in sinusoidal deformation. These perplexing aspects of this fluid were resolved by Prilutski *et al.*[107] who showed that the Oldroyd B model adequately represented the steady shear and dynamic data for these ideal elastic fluids. Furthermore, these investigators showed how several different fluids with similar properties could be formulated, and among these a solution of polyisobutylene (PIB) in polybutene (PB) has gained widespread use. Sridhar *et al.*[79] studied the extensional behaviour of such solutions and were able to predict velocity profiles in fibre spinning using the Oldroyd B model. This work clearly shows that the parameters entering the constitutive equation have the same magnitude in three different deformation fields.

Another fluid which exhibits similar ideal elastic properties is silicone oil although the level of elasticity is very low. The behaviour of silicone oils in extension has been investigated by Sridhar and Gupta[108] and the results are shown in Fig. 8.9. It is seen that near the nozzle the total deformation on the liquid is small and its behaviour is Newtonian as characterized by a Trouton's ratio of 3. Further down the spinline the deformation on the liquid increases and this leads to a much higher apparent extensional viscosity. The data in Fig. 8.9 show that the transition from Newtonian to elastic behaviour is smooth and depends on the extent of stretching imposed on the macromolecules. In contrast to the behaviour of melts, this fluid does not show a maximum in extensional viscosity.

The available data on suspensions are presented in Table 8.5. These experiments were motivated by the theoretical analysis of Batchelor[105] which predicted large increases in extensional viscosity due to the presence

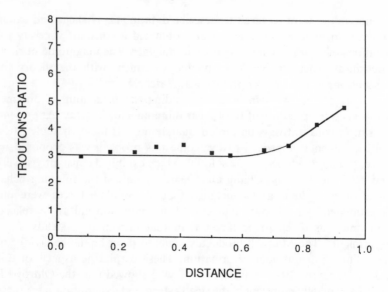

Fig. 8.9. Extensional viscosity of a weakly elastic liquid.[108]

of slender rods in Newtonian liquids. Over the range of concentrations used, the presence of solids does not significantly affect the shear viscosity. The studies using fibres have confirmed the predictions of the Batchelor theory at least qualitatively. The two studies on the suspension of beads have led to opposite conclusions regarding their effect on the apparent extensional viscosity. The reasons for this are not clear and require further experimentation.

TABLE 8.5
Extensional Viscosity of Suspensions

Suspension	Liquid	Stretch rate (s^{-1})	Results	Ref.
Glass fibres	Polybutene	0·1–10	$T_r \sim 25$	63
Glass fibres	Polybutene	0·1–2	T_r 17–260	72
Rayon fibres	Sugar solution	34–300	T_r 12–30	95
Glass fibres	Polybutene	0·5–3	T_r 3–50	109
Ballotini beads	PEO solution	1–25	Increase in η_E^+	104
Glass beads	PAA solution	1–4	Reduction in η_E^+	84

The emergence of novel materials such as liquid crystals has stimulated research into their behaviour in extension. Metzner and Prilutski[77] studied the extensional behaviour of a 40% solution of hydroxy-propylcellulose in glacial acetic acid. Their results are presented in Fig. 8.10. Also shown are the predictions of a theory proposed by Doi.[110] Figure 8.10 also includes data obtained on the same solution by T. Sridhar (unpublished work, 1986) using the pressure drop technique. The good agreement between the data from these two instruments is encouraging.

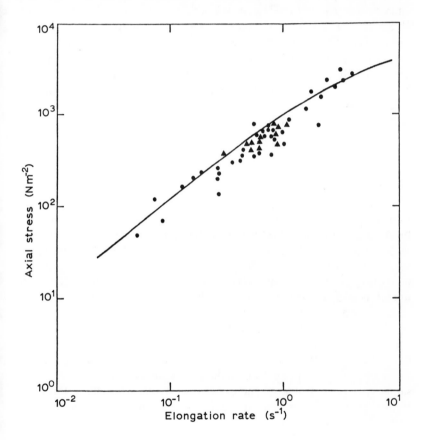

Fig. 8.10. Extensional viscosity of liquid crystalline fluid, comparison of data obtained in different instruments (ref. 77, and T. Sridhar, unpublished work, 1986).

8.6. CONCLUSIONS

A large number of techniques have been proposed for the measurement of extensional viscosity. The Trouton's ratio for Newtonian liquids is 3, but it increases by only an order of magnitude for polymer melts, and by as many as four orders of magnitude for dilute polymer solutions. This suggests that unusual flow effects due to large extensional viscosities are more likely to be encountered in polymer solutions than in polymer melts.

The techniques for polymer melts have achieved a degree of maturity and commercial instruments are available. There is nonetheless considerable scope for further improvements especially in simplifying the existing techniques and also in handling relatively lower viscosity materials. A variety of miscellaneous techniques have also appeared and some of these are extremely novel and interesting. These offer considerable simplicity but the data from these instruments have to be interpreted with considerable caution.

It is possible to use filament stretching techniques to obtain true extensional viscosity data for highly viscous melts provided that the total deformation is small and the deformation rates are low. For polymer solutions, low viscosity melts and high viscosity melts subject to high stretch rates, the extensional viscosity cannot be directly measured but must be inferred with the help of rheological models tested on the basis of transient data. In this regard, fibre spinning appears to be the most promising avenue, and it is the basis of the spinline viscometer which is the only commercial instrument for use with polymer solutions. Here significant progress has been made in the last few years on improving the measuring accuracy by simplifying the force measurement. There is an urgent need for adequate data on different fluids using the different techniques available. This would permit a closer examination of the validity and accuracy of the instruments; it would also allow testing of various constitutive equations that have been proposed in the literature so that a better understanding of polymeric fluid behaviour can emerge.

Finally, the effort involved in making accurate measurements of extensional viscosity is still large and explains the paucity of data in this area. In this sense, this measurement is a long way from reaching the status of shear viscosity measurements.

ACKNOWLEDGEMENTS

The authors wish to thank the National Science Foundation and the Australian Research Grants Scheme for supporting their individual research programs. The US–Australian Co-operative Science Program provided support for the collaborative effort. T. Sridhar wishes to thank the Department of Chemical Engineering, University of Delaware, where part of this chapter was written during a sabbatical.

REFERENCES

1. J. W. Hill and J. A. Cuculo, *J. Macromol. Sci., Rev. Macromol. Chem.*, 1976, **C14**, 107.
2. C. J. S. Petrie, *Elongational Flows*, Pitman, London, 1979.
3. D. C. Bogue, *Tensile Viscosity: a review*, Polymer Science and Engineering report No. 123, University of Tennessee, Knoxville, 1978.
4. J. M. Dealy, *J. Non-Newt. Fluid Mech.*, 1978, **4**, 9.
5. J. L. White, *J. Appl. Polym. Sci., Appl. Polym. Symp.*, 1978, **33**, 31.
6. F. N. Cogswell, *J. Non-Newt. Fluid Mech.*, 1978, **4**, 23.
7. J. L. White, *Polym. Eng. Rev.*, 1981, **1**, 297.
8. J. M. Dealy, *Rheometers for Molten Plastics*, Van Nostrand Reinhold, New York, 1982.
9. J. Meissner, *Chem. Eng. Comm.*, 1985, **33**, 159.
10. F. T. Trouton, *Proc. Roy. Soc. (Lond.)*, 1906, **A77**, 426.
11. K. Walters, *Rheometry*, Chapman and Hall, London, 1975.
12. J. M. Dealy, *Polym. Eng. Sci.*, 1971, **11**, 433.
13. R. L. Ballman, *Rheol. Acta*, 1965, **4**, 137.
14. J. F. Stevenson, *A.I.Ch.E.J.*, 1972, **18**, 540.
15. G. V. Vinogradov, B. V. Radushkevich and V. D. Fikhman, *J. Polym. Sci. (A2)*, 1970, **8**, 1.
16. J. Rhi-Sausi and J. M. Dealy, *Polym. Eng. Sci.*, 1976, **16**, 799.
17. P. K. Agrawal, W. -K. Lee, J. M. Lorntson, C. I. Richardson, K. F. Wissbrun and A. B. Metzner, *Trans. Soc. Rheol.*, 1977, **21**, 355.
18. F. N. Cogswell, *Plast. and Polym.*, 1968, **36**, 109.
19. J. M. Dealy, R. Farber, J. Rhi-Sausi and L. Utracki, *Trans. Soc. Rheol.*, 1976, **20**, 455.
20. G. V. Vinogradov, V. D. Fikhman and B. V. Radushkevich, *Rheol. Acta*, 1972, **11**, 286.
21. H. Munstedt, *Rheol. Acta*, 1975, **14**, 1077.
22. H. Mundstedt, *J. Rheol.*, 1979, **23**, 421.
23. J. Meissner, *Rheol. Acta*, 1969, **8**, 78.
24. J. Meissner, T. Raible and S. E. Stephenson, *J. Rheol.*, 1981, **25**, 1.
25. J. Meissner, *Trans. Soc. Rheol.*, 1972, **16**, 405.
26. J. Meissner, *Ann. Rev. Fluid Mech.*, 1985, **17**, 45.
27. O. Ishizuka and K. Koyama, *Polymer*, 1980, **21**, 164.
28. Y. Ide and J. L. White, *J. Appl. Polym. Sci.*, 1978, **22**, 1061.
29. C. W. Macosko and J. M. Lorntson, *Soc. Plast. Eng. Tech. Pap.*, 1973, **19**, 461.
30. A. E. Everage and R. L. Ballman, *J. Appl. Polym. Sci.*, 1976, **20**, 1137.
31. R. W. Connelly, L. G. Garfield and G. H. Pearson, *J. Rheol.*, 1979, **23**, 651.

32. T. Matsumoto and D. C. Bogue, *Trans. Soc. Rheol.*, 1977, **21**, 453.
33. J. Meissner, *Pure and Appl. Chem.*, 1975, **42**, 553.
34. H. M. Laun and H. Munstedt, *Rheol. Acta*, 1976, **15**, 517.
35. H. M. Laun and H. Munstedt, *Rheol. Acta*, 1978, **17**, 415.
36. H. Munstedt and H. M. Laun, *Rheol. Acta*, 1979, **18**, 492.
37. H. Munstedt, *J. Rheol.*, 1980, **24**, 847.
38. H. Munstedt and H. M. Laun, *Rheol. Acta*, 1981, **20**, 211.
39. T. Raible, A. Demarels and J. Meissner, *Polym. Bull.*, 1979, **1**, 397.
40. R. B. Bird, R. C. Armstrong and O. Hassager, *Dynamics of Polymeric Liquids*, Vol. 1, Wiley, New York, 1977.
41. W. R. Schowalter, *Mechanics of Non-Newtonian Fluids*, Pergamon Press, Oxford, 1978.
42. R. I. Tanner, *Engineering Rheology*, Clarendon Press, Oxford, 1985.
43. R. B. Bird, *Chem. Eng. Comm.*, 1982, **16**, 175.
44. A. Ziabicki, *Fundamentals of Fibre Formation*, Wiley, London, 1976.
45. Z. K. Walczak, *Formation of Synthetic Fibres*, Gordon and Breach, New York, 1977.
46. M. M. Denn, *Ann. Rev. Fluid Mech.*, 1980, **12**, 365.
47. A. Ziabicki and H. Kawai (Eds), *High Speed Fiber Spinning*, Wiley, New York, 1985.
48. E. F. Matthys and M. Khatami, paper presented at Winter Meeting of Society of Rheology, Santa Monica, California, 1987.
49. J. A. Spearot and A. B. Metzner, *Trans. Soc. Rheol.*, 1972, **16**, 495.
50. M. A. Matovich and J. R. A. Pearson, *Ind. Eng. Chem. Fund.*, 1969, **8**, 512.
51. N. Phan-Thien and B. Caswell, *J. Non-Newt. Fluid Mech.*, 1986, **21**, 225.
52. M. M. Denn, in *Computational Analysis of Polymer Processing*, J. R. A. Pearson and S. M. Richardson (Eds), Applied Science, London, 1983, p. 179.
53. C. D. Han, *Rheology in Polymer Processing*, Academic Press, New York, 1976.
54. C. D. Han, *Multiphase Flow in Polymer Processing*, Academic Press, New York, 1981.
55. F. N. Cogswell, *Polym. Eng. Sci.*, 1972, **12**, 64.
56. F. N. Cogswell, *Trans. Soc. Rheol.*, 1972, **16**, 383.
57. A. E. Everage and R. L. Ballman, *Nature*, 1978, **273**, 213.
58. E. D. Johnson and S. Middleman, *Polym. Eng. Sci.*, 1978, **18**, 963.
59. H. Munstedt and S. Middleman, *J. Rheol.*, 1981, **25**, 29.
60. T. Takaki and D. C. Bogue, *J. Appl. Polym. Sci.*, 1975, **19**, 419.
61. H. Nitschmann and J. Schrade, *Helv. Chim. Acta*, 1948, **31**, 297.
62. M. Zidan, *Rheol. Acta*, 1969, **8**, 89.
63. C. B. Weinberger and J. D. Goddard, *Int. J. Multiphase Flow*, 1974, **1**, 465.
64. K. M. Baid and A. B. Metzner, *Trans. Soc. Rheol.*, 1977, **21**, 237.
65. N. E. Hudson, J. Ferguson and P. Mackie, *Trans. Soc. Rheol.*, 1974, **18**, 541.
66. J. Ferguson and N. E. Hudson, *J. Phys. (E)*, 1975, **8**, 526.
67. M. Khagram, R. K. Gupta and T. Sridhar, *J. Rheol.*, 1985, **29**, 191.
68. R. Bragg and D. R. Oliver, *Nature Phys. Sci.*, 1973, **241**, 131.
69. D. R. Oliver and R. Bragg, *Rheol. Acta*, 1974, **13**, 830.
70. G. Astarita and L. Nicodemo, *Chem. Eng. J.*, 1970, **1**, 57.
71. T. Sridhar and R. K. Gupta, *Rheol. Acta*, 1985, **24**, 207.

72. J. Mewis and A. B. Metzner, *J. Fluid Mech.*, 1974, **62**, 593.
73. C. A. Moore and J. R. A. Pearson, *Rheol. Acta*, 1975, **14**, 436.
74. J. C. Chang and M. M. Denn, *J. Non-Newt. Fluid Mech.*, 1979, **5**, 369.
75. N. E. Hudson and J. Ferguson, *Trans. Soc. Rheol.*, 1976, **20**, 265.
76. G. R. McKay, J. Ferguson and N. E. Hudson, *J. Non-Newt. Fluid Mech.*, 1978, **4**, 89.
77. A. B. Metzner and G. Prilutski, *J. Rheol.*, 1986, **30**, 661.
78. M. L. Becraft and A. B. Metzner, *J. Rheol.*, in Press 1987.
79. T. Sridhar, R. K. Gupta, D. V. Boger and R. J. Binnington, *J. Non-Newt. Fluid Mech.*, 1986, **21**, 115.
80. D. R. Oliver, *Chem. Eng. J.*, 1975, **9**, 255.
81. D. R. Oliver and R. C. Ashton, *J. Non-Newt. Fluid Mech.*, 1976, **1**, 93.
82. D. Acierno, G. Titomanlio and L. Nicodemo, *Rheol. Acta*, 1974, **13**, 532.
83. D. Acierno, G. Titomanlio and R. Greco, *Chem. Eng. Sci.*, 1974, **29**, 1739.
84. L. Nicodemo, B. De Cindio and L. Nicolais, *Polym. Eng. Sci.*, 1975, **25**, 679.
85. S. T. J. Peng and R. F. Landel, *J. Appl. Phys.*, 1976, **47**, 4225.
86. R. T. Balmer and D. J. Hochschild, *J. Rheol.*, 1978, **22**, 165.
87. W. C. MacSporran, *J. Non-Newt. Fluid Mech.*, 1981, **8**, 119.
88. F. D. Martischius, *Rheol. Acta*, 1982, **21**, 288.
89. Y. Demay and J. F. Agassant, *J. Non-Newt. Fluid Mech.*, 1985, **18**, 187.
90. J. Mewis and G. De Cleyn, *A.I.Ch.E.J.*, 1982, **28**, 900.
91. R. C. Chan, PhD dissertation, State University of New York at Buffalo, 1988.
92. D. V. Boger, R. K. Gupta and R. I. Tanner, *J. Non-Newt. Fluid Mech.*, 1978, **4**, 239.
93. J. P. Tordella, *Trans. Soc. Rheol.*, 1957, **1**, 203.
94. A. B. Metzner and A. P. Metzner, *Rheol. Acta*, 1970, **9**, 174.
95. T. E. Kizior and F. A. Seyer, *Trans. Soc. Rheol.*, 1974, **18**, 271.
96. C. Balakrishnan and R. J. Gordon, *Proc. 7th Int. Congr. Rheol.*, Gothenburg, 1976, p. 265.
97. H. N. Nguyen, PhD thesis, Monash University, Australia, 1978.
98. J. C. Hsu and R. W. Flummerfelt, *Trans. Soc. Rheol.*, 1975, **19**, 523.
99. G. Pearson and S. Middleman, *A.I.Ch.E.J.*, 1977, **23**, 722.
100. G. G. Fuller, C. A. Cathey, B. Hubbard and B. E. Zebrowski, *J. Rheol.*, 1987, **31**, 235.
101. P. Schummer and K. H. Tebel, *J. Non-Newt. Fluid Mech.*, 1983, **12**, 331.
102. D. F. James, paper presented at Winter Meeting of Society of Rheology, Santa Monica, California, 1987.
103. K. P. Johnson, K. Walters and R. W. Williams, *J. Non-Newt. Fluid Mech.*, 1984, **14**, 173.
104. R. Buscall, D. J. Bye and I. S. Miles, *J. Non-Newt. Fluid Mech.*, 1985, **17**, 193.
105. G. K. Batchelor, *J. Fluid Mech.*, 1971, **46**, 813.
106. D. V. Boger, *J. Non-Newt. Fluid Mech.*, 1978, **3**, 87.
107. G. Prilutski, R. K. Gupta, T. Sridhar and M. E. Ryan, *J. Non-Newt. Fluid Mech.*, 1983, **12**, 233.
108. T. Sridhar and R. K. Gupta, *J. Non-Newt. Fluid Mech.*, in press 1988.
109. T. Sridhar and R. K. Gupta, *Proc. 4th Nat. Rheol. Conf.*, Adelaide, 1986, p. 185.
110. M. Doi, *J. Polym. Sci., Polym. Phys. Ed.*, 1980, **18**, 1005.

Chapter 9

Rotational Viscometry

ROBERT L. POWELL

Department of Chemical Engineering, University of California, Davis, California, USA

NOTATION: SYMBOLS NOT INCLUDED IN THE SOCIETY OF RHEOLOGY'S OFFICIAL NOMENCLATURE

a_c	fracture crack radius
Br	Brinkman number, eqn (9.88)
C_1, C_2	constants of integration, eqn (9.58)
$C_{M1}-C_{M5}$	Moore model parameters, eqn (9.100)
e	linear distance between cylinder axes
f_1, f_2	arbitrary functions arising from solution to eqn (9.59)
f_{instr}	instrumental frequency response
$\mathscr{F}$	total normal thrust, eqns (9.25) and (9.45)
$\mathscr{F}_i$	inertial contribution to total normal thrust, eqn (9.80)

h	gap in simple shearing flow, Fig. 9.1; gap between plates in parallel plate viscometer, Fig. 9.2.
h_c	gap in extended cone and plate geometry, Fig. 9.5(b)
h_R	gap at edge of cone and plate or parallel plate geometries
k_E	constant, eqn (9.92)
k_F	constant, eqn (9.79)
k_θ	thermal conductivity, eqn (9.88)
L	measuring length in concentric cylinder geometry
L_B	length between pressure taps in helical screw rheometer
L_{TS}, L_{BS}	distances between vanes and sample free surface and container bottom surface, respectively
L_v	length of vane rheometer
N_{1i}	inertial contribution to N_1, eqn (9.81)
p	hydrostatic pressure
p_a	atmospheric pressure
R	radius of cone and plate and parallel plate geometries, Fig. 9.2
R_B	barrel radius of helical screw rheometer
R_{cyl}	radius of cylinder containing sample for vane rheometer
Re	Reynolds number
R_i, R_o	radii of inner and outer cylinders, respectively, for concentric cylinder geometry, Fig. 9.4.
R_{in}	radius at which edge effects are important in cone and plate geometry
R_t	radius of truncated region of truncated cone and plate geometry, Fig. 9.5(a)
R_v	radius of vane rheometer
$R_1 - R_4$	radii of double concentric cylinder geometry, Fig. 9.6(c)
s	value of viscometric shear stress function at a particular shear rate
t_{appl}	duration of applied torque, Fig. 9.12
t_{max}	time to reach stress overshoot maximum
$\mathcal{T}$	torque, eqns (9.20) and (9.41)
$\mathcal{T}_{act}$, $\mathcal{T}_o$	actual and ideal torques, eqn (9.83)
$\mathcal{T}_{cp}$, $\mathcal{T}_{pp}$, $\mathcal{T}_{cc}$	transient torques for cone and plate, parallel plate and concentric cylinder geometries, respectively
$\mathcal{T}_m$	maximum torque in a vane rheometer experiment
$\hat{\mathcal{T}}$	Torque per unit length in concentric cylinder geometry, eqn (9.61)
V	velocity of moving plate in simple shearing flow, Fig. 9.1
Y	eqn (9.66)

α	cone angle
β	$(R_i/R_o)^2$
γ_{trans}	strain at which stress overshoot is observed
$\dot{\gamma}$	viscometric shear rate
$\dot{\gamma}_i$	shear rate at inner cylinder of Couette geometry, eqn (9.69)
$\dot{\gamma}_{\text{CF}}, \dot{\gamma}_{\text{CC}}$	critical shear rates for fracture and centrifugal expulsion, respectively
$\dot{\gamma}_{\text{EC}}$	shear rate in extended cone and plate geometry, eqn (9.102)
Γ	surface tension
δ	helix angle of screw in helical screw rheometer
Δ	thickness over which edge effects are important for cone and plate geometry, eqn (9.85)
θ_0, θ	reference and actual temperatures
θ_{max}	maximum temperature rise in cone and plate viscometer, eqns (9.89) and (9.90)
λ	Moore model function, eqn (9.101)
μ	Newtonian viscosity
ξ	coefficent appearing in viscosity–temperature relationship, eqn (9.91)
ρ	density
$\hat{\sigma}$	constitutive stress, eqn (9.1)
σ_e	shear stress acting on end of vanes, eqn (9.106)
σ_y	yield stress
τ_i	inertial time scale
ψ	eqn (9.77)
ω	angular velocity of fluid, Table 9.1
Ω	angular velocity of rotating member for cone and plate and parallel plate flows, Fig. 9.2
Ω_i, Ω_o	angular velocities of inner and outer cylinders, respectively, Fig. 9.4
$\Omega_{\text{CF}}, \Omega_{\text{CC}}$	critical angular velocities for fracture and centrifugal expulsion, respectively

9.1. INTRODUCTION

Rotational viscometry is usually used to measure the properties of fluids in flows which approximate a simple shearing motion (Fig. 9.1).[1-4] Such a flow can be effected in a fluid contained between two infinite parallel plates

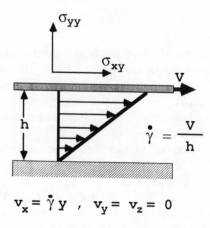

$$v_x = \dot{\gamma} y \quad , \quad v_y = v_z = 0$$

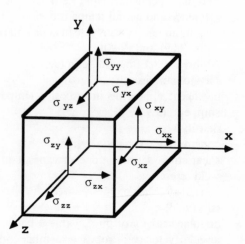

Fig. 9.1. Simple shearing flow. The bottom plate is fixed while the top plate moves parallel to it at a constant velocity; the stress components are also shown. Note that σ_{xz} and σ_{yz} are zero.

by fixing one and moving the second parallel to the first at a fixed speed. The shear rate is defined to be the plate velocity, V, divided by the gap spacing, h. Of the six components of the symmetric stress tensor, four are nonzero,[1-4] with σ_{xz} and σ_{yz} being zero. We assume that the materials under consideration are incompressible. The stress, $\boldsymbol{\sigma}$, can be decomposed into a hydrostatic pressure, p, which is not a material property, and a constitutive stress, $\hat{\boldsymbol{\sigma}}$:

$$\boldsymbol{\sigma} = -p\mathbf{I} + \hat{\boldsymbol{\sigma}} \tag{9.1}$$

The indeterminacy in the normal components of the stress due to the hydrostatic pressure means that only normal stress differences can be uniquely determined. Therefore three material properties completely characterize a general nonlinear fluid. Each property depends upon the shear rate, $\dot{\gamma} = V/h$. These properties consist of the shear stress function σ, the first normal stress difference, N_1, and the second normal stress difference, N_2 (see Fig. 9.1), where (see Table 9.2)

$$\sigma(\dot{\gamma}) = \sigma_{xy} \tag{9.2}$$

$$N_1(\dot{\gamma}) = \sigma_{xx} - \sigma_{yy} \tag{9.3}$$

$$N_2(\dot{\gamma}) = \sigma_{yy} - \sigma_{zz} \tag{9.4}$$

Rather than the shear stress function, the shear viscosity function, defined according to

$$\eta(\dot{\gamma}) = \sigma(\dot{\gamma})/\dot{\gamma} \tag{9.5}$$

is usually used, and in some cases it is convenient to define two normal stress functions $\psi_\alpha(\dot{\gamma}) = N_\alpha/\dot{\gamma}^2$ where $\alpha = 1, 2$.[4] Equations (9.2)–(9.4) define the constitutive properties for a very general class of fluids in viscometric flows.[1] These equations can be derived from the principles of continuum mechanics. Here our task begins with eqns (9.2)–(9.4).

Owing to its direct connection with the design of unit operations for processing viscoelastic materials,[5-7] measurements of the shear viscosity as a function of the shear rate predominate the literature on rheology. The first normal stress difference can also significantly affect such important phenomena as die swell (see Chapter 4) and the performance of lubricants.[8,9] Both σ and N_1 can be routinely measured using commercially available instruments. The second normal stress difference receives less attention and, as we shall see in Section 9.2, there are unique difficulties associated with its measurement. For many materials, it has been found to be nearly an order of magnitude smaller than and have the opposite sign to that of the first normal stress difference.[10]

Besides classical rotational viscometry, this chapter also describes newer experimental techniques aimed at elucidating the transient behavior of materials subjected to large time-dependent shearing deformations (Section 9.3.1). Such flow conditions correspond to those experienced by fluid elements in rapid processes, where materials are subjected to shear rates for short periods of time. The fluid, responding on its own time scale,

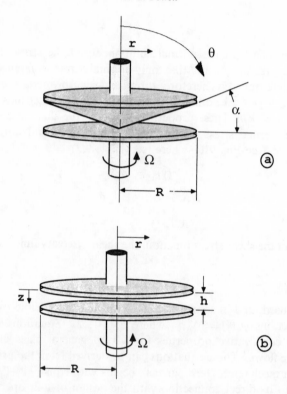

Fig. 9.2. (a) The cone and plate geometry; the plate rotates at a constant angular velocity while the cone is fixed. (b) The parallel plate geometry; the bottom plate rotates at a constant angular velocity while the upper plate is fixed.

generates time dependent stresses which correspond with the steady state stresses predicted by the viscometric functions only in the long time limit. Examples of such processes include high speed coating and processing of pulp fiber suspensions during papermaking.

Viscometer geometries that do not fit under the traditional classifications are discussed in Section 9.3.2. The vane rheometer and the helical screw rheometer may prove to be particularly valuable for measuring the properties of suspensions. Some of the problems faced in achieving an accurate determination of the yield stress are alleviated by the vane geometry, while the helical screw device potentially provides viscosity measurements of such difficult systems as settling slurries.

Special attention is given to what we choose to call applied stress rheometry (Section 9.3.3). This is also rotational rheometry based upon the simple shearing motion shown in Fig. 9.1. However, instead of the flow being due to the steady velocity of the upper plate, it is caused by the application of a constant shear stress at that plate. The distinction between the two techniques is similar to that between a 'hard' and a 'dead-weight' test in solid mechanics.[11] A hard test is an applied deformation experiment in which the stress is measured, corresponding to the imposition of the velocity boundary condition of Fig. 9.1. A dead-weight test is an applied stress test corresponding to a steady stress boundary condition in Fig. 9.1. The correspondence between results obtained from the two methods has engendered much controversy in the solid mechanics literature, and has led some experimentalists to believe that true determinations of material nonlinear behavior can only be derived from dead-weight tests:[11] 'hard testing machines, whatever their accuracy, are designed to force upon the specimen a prescribed strain history. The measured quantity is the stress history experienced by the loading elements in meeting the input recipe of the strain history. With dead-weight experiments, the stress is prescribed and the resulting measured strain history describes the accommodation of the material to the applied loads.' (ref. 11, p. 125) Under steady state conditions, the applied stress and applied deformation tests provide the same information for fluids. During the transient period, the applied stress test measures the creep compliance,[4] while the hard test measures stress growth or relaxation (see Section 9.3.1). Another feature of applied stress rheometry is that it may lend itself particularly well to the measurement of yield stress when used, for example, with the vane geometry.

TABLE 9.1

Flow fields and stresses for simple shearing flow and for each of the rheometers considered in Section 9.2

Flow	Coordinate system	Assumed velocity field	Derived shear rate	Viscometric stresses		
				$\sigma(\gamma)$	$N_1(\gamma)$	$N_2(\gamma)$
Simple shearing	(x, y, z)	$(v_x(y), 0, 0)$	V/h	σ_{xy}	$\sigma_{xx} - \sigma_{yy}$	$\sigma_{yy} - \sigma_{zz}$
Cone and plate	(r, θ, ϕ)	$(0, 0, r\omega(\theta))$	Ω/α	$\sigma_{\theta\phi}$	$\sigma_{\phi\phi} - \sigma_{\theta\theta}$	$\sigma_{\theta\theta} - \sigma_{rr}$
Parallel plate	(r, θ, z)	$(0, r\omega(z), 0)$	$r\Omega/h$	$\sigma_{\theta z}$	$\sigma_{\theta\theta} - \sigma_{zz}$	$\sigma_{zz} - \sigma_{rr}$
Concentric cylinder (small gap)	(r, θ, z)	$(0, r\omega(r), 0)$	$\dfrac{R_0 \Delta\Omega}{R_0 - R_i}$	$\sigma_{r\theta}$	$\sigma_{\theta\theta} - \sigma_{rr}$	$\sigma_{rr} - \sigma_{zz}$

9.2. CONVENTIONAL VISOMETERS

9.2.1. Cone and Plate

The cone and plate viscometer is usually used for measuring the shear viscosity and the first normal stress difference. Additionally, the normal stress combination $N_1 + 2N_2$ can be determined from the pressure distribution across the plate. However, these measurements require great care in minimizing or eliminating hole pressure errors (see Chapter 11).

TABLE 9.2
Velocity Gradient Tensor in Cartesian, Cylindrical and Spherical Coordinates[a]

Cartesian coordinates

$$\left\| \begin{array}{ccc} 2\dfrac{\partial v_x}{\partial x} & \dfrac{\partial v_y}{\partial x} + \dfrac{\partial v_x}{\partial y} & \dfrac{\partial v_x}{\partial z} + \dfrac{\partial v_z}{\partial x} \\[2mm] \cdot & 2\dfrac{\partial v_y}{\partial y} & \dfrac{\partial v_y}{\partial z} + \dfrac{\partial v_z}{\partial y} \\[2mm] \cdot & \cdot & 2\dfrac{\partial v_z}{\partial z} \end{array} \right\|$$

Cylindrical coordinates

$$\left\| \begin{array}{ccc} 2\dfrac{\partial v_r}{\partial r} & r\dfrac{\partial (v_\theta/r)}{\partial r} + \dfrac{1}{r}\dfrac{\partial v_r}{\partial \theta} & \dfrac{\partial v_r}{\partial z} + \dfrac{\partial v_z}{\partial r} \\[2mm] \cdot & \dfrac{2}{r}\left(\dfrac{\partial v_\theta}{\partial \theta} + v_r\right) & \dfrac{1}{r}\dfrac{\partial v_z}{\partial \theta} + \dfrac{\partial v_\theta}{\partial z} \\[2mm] \cdot & \cdot & 2\dfrac{\partial v_z}{\partial z} \end{array} \right\|$$

Spherical coordinates

$$\left\| \begin{array}{ccc} 2\dfrac{\partial v_r}{\partial r} & r\dfrac{\partial (v_\theta/r)}{\delta r} + \dfrac{1}{r}\dfrac{\partial v_r}{\partial \theta} & r\dfrac{\partial (v_\phi/r)}{\partial r} + \dfrac{1}{r\sin\theta}\dfrac{\partial v_r}{\partial \phi} \\[3mm] \cdot & \dfrac{2}{r}\left(\dfrac{\partial v_\theta}{\partial \theta} + v_r\right) & \dfrac{1}{r}\left[\sin\theta\dfrac{\partial}{\partial \theta}\left(\dfrac{v_\phi}{\sin\theta}\right) + \dfrac{1}{\sin\theta}\dfrac{\partial v_\theta}{\partial \phi}\right] \\[3mm] \cdot & \cdot & \dfrac{2}{r}\left[\dfrac{1}{\sin\theta}\dfrac{\partial v_\phi}{\partial \phi} + v_\theta \cot\theta + v_r\right] \end{array} \right\|$$

[a] The rate of deformation tensor is symmetric; the dots ($\cdot$) have been used for brevity.

TABLE 9.3
Conservation of Linear Momentum in Cartesian, Cylindrical and Spherical Coordinates

Rectangular cartesian coordinates

$$\rho\left(\frac{\partial v_x}{\partial t} + v_x \frac{\partial v_x}{\partial x} + v_y \frac{\partial v_x}{\partial y} + v_z \frac{\partial v_x}{\partial z}\right) = \frac{\partial \sigma_{xx}}{\partial x} + \frac{\partial \sigma_{xy}}{\partial y} + \frac{\partial \sigma_{xz}}{\partial z} + \rho b_x \quad (9.3.1)$$

$$\rho\left(\frac{\partial v_y}{\partial t} + v_x \frac{\partial v_y}{\partial x} + v_y \frac{\partial v_y}{\partial y} + v_z \frac{\partial v_y}{\partial z}\right) = \frac{\partial \sigma_{xy}}{\partial x} + \frac{\partial \sigma_{yy}}{\partial y} + \frac{\partial \sigma_{yz}}{\partial z} + \rho b_y \quad (9.3.2)$$

$$\rho\left(\frac{\partial v_z}{\partial t} + v_x \frac{\partial v_z}{\partial x} + v_y \frac{\partial v_z}{\partial y} + v_z \frac{\partial v_z}{\partial z}\right) = \frac{\partial \sigma_{xz}}{\partial x} + \frac{\partial \sigma_{yz}}{\partial y} + \frac{\partial \sigma_{zz}}{\partial z} + \rho b_z \quad (9.3.3)$$

Cylindrical coordinates

$$\rho\left(\frac{\partial v_r}{\partial t} + v_r \frac{\partial v_r}{\partial r} + \frac{v_\theta}{r} \frac{\partial v_r}{\partial \theta} - \frac{v_\theta^2}{r} + v_z \frac{\partial v_r}{\partial z}\right) = \frac{\partial \sigma_{rr}}{\partial r} + \frac{1}{r} \frac{\partial \sigma_{r\theta}}{\partial \theta} + \frac{\partial \sigma_{rz}}{\partial z}$$

$$+ \frac{1}{r}(\sigma_{rr} - \sigma_{\theta\theta}) + \rho b_r \quad (9.3.4)$$

$$\rho\left(\frac{\partial v_\theta}{\partial t} + v_r \frac{\partial v_\theta}{\partial r} + \frac{v_\theta}{r} \frac{\partial v_\theta}{\partial \theta} + \frac{v_r v_\theta}{r} + v_z \frac{\partial v_\theta}{\partial z}\right) = \frac{\partial \sigma_{r\theta}}{\partial r} + \frac{1}{r} \frac{\partial \sigma_{\theta\theta}}{\partial \theta} + \frac{\partial \sigma_{\theta z}}{\partial z}$$

$$+ \frac{2}{r}\sigma_{r\theta} + \rho b_\theta \quad (9.3.5)$$

$$\rho\left(\frac{\partial v_z}{\partial t} + v_r \frac{\partial v_z}{\partial r} + \frac{v_\theta}{r} \frac{\partial v_z}{\partial \theta} + v_z \frac{\partial v_z}{\partial z}\right) = \frac{\partial \sigma_{rz}}{\partial r} + \frac{1}{r} \frac{\partial \sigma_{\theta z}}{\partial \theta} + \frac{\partial \sigma_{zz}}{\partial z}$$

$$+ \frac{1}{r}\sigma_{rz} + \rho b_z \quad (9.3.6)$$

Spherical coordinates

$$\rho\left(\frac{\partial v_r}{\partial t} + v_r \frac{\partial v_r}{\partial r} + \frac{v_\theta}{r} \frac{\partial v_r}{\partial \theta} + \frac{v_\phi}{r\sin\theta} \frac{\partial v_r}{\partial \phi} - \frac{v_\theta^2 + v_\phi^2}{r}\right) = \frac{\partial \sigma_{rr}}{\partial r} + \frac{1}{r} \frac{\partial \sigma_{r\theta}}{\partial \theta}$$

$$+ \frac{1}{r\sin\theta} \frac{\partial \sigma_{r\phi}}{\partial \phi} + \frac{1}{r}(2\sigma_{rr} - \sigma_{\theta\theta} - \sigma_{\phi\phi} + \sigma_{r\theta}\cot\theta) + \rho b_r \quad (9.3.7)$$

$$\rho\left(\frac{\partial v_\theta}{\partial t} + v_r \frac{\delta v_\theta}{\partial r} + \frac{v_\theta}{r} \frac{\partial v_\theta}{\partial \theta} + \frac{v_\phi}{r\sin\theta} \frac{\partial v_\theta}{\partial \phi} + \frac{v_r v_\theta}{r} - \frac{v_\phi^2 \cot\theta}{r}\right) = \frac{\partial \sigma_{r\theta}}{\partial r} + \frac{1}{r} \frac{\partial \sigma_{\theta\theta}}{\partial \theta}$$

$$+ \frac{1}{r\sin\theta} \frac{\partial \sigma_{\theta\phi}}{\partial \phi} + \frac{1}{r}[3\sigma_{r\theta} + (\sigma_{\theta\theta} - \sigma_{\phi\phi})\cot\theta] + \rho b_\theta \quad (9.3.8)$$

(*continued*)

TABLE 9.3—contd.

$$\rho\left(\frac{\partial v_\phi}{\partial t} + v_r \frac{\partial v_\phi}{\partial r} + \frac{v_\theta}{r}\frac{\partial v_\phi}{\partial \theta} + \frac{v_\phi}{r\sin\theta}\frac{\partial v_\phi}{\partial \phi} + \frac{v_\phi v_r}{r} + \frac{v_\theta v_\phi}{r}\cot\theta\right)$$

$$= \frac{\partial \sigma_{r\phi}}{\partial r} + \frac{1}{r}\frac{\partial \sigma_{\theta\phi}}{\partial \theta} + \frac{1}{r\sin\theta}\frac{\partial \sigma_{\phi\phi}}{\partial \phi} + \frac{1}{r}(3\sigma_{r\phi} + 2\sigma_{\theta\phi}\cot\theta) + \rho b_\phi$$

$$(9.3.9)$$

In a typical cone and plate geometry (Fig. 9.2(a)) the cone is fixed while the plate is rotated at a constant angular velocity, Ω. The symmetry axes of the cone and the plate coincide and a spherical coordinate system is used to analyze the physical system (Table 9.1) wherein the equations of the cone and the plate are $\theta = \pi/2$ and $\theta = \pi/2 - \alpha$, respectively, α being the cone angle. We assume that the angular motion has persisted sufficiently long to eliminate transient effects associated with the start-up of the flow and that the velocity of the fluid contained between the cone and the plate is[2]

$$\mathbf{v} \approx (0, 0, r\omega(\theta)\sin\theta) \qquad (9.6)$$

Referring to Table 9.2, the shear rate corresponding to this velocity field is

$$\dot{\gamma} = \frac{d\omega}{d\theta}\sin\theta \qquad (9.7)$$

The conditions under which this velocity field is compatible with the conservation of linear momentum[†] are found by substituting eqn (9.6) into eqns (9.3.7)–(9.3.9) from Table 9.3:

$$-\rho r\omega^2\sin^2\theta = \frac{\partial\sigma_{rr}}{\partial r} - \frac{1}{r}(\sigma_{\theta\theta} + \sigma_{\phi\phi}) + \frac{2}{r}\sigma_{rr} \qquad (9.8)$$

$$-\rho r\omega^2\sin\theta\cos\theta = \frac{1}{r}\frac{\partial\sigma_{\theta\theta}}{\partial\theta} + \frac{1}{r}\cot\theta(\sigma_{\theta\theta} - \sigma_{\phi\phi}) \qquad (9.9)$$

$$0 = \frac{\partial\sigma_{\theta\phi}}{\partial\theta} + 2\sigma_{\theta\phi}\cot\theta \qquad (9.10)$$

[†] For all flows considered in this chapter, the conservation of mass imposes no restrictions on the assumed velocity fields beyond those imposed by the conservation of linear momentum.

Two assumptions are now made: (1) small cone angle, and (2) negligible fluid inertia. The experimental implications of these assumptions will be discussed in Sections 9.2.4.1 and 9.2.4.2, while here we consider their consequences in deriving formulae for relating measured quantities to the viscometric functions.

The assumption that the cone angle is small, $\alpha \approx 0$, means that the region of flow is confined to the narrow gap near $\theta = \pi/2$. To leading order, the trigonometric functions are approximated as $\sin\theta \approx 1$, $\cos\theta \approx 0$ and $\cot\theta \approx 0$. Neglect of fluid inertia is formally accomplished by setting $\rho = 0$.[2] For a Newtonian fluid, this is tantamount to having zero Reynolds number.[12,13] Under these conditions, eqns (9.8)–(9.10) become

$$0 = \frac{\partial \sigma_{rr}}{\partial r} - \frac{1}{r}(\sigma_{\theta\theta} + \sigma_{\phi\phi}) + \frac{2}{r}\sigma_{rr} \tag{9.11}$$

$$0 = \frac{\partial \sigma_{\theta\theta}}{\partial r} \tag{9.12}$$

$$0 = \frac{\partial \sigma_{\theta\phi}}{\partial \theta} \tag{9.13}$$

respectively. Using the relationships between the stress components and the viscometric functions given in Table 9.1, eqn (9.13) becomes

$$\frac{d\sigma}{d\dot\gamma} \frac{d^2\omega}{d\theta^2} = 0 \tag{9.14}$$

In general $d\sigma/d\dot\gamma \neq 0$, and hence

$$\frac{d^2\omega}{d\theta^2} = 0 \tag{9.15}$$

This is solved subject to the boundary conditions

$$\omega = \Omega \quad \theta = \frac{\pi}{2} \tag{9.16}$$

$$\omega = 0 \quad \theta = \frac{\pi}{2} - \alpha \tag{9.17}$$

These *no slip* boundary conditions assume that the fluid moves with the same velocity as the bounding surfaces.[2] Combining eqns (9.15)–(9.17) we obtain

$$\omega = \frac{\Omega}{\alpha}\left(\theta + \alpha - \frac{\pi}{2}\right) \tag{9.18}$$

The corresponding shear rate, eqn (9.7), is

$$\dot{\gamma} = \Omega/\alpha \tag{9.19}$$

Equation (9.19) shows that in the absence of fluid inertia, and for small cone angles, the fluid experiences a uniform shear rate. This contrasts with the capillary (Chapter 1) and parallel plate (Section 9.2.2) viscometers where the shear rate is non-uniform. Outside of this ideal cone and plate geometry only with a narrow gap Couette viscometer (Section 9.2.3) can a uniform shear rate be realized experimentally.

The viscosity at the set shear rate can be determined by measuring the torque exerted by the fluid on the cone, $\mathscr{T}$. This is related to the shear stress by

$$\mathscr{T} = \int_0^{2\pi} \int_0^R r^2 \sigma_{\theta\phi} \, dr \, d\phi \tag{9.20}$$

Since $\sigma_{\theta\phi} = \sigma(\dot{\gamma})$ is a constant, eqn. (9.20) can be integrated to obtain

$$\eta(\dot{\gamma}) = \sigma/\dot{\gamma} = \frac{3\mathscr{T}\alpha}{2\pi R^3 \Omega} \tag{9.21}$$

A typical experimental program using the cone and plate geometry consists of:

(i) choosing a geometry, i.e. fixing the plate radius and the cone angle;
(ii) choosing a value of shear rate;
(iii) rotating the plate at the corresponding value of angular velocity calculated using eqn (9.19);
(iv) measuring the torque once steady state is established;
(v) calculating the viscosity using eqn (9.21); and
(vi) repeating steps (ii)–(v) for all desired shear rates.

To relate the viscometric normal stress functions to measurable quantities, we combine eqn (9.11) and the definitions given in Table 9.1. We obtain

$$\frac{\partial \sigma_{rr}}{\partial r} = \frac{1}{r}(N_1 + 2N_2) \tag{9.22}$$

Following eqn (9.1), we divide the stress, σ_{rr}, into a constitutive part and a hydrostatic pressure:

$$\sigma_{rr} = -p + \hat{\sigma}_{rr} \qquad (9.23)$$

Since $\hat{\sigma}_{rr} = \hat{\sigma}_{rr}(\dot{\gamma})$ and $\dot{\gamma}$ is constant, eqn (9.22) becomes

$$-\frac{\partial p}{\partial \ln r} = N_1 + 2N_2 \qquad (9.24)$$

When plotted on a semi-logarithmic scale, the pressure as a function of the radial position should yield a straight line, the slope of which is $N_1 + 2N_2$. However, the routine application of this technique is limited by the hole pressure errors described in Chapter 11.

The most widely used technique for determining visometric normal forces is the total thrust method in which the total normal force exerted on the plate is measured. This is generally related to the normal stress, $\sigma_{\theta\theta}$, through

$$\mathscr{F} = -\int_0^R \int_0^{2\pi} \sigma_{\theta\theta} r \, dr \, d\phi \qquad (9.25)$$

Integrating eqn (9.25) requires a functional form for $\sigma_{\theta\theta}$ which is found by recognizing that

$$\frac{\partial \sigma_{rr}}{\partial r} = \frac{\partial \sigma_{\theta\theta}}{\partial r} \qquad (9.26)$$

and using this in eqn (9.22). Upon integrating the resulting expression from r to R, we obtain

$$\sigma_{\theta\theta}(R) - \sigma_{\theta\theta}(r) = (N_1 + 2N_2) \ln \frac{R}{r} \qquad (9.27)$$

Two additional assumptions are now required; (1) the free surface at $r = R$ is at atmospheric pressure, $\sigma_{rr}(R) = -p_a$; and (2) interfacial effects are absent. Referring to Table 9.1, these assumptions imply that

$$\sigma_{\theta\theta}(R) = N_2 - p_a \qquad (9.28)$$

Substituting eqns (9.27) and (9.28) into eqn (9.25) and integrating, we find

$$N_1 = 2\left(p_a + \frac{\mathscr{F}}{\pi R^2}\right) \qquad (9.29)$$

The application of eqn (9.29) is similiar to that of eqn (9.21), with the normal thrust now being the measured quantity. Both equations are widely used, but are subject to the limitations imposed by the assumptions in the derivation, particularly, small cone angle, negligible fluid inertia and edge effects. Possible errors resulting from these assumptions will be discussed in Section 9.2.4.

9.2.2. Parallel Plate

In the parallel plate, or torsional flow, viscometer (Fig. 9.2(b)) the sample is contained between two coaxial, parallel discs separated by a distance h; one of the discs rotates at a constant angular velocity, Ω, while the second is fixed. The measured quantities are the torque on the upper plate and the total normal force required to maintain a constant gap separation, which are related to the shear viscosity and the normal stress functions.

A cylindrical coordinate system is used (see Table 9.1) and it is assumed that the velocity has a single component

$$\mathbf{v} \approx (0, r\omega(z), 0) \tag{9.30}$$

where ω is the angular velocity of the fluid. This velocity field must satisfy the no-slip boundary conditions

$$\omega(0) = 0 \tag{9.31}$$

$$\omega(h) = \Omega \tag{9.32}$$

and the conservation of linear momentum, eqns (9.3.4)–(9.3.6) in Table 9.3. Assuming angular symmetry, these equations become

$$- \rho r \omega^2 = \frac{\partial \sigma_{rr}}{\partial r} + \frac{1}{r}(\sigma_{rr} - \sigma_{\theta\theta}) \tag{9.33}$$

$$0 = \frac{\partial \sigma_{\theta z}}{\partial z} \tag{9.34}$$

$$0 = \frac{\partial \sigma_{zz}}{\partial z} \tag{9.35}$$

Again, fluid inertia is neglected ($\rho = 0$) and, upon using the relationships given in Table 9.1, eqns (9.33) and (9.34) become

$$0 = \frac{\partial \sigma_{rr}}{\partial r} - \frac{1}{r}(N_1 + N_2) \tag{9.36}$$

$$0 = \frac{\partial \sigma}{\partial z} \tag{9.37}$$

Since σ, N_1 and N_2 are functions of $\dot{\gamma}$ only, eqn (9.37) implies that

$$\frac{d\sigma}{d\dot{\gamma}} \frac{\partial \dot{\gamma}}{\partial z} = 0 \tag{9.38}$$

and hence that

$$\frac{d^2\omega}{dz^2} = 0 \tag{9.39}$$

Solving this equation subject to eqns (9.31) and (9.32), we obtain

$$\omega = \frac{\Omega}{h} z \tag{9.40}$$

As with the cone and plate geometry, we seek a relationship between the viscometric shear stress, or viscosity function, and the torque which the fluid exerts on the plate. This is calculated using

$$\mathcal{T} = 2\pi \int_0^R r^2 \sigma_{\theta z} \, dr \tag{9.41}$$

where $\sigma_{\theta z} = \sigma(\dot{\gamma})$. A major departure now occurs between the cone and plate and parallel plate analyses. For the cone and plate case, the variation in the tangential velocity with radial distance is exactly compensated by the change in gap separation. Put in terms of simple shearing flow (Fig. 9.1), the cone and plate has a different 'V' and a different 'h' at each radial position, but each varies so as to maintain $\dot{\gamma}$ constant, with 'V' $= \Omega r$ and 'h' $= \alpha r$. For the parallel plate geometry, 'V' varies, but there is no offsetting change in the gap to maintain a constant shear rate.

We proceed with the analysis; by changing the variable of integration in eqn (9.41) from r to $\dot{\gamma} = (\Omega/h)r$

$$\dot{\gamma}_R^3 \mathcal{T} = 2\pi R^3 \int_0^{\dot{\gamma}_R} \dot{\gamma}^2 \sigma \, d\dot{\gamma} \tag{9.42}$$

where

$$\dot{\gamma}_R \equiv \frac{\Omega}{h} R \tag{9.43}$$

is the *edge shear rate*. Following the same procedure as used in the derivation for capillary rheometry (Chapter 1), eqn (9.42) is differentiated with respect to $\dot{\gamma}_R$, and upon rearranging we find

$$\eta(\dot{\gamma}_R) = \frac{\mathcal{T}}{2\pi R^3 \dot{\gamma}_R} \left(3 + \frac{d \ln \mathcal{T}}{d \ln \dot{\gamma}_R}\right) \tag{9.44}$$

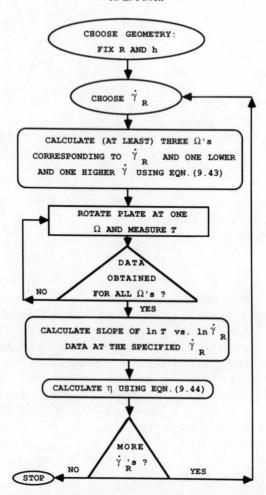

Fig. 9.3. Flow chart of a typical experimental program for measuring viscosity
using the parallel plate geometry.

The derivative on the right-hand side of this equation makes an experimental program using the parallel plate geometry for viscosity measurements fundamentally different from those with the cone and plate. Figure
9.3 shows details of a typical experimental program.

The value of the viscosity at a single shear rate should only be calculated
with eqn (9.44) after measuring the torque at (at least) three different shear

rates: the one of interest, one lower and one higher. Only then can the shape of the $\ln \mathscr{T}$ vs. $\ln \dot{\gamma}_R$ curve be estimated. The value of the viscosity will, if the test material remains homogeneous, be the same value that would be found with the cone and plate or capillary viscometer. Such a correspondence would provide a critical test as to whether the measured viscosities, as calculated from eqns (9.21) and (9.44), are real material properties, particularly for multiphase systems,[14-16] or whether the measuring geometry is creating some artifacts in the data.

To determine viscometric normal forces we calculate their relationship to the total normal thrust against the bottom plate:

$$\mathscr{F} = -\int_0^{2\pi} \int_0^R \sigma_{zz} r \, dr \, d\theta \tag{9.45}$$

To integrate this, we refer to Table 9.1 and find

$$\sigma_{rr} = \sigma_{zz} - N_2 \tag{9.46}$$

which is substituted into eqn (9.36) and integrated from 0 to r to obtain

$$\sigma_{zz}(r) = \sigma_{zz}(0) + N_2(\dot{\gamma}) + \int_0^{\dot{\gamma}} \frac{1}{\kappa} [N_1(\kappa) + N_2(\kappa)] \, d\kappa \tag{9.47}$$

Surface tension and edge effects are neglected, so that $\sigma_{rr}(R) = -p_a$; then, after evaluating eqn (9.47) at $r = R$ and using eqn (9.46), we find

$$-p_a = \sigma_{zz}(0) + \int_0^{\dot{\gamma}_R} \frac{1}{\kappa} [N_1(\kappa) + N_2(\kappa)] \, d\kappa \tag{9.48}$$

Subtracting eqns (9.47) and (9.48) yields

$$\sigma_{zz}(r) = -p_a + N_2(\dot{\gamma}) - \int_{\dot{\gamma}}^{\dot{\gamma}_R} \frac{1}{\kappa} [N_1(\kappa) + N_2(\kappa)] \, d\kappa \tag{9.49}$$

Substituting eqn (9.49) into eqn (9.45),[2,3] we find

$$\dot{\gamma}_R^2 \mathscr{F} = \pi R^2 \left(p_a + \int_0^{\dot{\gamma}_R} \dot{\gamma}(N_1 - N_2) \, d\dot{\gamma} \right) \tag{9.50}$$

Upon differentiating with respect to $\dot{\gamma}_R$ and rearranging:

$$N_1(\dot{\gamma}_R) - N_2(\dot{\gamma}_R) = \frac{2\mathscr{F}}{\pi R^2} \left(1 + \frac{1}{2} \frac{d \ln \mathscr{F}}{d \ln \dot{\gamma}_R} \right) \tag{9.51}$$

The combination of $N_1 - N_2$ at a single shear rate can only be determined if there are measurements of the normal thrust at (at least) three different

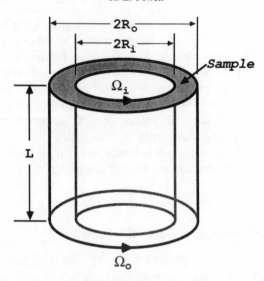

Fig. 9.4. The concentric cylinder geometry; the fluid is contained in the gap between two concentric cylinders which rotate at different angular velocities.

shear rates. The experimental procedure to be followed is similar to that discussed for eqn (9.44) with the total normal thrust rather than the torque being measured (see Fig. 9.3). Equations (9.29) and (9.51) provide, in principle, a means of finding N_2.[17] However, this method must be used with caution and, whenever possible, independent verification should be sought.

9.2.3. Concentric Cylinder

The concentric cylinder viscometer is generally used for shear viscosity measurements although it is possible to measure the primary normal stress difference.[18] Figure 9.4 shows the idealized system. The fluid is contained in the gap between two infinitely long concentric cylinders. The outer one rotates at a steady angular velocity, Ω_o, while the inner cylinder rotates at Ω_i, which is also constant. We use a cylindrical coordinate system wherein the inner and outer bounding surfaces of the fluid are at $r = R_i$ and $r = R_o$, respectively. The velocity of the fluid is assumed to have a component only in the θ-direction (Table 9.1)

$$\mathbf{v} \approx (0, r\omega(r), 0) \tag{9.52}$$

and the corresponding shear rate (Table 9.2) is

$$\dot{\gamma} = r \frac{d\omega}{dr} \tag{9.53}$$

The conditions under which eqn (9.52) represents a possible flow are found using eqns (9.3.4)–(9.3.6) in Table 9.3, which are

$$- \rho r \omega^2 = \frac{\partial \sigma_{rr}}{\partial r} + \frac{1}{r} (\sigma_{rr} - \sigma_{\theta\theta}) \tag{9.54}$$

$$0 = \frac{\partial \sigma_{r\theta}}{\partial r} + \frac{1}{r} \frac{\partial \sigma_{\theta\theta}}{\partial \theta} + \frac{2}{r} \sigma_{r\theta} \tag{9.55}$$

$$0 = \frac{\partial \sigma_{zz}}{\partial z} \tag{9.56}$$

We recall eqn (9.1) where $\sigma = \sigma(\dot{\gamma})$, and substitute into eqns (9.54) and (9.55). Then, upon differentiating the first of these with respect to θ and the second with respect to r, and equating the two expressions through $\partial^2 p / \partial r \partial \theta$, we obtain

$$\frac{d}{dr} \left(r \frac{\partial \sigma_{r\theta}}{\partial r} + 2\sigma_{r\theta} \right) = 0 \tag{9.57}$$

Solving this expression, we find

$$\sigma_{r\theta} = \frac{1}{2} C_1 + \frac{C_2}{r^2} \tag{9.58}$$

where C_1 and C_2 are constants of integration. The first of these is evaluated by substituting eqn (9.58) into eqn (9.55) and using eqns (9.53) and (9.1) to obtain

$$\frac{\partial p}{\partial \theta} = C_1 \tag{9.59}$$

or

$$p = C_1 \theta + f_1(r, z) \tag{9.60}$$

By eqn (9.56), $f_1(r, z) = f_2(r)$ only and eqn (9.60) says that the pressure is a multivalued function of the angular position, which is physically unrealistic, and hence that $C_1 = 0$. To evaluate C_2, we calculate the torque per cylinder length $\hat{\mathcal{T}}$, which acts at any radial position:

$$\hat{\mathcal{T}} = 2\pi r^2 \sigma_{r\theta} \tag{9.61}$$

Upon substituting eqn (9.58), we obtain

$$C_2 = \frac{\hat{\mathcal{T}}}{2\pi} \tag{9.62}$$

To use this result, note that $\sigma_{r\theta} = \sigma(\dot{\gamma})$, and we let $s = \sigma(\dot{\gamma})$ be the value of the function σ at a particular $\dot{\gamma}$ and define an inverse function

$$\dot{\gamma} = \sigma^{-1}(s) \tag{9.63}$$

Combining eqns (9.53), (9.58) and (9.62), we obtain

$$\frac{d\omega}{dr} = \frac{1}{r}\sigma^{-1}\left(\frac{\hat{\mathcal{T}}}{2\pi r^2}\right) \tag{9.64}$$

Integrating across the gap of the cylinders

$$\Delta\Omega \equiv \Omega_o - \Omega_i = -\frac{1}{2}\int_{s_i}^{s_o}\frac{1}{s}\sigma^{-1}(s)\,ds \tag{9.65}$$

Following Coleman et al.,[2] we consider a series of experiments in which $\Delta\Omega$ is varied, $\hat{\mathcal{T}}$ is measured, and the cylinder geometry, i.e. R_i and R_o, is fixed. Taking $\partial\Delta\Omega/\partial\hat{\mathcal{T}}$, we obtain

$$Y(s_i) \equiv 2M\frac{\partial\Delta\Omega}{\partial\hat{\mathcal{T}}} = \sigma^{-1}(s_i) - \sigma^{-1}(s_o) \tag{9.66}$$

Defining

$$\beta \equiv \frac{R_i^2}{R_o^2}$$

leads to

$$Y(\beta^n s_i) = \sigma^{-1}(\beta^n s_i) - \sigma^{-1}(\beta^{n+1} s_i) \tag{9.67}$$

Summing over n yields

$$\sum_{n=0}^{N} Y(\beta^n s_i) = \sigma^{-1}(s_i) - \sigma^{-1}(\beta^{N+1} s_i) \tag{9.68}$$

As $N \to \infty$, $\beta^N \to 0$ and, if the shear stress function is assumed to be continuous through $\dot{\gamma} = 0$, eqn (9.68) becomes

$$\sum_{n=0}^{\infty} Y(\beta^n s_i) = \sigma^{-1}(s_i) = \dot{\gamma}_i \tag{9.69}$$

In practice, this equation can be used if the series converges rapidly, i.e.

if $\beta \ll 1$. A typical experimental program for the large gap geometry would consist of:

(i) choosing a geometry, i.e. fixing R_i and R_o;
(ii) setting the angular velocity and measuring the torque on the inner or outer cylinder, then calculating $\hat{\mathcal{T}}$ by dividing the torque by the cylinder length;
(iii) calculating $2M(\partial\Delta\Omega/\partial M)$ for each measurement;
(iv) constructing a Y versus s_i $(=\hat{\mathcal{T}}/2\pi R_i^2)$ curve using the results from (iii);
(v) calculating $\dot{\gamma}_i$ using eqn (9.69) for all the data; and
(vi) calculating the viscosity using

$$\eta(\dot{\gamma}_i) = s_i/\dot{\gamma}_i \tag{9.70}$$

A much simplified methodology results as $\beta \rightarrow 1$. Then the integration of eqn (9.64) is written

$$\Delta\Omega = \int_{R_i}^{R_o} \frac{1}{r} \sigma^{-1}\left(\frac{\hat{\mathcal{T}}}{2\pi r^2}\right) dr \tag{9.71}$$

and the integrand is expanded about $r = R_i$. To leading order in the gap thickness we obtain

$$\Delta\Omega = \frac{R_o - R_i}{R_i} \sigma^{-1}(s_i) \tag{9.72}$$

The shear rate is now constant in the *narrow* gap with

$$\dot{\gamma} = \frac{R_i \Delta\Omega}{R_o - R_i} \tag{9.73}$$

This geometry approach permits an experimetnal program closely following that used for the cone and plate.

Since the shear rate is constant in the gap, so is the shear stress. Combining eqns (9.61) and (9.5), we obtain a formula for a single point determination of the viscosity:

$$\eta(\dot{\gamma}) = \frac{\hat{\mathcal{T}}(R_o - R_i)}{2\pi R_i^3 \Delta\Omega} \tag{9.74}$$

The total torque acting on the inner cylinder is measured, and $\hat{\mathcal{T}}$ is obtained by dividing this by the length of the cylinder, L.

An expression for the first viscometric normal stress can be found by integrating eqn (9.54) and using Table 9.1:

$$\Delta\sigma_{rr} = \sigma_{rr}(R_o) - \sigma_{rr}(R_i) = \int_{R_i}^{R_o} \left[\frac{1}{r} N_1 \left(\frac{\hat{\mathscr{T}}}{2\pi r^2}\right) - \rho r \omega^2\right] dr \quad (9.75)$$

Following Coleman *et al.*,[2] we define a corrected normal stress difference, $\Delta\sigma_{rr}^c$, which includes the centrifugal term $\rho r \omega^2$, such that

$$\Delta\sigma_{rr}^c = \int_{R_i}^{R_o} \frac{1}{r} N_1 \left(\frac{\hat{\mathscr{T}}}{2\pi r^2}\right) dr \quad (9.76)$$

By considering a series of measurements of $\Delta\sigma_{rr}$ and $\hat{\mathscr{T}}$, it is possible to calculate $\partial\Delta\sigma_{rr}^c/\partial\hat{\mathscr{T}}$, which is

$$2\hat{\mathscr{T}} \frac{\partial\Delta\sigma_{rr}^c}{\partial\hat{\mathscr{T}}} = \psi(s_i) \quad (9.77)$$

and

$$N_1(s_i) = \sum_{n=0}^{\infty} \psi(\beta^n s_i) \quad (9.78)$$

As with measurements of the viscosity, eqns (9.77) and (9.78) are only useful when $\beta \ll 1$. The experimental program required to implement this method is similar to that described for large gap measurements of the viscosity.

9.2.4. Sources of Errors

9.2.4.1. Fluid Inertia

In the derivations for the cone and plate and parallel plate geometries, the conservation of linear momentum is satisfied by neglecting fluid inertia. With the cone and plate geometry, fluid inertia has two effects. Firstly, even when the actual flow field is well approximated by eqn (9.18), the stress distribution across the plate will not be given by eqn (9.24). There is an inertial contribution to the pressure gradient:

$$\left.\frac{dp}{d \ln r}\right|_{\text{inertial}} = k_F \rho \Omega^2 r^2 \quad (9.79)$$

where k_F is a constant which has been predicted to be $1/3$[20] and 0.3 for small gaps.[13,21] This pressure gradient contributes

$$\mathscr{F}_i = -\frac{\pi \rho \Omega^2 R^4 k_F}{4} \qquad (9.80)$$

to the measured normal thrust.

Using eqn (9.29) to define an 'inertial normal force function', we find

$$N_{1i} = p_a - \tfrac{1}{2}\rho \Omega^2 R^2 k_F \qquad (9.81)$$

Kulicke *et al.*[19] experimentally determined k_F to be 0·3 to within 2·5% up to rotational speeds of $100 \, \text{s}^{-1}$, using Newtonian fluids having viscosities ranging from 1 mPa s to 0·6 Pa s. They also clearly showed the peril of neglecting inertial effects when testing samples having small N_1 (see references 3 and 22). First normal stress functions which appear to plateau and even to decrease at high shear rates actually increase monotonically when inertial effects are taken into account. Equation (9.80) can also be used to correct total thrust data for the parallel plate geometry. Again $k_F = 0·3$ has been determined experimentally.[19]

Fluid inertia can also modify the actual flow field, creating inflow towards the apex of the cone and outflow along the plate. This secondary flow gives rise to stresses in addition to those of the base flow which are reflected in the torque and normal thrust. Turian[13] has analyzed inertial effects in both a cone and plate and a parallel plate system for a Newtonian liquid. Defining the Reynolds number as

$$\text{Re} \equiv \frac{\rho \Omega R^2}{\mu} \qquad (9.82)$$

he showed that secondary flow contributes to the torque according to

$$\frac{\mathscr{T}_{act}}{\mathscr{T}_0} = 1 + \frac{3(\text{Re} \sin \alpha)^2}{4900} \qquad (9.83)$$

where $\mathscr{T}_{act}$ is the actual torque and $\mathscr{T}_0$ is the torque due to the basic, viscometric velocity field. Equation (9.83) predicts that fluid inertia can give rise to apparent shear thickening behavior. It agrees with experimental data[23] up to Reynolds numbers of 40. Turian's analysis has also been used by recent investigators[24] as a benchmark for testing alternative theoretical approaches.

Inertial effects on normal stress measurements are usually well described through eqns (9.79)–(9.81). There can be additional contributions: inertia-driven secondary flows. For small cone angles, if $0·15 \, \text{Re}^2 \ll 1$, they can be neglected.[13]

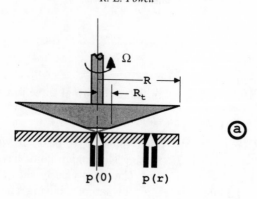

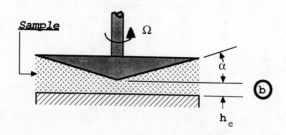

Fig. 9.5. (a) The truncated cone and plate geometry. (b) the extended cone and plate geometry.

In the concentric cylinder geometry, the principal inertial effect is to modify the measured pressure difference between the inner and outer cylinders, thereby influencing the normal force measurement, as reflected by the $\rho r \omega^2$ term in eqn (9.75). To evaluate precisely, the inertial correction $\omega(r)$ must be known. This can only be done by determining σ^{-1} so that eqn (9.64) can be integrated.

For a Newtonian fluid, secondary flow in the concentric cylinder will occur above a critical Taylor number[25]

$$\frac{\Omega R_{\mathrm{i}}^{1/2} \rho (R_{\mathrm{o}} - R_{\mathrm{i}})^{3/2}}{\mu} > 41 \tag{9.84}$$

if the inner cylinder is rotated. When the outer cylinder is rotated, the flow is stable.[25] Material viscoelasticity can be either stabilizing or destabilizing.[18]

9.2.4.2. Flow Geometry

The cone and plate geometry is usually configured with cones having angles less than 4° and which are slightly truncated (Fig. 9.5(a)). The theory of Section 9.2.1 assumes that the angle is 'small' and that the apex actually touches the plate. Furthermore, there is no allowance in the theory for the actual free surface at the edge other than that it is spherical and does not influence the flow field.

The finite cone angle and the free surface cause a deviation of the shear rate field near the edge from the idealized behavior as given by eqn. (9.19).[12,26,27] For a second-order fluid, having a constant viscosity and nonzero normal stress functions which depend upon the square of the shear rate,[28] Griffiths and Walters[12] showed that errors of less than 2% in the measured torques would result from using a cone angle 4° or smaller. For a Newtonian fluid in the truncated cone and plate geometry the thickness over which edge effects are significant, $\Delta = (R - R_{in})/R$ (where R_{in} is the radius at which numerical solutions for the finite cone[27] differ appreciably from the analytical solutions for the infinite cone[29]), depends upon the Reynolds number and the cone angle through

$$\Delta = \alpha[2 \cdot 9 - 2 \cdot 75 \log \text{Re} + 0 \cdot 725 (\log \text{Re})^2] \quad (9.85)$$

Hou's analysis[27] reveals that for a cone angle of 3°, even when $\text{Re} = 500$, the shear rate at the edge differs from the ideal one calculated using eqn (9.19) by less than 1%. A shear thinning material will show a greater tendency to deviate from the ideal flow although the percentage error in the shear stress field is less.[26] The combined effect is an error in the measured torque which is larger for a non-Newtonian fluid than for a Newtonian fluid.

Errors due to cone truncation are small, particularly for most commercial instruments for which $(R_t/R) \ll 1$ (Fig. 9.5(a)). Except in those particular circumstances where the truncation region is part of the measurement technique (see Section 9.3.2.1), it is usually ignored in the actual calculations of the viscometric functions, and the formulas of Section 9.2.1 are directly applied.

Edge effects in parallel plate measurements can be estimated using cone and plate results if we take $\sin \alpha = h/R$.[12] If $h/R < 0.075$, the error in the measured torque will be less than 2%.

The geometrical errors associated with the use of the concentric cylinder geometry are: (1) shear stresses exerted by the sample on the bottom surface of the inner cylinder which are not accounted for in the theory; and (2) nonideality of the flow in the cylindrical gap due to the finite extent of

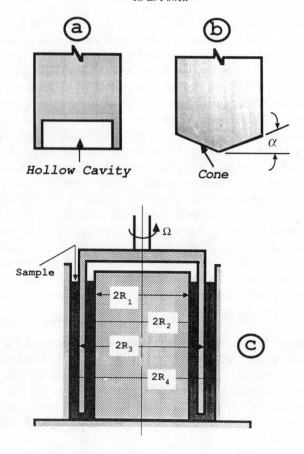

Fig. 9.6. Alternative concentric cylinder geometries. (a) Hollow cavity at the bottom for trapping an air bubble and reducing end effects. (b) Cone at the bottom for creating a cone and plate flow at the end. (c) Double concentric cylinder.

the cylinders. The two techniques for isolating the error due to fluid stresses acting on the bottom surface either eliminate the stresses or create a well defined flow between the inner and outer cylinders. The stresses can be eliminated or minimized by floating the sample on a substantially less viscous fluid than the one being tested and assuring that the bottom surface of the inner cylinder just comes into contact with this material. A variant of this method involves having an inner cylinder which has a hollow portion in the bottom (see Fig. 9.6(a)). Upon charging with the test sample an air bubble is trapped between the two flat surfaces which transmits negligible stresses. In the second alternative the region between the two flat surfaces is a cone and plate viscometer[30] (see Fig. 9.6(b)). This method is used for narrow gap concentric cylinder geometries, in which the flow field is characterized by a single shear rate, given by eqn (9.73). Ideally, the cone angle is machined to match this shear rate which, by eqn (9.13), requires that

$$\alpha = \frac{R_o - R_i}{R_i} \tag{9.86}$$

Another method, which is principally used to increase the accuracy of the concentric cylinder geometry, also minimizes the effect of shear stresses being transmitted across the bottom surfaces. The double concentric cylinder[31] has been especially promoted for use with applied stress rheometers. A schematic of this geometry is shown in Fig. 9.6(c). Test material is contained in the regions R_1–R_2 and R_3–R_4. Narrow gaps are always used, and the radii are machined so as to produce the same shear rates in both gaps, which by eqn (9.73) means that

$$\frac{R_2}{R_1} = \frac{R_4}{R_3} \tag{9.87}$$

Compared with the standard concentric cylinder configuration, this geometry has double the area over which shear stresses are measured, and effects due to the bottom surface of the inner cylinder are nearly eliminated. Care should be exercised to ensure that none of the sample fills the upper cavity between the two flat surfaces.

The finite length of the cylinders affects measurements to the extent that the flow fields at the ends are not ideal. Making measurements using different length cylinders provides the most straightforward means of exploring the consequences of these effects. If the inner cylinder is rotated and it extends above the fluid, an attempt should be made to quantify any change in the effective area over which shear stresses are transmitted due to rod climbing, while recognizing that rod climbing itself implies the existence of a non-viscometric flow.[32,33] An alternative procedure involves the use of guard rings which isolate the measuring section away from the ends.[2]

9.2.4.3. *Viscous Heating*

Energy generation due to stress working can give rise to temperature changes in a sample and lead to anomalous values of the measured viscosity. Viscous heating effects are greatest at high shear rates or for high viscosity fluids. Chapter 5 provides a comprehensive analysis of the effects of viscous heating. Here we use the specific example of the cone and plate geometry to discuss its effects on viscometric measurements.

Theoretical estimates of viscous heating have been made by Turian and Bird,[34] Klijn et al.[35] and Winter.[36,37] The critical parameter is the Brinkman number, Br, defined as

$$\text{Br} = \mu V^2 / k_\theta \theta_0 \qquad (9.88)$$

where V is characteristic velocity, k_θ is thermal conductivity and θ_0 is a reference temperature. These theories differ according to (i) the thermal boundary conditions assigned at the surfaces of the cone and the plate, (ii) the temperature dependence of the thermal conductivity and the viscosity, and (iii) whether the problem is posed as an initial value problem or a steady state solution is sought at the outset. For cone and plate rheometers operating at steady state with constant temperature boundaries, the maximum temperature can be estimated[34] using either

$$\theta_{\max} = \theta_0[1 + (1/8)\text{Br}] \qquad (9.89)$$

or

$$\theta_{\max} = \theta_0[1 + (1/\xi)\ln(1 + \text{Br}\,\xi/8)] \qquad (9.90)$$

where the characteristic velocity, V in eqn. (9.88), is $R\Omega$ and ξ is the coefficient appearing in the temperature–viscosity relationship, viz.

$$\mu/\mu_0 = \exp[-\xi(\theta - \theta_0)/\theta_0] \qquad (9.91)$$

μ_0 being the viscosity at θ_0. Equation (9.89) was derived assuming that both viscosity and thermal conductivity are polynomials in temperature, while in deriving eqn (9.90) the thermal conductivity was constant and the viscosity varied according to eqn (9.91). Turian and Bird[34] showed that both eqns (9.89) and (9.90) could estimate experimental data when temperature changes are small. In an experimental program it is desirable to take data before viscous heating can become appreciable. Predictions of this time scale have been obtained by Klijn et al.[35] and Winter.[36,37]

9.2.4.4. Sample Instability

Besides secondary flows, which in the case of the concentric cylinder geometry result from flow instability, two other instabilities are sample fracturing[38,39] and centrifugal expulsion.[40] Each of these can have catastrophic effects on rheological measurements.

Sample fracturing in the cone and plate and the parallel plate geometries consists of the propagation of a 'crack' from the edge, i.e. the sample/air interface, inward. During an experiment, it might be detected either visually or by observing a decrease in the measured torque with time. Hutton's analysis, based on an elastic energy approach,[38,39] predicts that sample fracture occurs at a critical shear rate $\dot{\gamma}_{CF}$, corresponding to a critical rotational speed, Ω_{CF}, at which

$$N_1 = k_E \Gamma / h_R \tag{9.92}$$

with

$$\dot{\gamma}_{CF} \equiv \Omega_{CF} R / h_R \tag{9.93}$$

where Γ is the surface tension, h_R is the gap at the edge of the geometry, and k_E is a constant which was found to be 24 or 36.[39]

Tanner and Keentok[40] provided independent theoretical and experimental evidence that eqn (9.92) is a satisfactory criterion. They analyzed the growth of a crack in a second-order fluid[28,41] using fracture mechanics, and showed that sample fracture was governed by the magnitude of the second normal stress difference. Their criterion is

$$|N_2| > 2\Gamma / 3a_c \tag{9.94}$$

where a_c is the radius of the (semicircular) crack. This expression can be made to correspond to eqn (9.92) when $|N_2|N_1$ is equal to a constant.[40]

Sample expulsion due to centrifugal forces is possible for both Newtonian and viscoelastic fluids. In the latter case, this mechanism competes with sample fracturing to limit the highest shear rate at which reliable data can be obtained. Tanner and Keentok[40] argue that a model based upon the Newtonian fluid can provide reasonable estimates of the critical shear rate for centrifugal expulsion, $\dot{\gamma}_{CC}$, even for viscoelastic fluids where radial stresses are present. For the cone and plate and parallel plate geometries, they found

$$\dot{\gamma}_{CC} > \sqrt{\frac{20\Gamma}{3\rho(\alpha R)^3}} \tag{9.95}$$

and

$$\dot{\gamma}_{CC} = \frac{\Omega_{CC} R}{h} > \sqrt{\frac{20\Gamma}{3\rho h^3}} \tag{9.96}$$

respectively, where Ω_{CC} is the critical speed for centrifugal expulsion.

The equations of this section provide *a priori* estimates of the highest shear rate at which data can be obtained without catastrophic material instabilities affecting the measurements. Although there has been some experimental verification, these models should be viewed as semi-quantitative, particularly since they do not address the complications of describing material properties in non-viscometric flows.

9.2.4.5. Material Effects

The nature of the sample itself can provide for a variety of experimental difficulties including: slippage at the fluid/solid interface, sample inhomogeneity, shear-induced particle migration, particle bridging across geometry members, trapped air bubbles, and sample evaporation.

Slippage at solid surfaces does not appear to be of principal concern for polymeric fluids.[2] For flows of suspensions there is evidence that a particle depletion layer exists near solid boundaries,[42-44] which could be interpreted as slippage of the sample along a suspending fluid layer. In gels there is also evidence that a water layer exists near solid boundaries.[45] Special precautions are required to ensure that the idealized applied shearing deformation is being effected in the entire sample. For suspensions of solid particles a good approach is to obtain data using different viscometer geometries. Studies with suspensions of spherical particles,[14] suspensions of rod-like particles[15,46,47] and particulate filled polymer melts[16] indicate that, if the ratio of the edge gap to longest particle dimensions is greater than 3, the effect of viscometer geometry, and hence bounding surfaces, should be small. A similar result has been obtained using an entirely different technique, falling ball rheometry, to study suspensions of rod-like particles.[48,49] When the diameter of the container is three times the length of the rods, no boundary effects are observed.[49] Greater accuracy may require larger characteristic viscometer gap to characteristic particle length ratios. For spherical particle suspensions, geometrical effects have been observed in capillary flow even when the tube diameter is nearly 20 times as large as the particle diameter.[50]

In systems where the existence of a low viscosity layer near a solid boundary is a persistent problem, such as with gels[45] and pulp suspensions,[44] this layer can be disrupted by roughening the surfaces. Proven methods include coating the surfaces with sand using lacquer or fixing a piece of sandpaper to the surface. In cases where the sample is very cohesive, it can be attached to the solid surfaces using adhesive.[45]

Suspensions of solid particles can exhibit effects such as shear-induced particle migration, sedimentation, and particle bridging. The last of these will most likely occur with the cone and plate geometries where the cone truncation commonly results in gaps of less than 50 μm at the apex. The presence of even a few particles having a similar diameter as the cone gap can lead to asymmetric torque measurements.[51] Use of the parallel plate geometry circumvents this problem but creates the possibility of particle migration due to the nonuniform shearing field.[52] Such effects have been highlighted by the recent work of Leighton and Acrivos[53] which demonstrates that torque transients found by Gadala-Maria and Acrivos[54] in concentrated suspensions of spheres may be due to shear-induced diffusion which results in particle migration.

Sedimentation effects will be significant when the density difference between the particle and the suspending fluid is large, the suspending fluid viscosity is small, or the particles are large. These effects can be estimated by calculating the sedimentation velocity for a single particle (ref. 55, eqn (4.9.20)). If the velocity is sufficiently fast, special instruments may be required to maintain a uniform sample, such as using a helical screw rheometer (Section 9.3.2.3) or a concentric cylinder geometry which provides for pumping the suspension out of the gap, through a mixer, and back into the gap while tests are underway.[56]

Another mechanism for phase separation is the presence of trapped air bubbles at one of the bounding surfaces. Air bubbles can also cause experimental difficulties when they are too small to migrate under the force of gravity and are trapped in the sample. Non-volatile samples can be exposed to a vacuum immediately prior to testing, although in highly viscous materials bubble growth and expulsion may be possible only under prohibitively high vacuum or over very long times. Centrifugation may be used for single-phase materials to the same end.

Sample evaporation is particularly troublesome for suspensions or solutions with high concentrations of particles or solute. A suspension of spheres at a volume loading above 0·6 will undergo a large increase in the viscosity[57] with even a small decrease in the solvent. One method of controlling evaporation is to coat the sample/air interface with a layer of a low volatility, relatively non-viscous oil.[58] For the cone and plate and parallel plate geometries, gravity will cause the film to drain and it will require periodic replenishment. The concentric cylinder geometry is well suited for controlling evaporation by this method, since the oil can be floated on the sample/air interface, creating a stable barrier. Other measures that can help alleviate evaporation include humidifying the sample environment and eliminating direct air flow through the test chamber.

9.2.4.6. *Experimental Effects*

Errors arising from the equipment can be due either to the inherent difficulties associated with a particular instrument or to poor calibration, machining or alignment.

For the cone and plate and parallel plate geometries, alignment errors result from the surfaces in contact with the fluid not being parallel or by having the symmetry axes of each member not coincident. One manufacturer[59] recommends maintaining parallelism to within ± 0.00025 cm and concentricity to within ± 0.00125 cm. With the concentric cylinder geometry, one member may be tilted relative to the second or their axes may be misaligned. The latter has been studied quite extensively in connection with the journal bearing problem. Beris *et al.*[60] have shown that small axial misalignment will not affect the measured torque since the induced shear stress error varies periodically with the angular position. When integrated over the surface of the inner cylinder, this error averages to zero. However, even for small values of the dimensionless cylinder eccentricity, $e/(R_o - R_i)$, where e is the linear distance between the two cylinder axes, flow separation could occur at the outer cylinder for sufficiently large Deborah numbers.

Geometrical imperfections due to machining errors have been extensively analyzed by Cheng[61] who reported on the accuracy of machining cones for the Weissenberg rheogoniometer. Similar studies have not appeared for other manufacturers, and it is not known whether the improvements in machining technology over the past 20 years have had any impact on the quality of cones produced for the Weissenberg rheogoniometer.

Another error which can occur in long-term testing or with the use of specialized transducers is caused by mechanical or electrical drift, which could be misinterpreted as a long-term stress transient due to the sample. With applied stress rheometers the problem is particularly acute since long time measurements are often desired. In these instruments imbalance can occur from slight angular variations in the air flow within the air bearing or from small asymmetries in the geometries. The first problem can usually be adjusted with the facilities provided by the manufacturer. Geometrical asymmetries can be compensated by dynamic balancing[62] accomplished using a collar fitted over the shaft which has holes at equal angular spacings for set screws. Using screws of various densities, e.g. steel and teflon, the system is balanced so that no changes in angular velocity are detected over the course of a rotation.

The use of fast response piezoelectric transducers can lead to significant problems from electrical drift.[63,64] When charge amplifiers are used for the measurements, this problem can be somewhat alleviated by maintaining clean electrical contacts, and using low-loss cables. A better method is to measure the charge directly, e.g. using electrometers.[63] In either case the drift is generally linear with time, which allows for the possibility of determining the rate of drift and estimating the contribution of this error to measurements.

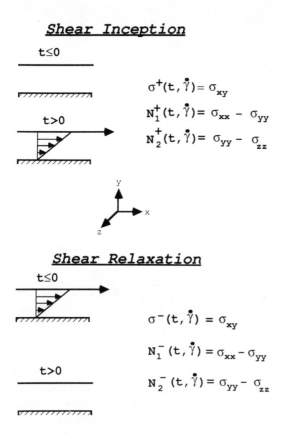

Fig. 9.7. Shear inception and shear relaxation experiments and their material functions. For shear inception, the sample is initially at rest, and at $t = 0$ shear flow is initiated. For shear relaxation, the sample is undergoing steady shear flow up to $t = 0$, after which flow ceases. Material properties are measured for $t > 0$.

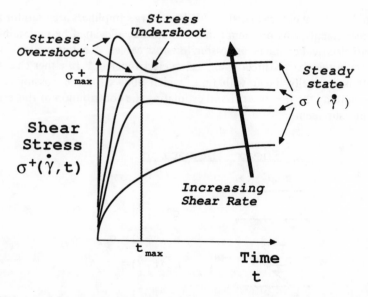

Fig. 9.8. Schematic of stress growth behavior found for polymeric fluids.

9.3. NOVEL RHEOMETRICAL FLOWS

9.3.1. Transient Flow Viscometry

9.3.1.1. Introduction

The three viscometric functions fully characterize a material in steady shearing flows in the absence of yielding and time dependent material behavior. They do not provide any information about the unsteady state response of a material. This is usually inferred from oscillatory rheometry (see Chapter 10) which characterizes material response to small deformations. While such experiments are a good probe of material microstructure they do not provide insight into stresses which are generated by large time dependent deformations. For this purpose there has been considerable effort to develop the experimental methodology for performing measurements in transient shearing flows, particularly shearing inception and cessation.

In the shearing inception experiment, the sample is initially at rest and at $t = 0$ it is forced to undergo a steady shearing flow (Fig. 9.7). Three material properties,[4] which are functions of both the shear rate and time, govern the stress response: σ^+, the shear stress growth function, and N_1^+

and N_2^+, the first and second normal stress growth functions, respectively. Shearing cessation is the instantaneous stopping of a steady shearing flow. There are three material properties governing the stress relaxation of the material, each of which is a function of the prior shear rate and the time after cessation: σ^-, N_1^-, N_2^-.

There are several recent reveiws of transient shearing flow measurements and experimental methodology.[65-67] Our emphasis is on the measurement of the shear stress growth function, which has been the most widely measured transient shearing property for fluid-like materials. Stress relaxation measurements are more common for solid-like materials, and many factors bearing upon stress growth measurements in liquids also apply to stress relaxation measurements. Also, we do not focus on the normal stress growth functions. As with the steady shearing measurements, the time dependent normal force measurements are more susceptible to experimental design imperfections than the shearing measurements.

For polymeric liquids (for some representative recent papers see references 68-72) and for some suspensions,[15,63,74] behavior such as that illustrated in Fig. 9.8 is found. At low shear rates, upon application of shearing, the shear stress increases monotonically, reaching a maximum, steady state value at long times. At higher shear rates, 'stress overshoot' is observed, wherein the stress increases initially but then reaches a maximum before decaying and finally leveling off to a steady state. At still higher shear rates there are strong indications[69] that, after the maximum is reached, the stress decays through a minimum 'stress undershoot' and then increases to the final steady state value. Other materials, such as concentrated suspensions of spherical particles,[54] show different time dependencies which can include both a short time and a long time response. These can be due to microstructural rearrangement or shear-induced diffusion across streamlines.[53] It is also possible that the material is thixotropic, changing properties with the duration of shearing.

9.3.1.2. Theory

Theoretical relationships between measured quantities and material properties are based upon the assumption that the flows shown in Fig. 9.7 can be realized in the laboratory. For shearing inception, one boundary accelerates instantaneously to a constant velocity and simple shearing flow is established immediately. The corresponding condition for the shear relaxation experiment is that the moving plate is brought to rest instantaneously, stopping the motion of the test material. Under the additional assumptions made in Sections 9.2.1–9.2.3, these time dependent flows satisfy the dynamical equations. The methodologies used in those sections allow relationships between time dependent torques and the transient shear stress functions to be determined. Denoting σ^+ and σ^- by $\sigma(t, \dot{\gamma})$, these relationships are

Cone and plate

$$\sigma(t, \dot{\gamma}) = \frac{3\mathcal{T}_{cp}}{2\pi R^3} \tag{9.97}$$

Parallel plates

$$\sigma(t, \dot{\gamma}) = \frac{\mathcal{T}_{pp}}{2\pi R^3} \left(3 + \frac{\partial \ln \mathcal{T}_{pp}}{\partial \ln \dot{\gamma}_R} \bigg|_{t \text{ fixed}} \right) \tag{9.98}$$

Concentric cylinders (narrow gap)

$$\sigma(t, \dot{\gamma}) = \frac{\mathcal{T}_{cc}}{2\pi R_i^2 L} \tag{9.99}$$

The time dependent torques developed in the cone and plate, parallel plates and concentric cylinders geometries are denoted by $\mathcal{T}_{cp}$, $\mathcal{T}_{pp}$ and $\mathcal{T}_{cc}$, respectively. Equations (9.97)–(9.99) are essentially the same as eqns (9.21), (9.44) and (9.74), except that $\mathcal{T}_{cp}$, $\mathcal{T}_{pp}$ and $\mathcal{T}_{cc}$ are functions of both shear rate and time, and the steady state expressions must be converted from equations for viscosity to equations for the viscometric shear stress. This difference alters eqn (9.98) from its corresponding steady state formula by having the total derivative in eqn (9.44) become a partial derivative with t held fixed. Measurements of the transient shear stress functions using the parallel plate geometry require that torque versus time data are obtained at (at least) three different shear rates: the shear rate of interest and two bracketing it. These data are used to construct curves so that $(\partial \ln \mathcal{T}_{pp}/\partial \ln \dot{\gamma}_R)_{t \text{ fixed}}$ can be calculated and used in eqn (9.98). This process can be quite tedious but, when used in conjunction with transient data in the cone and plate geometry, it provides an independent verification of the behavior of polymeric fluids.[69] Also, the parallel plate geometry has much greater application to the rheology of filled systems owing to the control of the gap-to-particle size ratio that is possible.

9.3.1.3. Experimental Methods and Sources of Errors
The two principal experimental issues to consider when performing transient flow measurements are the time response of the measuring system, viz. the rheometer and recording equipment, and the dependence of the

measurement upon viscometer geometry. Related concerns are the instrument compliance (e.g. the amount the gap between the cone and the plate changes due to normal forces which develop during shearing) and edge effects.

Since the property being measured is a function of time, the instrument being used for the measurement must respond faster than the shortest time scale of interest. For accurate determinations of stress overshoot, the frequency response of the instrument should be $f_{instr} \gg 1/t_{max}$ (see Fig. 9.8). With polymeric liquids, a good rule-of-thumb for making *a priori* estimates of t_{max} is $t_{max} = \gamma_{trans}/\dot\gamma$. For shear rates less than $50\,s^{-1}$, γ_{trans} is a constant which has been experimentally determined for a number of fluids to be between 2 and 3.[69,71,72,75] At higher shear rates, $\gamma_{trans} > 3$.[69,71] Suspensions of highly concentrated spherical particles[54] and short fibers[15] in Newtonian fluids have values of γ_{trans} of about 5. At shear rates of $10\,s^{-1}$ and greater, the time response of the instrument should therefore be much less than 200 ms. This criterion can be met by eliminating or minimizing three main sources of error which include (1) the start-up time of the driving member of the viscometer geometry (i.e. the length of time it takes for the angular velocity to reach its steady state value), (2) the time response of the stress measuring transducer and its associated electronics, and (3) the time response of the data acquisition system. A potential additional limitation is the inertial time scale of the fluid, i.e. the time to develop steady state flow in an otherwise ideal viscometer. This time scale is $\tau_i = \rho h^2/\mu$ for Newtonian fluids, implying that $\tau_i \approx 10^{-5}\,s$, for a fluid of viscosity 100 Pa s in a typical viscometer geometry.

With most rheological instrumentation, item (1) is essentially fixed by the manufacturer's design. However, the information necessary to evaluate its potential effect is not usually given. Crawley and Graessley[76] and Chan and Powell[63] comprehensively characterized the relevant instrument parameters for Weissenberg rheogoniometers.

Developing fast time response stress transducers or carefully evaluating the possible effects of using factory-supplied stress measuring systems has received the most attention. Lockyer and Walters[77] showed that with a torsion bar based stress measuring system, which requires finite angular deflections, 'stress overshoot' could be observed for a Newtonian fluid, where it is essentially a 'ringing' of the stress measuring assembly. The two pioneering experimental studies using rheogoniometers were by Meissner[78] and Lee et al.[79] Meissner[78] developed a 'stiffened' torque and normal force measuring system based upon the existing linear variable displacement transducers. This approach has been followed by Zapas and

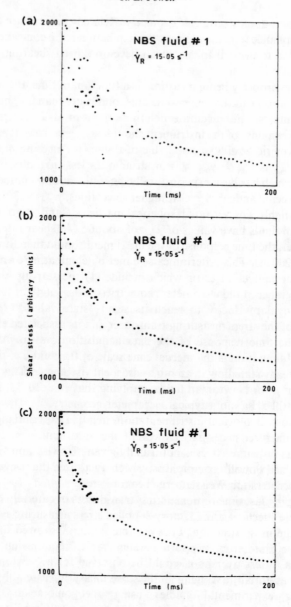

Fig. 9.9. Averaging of stress relaxation data to decrease noise. Seven experiments are run at the same shear rate and stored digitally: (a) the first run; (b) average of three data sets; (c) average of seven data sets.

Phillips,[72] Kee and Carreau[80] and Lewis and Shoemaker[81] who also showed that the transducer electronics may influence measurements by imposing their own time response on the detected signal. Lee *et al.*[79] retrofitted their rheogoniometer with piezoelectric measuring transducers having a time response of approximately 10^{-5} s. These transducers undergo small deflections upon the application of stresses ($< 1 \mu$m), and therefore they have the additional advantage of minimizing any changes in the viscometer geometry. During transient experiments, the charge generated by the applied stress is detected using a charge amplifier[63,79,82,83] which itself has a very short time response. The principal disadvantage of the piezoelectric transducer is signal drift due to charge leakage which makes long time steady state measurements difficult. Chan and Powell[63] found that this was reduced by measuring the charge directly using an electrometer.

The limitation imposed by the data logging device is, today, easily overcome by using a microcomputer-based data acquisition system.[63,73,81] For example, Chan and Powell[63] developed an inexpensive data acquisition system capable of time domain resolution of 0·5 ms which was achieved by sampling at frequencies up to 4 kHz. An additional, and potentially even greater, advantage of a microcomputer-based instrument over an analog system is that data are available in a form which can be processed directly. Ganani *et al.*[84] demonstrated that the signal-to-noise ratio for a set of transient data can be dramatically increased by averaging several sets of data obtained under the same shearing conditions. Figure 9.9 shows the results of such an averaging technique. The data at the top of Fig. 9.9 are the result of a single stress relaxation experiment, while the next two frames demonstrate the result averaging over three and seven repetitions, respectively. The digitized data can be readily operated upon by other data smoothing procedures, such as a three-point quadratic fit. The smoothed, digital data can be directly fitted to functional equations,[73,85,86] further streamlining the process of determining parameters in constitutive equations.

With computer control as well as computerized data acquisition it also becomes possible to execute more complicated shearing histories, such as those used by Gadala-Maria and Acrivos[54] and Moore.[86] Shearing initiation and data acquisition can be precisely linked. The acquired data can be fitted directly to a model, such as that proposed by Moore[86] for thixotropic materials. His model requires fitting data to a system of the form

$$\sigma^+ = \dot{\gamma}[C_{M5} + C_{M3}\{\lambda - (\lambda - C_{M4}) \exp\left[-(C_{M1} + C_{M2}\dot{\gamma})t\right]\}]$$
(9.100)

where

$$\lambda = \frac{C_{M1}}{C_{M1} + C_{M2}\gamma} \tag{9.101}$$

and C_{M1} to C_{M5} are constants.

Such a model cannot describe polymeric fluids having characteristic times associated with stress build-up. It does appear to describe some suspensions, particularly clays.[86] However, caution should be exercised, because modern techniques indicate that even suspensions may exhibit a stress growth time scale.[15,54] Equations (9.100) and (9.101) might adequately model materials when the stress maximum is reached almost instantaneously, and there is a period of stress decay to equilibrium. In that case, the digitized data could be used to determine C_{M1} to C_{M5} as follows: (1) calculate C_{M3} and C_{M1} from the initial value of σ^+; (2) perform a linear least-squares fit of $\ln[\sigma^+ - \sigma(\dot{\gamma})]$ versus t, at different shear rates, to find C_{M1} and C_{M2}; (3) determine C_{M5} by measuring $\sigma(\dot{\gamma})$ at a sufficiently high shear rate so that no shear dependence is observed; (4) calculate C_{M3} from steady state measurements; (5) use the result of step (1) to determine C_{M4} independently.

The effect of measurement geometry has been studied by comparing measurements of σ^+ and σ^- obtained using the cone and plate geometry with various cone angles[76,78] and using both the parallel plate and the cone and plate geometries.[69] For cone angles up to 8°, the transient shear stress response was dependent upon geometry, although the differences are generally within the measuring errors. Ganani and Powell[69] showed that the parallel plate geometry yielded transient shear stress data which, to within experimental error, overlapped data obtained using a 1° cone. The operational difficulty in using eqn (9.98), which was discussed in Section 9.3.1.2, makes parallel plates the geometry of choice only when the ability to vary the gap spacing is desired.[15]

9.3.2. Other Geometrical Configurations

9.3.2.1. Alternative Cone and Plate Geometries

The extended cone and plate geometry suggested by Jackson and Kaye[87] (see Fig. 9.5(b)) provides a method for determining the second normal stress function from total thrust normal force measurements. As opposed to the usual cone and plate flow (Section 9.2.1), the apex of the cone does not touch the plate. Rather, there is a finite distance between the apex and the plate, which is called h_c. Marsh and Pearson[88] showed that the characteristic shear rate is

$$\dot{\gamma}_{EC} = \frac{R\Omega}{h_c + R \tan \alpha} \tag{9.102}$$

and that

$$N_2(\dot{\gamma}_{EC}) = \left[\frac{\mathscr{F}}{R^2}\left(2 - \frac{\partial \ln \mathscr{F}}{\partial \ln h_c}\right) + N_1(\dot{\gamma}_{EC})\right]\frac{\Omega}{\Omega - \dot{\gamma}_{EC} \tan \alpha} \tag{9.103}$$

Using eqn (9.103), values of N_2 at $\dot{\gamma}_{EC}$ can be determined if N_1 is known in advance, for example by performing total thrust measurements with the usual cone and plate geometry (see Section 9.2.1). The partial derivative is taken with the angular velocity fixed, and it is evaluated at a particular gap separation. The experimental procedure to be followed in implementing this technique consists of measuring the total thrust as a function of the gap separation, calculating $(\partial \ln \mathscr{F}/\partial \ln h_c)$ and then using eqn (9.103) to find N_2. The value of the gap separation to be used in the calculation of N_2 should be determined as part of the experimental program. Jackson and Kaye[87] showed that good results could be obtained by extrapolating to $h_c = 0$, for which eqn (9.103) does not apply[88] and it is necessary to use

$$N_2(\dot{\gamma}) = -\frac{\tan \alpha}{R}\frac{d\mathscr{F}}{dh_c}\bigg|_{h_c=0} - \frac{dN_1}{d\dot{\gamma}} \tag{9.104}$$

In the expression, $\dot{\gamma}$ is the shear rate in a cone and plate viscometer (see eqn (9.19)), which is the value of $\dot{\gamma}_{EC}$ obtained from eqn (9.102) when $h_c = 0$ and α is small.

The truncated cone and plate geometry[27,89] provides another means of measuring normal stresses using a modified form of the cone and plate. This configuration (see Fig. 9.5(a)) is used in conjunction with pressure distribution rather than total thrust measurements. The flow in the gap is assumed to be the same as that for the parallel plates in the truncation region and for the cone and plate in the conical region, with a smooth transition between them. These assumptions have been shown valid for Newtonian[27] and shear thinning[26] fluids, and serve to validate Lodge's[89] analysis which showed that

$$N_2 = (N_1 + 2N_2) + \dot{\gamma}\frac{d}{d\dot{\gamma}}[(N_1 + 2N_2)(\ln(R/R_t)) - p(0)] \tag{9.105}$$

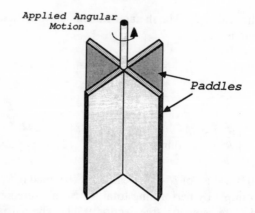

Applied Angular
Motion

Paddles

Fig. 9.10. Schematic of vanes for vane rheometer.

with the shear rate given by eqn (9.19). The quantity $(N_1 + 2N_2)$ is determined from measurements of $p(r)$ in the conical region (see Section 9.2.1) and $p(0)$ which is the pressure at the center of the plate.

9.3.2.2. Vane Rheometer

The vane rheometer has recently been shown to be a useful device for the measurement of yield stress in concentrated suspensions[90,91] and greases.[92] As described by Boger and his co-workers,[90,91] this method uses a four-bladed vane such as that shown schematically in Fig. 9.10. The vane is rotated at a constant angular velocity of less than 10 rpm and the torque acting on the vane is recorded.[90,91] As the vane rotates, the torque increases until it reaches a maximum, corresponding to the yield point, and then decays to steady state.

Assuming that effects due to the upper free surface and the container boundaries are negligible and that shearing occurs along a cylindrical surface of radius R_v and along flat surfaces of radius R_v, where R_v is the radius of the vanes, Dzuy and Boger[91] showed that the maximum torque is

$$\mathscr{T}_m = 2\pi R_v^2 L_v \sigma_y + 4\pi \int_0^R \sigma_e r^2 dr \qquad (9.106)$$

Here σ_y is the yield stress, L_v is the length of the vane and σ_e is the unknown shear stress distribution along the top and bottom, flat shearing surfaces. When σ_e is assumed to be known and equal to the yield stress, eqn (9.106) assumes the simplified form

$$\mathscr{T}_m = 2\pi R_v^3 (L_v/R_v + 2/3)\sigma_y \qquad (9.107)$$

From this expression the yield stress is calculated directly. To use eqn (9.106) we recognize that, for a given vane radius, the second term is constant. Measurements of the maximum torque for vanes of varying lengths should result in a linear relationship between $\mathscr{T}_m$ and L_v the slope of which is related to the yield stress. Yield stress values obtained using both equations agree well with values found by more 'conventional' techniques for determining the yield stress.[91]

This method has been revived by rheologists relatively recently, and there are few studies that demonstrate the problems associated with applying it to a wide variety of materials. Boger and his co-workers[90,91] have provided design criteria under which reliable measurements can be obtained for red muds (bauxite residue slurries), and suspensions of titanium dioxide, uranium oxide and brown coal. These include: $L_v/R_v < 7$, $R_{cyl}/R_v > 2$, $L_{TS}/R_v > 2$, and $L_{BS}/R_v > 1$, where R_{cyl} is the radius of the cylindrical container holding the sample, L_{TS} is the distance between the top surface of the vanes and the free surface of the sample, and L_{BS} is the distance between the vanes and the bottom surface of the container. Finally, we also note that the technique, as recently pursued,[90–92] uses a hard testing machine (see Sections 9.1 and 9.3.3) for measuring the yield stress. The technique also needs to be pursued with an applied stress device with a focus upon recently raised issues regarding the determination of yield stresses.[93,94]

9.3.2.3. Helical Screw Rheometer

The helical screw rheometer recently proposed by Kraynik and his co-workers[95,96] appears to offer advantages for use at high temperatures and pressures, with chemically reacting systems having a time varying viscosity, with suspensions, and as a process monitoring device. The instrument (see Fig. 9.11) is essentially a single-screw extruder having minimal flight clearance operating with a closed discharge. Two measurements are made: the angular velocity of the screw, and the pressure difference along two transducers located in the wall of the barrel. As the screw turns and the flights pass under the pressure transducers, a periodic pressure is recorded. The average pressure difference along the barrel, p, measured over several cycles, is related to the angular pressure gradient through

$$\Delta p = [L_B(\partial p/\partial\theta)]/(R_B \tan \delta) \qquad (9.108)$$

where L_B is the length along the barrel, R_B is the barrel radius and δ is the

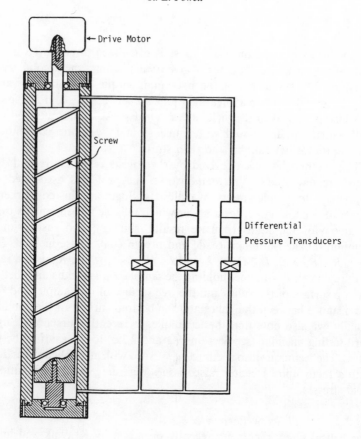

Fig. 9.11. Helical screw rheometer (courtesy of Dr Kraynik, Sandia National Laboratories).

helix angle of the screw. Kraynik *et al.*[95,96] showed that the angular pressure gradient could, in turn, be related to the parameters of specific constitutive relations, including the power law, Ellis, and Bingham models. In subsequent theoretical developments[97] the necessity of assuming any particular form of the constitutive relation in obtaining measurements of the shear viscosity versus shear rate has been eliminated.

9.3.3. Applied Stress Rheometry

When operating at steady state with standard rotational geometries, applied stress rheometers can yield the same information as rheometers

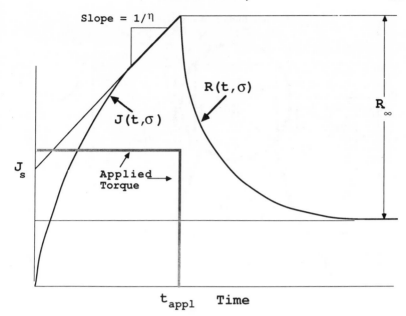

Fig. 9.12. Schematic of results from a creep and recovery test.

having fixed rotational speeds. The derivations in Section 9.2 apply except that, for applied stress rheometers, the shear stress is the independent variable, and the angular velocity or shear rate is measured.

The principal difference between the 'hard' machine and the applied stress rheometer (see Section 9.1) is realized when transient tests are performed. Section 9.3.1 described the transient test for the 'hard' device in which the test material is subjected to a sudden change in the shear rate and the time dependent stresses are measured. The corresponding experiment in an applied stress rheometer has the sample experience a sudden change in the shear stress imposed by one of the solid boundaries, with the resulting time dependent shear rate being measured. It is assumed that the applied shear stress instantaneously establishes a time dependent simple shearing flow (see Fig. 9.1). Figure 9.12 shows a typical result of such an experiment which is cast in terms of the creep compliance $J(t, \sigma) = \gamma/\sigma$, where γ is the strain. Initially the material exhibits time dependent behavior in which the shear rate is uniform across the gap but varies with time. At the longest times, the shear rate is constant and $J(t, \sigma)$ is linear. In this terminal region

$$J(t, \sigma) = J_s(\sigma) + t/\eta \qquad (9.109)$$

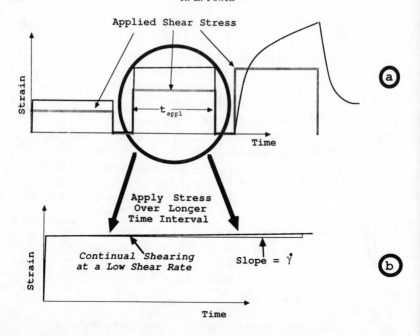

Fig. 9.13. Schematic of possible results from a series of creep tests aimed at measuring yield stress.

The property $J_s(\sigma)$ is the steady state compliance which depends upon the shear stress and which tends to a constant value as $\sigma \to 0$.[4,98] Another test often performed using an applied stress rheometer is the recoil test, which is also shown schematically in Fig. 9.12. The stress is applied up to time t_{appl}, at which point it is relieved. An elastic material then tends to recover some of the deformation, which is seen experimentally as a decrease in the total strain. The recoil function, $R(t, \sigma) = [\gamma(0) - \gamma(t)]/\gamma(0)$, is measured as well as the ultimate recoil, $R_\infty = \lim_{t \to \infty} R(t, \sigma)$. At sufficiently low values of the shear stress, for polymeric fluids, this property also approaches a constant value, with

$$\lim_{\sigma \to 0} J_s(\sigma) = \lim_{\sigma \to 0} R_\infty(\sigma) \tag{9.110}$$

Equation (9.110) provides a good means of checking results from an applied stress rheometer.[98,99] Other considerations for the use of such devices with polymeric fluids can be found in the papers of Plazek and his co-workers.[100,101]

The applied stress rheometer is an ideal instrument for yield stress determinations, when used with the standard geometries of Sections 9.2.1–9.2.3 or with a vane attachment (Section 9.3.2.2). Experimental programs can be designed in which increasing amounts of stress are applied over some time interval until 'yield' is detected. Two problems can arise from such a protocol. If two stresses are applied, σ_1 and σ_2 where $\sigma_2 > \sigma_1$, and yield is detected at σ_2 but not at σ_1, then it is considered that the yield point has been bracketed. Attempting to narrow the range between σ_1 and σ_2 may require waiting for several hours before the sample has had time to rebuild whatever structure it may have had before yield occurred.

The second problem is partly experimental and partly material. Figure 9.13 shows a schematic of the possible results of an experimental program meant to determine the yield stress. In all experiments the duration of the applied stress is t_{appl}. For the lowest stress, the sample reaches an equilibrium strain, with no additional, measurable deformation occurring. At the highest applied stress, flow occurs. In the middle, there is some question as to whether flow has taken place, i.e. whether the material has yielded. Extending the duration of the applied stress could reveal a curve such as that shown in Fig. 9.13(b). Here we clearly observe flow over a very long time, which implies that, at very low shear rates, the sample has a very high viscosity.[93] Measuring yield stress requires the test duration, which if too short may result in a high viscosity fluid being disguised as a material with a yield stress. When precision is desired, and long tests are to be performed, sample stability and electrical and mechanical drift (Section 9.2.4.6) can be the limiting factor.

REFERENCES

1. C. Truesdell and W. Noll, *Handbuch der Physik*, Vol. IIIA, Springer-Verlag, New York, 1965.
2. B. D. Coleman, H. Markovitz and W. Noll, *Viscometric Flows of Non-Newtonian Fluids*, Springer Tracts in Natural Philosophy, Vol. 5, Springer-Verlag, New York, 1966.
3. K. Walters, *Rheometry*, Chapman and Hall, London, 1975.
4. R. B. Bird, R. C. Armstrong and O. Hassager, *Dynamics of Polymeric Liquids*, Vol. 1, Fluid Mechanics, Wiley, New York, 1977.
5. J. R. A. Pearson, *Mechanics of Polymer Processing*, Elsevier Applied Science, London, 1985.
6. Z. Tadmoor and C. Gogos, *Principles of Polymer Processing*, Wiley, New York, 1979.
7. S. Middleman, *Fundamentals of Polymer Processing*, McGraw-Hill, New York, 1977.

Oliver and R. C. Ashton, *J. Non-Newt. Fluid Mech.*, 1980, **7**, 369.
9. D. R. Oliver and M. Shahidullah, *J. Non-Newt. Fluid Mech.*, 1983, **13**, 93.
10. M. Keentok, A. G. Georgescu, A. A. Sherwood and R. I. Tanner, *J. Non-Newt. Fluid Mech.*, 1980, **6**, 303.
11. J. F. Bell, *Handbuch der Physik*, Vol VIA/1, Springer-Verlag, New York, 1974.
12. D. F. Griffiths and K. Walters, *J. Fluid Mech.*, 1970, **42**, 379.
13. R. M. Turian, *Ind. Eng. Chem. Fund.*, 1972, **11**, 361.
14. D. Chan and R. L. Powell, *J. Non-Newt. Fluid Mech.*, 1984, **15**, 165.
15. E. Ganani and R. L. Powell, *J. Rheol.*, 1986, **30**, 995.
16. Y. Chan, J. L. White and Y. Oyanagi, *J. Rheol.*, 1978, **22**, 507.
17. M. Keentok and R. I. Tanner, *J. Rheol.*, 1982, **26**, 301.
18. J. M. Broadbent and A. S. Lodge, *Rheol. Acta*, 1971, **10**, 557.
19. W. M. Kulicke, G. Kiss and R. S. Porter, *Rheol. Acta*, 1977, **19**, 568.
20. N. Adams and A. S. Lodge, *Phil. Trans. Roy. Soc.* (London), 1964, **A256**, 1068.
21. K. Walters and N. D. Waters, in *Polymer Systems: Deformation and Flow*, R. E. Wetton and R. W. Whorlow (Eds), Macmillan, London, 1968, pp. 211–35.
22. J. M. Dealy, *Rheometers for Molten Plastics*, Van Nostrand Reinhold, New York, 1982.
23. D. C.-H. Cheng, *Chem. Eng. Sci.*, 1968, **23**, 895.
24. G. Heuser and E. Krause, *Rheol. Acta*, 1979, **18**, 553.
25. P. G. Drazin and W. H. Reid, *Hydrodynamic Stability*, Cambridge University Press, Cambridge, 1984.
26. D. J. Paddon and K. Walters, *Rheol. Acta*, 1979, **18**, 565.
27. T. H. Hou, *Rheol. Acta*, 1981, **20**, 14.
28. B. D. Coleman and H. Markovitz, *J. Appl. Phys.*, 1964, **35**, 1.
29. M. J. King and N. D. Waters, *Rheol. Acta*, 1970, **9**, 164.
30. M. Mooney and R. H. Ewart, *Physics*, 1934, **5**, 350.
31. F. Moore and L. J. Davies, *Trans. Brit. Ceram. Soc.*, 1956, **55**, 313.
32. D. D. Joseph and G. S. Beavers, *Arch. Rat. Mech. Anal.*, 1973, **49**, 321, 381.
33. G. S. Beavers and D. D. Joseph, *J. Non-Newt. Fluid Mech.*, 1979, **5**, 323.
34. R. M. Turian and R. B. Bird, *Chem. Eng. Sci.*, 1963, **18**, 689.
35. P.-J. Klijn, J. Ellenberger and J. M. H. Fortuin, *Rheol. Acta*, 1979, **18**, 303.
36. H. H. Winter, *Rheol. Acta*, 1972, **11**, 216.
37. H. H. Winter, *Int. J. Heat Mass Trans.*, 1971, **14**, 1203.
38. J. F. Hutton, *Proc. Roy. Soc.* (London), 1965, **A287**, 222.
39. J. F. Hutton, *Rheol. Acta*, 1969, **8**, 54.
40. R. I. Tanner and M. Keentok, *J. Rheol.*, 1983, **27**, 47.
41. W. O. Criminale, J. L. Ericksen and G. L. Filbey, *Arch. Rat. Mech. Anal.*, 1958, **1**, 410.
42. O. L. Forgacs, A. A. Robertson and S. G. Mason, *Pulp and Paper Mag. Can.*, 1958, **59**, 117.
43. V. Vand, *J. Phys. Coll. Chem.*, 1948, **52**, 277.
44. N. Thalen and D. Wahren, *Svensk Papperstidning*, 1964, **67**, 1.
45. L. L. Navickis and E. B. Bagley, *J. Rheol.*, 1983, **27**, 519.
46. M.A. Nawab and S.G. Mason, *J. Phys. Chem.*, 1958, **62**, 1248.

47. W. R. Blakney, *J. Coll. Interface Sci.*, 1966, **22**, 324.
48. A. L. Graham, L. A. Mondy, M. Gottlieb and R. L. Powell, *Appl. Phys. Lett.*, 1987, **50**, 127.
49. W. M. Milliken, M. Gottlieb, A. L. Graham, L. A. Mondy and R. L. Powell, submitted for publication.
50. V. Seshadri and S. P. Sutera, *J. Coll. Interface Sci.*, 1968, **27**, 101.
51. A. C. Li, W. J. Milliken, R. L. Powell and J. C. Slattery, submitted for publication.
52. T. E. Karis, D. C. Prieve and S. L. Rosen, *J. Rheol.*, 1984, **28**, 381.
53. D. G. Leighton and A. Acrivos, *J. Fluid Mech.* (in press).
54. F. Gadala-Maria and A. Acrivos, *J. Rheol.*, 1980, **24**, 799.
55. G. K. Batchelor, *An Introduction to Fluid Dynamics*, Cambridge University Press, Cambridge, 1967.
56. F. Ferrini, D. Ercolani, B. de Cindio, L. Nicodemo, L. Nicolais and S. Ranaudo, *Rheol. Acta*, 1979, **18**, 289.
57. D. J. Jeffrey and A. Acrivos, *A.I.Ch.E.J.*, 1976, **22**, 417.
58. D. V. Boger and A. V. R. Murthy, *Trans. Soc. Rheol.*, 1969, **13**, 405.
59. Instruction manual: *The Weissenberg Rheogoniometer Model R20*, Sangamo Weston Controls, Bognor Regis, Sussex, 1987.
60. A. Beris, R. C. Armstrong and R. A. Brown, *J. Non-Newt. Fluid Mech.*, 1983, **13**, 109.
61. D. C.-H. Cheng, *Rheol. Acta*, 1968, **7**, 85.
62. D. Cohen, L. Rakesh and R. L. Powell, presented at 57th Annual Meeting of the Society of Rheology, Ann Arbor, Michigan, 1985.
63. D. Chan and R. L. Powell, *J. Rheol.*, 1984, **28**, 449.
64. J. Lerthanapredakul, Phd dissertation, Washington University, St. Louis, Missouri, 1983.
65. E. Ganani, PhD dissertation, Washington University, St. Louis, Missouri, 1984.
66. C. F. Shoemaker and J. L. Lewis, to appear in *Encyclopedia of Fluid Mechanics*, Vol. 7, N. P. Cheremisinoff (Ed.) Gulf, 1988.
67. D. S. Soong, *Rubber Chem. Technol.*, 1981, **54**, 641.
68. P. Attané, J. M. Pierrard and G. Turrel, *J. Non-Newt. Fluid Mech.*, 1985, **18**, 295.
69. E. Ganani and R. L. Powell, *J. Rheol.*, 1985, **29**, 931.
70. P. R. Soskey and H. H. Winter, *J. Rheol.*, 1984, **28**, 625.
71. E. V. Menezes and W. W. Graessley, *J. Polym. Sci., Polym. Phys. Ed.*, 1982, **20**, 1817.
72. L. J. Zapas and J. C. Phillips, *J. Rheol.*, 1981, **25**, 405.
73. S.-F. Lin and R. S. Brodkey, *J. Rheol.*, 1985, **29**, 147.
74. M.-C. Yang, L. E. Scriven and C. W. Macosko, *J. Rheol.*, 1986, **30**, 1015.
75. K. Osaki, S. Ohta, M. Fukuda and M. Kurata, *J. Polym. Sci., Polym. Phys. Ed.*, 1976, **14**, 1701.
76. R. L. Crawley and W. W. Graessley, *Trans. Soc. Rheol.*, 1977, **21**, 19.
77. M. A. Lockyer and K. Walters, *Rheol. Acta*, 1976, **15**, 179.
78. J. Meissner, *J. Appl. Polym. Sci.*, 1972, **16**, 2877.
79. K. H. Lee, L. G. Jones, K. Pandalai and R. S. Brodkey, *Trans. Soc. Rheol.*, 1970, **14**, 555.

80. D. De Kee and P. J. Carreau, *J. Rheol.*, 1984, **28**, 109.
81. J. L. Lewis and C. F. Shoemaker, *Rheol. Acta*, 1985, **24**, 58.
82. R. W. Higman, *Rheol. Acta*, 1973, **12**, 533.
83. P. Attané, P. Le Roy and G. Turrel, *J. Non-Newt. Fluid Mech.*, 1980, **6**, 269.
84. E. Ganani, D. Chan and R. L. Powell, *Proc. Ann. Tech. Conf. Soc. Plastics Engrs*, New Orleans, Louisiana, 1984, p. 346.
85. P. Attané, G. Turrel. J. M. Pierraid and P. J. Caneau, *J. Rheol.*, 1988, **32**, 23.
86. F. Moore, *Trans. Brit. Ceram. Soc.*, 1959, **58**, 470.
87. R. Jackson and A. Kaye, *Brit. J. Appl. Phys.* 1966, **17**, 1355.
88. B. D. Marsh and J. R. A. Pearson, *Rheol. Acta*, 1968, **7**, 326.
89. A. S. Lodge, *Rheol. Acta*, 1971, **10**, 554.
90. Q. D. Nguyen and D. V. Boger, *J. Rheol.*, 1983, **27**, 321.
91. N. Q. Dzuy and D. V. Boger, *J. Rheol.*, 1985, **29**, 335.
92. M. Keentok, J. F. Milthorpe and E. O. Donovan, *J. Non-Newt. Fluid Mech.*, 1985, **17**, 23.
93. H. A. Barnes and K. Walters, *Rheol. Acta*, 1984, **24**, 323.
94. D. C.-H. Cheng,*Rheol. Acta*, 1986, **25**, 542.
95. A. M. Kraynik, J. H. Aubert, R. N. Chapman and D. C. Gyure, *Proc. Ann. Tech. Conf. Soc. Plastics Engrs.*, New Orleans, 1984, p. 405.
96. A. M. Kraynik, J. H. Aubert and R. N. Chapman, *Proc. IXth Int. Congr. Rheol.*, 1984, **4**, 77.
97. A. M. Kraynik, L. Romero, M. Baer and M. Dillon, presented at 58th Annual Meeting Soc. Rheol., Tulsa, Oklahoma, 1986.
98. L. Rakesh, R. Lam and R. L. Powell, *J. Polym. Sci., Polym. Phys. Ed.*, 1985, **23**, 1263.
99. C. P. Wong and G. C. Berry, *Polymer*, 1979, **20**, 229.
100. D. J. Plazek, *Meth. Exp. Phys.*, 1980, **16c**, 1.
101. D. J. Plazek, *J. Polym. Sci. (A-2)*, 1968, **6**, 621.

Chapter 10

Oscillatory Rheometry

GÉRARD MARIN

Laboratoire de Physique des Matériaux Industriels, Université de Pau et des Pays de l'Adour, Pau, France

NOTATION

a, a_0	deformation and maximum deformation, eqn (10.2)
A	shape factor, eqns (10.20), (10.22), (10.25)–(10.30)
B	spring constant, eqn (10.20)
B	torsional rigidity, eqns (10.33)–(10.36)
C_y	couple in Kepes balance rheometer, eqn (10.48)

d	offset distance in orthogonal rheometer
E_{st}, E_d	storage and loss moduli, eqns (10.10) and (10.11) respectively
G_N^0	Plateau modulus of entangled polymers
h	cylinder length, eqns (10.26)–(10.29)
I	moment of inertia, eqns (10.67)–(10.72)
K	instrument compliance, eqns (10.92)–(10.95)
n	number of peaks counted in logarithmic decrement, eqn (10.66)
S	surface area of upper face, eqn (10.1)
T_f	frictional couple, eqn (10.47)
α	inertia effect, eqn (10.80)
λ	instrument constant, eqns (10.50b)–(10.58)
σ^-, $\sigma^+(t)$	stress relaxation and stress growth functions
τ_0	terminal relaxation time
ϕ	phase difference, eqn (10.2)

Oscillatory tests belong to the general framework of dynamic measurements in which usually both stress and strain vary harmonically with time. In most cases, the relevant strains or strain rates are small enough to stay within the limits of linear viscoelasticity. From a theoretical point of view, this simplification avoids the use of complex non-linear theories; the mathematical theory of linear viscoelasticity[1] constitutes a convenient and accurate analytical tool to analyse the experimental data. So this family of rheological techniques may be defined as 'mechanical spectroscopy', and the mathematical formalism of the usual spectroscopic method of physics and physical chemistry may be applied to dynamic mechanical experiments (see Section 10.2.5).

The dynamic properties of viscoelastic materials are of considerable practical interest, as the processability of these materials can often be directly related to the 'viscous' and 'elastic' parameters derived from such measurements. In the case of thermostable materials, the dynamic properties can yield insight into the microstructure of the material under study, as well as the conventional methods of physical chemistry.[2] This class of rheological experiments may also offer convenient methods to determine the thermodynamic transition temperatures, when measurements are made as a function of temperature. In the case of non-thermostable materials the evolution of the dynamic viscoelastic properties as a function of time reflects changes in the molecular structure. Consequently these techniques are to be considered in a wide range of applications, from the conventional rheological methods in the frequency domain to sophisticated transient experiments designed to characterize, for example, the kinetics of chemical reactions in the molten (condensed) state.

10.1. INTRODUCTION: MATERIAL FUNCTIONS DERIVED FROM OSCILLATORY MEASUREMENTS

Let us consider that a sinusoidal force $F = F_0 \cos \omega t$ is applied to the upper face of a parallelepipedic block of viscoelastic material (Fig. 10.1), where F_0 is the amplitude of the force and ω is the angular frequency ($\omega = 2\pi f$) of the applied force. We will assume here that h is small, so that we may neglect the inertia forces and assume that the strain is the same at all points. In that case, the stress σ is

$$\sigma = \frac{F}{S} = \frac{F_0}{S} \cos \omega t = \sigma_0 \cos \omega t \qquad (10.1)$$

where S is the surface of the upper face.

The application of harmonic stress does not result instantaneously in a harmonic strain; at small frequencies, the steady state is reached after a time of the order of magnitude of the longest relaxation time of the material under study. Once the steady state is reached, the deformation a is

$$a = a_0 \cos (\omega t - \phi) \qquad (10.2)$$

and the strain, assumed to be the same within the sample, is

$$\gamma = \frac{a_0}{h} \cos (\omega t - \phi) = \gamma_0 \cos (\omega t - \phi) \qquad (10.3)$$

where a_0 is the amplitude of the deformation.

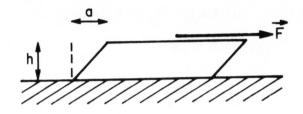

Fig. 10.1. Dynamic shearing of a thin parallelepipedic block.

For perfect solid behaviour, the stress is in phase with the strain ($\phi = 0$); in the case of a purely viscous liquid, the strain is in quadrature with the stress ($\phi = 90°$).

At large amplitudes, harmonic stresses do not usually result in harmonic strains (and vice versa); large amplitude periodic deformations are mainly used to test constitutive equations and/or molecular models, but are not of the same practical interest as other non-linear experiments such as steady shearing or transient experiments (before and after steady state) in the field of applied rheology. In the case of small deformations, i.e. within the framework of linear viscoelasticity, the phase lag ϕ and the ratio γ_0/σ_0 (peak strain/peak stress) are material properties, i.e. are constant at a given frequency.

As we will be dealing with differential equations of harmonic functions, it is more convenient to use complex functions. The complex stress may be defined as

$$\sigma^* = \sigma_0 \exp(j\omega t) \tag{10.4}$$

and the complex strain will be

$$\gamma^* = \gamma_0 \exp[j(\omega t - \phi)] = \gamma_0 \exp(j\omega t)\exp(-j\phi) \tag{10.5}$$

The true stress σ is the real part of the complex stress

$$\sigma = \mathscr{R}(\sigma^*) = \mathscr{R}[\sigma_0 \exp(j\omega t)] \tag{10.6}$$

whereas the true strain is

$$\gamma = \mathscr{R}(\gamma^*) = \mathscr{R}\{\gamma_0 \exp[j(\omega t - \phi)]\} \tag{10.7}$$

We are now ready to define the three complex functions that relate the stress to the strain or rate of strain. These material functions of linear viscoelasticity are *not* independent, and it is easy to derive each one from another through simple algebraic relations. When using complex functions, time appears as $\exp(j\omega t)$ in the stress or strain expression, so their ratio will only be a function of the circular frequency ω.

10.1.1. The Complex Shear Modulus
The complex shear modulus, $G^*(\omega)$,

$$G^*(\omega) = \frac{\text{complex stress}}{\text{complex strain}} = \frac{\sigma^*}{\gamma^*} = G'(\omega) + jG''(\omega) \tag{10.8}$$

where $j = \sqrt{-1}$. $G^*(\omega)$ may be experimentally determined from oscillatory measurements at a given strain amplitude. The real part of this function is called the 'storage' modulus, $G'(\omega)$, and gives the in-phase stress to strain ratio. The imaginary part of the complex modulus, $G''(\omega)$, is the out-of-phase stress to strain ratio.

From an energy viewpoint, the total elastic energy stored within a full cycle is zero:

$$E = \oint G'\gamma \, d\gamma = 0 \tag{10.9}$$

However, the maximum elastic energy is stored during a quarter cycle:

$$E_{st} = \int_0^{\gamma_0} G'\gamma \, d\gamma = \frac{1}{2} G' \gamma_0^2 \tag{10.10}$$

Within the same period, the dissipated energy is

$$E_d = \int_0^{\gamma_0} G'' \frac{\dot{\gamma}}{\omega} \, d\gamma = \frac{1}{4} \pi G'' \gamma_0^2 \tag{10.11}$$

where $\dot{\gamma}$ is the rate of strain. Hence the ratio of the dissipated energy to the stored energy during a quarter cycle is

$$\frac{E_d}{E_{st}} = \frac{\pi}{2} \frac{G''}{G'} = \frac{\pi}{2} \tan\phi \tag{10.12}$$

We have displayed on Fig. 10.2 the schematic variation of the complex shear modulus of a high molecular weight polymer having a narrow distribution of molecular weights as a function of circular frequency ω. At the lowest frequencies (terminal region of relaxation), the double logarithmic plot of $G'(\omega)$ and $G''(\omega)$ gives limiting slopes of 2 and 1 respectively; within this domain of relaxation, the behaviour of the material is mainly liquid behaviour ($G' \ll G''$), and three parameters may be derived from this analysis: (i) the zero-shear viscosity, η_0; (ii) the limiting compliance, J_e^0; (iii) the 'terminal' relaxation time, $\tau_0 = \eta_0 J_e^0$.[2]

At intermediate frequencies, the real part of the complex modulus is nearly constant ($G'(\omega) \approx G_N^0$), showing quasi-elastic behaviour: the temporary network of entanglements formed in a melt of long macromolecular chains appears to be permanent in that time (or frequency) scale. The values of the parameters η_0, J_e^0, τ_0 and G_N^0 yield direct insight into the molecular structure of these materials. Increasing frequency enables one to focus on smaller parts of the molecules, and the behaviour observed at high frequencies characterizes the relaxation of small parts of the molecule (i.e. a few monomeric units); the glassy modulus, G_g, measured at high

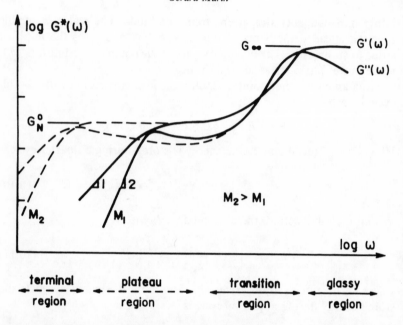

Fig. 10.2. Schematic diagram of the complex shear modulus of a bulk polymer as a function of frequency; M is the polymer molecular weight.

frequencies is of the same order of magnitude for all organic materials ($\sim 10^9\,\text{Pa}$), and ultrasonic methods are more suitable in this frequency range than oscillatory rheometry. One can locate the limit of applicability of oscillatory rheometry in the transition region between the rubbery behaviour and the glassy behaviour ($\omega \approx 100\text{--}1000\,\text{rad s}^{-1}$).

10.1.2. The Complex Compliance

The complex compliance, $J^*(\omega)$, is defined as

$$J^*(\omega) = \frac{\text{complex strain}}{\text{complex stress}} = \frac{\gamma^*}{\sigma^*}$$

$$= \frac{1}{G^*(\omega)} = J'(\omega) - jJ''(\omega) \qquad (10.13)$$

J^* is the reciprocal of the complex modulus G^*; it can be derived from oscillatory measurements at a given stress amplitude. Otherwise the compliance $J^*(\omega)$ may be calculated from the corresponding values of $G'(\omega)$

and $G''(\omega)$ through the equations

$$J' = \frac{G'}{G'^2 + G''^2} \tag{10.14a}$$

$$J'' = \frac{G''}{G'^2 + G''^2} \tag{10.14b}$$

Conversely

$$G' = \frac{J'}{J'^2 + J''^2} \tag{10.15a}$$

$$G'' = \frac{J''}{J'^2 + J''^2} \tag{10.15b}$$

In the case of a viscoelastic liquid, it may be useful to define a 'retardational' compliance:

$$J_r^*(\omega) = J^*(\omega) - \frac{1}{j\omega\eta_0} \tag{10.16}$$

where η_0 is the zero-shear viscosity of the liquid under study; hence

$$J_r'(\omega) = J'(\omega) \tag{10.17a}$$

$$J_r''(\omega) = J''(\omega) - \frac{1}{\omega\eta_0} \tag{10.17b}$$

This way of analysing the data allows us to separate the viscoelastic retarded behaviour from the viscous flow.[3] Typical variations of $J'(\omega)$ and $J''(\omega)$ for a polymer melt are given in Section 10.2.5 (Fig. 10.13). The parameters of linear viscoelasticity (η_0, J_e^0, τ_0) described in Section 10.1.1 can also be derived from an analysis in terms of the complex compliance $J^*(\omega)$. In Fig. 10.3, the *retardational* compliance $J_r^*(\omega)$ is plotted in the complex plane (imaginary part $J_r''(\omega)$ as a function of the real part $J'(\omega)$), which is the mechanical analogy of the Cole–Cole diagram for complex dielectric permittivity. This *linear* plot is much more sensitive to structural changes in the test samples than the usual double-logarithmic plots of either $J^*(\omega)$ or $G^*(\omega)$. The two retardation domains observed on Fig. 10.3 may be directly related to the molecular characteristics of the material under study.[4]

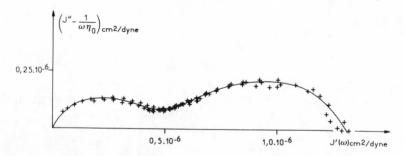

Fig. 10.3. Complex retardational compliance in the complex plane for a high molecular weight polymer (polystyrene; $M = 390\,000$).[4]

10.1.3. The Complex Viscosity

The complex viscosity, $\eta^*(\omega)$, is defined as

$$\eta^*(\omega) = \frac{\text{complex stress}}{\text{complex rate of strain}} = \frac{\sigma^*}{\dot{\gamma}^*(\omega)} = \frac{G^*(\omega)}{j\omega}$$

$$= \eta'(\omega) - j\eta''(\omega) \tag{10.18}$$

Hence

$$\eta' = \frac{G''}{\omega} \tag{10.19a}$$

$$\eta'' = \frac{G'}{\omega} \tag{10.19b}$$

The variations of $\eta'(\omega)$ and $\eta''(\omega)$ as a function of frequency have been plotted on Fig. 10.4 for the same sample as in Section 10.1.2. A linear plot of the same functions in the complex plane is shown in Fig. 10.5. An analysis in terms of complex viscosity focuses mainly on the terminal region of relaxation, and the viscoelastic parameters of that particular relaxation domain are easily derived from the Cole–Cole analysis,[5,6] whereas these domains are strongly coupled in the conventional logarithmic curves of the shear modulus $G^*(\omega)$.

10.2. TEST METHODS IN OSCILLATORY RHEOMETRY

The test methods used in oscillatory rheometry fall into two categories. The balance rheometer and the orthogonal rheometer are the most

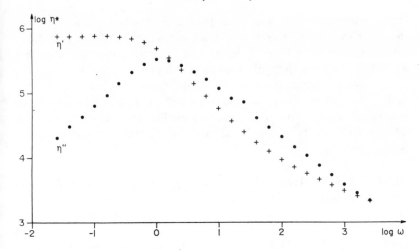

Fig. 10.4. Real and imaginary parts of the complex viscosity as a function of frequency (polystyrene; $M = 110\,000$; $T = 160\,°C$).

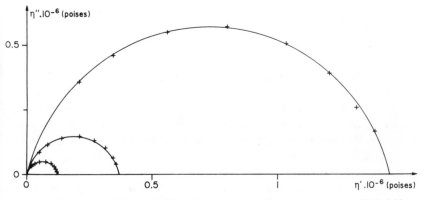

Fig. 10.5. Cole–Cole plot of complex viscosities at various temperatures (156, 166, and 176 °C) for the same sample as in Fig. 10.4.

popular instruments of the category that involves a steady rotation of boundary surfaces at the same angular velocity; they are described in Section 10.2.2. The other category, which we shall refer to as *conventional rheometers* after Walters,[7] may be divided into two groups. Most instruments operate at controlled angular or linear harmonic displacement; this group may be referred to as *controlled strain rheometers*. Fewer rheometers operate with a controlled harmonic torque (rotary rheometers) or force (linear displacement rheometers) applied to a boundary surface; these are the *controlled stress rheometers*. Controlling the stress (torque/force) rather than the strain (angular/linear displacement) may be useful, especially when dealing with highly non-linear samples or materials presenting a yield point; however, this method requires more complicated electronics in the drive system. The controlled strain and controlled stress rheometers belong, however, to the same group of oscillatory rheometers, as far as linear viscoelasticity is concerned, and such methods are described in Section 10.2.1.

10.2.1. Controlled Torque (Force) and Controlled Displacement Methods

The main experimental arrangements for liquids are presented schematically in Fig. 10.6. The diagrams (a)–(c) present the same experimental geometries as those used for steady shearing flows: the cone–plate (a), parallel plates (b), and coaxial cylinders (Couette flow) geometries (c). In that case, a harmonic displacement is generated at one of the boundary surfaces, while the torque is measured on the other. In the schematic diagrams (a)–(c), the drive system is located on the upper part while the torque is measured on the lower part. In the newest generation of instruments, the angular displacement of the torque measurement part is negligible, and maximum angular stiffness is desired. Furthermore, a large axial stiffness is now achieved on the cone–plate and parallel plates instruments, in order to avoid widening of the sample gap under the effect of the high normal forces developed in highly viscoelastic liquids (see Section 10.2.6).

For the older generation of instruments, the oscillation of the controlled displacement surface generates a harmonic displacement of the other surface, that is generally the upper part supported by a torsion wire or an equivalent elastic device. The theory for this type of instrument will be presented at the end of this section.

When a harmonic torque or force of amplitude T_0 is applied to the mobile boundary of inertia I (Fig. 10.6(a–c)) or mass M (Fig. 10.6(d–f)), the displacement θ^* (either angular or linear) will become harmonic, and the equation of motion will be

$$T^*(\omega; t) = T_0 \exp(j\omega t) = I\frac{\mathrm{d}^2\theta^*}{\mathrm{d}t^2}$$

$$+ [AG^*(\omega) + B]\theta^*(\omega) \qquad (10.20)$$

where A is a shape factor depending on the test geometry; the mass M replaces the moment of inertia in cases (d)–(f). In some situations the mass

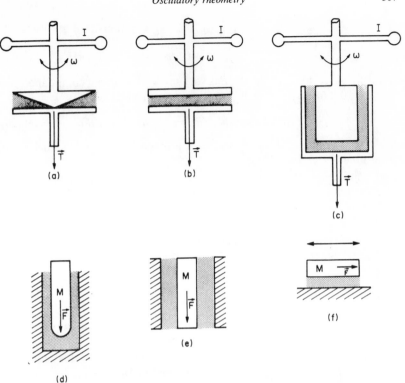

Fig. 10.6. The main geometries used in dynamics tests for viscoelastic liquids: (a) cone–plate; (b) parallel plates, torsion; (c) concentric cylinders, rotation; (d) annular pumping; (e) concentric cylinders, axial motion; (f) 'sandwich' rheometer.

M is acted on by a torsion wire (a–c) or a spring (d–f), producing a force (torque) $B\theta^*$. When the steady state is reached, the solution of eqn (10.20) is

$$\theta^*(\omega; t) = \theta_0 \exp[j(\omega t - \phi)] \tag{10.21}$$

where θ_0 is the displacement amplitude and ϕ is the phase lag. So, dividing eqn (10.20) by $\exp(j\omega t)$:

$$T_0 = -I\omega^2\theta_0\exp(-j\phi) + [AG^*(\omega) + B]\theta_0\exp(-j\phi) \tag{10.22}$$

or

$$T_0 \exp (j\phi) = \theta_0(-I\omega^2 + AG^* + B) = \theta_0$$
$$\times (-I\omega^2 + AG' + B + jAG'') \quad (10.23)$$

In the most recent instruments, B is very small (instrument compliance; see Section 10.2.6) and I is negligible at low frequencies, so

$$T_0 \exp (j\phi) = \theta_0 AG^* = \theta_0 A(G' + jG'') \quad (10.24)$$

So, a measurement of T_0, θ_0 and ϕ at a given frequency is sufficient to determine $G'(\omega)$ and $G''(\omega)$.

We shall now discuss the various test geometries (Fig. 10.6(a–f)) and give the relevant shape factor A in each case.

10.2.1.1. Cone–Plate
The test material is held between a plate of radius **R** and a cone of angle α_0 (Fig. 10.6(a))

$$A = \frac{2\pi R^3}{3\alpha_0} \quad (10.25)$$

This equation is valid only at cone-angle values small enough (typically 1–10°) to obtain a laminar flow. The availability of a constant shear rate at all points in the material is the most interesting feature of this geometry, especially when working on highly non-Newtonian systems, such as high molecular weight polymers or polyphasic systems.

10.2.1.2. Parallel Plates
The test piece is a cylindrical flat rod of radius **R** and thickness h:

$$A = \frac{\pi R^4}{2h} \quad (10.26)$$

In parallel plate geometry (Fig. 10.6(b)) the shear deformation is maximum at the plate edge and zero at the centre, so the shear rate is not uniform at all points in the material; as a consequence, one has to check carefully that the amplitude of the input motion is small enough to verify the linearity hypothesis. This geometry has however several advantages: for high viscosity materials it may be difficult to squeeze the sample between a cone and plate in the Section 10.2.1.1 geometry, and parallel-plate geometry is a convenient alternative. In the same way, when working on thermosetting or crosslinking materials, it is easier to remove a sample from a parallel-plate set-up once the experiment has been completed.

10.2.1.3. Concentric Cylinders

In the case of oscillatory shearing between two concentric cylinders (Fig. 10.6(c), the inner cylinder of radius R_1 and length h is given forced harmonic oscillations about its axis while the resultant harmonic torque is measured on the outer cylinder of the same length and radius R_2. The shape factor is the same as for a Couette flow:

$$A = 4\pi h \frac{R_1^2 R_2^2}{R_2^2 - R_1^2} \tag{10.27}$$

10.2.1.4. Annular Pumping

The annular pumping geometry is given on Fig. 10.6(d); the sample is located between two concentric cylinders, the closed bottom of the outer cylinder acting as a fluid reservoir. The up and down motion of the inner cylinder compresses and forces the sample up the annulus. If the reservoir is sufficiently large to neglect shear below the inner cylinder, the shape factor is[8]

$$A = \frac{2\pi h}{\ln\left(\dfrac{R_2}{R_1}\right) - \dfrac{R_2^2 - R_1^2}{R_2^2 + R_1^2}} \tag{10.28}$$

In the case of highly viscoelastic materials such as polymer melts, the shear and elongation occurring at the edge of the inner cylinder may have drastic effects on the measured forces, and the results obtained with this type of geometry are to be regarded mainly as qualitative.

10.2.1.5. Concentric Cylinders; Axial Motion

The edge effects are better mastered in the case of axial motion of the inner cylinder of a coaxial cylinder system, the sample being located within the gap between the cylinders without being pushed up by the inner cylinder (Fig. 10.6(e)):

$$A = \frac{2\pi h}{\ln\left(R_2/R_1\right)} \tag{10.29}$$

The drawback of this geometry is that its application is limited to high viscosity materials, so that surface tension holds the sample within the gap. Otherwise the gap has to be very small and perfect alignment of the two cylinders has to be achieved.

10.2.1.6. The 'Sandwich' Rheometer

The simplest geometry (Fig. 10.6(f)) for oscillatory shear is not the easiest to set up and to use, because of the importance of edge effects and the difficulty in building rigid instruments (the normal forces developed in shearing tend to increase the gap **h**) with a perfectly linear harmonic motion; this geometry is the only one, among the six presented here, having no symmetry of revolution about the axes of forces or torques. Neglecting the edge effects, the shape factor is

$$A = S/h \qquad (10.30)$$

where S is the effective surface area of the sample and h is the gap.

For the first generation rotary rheometers, one of the boundary surfaces is oscillated with a known angular amplitude while the angular motion of the other surface is measured, that surface being generally the upper one supported by a torsion wire or an elastic device with a calibrated elastic constant. The oscillatory motion of the driven part is measured by its angular position:

$$\theta_1^*(\omega; t) = \theta_1 \exp(j\omega t) \qquad (10.31)$$

On reaching the steady state, the suspended part will oscillate at the same frequency with an angular position θ_2^* generally out of phase with θ_1^*:

$$\theta_2^*(\omega; t) = \theta_2^* \exp[j(\omega t + \phi)] \qquad (10.32)$$

where ϕ is the phase lead of the suspended member. The equivalent of eqn (10.20) in that case will be

$$B\theta_2^* + I\frac{d^2\theta_2^*}{dt^2} = AG^*(\theta_1^* - \theta_2^*) \qquad (10.33)$$

where B is the torsional rigidity of the torsion wire. Dividing eqn (10.33) by $\exp(j\omega t)$, we can write

$$(B - I\omega^2)\theta_2 \exp(j\phi) = AG^*[\theta_1 - \theta_2 \exp(j\phi)] \qquad (10.34)$$

and

$$G^*(\omega) = \frac{B - I\omega^2}{A} \frac{\theta_2 \exp(j\phi)}{\theta_1 - \theta_2 \exp(j\phi)} \qquad (10.35)$$

so

$$G'(\omega) = \frac{B - I\omega^2}{A} \frac{(\theta_2/\theta_1)(\cos\phi - \theta_2/\theta_1)}{(\theta_2/\theta_1)^2 - 2(\theta_2/\theta_1)\cos\phi + 1} \qquad (10.36a)$$

$$G''(\omega) = \frac{B - I\omega^2}{A} \frac{(\theta_2/\theta_1)\sin\phi}{(\theta_2/\theta_1)^2 - 2(\theta_2/\theta_1)\cos\phi + 1} \qquad (10.36b)$$

10.2.2. The Orthogonal Rheometer, the Balance Rheometer, and New Rheometer Designs

For conventional rheometers, the complex functions of linear viscoelasticity are determined by subjecting the sample to a harmonic motion of small amplitude. However, it is not necessary to create an unsteady motion to determine G^*, J^* or η^*: some new geometries have been recently offered that generate flows involving a steady rotation of the sample, but for which fluid elements are subjected to a small harmonic deformation. The most commonly used of this class of geometries are the ERD (eccentric rotating discs) rheometer and the tilted sphere (balance rheometer), both being available in recent commercial instruments (see Chaper 13).

Besides the basic interest in original flow situations, there are other reasons for interest in this type of rheometer:

(a) In the case of a Newtonian fluid, an exact solution of the full Navier–Stokes equations, including inertia, can be derived;[7] for a viscoelastic material, the governing equations of motion are the Navier–Stokes equations with complex viscosity replacing Newtonian viscosity.

(b) The real and imaginary parts of the complex functions of viscoelasticity can be obtained separately, as the basic principle of these instruments is to measure forces or torques in two perpendicular directions, without the need for determining a phase lag as in conventional rheometers; the precise measurement of a phase lag (especially when $\phi \approx 0$ and $\phi \approx 90°$) involves a complex electronic network that may introduce unwanted phase shifts, so in principle these new geometries should give better resolution.

10.2.2.1. The Orthogonal Rheometer

The orthogonal rheometer or ERD (eccentric rotating discs) rheometer was introduced by Gent[9] in 1960 and then popularized by Maxwell.[10] The test geometry consists of two parallel plates rotating at the same angular velocity ω. The two normal axes of the plates are parallel but not coincident; the distance d between the two axes is small compared with the gap between the plates h (see schematic diagram on Fig. 10.7). The two components of the force, along the offset d, and perpendicular to that direction, are measured as a function of frequency. From these forces G^*, η^* or J^* can be determined.

Gérard Marin

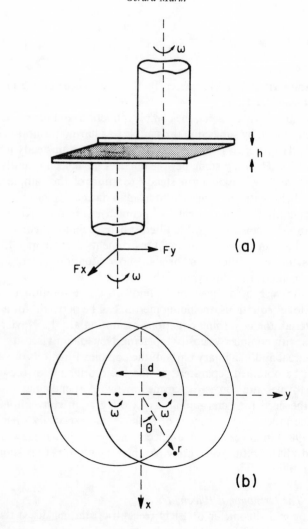

Fig. 10.7. The orthogonal (or ERD: eccentric rotating discs) rheometer: (a) vertical cross-section; (b) view from above.

For a purely elastic body, it is easy to derive the constant force F_y created along the y-axis by a displacement d of the upper face of a rod of radius R and length h:

$$F_y = -G\pi R^2 \frac{d}{h} \qquad (10.37)$$

where G is the shear modulus of the elastic rod. Rotation of both discs through the same angle (or at the same angular velocity) will create no other force, as there is no torsion of the cylinder. Let us now consider a purely viscous material. A fluid element on the lower plate will have a velocity v_y along the y-axis:

$$v_y = \omega x \tag{10.38a}$$

if the origin of the axes is chosen in the plane of the lower disc, midway between the disc axes; see the schematic diagram Fig. 10.7(b). Thus the component of the velocity along the x-axis is

$$v_x = -\omega \left(y + \frac{d}{2} \right) \tag{10.38b}$$

In the same way, for a fluid particle located on the upper disc:

$$v_y = \omega x \tag{10.39a}$$

$$v_x = -\omega \left(y - \frac{d}{2} \right) \tag{10.39b}$$

Consequently, the strain rate is zero in the y direction, and the strain rate in the x direction is

$$\dot{\gamma}_x = \omega \frac{d}{h} \tag{10.40}$$

So the force F_x exerted in the x direction for a purely viscous fluid is

$$F_x = -\pi R^2 \eta \omega \frac{d}{h} \tag{10.41}$$

where η is the fluid viscosity.

This simple demonstration shows how this geometry can give, by the measurement of two separate forces (F_x and F_y), the 'elastic' and 'viscous' response of materials. A more rigorous demonstration for the case of viscoelastic material may be presented[7] in a cylindrical coordinate system (r, θ, z) with the same origin of axes as before (lower plate midway between axes). In this coordinate system, the appropriate velocity distribution for ERD flow is

$$v_r = \frac{\omega d}{h} \left(z - \frac{h}{2} \right) \cos \theta \tag{10.42a}$$

$$v_\theta = r\omega - \frac{\omega d}{h}\left(z - \frac{h}{2}\right)\sin\theta \qquad (10.42b)$$

$$v_z = 0 \qquad (10.42c)$$

The relevant stress components σ_{zr} and $\sigma_{z\theta}$ are

$$\sigma_{zr} = \frac{d}{h}\left(G'\sin\theta + G''\cos\theta\right) \qquad (10.43a)$$

$$\sigma_{z\theta} = \frac{d}{h}\left(G'\cos\theta - G''\sin\theta\right) \qquad (10.43b)$$

We are now able to calculate the two components of the tangential force acting on the lower plate:[7]

$$F_x = -\int_0^R \int_0^{2\pi} [\sigma_{rz}\cos\theta - \sigma_{z\theta}\sin\theta]r\,d\theta\,dr \qquad (10.44a)$$

$$F_y = -\int_0^R \int_0^{2\pi} [\sigma_{rz}\sin\theta + \sigma_{z\theta}\cos\theta]r\,d\theta\,dr \qquad (10.44b)$$

So

$$F_x = -\frac{d}{h}\pi R^2 G'' \qquad (10.45a)$$

and

$$F_y = -\frac{d}{h}\pi R^2 G' \qquad (10.45b)$$

which are the same as the 'intuitive' equations (10.37) and (10.41). These equations may be condensed in a complex form:

$$\overline{F^*(\omega)} = F_x - jF_y = -\frac{d\pi R^2}{jh}G^*(\omega) \qquad (10.46)$$

So the forces F_x and F_y may be directly converted into dynamic data.

The above theory assumes that both discs are rotating with the same angular velocity ω; in experimental devices, one disc is driven while the other rotates freely and follows through viscous drag. In practice there is a slight difference in the speeds of the discs: the stresses produced by the flow will cause equal and opposite forces F_{x1} and F_{x2} to act on the axes of the lower and upper disc respectively. Thus, a net torque dF_x will act about the axis of the lower disc (free to rotate). To balance this torque, the free disc rotates in fact at a slightly smaller angular velocity, causing a small torsional flow to occur. In addition, there is a frictional couple T_f due to the friction of the free rotating disc bearing. The velocity lag Δw has been calculated for a viscoelastic liquid by Davis and Macosko,[11] using the Lodge integral constitutive equation (i.e. a reasonable viscoelastic model in the linear domain):

$$\frac{\Delta\omega}{\omega} = 2\left(\frac{d}{R}\right)^2 \frac{\eta'(\omega)}{\eta_0} + \frac{2T_f h}{\pi R^4 \eta_0} \tag{10.47}$$

where η' is the real part of the complex viscosity at frequency ω, and η_0 is the zero-shear viscosity. For a Newtonian fluid, $\eta' = \eta_0$. In commercial instruments, the friction torque T_f is minimized by using an air bearing. The intrinsic lag is negligible for high viscosity liquids in the linear range when the ratio d/R is small, but should be taken into account for low viscosity materials and at large deformations (non-linear behaviour).

10.2.2.2. *The Kepes Balance Rheometer*
The basic principle of the balance rheometer is very similar to that of the orthogonal (ERD) rheometer. It was introduced by Kepes[12] in 1968. Consider a test material located between two concentric spherical surfaces, the inner sphere having a radius R_1 and the outer sphere a radius R_2. If the two spheres are rotating about the same axes Oz at the same angular velocity ω, the sample is unsheared and experiences steady rigid body rotation. If the outer sphere is now tilted by an angle α (see Fig. 10.8), the sample will experience rigid body rotation plus dynamic shearing. For a purely elastic material, the resulting couple exerted on the inner sphere will tend to 'realign' the axes; this couple about the y-axis, C_y, may be derived from the general eqns (10.58a) and (10.58b) in the case of purely elastic material ($G' = G$ and $G'' = 0$):

$$C_y = 8\pi\alpha \frac{R_1^3 R_2^3}{R_2^3 - R_1^3} G \tag{10.48}$$

where G is the shear modulus of the elastic material; in that case, the couple C_x acting about the x-axis is zero.

The theory of the instrument has been developed by Yamamoto,[13] leading to eqn (10.58) with the (unnecessary) assumption that the gap $(R_2 - R_1)$ is small, and by Jones and Walters.[14] In the case of a viscoelastic material, we will use the spherical polar coordinate system (r, θ, ϕ) shown in Fig. 10.8(b):

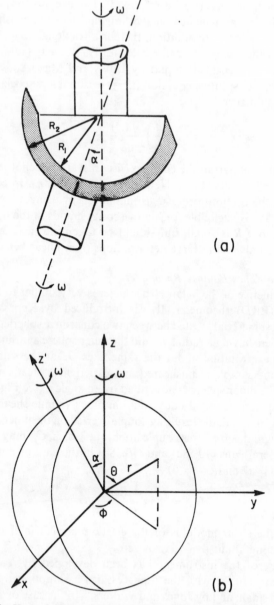

Fig. 10.8. The Kepes balance rheometer: (a) vertical cross-section; (b) coordinate system for the balance rheometer.

$$x = r \sin\theta \cos\phi \qquad (10.49)$$

$$y = r \sin\theta \sin\phi$$

$$z = r \cos\theta$$

The velocity distribution for a sample located between $r = R_1$ and $r = R_2$ is

$$v_r = 0 \qquad (10.50a)$$

$$v_\theta = -f(r) \sin\phi$$

$$v_\phi = \omega r \sin\theta - f(r) \cos\theta \cos\phi$$

where

$$f(r) = \lambda\alpha\omega \left(r - \frac{R_1^3}{r^2} \right) \qquad (10.50b)$$

and

$$\lambda = \frac{R_2^3}{R_2^3 - R_1^3} \qquad (10.51)$$

the relevant stress components are

$$\sigma_{r\theta} = \sigma_{\theta r} = 3\alpha\lambda(G' \cos\phi - G'' \sin\phi) \frac{R_1^3}{r^3} \qquad (10.52a)$$

$$\sigma_{r\phi} = \sigma_{\phi r} = -3\alpha\lambda(G' \sin\phi + G'' \cos\phi) \frac{R_1^3}{r^3} \cos\theta \qquad (10.52b)$$

We will now calculate the forces and the couples acting on the inner sphere. In the commercial instrument the test geometry is a spherical bob placed in a hemispherical cup (Fig. 10.8(a)), so we have to consider the resultant forces and torques acting on the lower half of a sphere (θ has to be integrated between $\pi/2$ and π). The forces F_x and F_y acting on the inner hemisphere are

$$F_x = R_1^2 \int_0^{2\pi} \int_{\pi/2}^{\pi} [\sigma_{rr} \sin\theta \cos\phi + \sigma_{r\theta} \cos\theta \cos\phi - \sigma_{r\phi} \sin\phi]$$

$$\times \sin\theta \, d\theta \, d\phi \qquad (10.53a)$$

$$F_y = R_1^2 \int_0^{2\pi} \int_{\pi/2}^{\pi} [\sigma_{rr} \sin \theta \sin \phi + \sigma_{r\theta} \cos \theta \sin \phi + \sigma_{r\phi} \cos \phi]$$

$$\times \sin \theta \, d\theta \, d\phi \qquad (10.53b)$$

Integration of eqns (10.53a) and (10.53b) gives

$$F_x = -3\pi\lambda\alpha R_1^2 G' \qquad (10.54a)$$

$$F_y = 3\pi\lambda\alpha R_1^2 G'' \qquad (10.54b)$$

So the measurements of the forces F_x and F_y, perpendicular to the axis of rotation of the inner sphere, and acting respectively in the plane of axes of the two hemispheres and the perpendicular direction, lead to the dynamic parameters

$$G'(\omega) = \frac{-F_x}{3\pi\lambda\alpha R_1^2} \qquad (10.55a)$$

$$G''(\omega) = \frac{F_y}{3\pi\lambda\alpha R_1^2} \qquad (10.55b)$$

We may define, as above (Section 10.2.1.1), a complex force $F^*(\omega) = F_x + jF_y$ and its conjugate $\overline{F}^*(\omega)$; hence

$$\overline{F^*(\omega)} = F_x - jF_y = -3\pi\lambda\alpha R_1^2 G^*(\omega) \qquad (10.56)$$

which is similar to eqn (10.46) for the ERD geometry. In the commercial instrument, the couples (instead of the forces) acting about the x and y axes are measured:

$$C_x = -R_1^3 \int_0^{2\pi} \int_{\pi/2}^{\pi} [\sigma_{r\theta} \sin \phi + \sigma_{r\phi} \cos \theta \cos \phi]$$

$$\times \sin \theta \, d\theta \, d\phi \qquad (10.57a)$$

$$C_y = R_1^3 \int_0^{2\pi} \int_{\pi/2}^{\pi} [\sigma_{r\theta} \cos \phi + \sigma_{r\phi} \cos \theta \sin \phi$$

$$\times \sin \theta \, d\theta \, d\phi \qquad (10.57b)$$

Integration of these two equations gives

$$C_x = 4\pi R_1^3 \alpha\lambda G'' \qquad (10.58a)$$

$$C_y = 4\pi R_1^3 \alpha\lambda G' \qquad (10.58b)$$

These equations indicate that measurements of couples C_x and C_y acting about the x and y axes immediately give the linear viscoelastic functions $G'(\omega)$ and $G''(\omega)$.

10.2.2.3. New Rheometers

Other designs, involving steady motion instead of harmonic displacement or rotation, have been presented. However, these new geometries are far less popular than the balance rheometer or the ERD rheometer, mainly because of the importance of artifacts and edge effects on the measurements. These geometries have been thoroughly described by Walters *et al.*;[15,16,7] they are the eccentric cylinder, the displaced sphere, the tilted cone and the tilted cylinder geometries. The eccentric cylinder geometry is the only one that has experienced any significant experimentation, being available as an option for the Weissenberg rheogoniometer. The schematics of these designs are given on Fig. 10.9(a–d), and other designs derived from the same basic idea may be presented. For these instruments, the forces (or couples) measured may be immediately converted into relevant complex modulus (or complex viscosity) data; the equations giving $G^*(\omega)$ from the forces F_x and F_y are similar to those obtained for the balance rheometer or the ERD rheometer.[15]

(a) Eccentric cylinder rheometer (Fig. 10.9(a)). The fluid is contained between eccentric cylinders which rotate at the same angular velocity.

$$\overline{F^*(\omega)} = F_x - jF_y = \frac{4\pi hd}{j\left(\ln \dfrac{R_2}{R_1} - \dfrac{R_2^2 - R_1^2}{R_2^2 + R_1^2}\right)} G^*(\omega) \quad (10.59)$$

where R_1 and R_2 are the cylinder radii ($R_2 > R_1$), h is their length and d the small displacement of the axis of the inner cylinder.

(b) Displaced sphere rheometer (Fig. 10.9(b)). The test fluid is contained between two spheres rotating with the same angular velocity ω about their axes which are parallel but not coincident.

$$\overline{F^*(\omega)} = F_x - jF_y = \frac{24\pi dR_2(\beta^5 - 1)}{j(\beta - 1)^4(4\beta^2 + 7\beta + 4)} G^*(\omega) \quad (10.60)$$

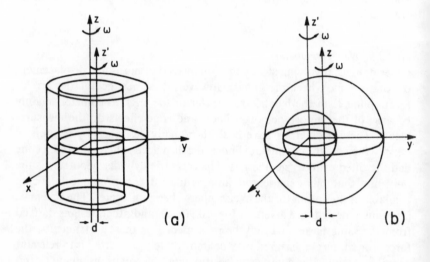

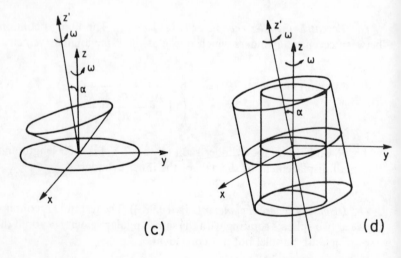

Fig. 10.9. Schematic diagrams of new rheometers: (a) eccentric cylinder; (b) displaced sphere; (c) tilted cone; (d) tilted cylinder.

where R_1 and R_2 are the cylinder radii $(R_2 > R_1)$, $\beta = R_2/R_1$ and d is the small displacement between the centres of the spheres.

(c) Tilted cone rheometer (Fig. 10.9(c)). It is basically the cone–plate geometry in which the cone is tilted through a small angle α.

$$\overline{F^*(\omega)} = F_x - jF_y = \frac{1}{2} \pi R^2 \alpha f(\theta) G^*(\omega) \qquad (10.61)$$

where R is the radius of the plate and $f(\theta)$ a function of the cone angle θ that has been tabulated[14] for θ values ranging from $1°$ to $10°$.

(d) Tilted cylinder rheometer (Fig. 10.9(d)). The test fluid is contained between cylinders of radii R_1 and R_2 $(> R_1)$ rotating with the same angular velocity ω. One cylinder is tilted through a small angle α from an initial position where the cylinders are coaxial.

$$\overline{F^*(\omega)} = F_x - jF_y = \frac{2\pi\alpha h^2 G^*(\omega)}{j[(\beta^2 - 1)/(\beta^2 + 1) - \ln \beta]} \qquad (10.62)$$

where $b = R_2/R_1$ and h is the cylinder length.

These equations may be modified to take into account the large end effects occurring with viscoelastic materials,[16] but it seems difficult to account for these numerous and irregular effects theoretically[17] in the case of highly viscous materials.

10.2.3. Free Oscillation Rheometers

The experiments involving free oscillations are a simpler alternative for measuring complex viscosity, because only displacement is measured. In general, these experiments are easier to perform than those in the forced-oscillation situation described above; the result of this simplification is a considerable reduction in the available frequency range, and the experimental results are much more difficult to interpret rigorously. The free oscillation method has mainly been used for solids or solid-like materials (like gels or very high viscosity liquids), but there are many situations in which free oscillation experiments may be valuable, such as the rheological characterization of liquid to solid transitions, e.g. sol–gel transition of elastomers or thermosetting materials.

In most applications, the basic experimental set-up is a simple torsion pendulum, the sample test geometries being the same as described in

Section 10.2.1 (Fig. 10.6(a–c)). An inertia member is fixed to the axis of rotation and imposes a torque on the sample when an angular displacement is given. When the inertia member is released, the system experiences free torsional oscillations with a frequency depending on (i) the inertia and the elastic features of the system, and (ii) the viscoelastic properties of the sample. A typical set-up for liquids may be found in reference 18.

For this class of rheometers, the instrument member supporting the rotating mass undergoes damped harmonic oscillations that are recorded to measure the frequency (ω) and the logarithmic decrement (D); see Fig. 10.10(a). In the linear viscoelastic domain, the angular displacement θ is damped as

$$\theta = \theta_0 \cos \omega t \exp(-dt) \tag{10.63}$$

It is convenient to use the complex notation

$$\theta^*(\omega; t) = \theta_0 \exp(j\omega t) \exp(-dt) = \theta_0 \exp[(j\omega - d)t] \tag{10.64}$$

where $\omega = 2\pi/T$ and T is the period of the harmonic motion. The logarithmic decrement is the absolute value of the slope of θ_i as a function of i, the index of the successive peaks $\theta_0, \theta_1, \ldots, \theta_i, \ldots, \theta_n$; see Fig. 10.10(a). Then

$$D = dT = \ln\left(\frac{\theta_i}{\theta_i + 1}\right) \tag{10.65}$$

A rough determination of the logarithmic decrement may be obtained by measuring the amplitude of only two peaks (generally θ_1 and another peak θ_n), so

$$D = \frac{1}{n-1} \frac{\theta_1}{\theta_n} \tag{10.66}$$

However, this determination is less precise than a graph of $(\log \theta_i; i)$; besides, the linearity of this graph will eventually confirm the internal consistency of the analysis.

Referring to eqn (10.20), the equation of motion for free oscillation is

$$O = I \frac{d^2\theta^*}{dt^2} + [AG^*(\omega) + B]\theta^* \tag{10.67}$$

In order to solve this equation, it is common to assume η' and $G' = \eta''/\omega$ are constant. It is important to point out that this assumption is often very approximate, e.g. for high molecular weight polymers in the terminal region of relaxation. However, it may be a reasonable assumption in the

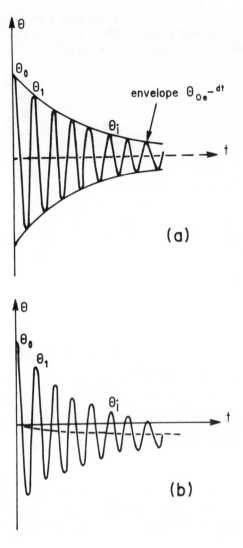

Fig. 10.10. Trace of the damped motion of the displaced member of a free oscillation rheometer [(b) decay accompanied by creep recovery].

case of solid-like material, e.g. polymers in the rubbery plateau region and crosslinking material at the onset of the liquid to solid transition. Following this assumption, eqn (10.67) may be solved as follows:

$$\theta^*(\omega; t) = \theta_0 \exp(-dt)\exp[j(\omega t + \phi)] \tag{10.68a}$$

with

$$d = A\eta'/2I \tag{10.68b}$$

$$\omega^2 = \frac{AG' + B}{I} - d^2 \tag{10.68c}$$

This solution applies if $4I(AG' + B) > A^2\eta'^2$. So, in the case of highly viscous materials, one has to make I large or/and add a spring in order to decrease the rate of decay, if this method is chosen.

In order to evaluate the effects of frictional losses of the torsion wire and the mobile parts of the system, we may solve eqn (10.67) exactly in the case of a purely viscous material, introducing a factor n that includes these frictional losses:

$$O = I\frac{d^2\theta^*}{dt^2} + A(\eta + n)\frac{d\theta^*}{dt} + B\theta^* \tag{10.69}$$

Thus the equation of the free motion in air (without sample) will be

$$O = I\frac{d^2\theta^*}{dt^2} + An\frac{d\theta^*}{dt} + B\theta^* \tag{10.70}$$

The solution of this differential equation with constant coefficients is

$$\theta^*(\omega; t) = \theta_0 \exp(-d_0 t)\exp(j\omega_0 t) \tag{10.71a}$$

with

$$d_0 = An/2I \tag{10.71b}$$

$$\omega_0^2 = \frac{B}{I} - d_0^2 \tag{10.71c}$$

where ω_0 is the natural frequency of free oscillations of the instrument. It is now straightforward to solve the complete equation of motion (including sample viscosity η; eqn (10.69)):

$$\theta^*(\omega; t) = \theta_0 \exp(-dt)\exp(j\omega t) \tag{10.72a}$$

with

$$d = \frac{A(n + \eta)}{2I} = d_0 + \frac{A\eta}{2I} \quad (10.72b)$$

$$\omega^2 = \frac{B}{I} - \frac{A^2(\eta + n)^2}{4I^2} = \omega_0^2 - \frac{\eta n A^2}{2I^2} - \frac{\eta^2 A^2}{4I^2} \quad (10.72c)$$

This last equation reveals that ω has to be different from the natural frequency ω_0, and this places limits on the sample dimensions and instrument constants (I, n), for a given material. This also explains why the most efficient instruments are generally designed specifically for free oscillation testing, and one has to bear in mind these limitations when performing free oscillation tests with instruments designed primarily for forced oscillation testing.

In the case of viscoelastic liquids, the trace of the damped motion may be of the form of Fig. 10.10(b) when the time of application of the initial deformation is not small compared with the relaxation time of the sample; some flow occurs during the initial deformation, and creep recovery is occurring simultaneously with oscillations. This may be avoided either by making the initial deformation quasi-impulsive or by beginning the experiment by a series of forced oscillations before allowing them to decay.

10.2.4. Resonant Methods

Using the general equation for forced oscillations, eqn (10.23), the oscillation amplitude θ_0 can be written as

$$\theta_0 = \frac{T_0 \exp{(j\phi)}}{-I\omega^2 + AG^* + B} \quad (10.73)$$

The magnitude of the denominator is

$$|-I\omega^2 + AG^* + B| = [(AG' + B - I\omega^2)^2 + (AG'')^2]^{1/2} \quad (10.74)$$

At *resonance*, this quantity falls to a minimum: θ_0 becomes large and easily measurable; G' and G'' at resonance are given by

$$G' = \frac{I\omega^2 - B}{A} \quad (10.75a)$$

$$G'' = \frac{T_0}{A\theta_0} \quad (10.75b)$$

This method is *a priori* simple and easy to handle, when resonance is determined by varying frequency. The other method (varying I: mass or inertia of the measuring system) is cumbersome experimentally but better theoretically. However, the ability to change I is necessary in order to set resonance within the available frequency range, for a given family of materials. The drawbacks of this method are of the same kind as for the free oscillation method: the available frequency range is limited. Besides, the method of obtaining G' and G'' by varying frequency is open to criticism; G' and G'' are a function of frequency, and the denominator of eqn (10.73) is not necessarily a minimum when its real part is zero, unless G' and G'' are changing slowly with frequency or the loss modulus G'' is low. The advantage of this method is that, like the free oscillation method, it does not require phase shift measurements. Designs and references to resonant apparatus for viscoelastic solids and liquids may be found in Ferry's classic book.[2] Silberberg and Mijnlieff[19] have described a Couette (concentric cylinder) rheometer designed specifically for viscoelastic liquids.

10.2.5. Time Domain Mechanical Spectroscopy (TDMS)

Spectroscopy methods are used in a large number of analytical tests of physics and physical chemistry, and the availability of fast electronic systems has enabled considerable experimental breakthroughs in that area. The ability to convert time domain data (transient experiments) into frequency domain data (dynamic experiments) may now be achieved efficiently thanks to powerful hardware and software (FFT algorithms). The mathematical theory of linear viscoelasticity[1] is the rheological analogue of basic theories of other spectroscopy methods, the general formalism being basically the same. Unfortunately this powerful analytical tool has seldom been used by rheologists, despite its considerable possibilities. The principle of time domain spectroscopy is to convert a transient signal into a frequency-dependent complex function, through a Fourier-like transform. The advantage of the method is a large saving in experimental time compared with regular frequency domain experiments. The drawbacks of the method are two-fold:

(1) Generally, the frequency domain data obtained by time domain spectroscopy are less accurate than those from direct measurements in the frequency domain, unless an average is made over a large number of experiments (losing in that case the saving in time).

(2) The frequency domain data are obtained in most cases at a limited range of frequencies, depending mainly on the sampling time and the accuracy of the transient signal.

In the case of rheological experiments, this means that it is possible to convert relaxation or creep experiments into complex shear modulus or complex compliance data.

10.2.5.1. *Complex Compliance from Creep Experiments*

We have plotted in Fig. 10.11 the schematic diagram of the creep response of a viscoelastic material. A constant stress (corresponding to a constant torque in a rotary rheometer) is applied at time $t = 0$. The system exhibits an instantaneous response J_∞ ($J_\infty \approx 10^{-9} \, \mathrm{m}^2 \mathrm{N}^{-1}$ for most organic glasses) that is negligible compared with the compliance value in the

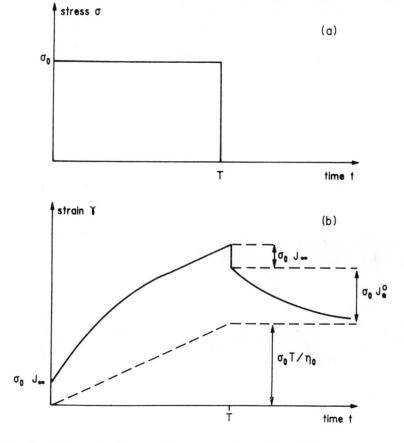

Fig. 10.11. Schematic diagram of a creep experiment (a), and the creep response of a viscoelastic material (b).

terminal region of relaxation (large times). Then the system exhibits a retarded elastic response as well as steady viscous flow:

$$J(t) = J_\infty + \frac{t}{\eta_0} + J_r(t) \qquad (10.76)$$

$J_r(t)$ is the retardational contribution to the creep function. The mathematical theory of linear viscoelasticity demonstrates that the complex compliance may be expressed in terms of the creep function:[1]

$$J^*(\omega) = J_\infty + \frac{1}{j\omega\eta_0} + \int_0^\infty \frac{dJ_r(t)}{dt} \exp(-j\omega t) \, dt \qquad (10.77)$$

The derivation of the complex compliance from the creep function, although rarely used by rheologists, has been employed mainly as a refined technique to study the viscoelastic properties of well defined materials; the creep rheometers were mainly fundamental research-oriented instruments that were very accurate but difficult to use as a standard tool of rheological characterization, unlike the popular oscillatory instruments. However,

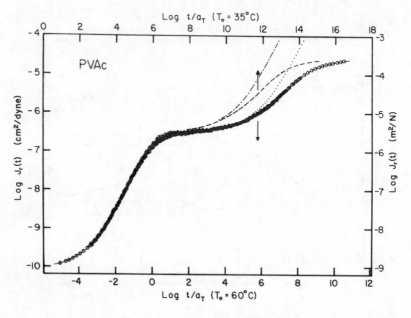

Fig. 10.12. Creep response of a viscoelastic material (polyvinylacetate; $M = 6.5 \times 10^5$; $T = 60\,°C$); data from Plazek.[20]

some commercial creep rheometers have recently become available, and the TDMS/creep method could easily be implemented on these instruments. We show in Fig. 10.12 the creep data obtained by Plazek *et al.*[18] on a polyvinylacetate sample. The curve covers a wide range of times because of the use of the time/temperature equivalence. The complex compliance curves in Fig. 10.13 have been calculated from the creep curve through intermediate calculation of the distribution of retardation times ('retarda-

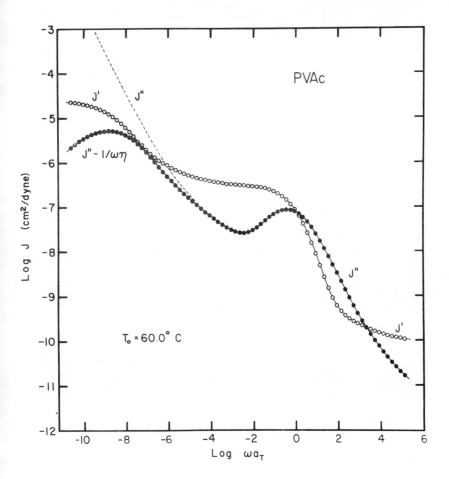

Fig. 10.13. Real and imaginary parts of complex compliance derived from the transient data of Fig. 10.12 (from Plazek[20]).

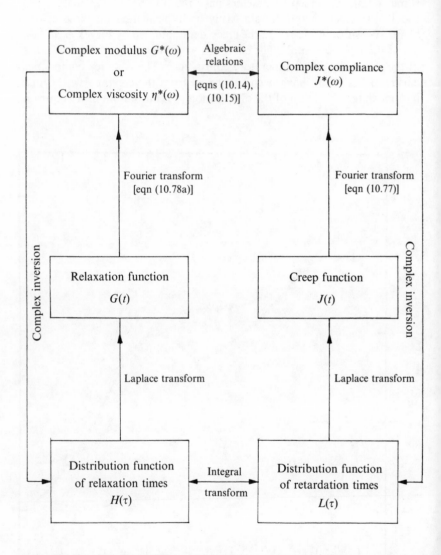

Fig. 10.14. Interrelations between the various functions of linear viscoelasticity (after Gross[1]).

tion spectrum'), but this step is theoretically unnecessary as shown by eqn (10.77) and Fig. 10.14. A complete description of the interrelations between the various viscoelastic functions and spectra may be found in references 1 and 2; a schematic diagram is given in Fig. 10.14.

10.2.5.2. Complex Shear Modulus from Stress Growth Experiments

Most rotary rheometers designed for steady shearing experiments are *strain rheometers*, i.e. the angular deformation is controlled rather than the torque (*stress rheometers*). A constant shear rate $\dot{\gamma}_0$ is applied at time $t = 0$, and the stress is made to increase, its steady value giving the viscosity ($\sigma = \sigma_0$) (see Fig. 10.15) which is a function of shear rate at high shear rates for non-Newtonian fluids. The transient function $\sigma(t)$ is one of the key functions used for testing non-linear constitutive equations. This $\sigma(t)$ function may be used *in the linear region* (low shear rates) to derive the complex viscosity through a Fourier transform:[1,21]

$$\eta^*(\omega) = \int_0^\infty G(t) \exp(-j\omega t)\, dt \qquad (10.78a)$$

with

$$G(t) = \frac{1}{\dot{\gamma}}\left(\frac{d\sigma^+(t)}{dt}\right) \qquad (10.78b)$$

The stress relaxation function $\sigma^-(t)$ after cessation of flow at time t may also be used:

$$G(t) = -\frac{1}{\dot{\gamma}}\left(\frac{d\sigma^-(t)}{dt}\right) \qquad (10.79)$$

These equations may also be written in terms of shear modulus as $G^*(\omega) = j\omega\eta^*$.

The angular acceleration (or deceleration) of the most recently available commercial rotary rheometers is high enough to consider the application (or stopping) of flow as instantaneous compared with the relaxation times of highly viscoelastic materials such as polymer melts. A comparison of the data obtained at one temperature with the TDMS method with data obtained from conventional oscillatory rheometry is plotted in Fig. 10.16 for a commercial polymer.[21] The available frequency range covered by TDMS depends on the quality of the step signal for shear rate (i.e. the angular acceleration of the rheometer), the sampling time of the transient signal and the accuracy of the measurement. In any case, the frequency range is smaller for TDMS than for the conventional frequency sweep, but

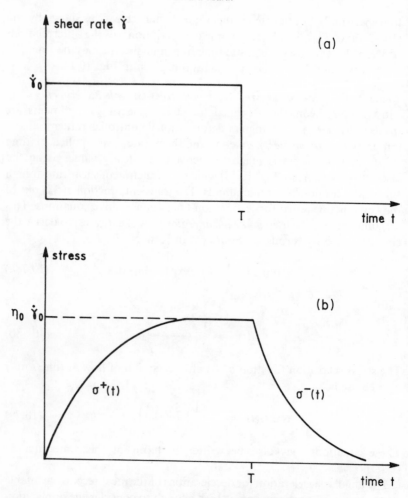

Fig. 10.15. Schematic diagram of start-up, then cessation of flow (a) and the response of a viscoelastic material (b).

the saving in time is considerable (it is easily ten times faster). Thus the TDMS method may be used for the study of fast degrading or chemically active materials. It is easy to put a sample in a rotary rheometer and do start-up shearings at regular time intervals. The Fourier transforms of the successive $\sigma(t)$ curves are 'snapshots' of $G^*(\omega)$ as a function of time, which provide a rheological survey of the chemical evolution of the system.

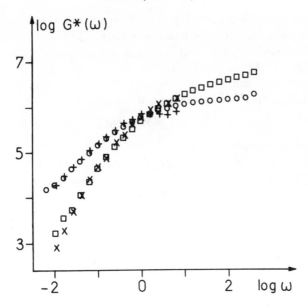

Fig. 10.16. Comparison of the shear complex moduli obtained from frequency sweep (●, □) and from Fourier transform of stress relaxation after cessation of flow (+, ×) (polymethylmethacrylate; $T = 200\,°C$).[21]

10.2.6. Sources of Errors

10.2.6.1. Inertia Effects

All the theories developed in the above sections assume the absence of fluid inertia. This is a reasonable assumption for the high viscosity liquids usually characterized in oscillatory rheometry, as the maximum frequency reached by the family of instruments described above is of the order of 100 Hz. For low viscosity liquids, the inertia effects may be non-negligible at the highest frequencies. However, it must be stressed that these liquids (also referred to as 'thin fluids') generally have Newtonian (non-elastic) behaviour in this frequency range; owing to their small relaxation times, frequencies in the kHz and MHz range are certainly more suitable in the determination of their viscoelastic behaviour. Oscillatory rheometry is *not* the most appropriate technique for studying the viscoelasticity of these materials; ultrasonic rheology is a more adequate technique to cover the distribution of relaxation times of low viscosity materials such as oils or oligomers. These ultrasonic techniques have been extensively developed, both experimentally and theoretically, by Lamb and coworkers, and a review of these ideas may be found in reference 3.

As far as oscillatory rheometry is concerned, inertia effects can be taken into account in the theories leading to analytical solutions in some cases, and involving numerical analysis in others. Generally speaking, the inertia effects are governed by the complex function[7]

$$\alpha^2 = -j\omega\rho/\eta^*(\omega) \qquad (10.80)$$

where ρ is the sample density.

In the case of oscillatory shearing between parallel plates (see Section 10.2), inertia effects are governed by the product αh,[7] so they can be reduced by lowering the gap h between the plates. In the *absence* of fluid inertia, eqn (10.35) may be rewritten, taking Walter's formalism:[7]

$$\frac{\theta_1 \exp(-j\phi)}{\theta_2} = 1 - \frac{j}{\eta^*} S \qquad (10.81)$$

where

$$S = \frac{2h(B - I\omega^2)}{\pi R^4 \omega} \qquad (10.82)$$

When inertia effects are *included* in parallel plate geometry, this equation becomes[7]

$$\frac{\theta_1 \exp(-j\phi)}{\theta_2} = \cos(\alpha h) + \frac{S}{\rho h^2 \omega} \alpha h \sin(\alpha h) \qquad (10.83)$$

When αh is small, eqn (10.83) may be expanded in series of powers of αh. In any case, α (and hence η^*) can be determined from a knowledge of the amplitude ratio θ_1/θ_2 and the phase lag ϕ.

The exact solution is more complicated in the case of coaxial cylinder geometry and cone–plate geometry, involving Bessel functions with complex arguments, requiring cumbersome methods to obtain $\eta^*(\omega)$, for the experimentalist. Simpler corrections may be derived, at small annular gap values in the case of the concentric-cylinder geometry, and at small α values in the case of the cone–plate geometry.[7] From the standpoint of inertia effects, this means that all the conventional geometries may be used with high viscosity liquids at the moderate frequencies covered by oscillatory rheometry; for low viscosity materials, the use of parallel-plate geometry facilitates corrections to take inertia effects into account.

Concerning the new rheometers, the effects of inertia are difficult to investigate in the case of the Kepes balance rheometer, but these effects are very small in the case of couple measurements.[7] In the case of the orthogonal rheometer, the modified expression for the complex force $F^*(\omega)$ (eqn (10.46)) is

$$\overline{F^*(\omega)} = F_x - jF_y = -\frac{d\pi R^2}{j} G^*(\omega) \frac{\alpha[1 + \cosh(\alpha h)]}{\sinh(\alpha h)} \quad (10.84)$$

If αh is small, the hyperbolic functions may be expressed in powers of αh:[7]

$$\overline{F^*(\omega)} = F_x - jF_y = -\frac{d\pi R^2}{jh} G^*(\omega) \left(1 + \frac{\alpha^2 h^2}{12} - \frac{\alpha^4 h^4}{720}\right) (10.85)$$

So α (and hence $\eta^*(\omega)$) can be determined from a knowledge of the forces F_x and F_y in the ERD mode, in the case of non-negligible fluid inertia.

10.2.6.2: Non-linear Effects

The instruments described above are mainly used under conditions where strains are small enough to be in the domain of linear viscoelasticity. These instruments are also capable of applying large deformations, but most studies involving oscillatory rheometry at large strain amplitudes are fluid-mechanics oriented; it is one of the various flow situations explored to test non-linear constitutive equations, rather than a systematic rheological characterization of viscoelastic materials. Another way of using oscillatory tests to investigate non-linear behaviour is the superimposition of small oscillatory shearing on a steady flow. These experiments show the evolution of the distribution of relaxation times as a function of shear rate, and non-linear phenomenological models may give a good description of the behaviour of viscoelastic fluids in that particular flow situation. From a purely rheological point of view, a good survey of these types of test may be found in reference 7. Other types of superposition may be envisaged in the new-rheometers geometries (Section 10.2.2.3), harmonically displacing the axes of rotation in the various directions, or rotating the axes at different angular speeds.

However, in most applications non-linear effects are unwanted and the linearity assumption should be tested before analysing the data. Furthermore, the angular displacement should be decreased as frequency is increased, in order to obtain measurable torque values at low frequencies and to remain in the linear region at the highest frequencies. A typical sign of non-linearity is a discontinuity in the $G'(\omega)$ and $G''(\omega)$ curves occurring at a frequency where the strain amplitude has been changed.

10.2.6.3. Instrument Stiffness

Neglecting or underestimating instrument compliance is certainly the prime cause of error in the measurement of the viscoelastic parameters in oscillatory rheometry. High molecular weight polymers go from a liquid-like behaviour at low frequencies to a solid-like behaviour at the highest frequencies, and the modulus values in the transition and glassy region (see Fig. 10.2) may reach 10^8–10^9 N m^{-2}; few rotary rheometers are stiff enough to measure such high modulus levels. The instrument compliance effects may also be important in the case of 'thin fluids' made up of small molecules, especially when working close to their glass transition temperatures. As a consequence, particular attention should be paid to correction for instrument compliance, in order to determine the physical parameters from oscillatory rheometry measurement. Neglecting this correction may lead to measuring the stiffness of the instrument instead of the modulus of the sample, especially at high frequencies. On account of the increasing popularity of rotary rheometers, we will describe the various ways of evaluating instrument stiffness and how to use the compliance value to correct the experimental data to derive the correct values of the complex shear modulus.

(a) Compliance correction in oscillatory, rotary rheometry. In the most recent rotary rheometers, a harmonic deformation is exerted on one part of the instrument while the harmonic couple is recorded by a measuring cell containing a torque transducer. These instruments are very stiff, allowing a very small angular deformation of the torque measuring system, unlike the torsion bars (or equivalent systems) of the older instruments. Nevertheless the angular deformation (torsion) of the measuring system is not negligible at high modulus levels of the test sample, so the real deformation experienced by the sample is *not* the applied deformation. The apparent modulus G_a^* (neglecting instrument compliance) may be derived from eqn (10.24):

$$G_a^* = \frac{T_0 \exp(j\phi)}{\theta_0 A} \tag{10.86}$$

where T_0 is the amplitude of the torque, θ_0 the amplitude of the applied angular displacement, A the shape factor of the given geometry and ϕ the phase lag between torque and angular displacement.

It is reasonable to assume that the compliance effect is mainly a purely elastic contribution, so the real deformation $\theta_r^*(\omega; t)$ exerted on the sample is

$$\theta_r^*(\omega; t) = \theta_0 \exp[j(\omega t - \phi)] - KT_0 \exp(j\omega t) \qquad (10.87)$$

where K is the compliance of the instrument (rad $N^{-1} m^{-1}$ in SI units; rad dyn^{-1} cm^{-1} in cgs units). So the true complex shear modulus $G_t^*(\omega)$ of the sample is

$$G_t^*(\omega) = \frac{T_0 \exp(j\phi)}{\theta_0 A - KT_0 A \exp(j\phi)} \qquad (10.88)$$

This equation may also be transformed as

$$G_t'(\omega) = \frac{G_a' C_1 + G_a'' C_2}{C_1^2 + C_2^2} = \frac{G_a' - KA|G_a^*|^2}{C_1^2 + C_2^2} \qquad (10.89)$$

and

$$G_t''(\omega) = \frac{G_a'' C_1 + G_a' C_2}{C_1^2 + C_2^2} = \frac{G_a''}{C_1^2 + C_2^2} \qquad (10.90)$$

with

$$C_1 = 1 - KA|G_a^*|\cos\phi = 1 - KAG_a'$$
$$C_2 = KA|G_a^*|\sin\phi = 1 - KAG_a'' \qquad (10.91)$$
$$|G_a^*| = (G_a'^2 + G_a''^2)^{1/2}$$

So the corrected values of $G'(\omega)$ and $G''(\omega)$ may be easily calculated from the applied deformation and torque values, once the values of K is known. Two different methods may be used to measure the instrument compliance value K:

(1) The mechanical method consists of making a direct measurement of the stiffness. A static torque is applied to the instrument members at the sample level, and the corresponding angular displacement is measured; this measurement may be very precise when using an optical method. The measurement of K is however a static measurement, and the compliance value may be different (but of the same order of magnitude) when oscillating one instrument member.

(2) The numerical method involves measurements of G' and G'' on a given material, but at various A values, i.e. using plates of different radii or different cone angles. Several least-squares methods may be used; the simplest may be to linearize the problem using the function G_a'/G_a'':

$$\frac{G'_a}{G''_a} = \frac{G'_t}{G''_t} + KA\,\frac{|G^*_a|^2}{G''_a} \tag{10.92}$$

The ratio G'_t/G''_t is a constant at a given frequency, so a plot of (G'_a/G''_a) as a function of $A(|G^*_a|^2)/G''_a$ (at various cone angle values, e.g. in cone-plate geometry) gives the value of K. By this method the initial hypothesis that the stiffness correction is a purely elastic contribution, independent of angular frequency ω, can also be verified.

(b) Compliance correction in the ERD geometry. The forces F_x and F_y in the ERD experiment are measured by transducers that do not have a negligible deflection at high values of the forces. This, along with the fact that the plates and spindles are not perfectly rigid, can cause a shift in both the magnitude and direction of the imposed eccentricity d_a, so the true eccentricity $d(d = d_a - d_k$, where d_k is the deformation due to instrument compliance) should be included into the ERD equation. Furthermore, the F_x forces also impose an eccentricity in the x direction. Through a calculation similar to that developed in section (a) for the compliance effects in torsion, the true modulus values in the ERD model are

$$G'_t = \frac{G'_a\left(1 - K\,\dfrac{\pi R^2}{h}\,\dfrac{|G^*_a|^2}{G'_a}\right)}{\left(1 - K\,\dfrac{\pi R^2}{h}\,G'_a\right)^2 + \left(K\,\dfrac{\pi R^2}{h}\,G''_a\right)^2} \tag{10.93}$$

and

$$G''_t = \frac{G''_a}{\left(1 - K\,\dfrac{\pi R^2}{h}\,G'_a\right)^2 + \left(K\,\dfrac{\pi R^2}{h}\,G''_a\right)^2} \tag{10.94}$$

where K is the instrument compliance ($\mathrm{m\,N^{-1}}$ in SI units; $\mathrm{cm\,dyn^{-1}}$ in cgs units), and $G^*_a(\omega)$ is the apparent complex shear modulus assuming no compliance effects.

In the same way as for compliance effects in torsion, the compliance in the x and y directions in the ERD geometry can be either measured applying static forces in the x and y directions on the upper and lower discs, or evaluated numerically by a least-squares method after running ERD experiments at various gap settings (h) or disc radii values (R). This method should be preferred, as it gives the true 'dynamic' compliance values. The form of eqns (10.93) and (10.94) shows that changing the eccentricity value d does *not* lead to the compliance value. The best method is to vary the gap h using the same sample, since changing the plate diameter (and then using different plates) could change the overall compliance value.

It is possible to derive for the ERD geometry an equation equivalent to eqn (10.92):

$$\frac{G'_a}{G''_a} = \frac{G'_t}{G''_t} + K\frac{\pi R^2}{h}\frac{|G^*_a|^2}{G''_a} \tag{10.95}$$

and use a linear regression analysis method to derive K.

A comparison of the compliance effects on the most recent commercial instruments shows that the compliance correction is larger in the ERD mode than in oscillatory and rotary rheometry at the same modulus levels.

10.3. APPLICATIONS TO POLYPHASIC SYSTEMS

The properties of composite materials are determined by (i) the properties of the components, (ii) the shape and size of the dispersed phase, and (iii) the structure and properties of the interface between the two main phases.

Measurements of the dynamic mechanical properties on polyphasic systems in the fluid state lead to interesting information on both the structure and the processability of the system; furthermore these measurements may be correlated with the final properties of the material such as impact strength or phase adhesion in the case of polymer blends. The main advantage of performing dynamic measurements at small strain or stress levels is that the microstructure of the system is usually well defined and stable throughout the experiment. This is not the case for the usual steady flow experiments, such as capillary rheometry; while flowing through a die, for example, the dispersed phase of a polymer blend is strongly deformed along the capillary wall, but it is much less oriented in the vicinity of the centre. The microstructure of the sample is not homogeneous in the sample cell and changes with the shear rate, so a fine characterization of the structure/properties relationship seems difficult to achieve in that case. On the contrary, small oscillation measurements are quasi-equilibrium tests in which the sample maintains its microstructure. However, one has to be aware that polyphasic systems are strongly non-

Newtonian, and the linearity tests have to be made carefully in that case. The cone–plate geometry, where small strain levels may be achieved while keeping a constant shear rate throughout the sample, seems particularly appropriate to polyphasic systems. Non-linear effects would be more difficult to control in parallel-plate geometry, where the shear rate is not uniform from the centre to the edge.

When it is important to characterize materials that may be strongly anisotropic in flow, such as triblock copolymers, fibre reinforced materials, or liquid crystalline polymers, it may be interesting first to pre-orient the material in steady shearing between cone and plate in a rotary rheometer, then perform small oscillation dynamic measurements on the oriented sample. Comparison with the data observed on the un-oriented (isotropic) sample may lead to interesting conclusions on the physical properties of the material.

10.3.1. Particle-filled Materials
In the case of material filled with rigid particles and fillers, the analysis of experimental data may be the same as for one-component systems; these materials may be considered as thermorheologically simple materials, so the time temperature equivalence may be applied, i.e. changing temperature is equivalent to changing frequency. The theories of composite systems, relating the mechanical properties of the composite material to the system composition and the individual properties of the components, have been elaborated in terms of either viscosities or elastic moduli; these theories may be extended to the viscoelastic response by application of the 'correspondence principle', that is by substitution of complex viscosities or moduli for shear viscosities or moduli.

A large number of theories predicting the moduli of composites are related to theories of the viscosity of particle-filled liquids. The basic theory is Einstein's equation[23] for the viscosity of a suspension of rigid spherical particles in very dilute concentrations. A large number of equations have been proposed to extend Einstein's law up to moderate and high concentration, such as Mooney's[24] equation which is widely used for many kinds of suspensions. For elastic materials containing spherical particles of any modulus, the Kerner[25] model and its derivatives[26] may be used to calculate the modulus of a composite. These theories indicate that the modulus of a composite material should be independent of the size of the filler particles. However, the experimental data show an increase in modulus (or viscosity) as the particle size decreases. Interfacial properties play an important role there, and this demonstrates that the properties of the interface as well as the distribution of particle size should also be known in order to obtain a high level of correlation between the composite structure and its viscoelastic properties.

10.3.2. Polymer Blends and Block Copolymers

Non-compatible (A + B) polymer blends are constituted with a B phase dispersed within an A matrix, plus usually an interphase that may be a compatible A–B interphase or A–B copolymer that has either been added or chemically formed during the process. Most technical and high impact polymers have the interphase that gives good adhesion between the matrix and the discontinuous phase and good control of the dispersed phase, leading to improved mechanical and thermal properties. Incompatible polyblends are *not* thermorheologically simple materials, and their dynamic mechanical properties, when measured at a wide range of frequencies, can exhibit three relaxation domains: a relaxation domain due to the A matrix (which may be modified by some B content), a domain due to the dispersed B phase (which may be modified by some A content), and a domain due to relaxation of the interphase. These different relaxation domains are usually coupled, because of the broad distribution of relaxation times for each component. However, these relaxation domains may be separate when the relaxation times of the components differ by one or several orders of magnitude. Each relaxation domain shifts differently with temperature, so the time/temperature equivalence cannot be used theoretically in that case, unless a different shift is applied for each relaxation domain. When working in a limited range of temperature and when the viscosity activation energy or WLF parameters are not too

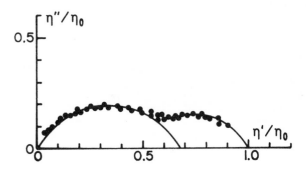

Fig. 10.17. Cole–Cole plot of complex viscosities for a ternary blend (polystyrene/ polycarbonate/tetramethylpolycarbonate).[22]

different, time/temperature superposition may however be used as a first approximation, without the physical meaning it has for homopolymers or compatible blends. One of the main features of the viscoelastic behaviour of polymer blends or copolymers is the additional low-frequency relaxation domain (compared with homopolymers) due to the relaxation of macromolecules trapped at the interphase (technical polyblends) or chemically linked to the dispersed phase (block copolymers). Figure 10.17 shows a plot of the complex viscosities of a ternary blend; the additional low frequency relaxation domain (compare Fig. 10.17 with Fig. 10.5) is due to the viscoelastic behaviour at the interphase, resulting in large values of relaxation times and viscosities. Clearly it appears that the low frequency behaviour in oscillatory rheometry is an important feature of multiphase systems, which usually have large relaxation times and sometimes exhibit solid-like behaviour at the lowest frequencies. As far as analysis of data is concerned, mechanical coupling models such as that of Takayanagi *et al.*[27] can be regarded as generalizations of the familiar analogue models of viscoelasticity using springs and dashpots, and provide a convenient way to relate the properties of a multiphase system to the properties of the individual components.[28]

REFERENCES

1. B. Gross, *Mathematical Structure of the Theories of Linear Viscoelasticity*, Hermann, Paris, 1953.
2. J. D. Ferry, *Viscoelastic Properties of Polymers*, Wiley, New York, 1970.
3. G. Harrison, *The Dynamic Properties of Supercooled Liquids*, Academic Press, London, 1976.
4. G. Marin and W. W. Graessley, *Rheol. Acta,* 1977, **16,** 527.
5. G. Marin, J. J. Labaig and P. Monge, *Polymer,* 1975, **16,** 223.
6. J. P. Montfort, G. Marin and P. Monge, *Macromolecules,* 1984, **17,** 1551.
7. K. Walters, *Rheometry*, Chapman and Hall, 1975.
8. W. Philipoff, in *Physical Acoustics*, Vol. IIB, W. P. Mason (Ed.), Academic Press, New York, 1965.
9. A. N. Gent, *Brit. J. Appl. Phys.,* 1960, **11,** 165.
10. B. Maxwell and R. P. Chartoff, *Trans. Soc. Rheol.,* 1965, **9,** 41.
11. W. M. Davis and C. Macosko, *A.I.Ch.E.J.,* 1974, **20,** 600.
12. A. Kepes, 5th Congress on Rheology, Kyoto, 1968.
13. M. Yamamoto, *Jap. J. Appl. Phys.,* 1969, **8,** 152.
14. T. E. R. Jones and K. Walters, *Brit. J. Appl. Phys. (J. Phys. D.),* 1969, **2,** 815.
15. T. N. G. Abbot, G. W. Bowen and K. Walters, *J. Phys. (D.),* 1971, **4,** 190.
16. J. M. Broadbent and K. Walters, *J. Phys. (D.),* 1971, **4,** 1869.
17. G. W. Bowen, J. M. Broadbent and K. Walters, *J. Phys. (D.),* 1973, **6,** 83.

18. D. J. Plazek, *Trans. Soc. Rheol.,* 1958, **2,** 39.
19. A. Silberberg and P. J. Mijnlieff, *J. Polym. Sci. (A2),* 1970, **8,** 1089.
20. D. J. Plazek, *Polymer J.,* 1980, **12,** 1.
21. G. Marin, J. Peyrelasse and P. Monge, *Rheol. Acta,* 1983, **22,** 476.
22. C. Belaribi, G. Marin and P. Monge, *Eur. Polym. J.,* 1986, **6,** 487.
23. A. Einstein, *Ann. Physik,* 1905, **17,** 549; 1907, **19,** 289.
24. M. Mooney, *J. Colloid Sci.,* 1951, **6,** 162.
25. E. H. Kerner, *Proc. Phys. Soc.,* 1966, **B69,** 808.
26. L. E. Nielsen, *Mechanical Properties of Polymers and Composites,* Marcel Dekker, New York, 1974.
27. M. Takayanagi, H. Harima and Y. Iwata, *J. Soc. Mater. Sci. Japan,* 1963, **12,** 389.
28. D. R. Paul and S. Newman, *Polymer Blends,* Academic Press, New York, 1978.

Chapter 11

Normal Stress Differences from Hole Pressure Measurements

A. S. LODGE

The University of Wisconsin–Madison Engine and Rheology Research Centers, Department of Engineering Mechanics, and Engineering Experiment Station, Madison, Wisconsin, USA

NOTATION

$a(T)$	time–temperature shift function
b	hole diameter or slit width parallel to main flow direction
h_i^2	diagonal components of metric tensor for the coordinate system y_i of Fig. 11.6
h, w	height and width of slit die cross-section
L^*	defined by eqn (11.40)
n	d log P_e^*/d log σ
N_3, β	$N_1 + 2N_2, -N_2/N_1$
$P_{1,av}, P_2, P_3$	pressures measured with flush-mounted and two hole-mounted transducers

P^*	$P_{1,av} - P_2$ ('hole pressure')
P^*_f	contribution to P^* from finite width effects in flush-mounted transducer
P^*_i, P^*_e	inertial and elastic contributions to P^*
P^*_N	value of $P^* - P^*_f$ for a Newtonian liquid
p_{ij} ($i = 1, 2, 3$)	physical components of stress for the orthogonal coordinate system y_i
r, R	distance from axis, and gap radius in cone–plate rheometer
Re	$\rho b h \dot{\gamma}/(4\eta)$ (Reynolds number)
T	absolute temperature
X_r	$\rho_o T_o X/(\rho T)$ ($X = \sigma$, σ_p, N_i, P^*_e: 'reduced stress')
z	distance between holes
$\dot{\gamma}_a$	approximate wall shear rate in slit die rheometer
$\dot{\gamma}_r$	$\dot{\gamma}a(T)$ ('reduced shear rate')
η, η_s	solution or melt viscosity, solvent viscosity
η_{rel}	η/η_s (relative viscosity)
ρ_{ij}	principal radii of curvature for the y_i coordinate surfaces of Fig. 11.6
ρ, ρ_o	densities at temperatures T, T_o
σ, $\dot{\gamma}$, N_1, N_2	shear stress, shear rate, 1st and 2nd normal stress differences in unidirectional shear flow
σ_p	$\sigma - \eta_s\dot{\gamma}$ (polymer contribution to shear stress)

11.1. ORIGIN OF THE HOLE PRESSURE

Near the mouth of a liquid-filled hole in a rigid wall over which liquid undergoes shear flow, the stream surfaces are curved, appearing convex when viewed from the hole base (Fig. 11.1). For the particular case of creeping flow of a Newtonian liquid past the mouth of a transverse slot,[1] the local stream surfaces are symmetric with respect to reflection in the hole center plane (Figs. 11.1, 11.6(a)). As the Reynolds number Re is increased from zero, asymmetry develops,[3] with the stream surfaces being deflected in the flow direction in the sense shown in Fig. 11.6(b). For non-Newtonian liquids,[2,3] similar stream surface patterns are found, but there is, in addition, a tendency for the asymmetry to develop in the opposite direction, presumably due in some way to the elasticity of the liquid, or to the shear rate dependence of viscosity. Near the hole mouth, there is a dividing stream surface separating the liquid into two zones; between this surface and the hole base, one or more vortices occur, and the fluid velocities are very small.

At the base of a sufficiently deep hole (through which no liquid flows), the velocity gradient will be nearly zero and consequently the pressure P_2 exerted by the liquid on the hole base will be nearly uniform. We are interested in the differences

$$P^* := P_{1,av} - P_2 \quad \text{and} \quad P^{**} := P_1 - P_2 \quad (11.1)$$

between P_2, a pressure P_1 which the liquid would exert on the wall if the hole were filled in, and an average pressure $P_{1,av}$ which would be recorded by a pressure transducer mounted flush with a rigid wall opposite the hole axis (Fig. 11.2). It is understood that static pressure fields due to gravity

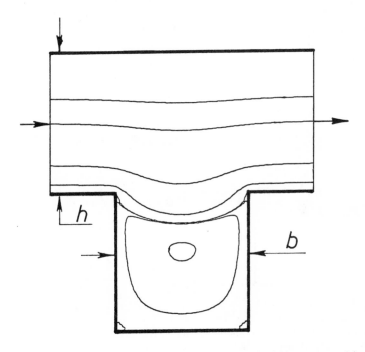

Fig. 11.1. Streamlines for an incompressible Newtonian liquid in pressure-driven two-dimensional creeping flow past the mouth of a liquid-filled transverse slot calculated by Trogdon and Joseph[1] by means of matched eigenfunction expansions. Slot width b, die height h, and slot depth are equal. The streamlines and speed field have symmetry with respect to reflection in the slot center plane.

are subtracted, and do not affect $P*$ or $P**$. We shall be concerned mainly with the case in which the hole mouth is a transverse slot of width b (measured parallel to the main flow direction) or a circle of diameter b.

In unidirectional shear flow, the stress at a point is determined, to within an additive isotropic stress, by the shear stress σ and the first and second normal stress differences N_1 and N_2. It is well known[4] that in rotational rheometers (such as the cone/plate or concentric cylinder rheometers) shear surface curvatures combine with N_1- and N_2-fields to generate wall pressure distributions whose measurement enables one to determine N_1 and N_2 under suitable conditions.

For flow past a hole, the question arises whether the combination of hole-induced stream surface curvature and main-shear-flow-induced normal stress difference fields can be used to estimate N_1 and N_2 from measured values of $P*$ or $P**$. If it can, such methods could give on-line measurements of N_1 and N_2 and measurements at higher shear rates than those attainable in rotational rheometers. It is possible that the presence of the hole might perturb the unidirectional shear flow, but if the hole is small enough ($b \ll h$, where h denotes the separation between the die walls) this perturbation might have a negligible effect on the flow history while giving enough shear surface curvature to generate measurable pressure differences.

Figure 11.3 gives a schematic diagram showing the presence of an N_1 field, tangential to the shear surfaces; a force balance on the liquid

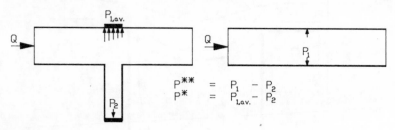

$$P** = P_1 - P_2$$
$$P* = P_{1,av.} - P_2$$

Fig. 11.2. Definition of hole pressures $P**$ and $P*$. A liquid undergoes unidirectional shear flow between two horizontal walls (right) and exerts a pressure P_1 at a point on one wall. At this point, a deep hole is inserted (left) and filled with liquid which exerts a pressure P_2 on the closed base. A pressure transducer mounted flush with the opposite wall with center on the hole centerline records an average pressure $P_{1,av.}$. Upstream (and downstream) boundary conditions are the same for the two cases; the flow can be generated either by a pressure gradient or by relative motion of the walls. The definition can be extended by allowing the two parallel horizontal walls to be curved.

enclosed by the dashed lines shows[10] that, figuratively speaking, forces associated with N_1 tend to pull the liquid out of the hole, but since this is not possible they generate a difference P^* between $P_{1,av}$ and P_2 such that P^* should increase monotonically with increasing N_1. Two questions now arise: can we subtract any inertial contributions to P^* which might occur, and is there a discoverable universal relation between P^* and N_1 (which can be used to determine N_1 from measured values of P^*)? We consider inertial effects first.

11.2. NEWTONIAN LIQUID HOLE PRESSURES

For an incompressible, homogeneous Newtonian liquid in isothermal flow which is fully developed upstream from the hole mouth, it is possible to see, from dimensional analysis, that the stream surface curvature field is determined by the geometry and by the Reynolds number **Re**, provided that gravity does not affect the velocity field. This would be the case, for example, for flow between parallel walls, one of which contains the hole, when, say, the upstream velocity profile is specified to be parabolic; for

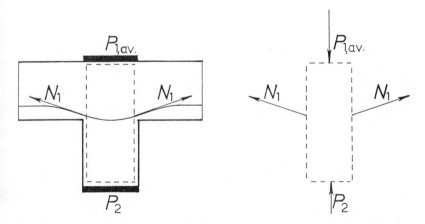

Fig. 11.3. Origin of the elastic contribution to hole pressure: equilibrium of forces acting on the region of liquid enclosed by dashed lines shows that a first normal stress difference field N_1 acting tangentially to curved shear lines will generate a positive value of $P^* = P_{1,av} - P_2$ which will increase monotonically with increase of N_1. In certain limiting cases (e.g. for creeping flow of a Second Order Fluid), symmetry requires that tangential components of traction acting on the vertical dashed faces will cancel each other.

deep holes, the only dimensionless quantities involved are Re, b/h, and ρ_{ij}/h, where ρ_{ij} denote the local principal radii of curvature of the stream surface.

We shall use the notation $P^* = P^*_N$ to label the hole pressure for a Newtonian liquid. For creeping flow (Re = 0), it can be shown,[10] by making use of the symmetry of the stream surfaces, that $P^*_N = 0$ (see below). When Re > 0, we know of no analytical expression for P^*_N. From dimensional analysis, we can expect a relation of the form

$$P^*_N = \sigma f(\text{Re}, b/h) \tag{11.2}$$

where σ denotes the value of shear stress at the wall, unperturbed by the hole, and $f(\ )$ is a dimensionless unknown function. Because we are assuming that the flow is fully developed at the hole, the upstream die length will not occur in eqn (11.2). We are also assuming that the hole depth is so great that it does not occur in eqn (11.2); for this and other reasons, it is clearly essential that there should be no net flow through the hole, otherwise its depth must be included in eqn (11.2).

The function $f(\ )$ has been estimated by numerical analysis for the case of a transverse slot[5] and a circular hole.[6] Comparisons with measured values[7,8] are shown in Figs 11.4 and 11.5. It is seen that there is reasonable agreement at lower and some disagreement at higher values of Re. The non-zero P^*_N owes its existence to stream surface asymmetry generated by inertial forces; the actual value of P^*_N obtained with a given apparatus could, therefore, be influenced as well by any additional asymmetry generated by unequal hole edges. For these transverse slot measurements,[7] the slots used were so narrow (40–50 μm) that it was not possible to be sure that the edges were substantially equivalent to one another, so the disagreement might be explicable in these terms. Considering the difficulty of measurement and the fact that there are no adjustable parameters involved in the comparisons, the agreement shown is encouraging and gives reason for placing confidence in the methods of measurement.

Here and throughout, we use the following definition of Reynolds number:

$$\text{Re} = \rho b h \dot\gamma^2 / (4\sigma) \tag{11.3}$$

where $\dot\gamma$ denotes the value of shear rate at the wall, unperturbed by the hole, and ρ denotes the density. The advantage of this choice is that, from computations, the following simple relation is approximately valid[5] for a range of values of b:

Transverse slot: $P^*_N = -0.033\sigma \text{ Re} \ (b < 0.8h; \text{ Re} < 2b/h)$ (11.4)

For a circular hole, measurements[8] give the result

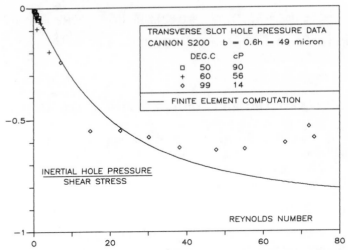

Fig. 11.4. Values of P_N^*/σ for a Newtonian liquid (Cannon S200) flowing over a transverse slot measured by Lodge[7] at 50 °C, 60 °C, and 99 °C for a range of values of Reynolds number Re $= \rho bh\dot{\gamma}/(4\eta)$. The curve represents values computed by Jackson and Finlayson.[5] No adjustable parameters are involved. The measured and calculated values agree up to, but not above, Re $= 30$.

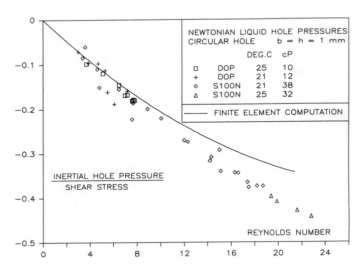

Fig. 11.5. Values of P_N^*/σ for Newtonian liquids (dioctyl phthalate and a base oil S100-N) flowing past a circular hole measured by Tong[8] for a range of values of Reynolds number Re $= \rho bh\dot{\gamma}/(4\eta)$. The curve represents values for an incompressible Newtonian liquid for the case $b = h$ computed by Crochet *et al.*;[6] no adjustable parameters are involved. Measured and computed values agree for Re < 6.

Circular hole: $P_N^* = -0.024\sigma \, \text{Re} \ (b = h; \, \text{Re} < 8)$ (11.5)

Computation[6] gives the same result for $\text{Re} = 1.07$; for $\text{Re} = 5.33$, the factor 0.024 is replaced by 0.023.

11.3. SECOND ORDER FLUID: CREEPING FLOW ANALYSIS

For steady, creeping, isothermal flow of a homogeneous, incompressible, Second Order Fluid past a deep, transverse slot, Tanner and Pipkin[10] have given an approximate analysis, valid for small slot widths ($b \ll h$), leading to the remarkably simple result

Transverse slot: $P^* = N_1/4 \qquad (P_i^* = 0)$ (11.6)

where N_1 denotes the value of the first normal stress difference at the wall, unperturbed by the hole. The 'switching on' of the non-Newtonian terms in the Second Order Fluid constitutive equation leaves the Newtonian velocity field unchanged[12] but changes the stress field and hence, in particular, the pressures $P_{1,\text{av}}$ and P_2. We use P_i^* to denote the inertial contribution to hole pressure (assuming that it can be separately identified); for a Newtonian liquid, $P_i^* = P_N^*$.

For most polymeric liquids (with the possible exception of certain 'liquid crystals'), $N_1 > 0$. It follows from eqn (11.6) that $P^* > 0$, and is thus opposite in sign to P_N^*. It is noteworthy that eqn (11.6) predicts that P^* should be independent of b; this again contrasts with the Newtonian case for $\text{Re} > 0$.

A similar approximate analysis by Kearsley[11] for creeping, rectilinear shear flow parallel to a narrow slot gives the result

Parallel slot: $P^* = -N_2/2 \qquad (P_i^* = 0)$ (11.7)

The derivations of eqns (11.6) and (11.7) are made possible by the fact that, for creeping flow of a homogeneous Second Order Fluid, the non-Newtonian terms can be equilibrated by pressure fields for 2-dimensional flow[12] and for rectilinear flow.[13] For the hole geometries considered, the Newtonian flow symmetry is such that $\sigma = p_{xy}$ is an even function of x in a neighborhood of the hole centerline ($=$ the y-axis of a rectangular Cartesian coordinate system with the x-axis parallel to the streamlines of the unperturbed flow); on the hole centerline, it follows that $\partial\sigma/\partial x = 0$ and hence that $\partial p_{yy}/\partial y = 0$. Thus p_{yy} has equal values at the hole base and at a point far above the hole where a negligible disturbance is assumed. It is this assumption which makes the analysis approximate, valid for small holes. Here, p_{xy} and p_{yy} denote Cartesian stress components.

The restrictions to 2-dimensional or rectilinear flow can be lifted[14] for the subset of homogeneous, incompressible Second Order Fluids for which

$$\beta := -N_2/N_1 = 1/2 \qquad (11.8)$$

In this case, we have

$$N_1/4 = -N_2/2 = (N_1 - N_2)/6 \qquad (\beta = 1/2) \qquad (11.9)$$

and so the transverse and parallel slot results (11.6) and (11.7) are the same. It also follows that these results apply to holes of any symmetric cross-section such that the Newtonian velocity field has the required symmetry; in particular, for a circular hole, we may write the result (for later comparison) in the form

$$Circular\ hole: P^* = (N_1 - N_2)/6 \qquad (\beta = 1/2; P_i^* = 0)$$

$$(11.10)$$

Because it predicts zero stress relaxation, the Second Order Fluid constitutive equation applies to no known non-Newtonian polymeric liquid. However, if the flow is globally a unidirectional shear flow, a wide class of constitutive equations can be reduced[15,16] to an equation of tensorial form similar to that of the Second Order Fluid but with coefficients which are not constants (in general) but scalar functionals of shear rate; if, in addition, for a given liquid under a limited range of shear rates, these coefficients do not vary very much, then one might be justified in hoping[13] that the Second Order Fluid analysis of hole pressures might furnish a useful approximation. Tanner and Pipkin gave measurements of hole pressure which did, in fact, agree reasonably well with this analysis.[10] We give additional data below.

11.4. HIGASHITANI–PRITCHARD CREEPING FLOW ANALYSIS

In an attempt to estimate hole pressures without assuming any particular form of constitutive equation, Higashitani and Pritchard[17,18,24] introduced certain assumptions which enabled them to analyze in more detail the force balance shown in Fig. 11.3 (according to which P^* should increase monotonically with N_1). The hole cross-section can be circular, or rectangular with its narrow axis parallel to or perpendicular to the main flow direction, or, indeed, any other shape having sufficient symmetry. Their assumptions may be expressed as follows:

(A) The flow is everywhere a unidirectional shear flow, with Re = 0.
(B) An orthogonal system of curvilinear space coordinates y_i exists with the y_1-curves as shear lines and the y_2-surfaces as shear surfaces (Fig. 11.6(a)).
(C) The hole centerline (a y_2-curve, with $y_1 = y_3 = 0$, say) is straight, and the shear surfaces and speed field have symmetry with respect to reflection in a plane $y_1 = 0$ through the centerline perpendicular to the main flow direction.
(D) At all points on the hole centerline, $\partial p_{11}/\partial y_1 = \partial p_{12}/\partial y_1 = 0$, where p_{ij} denote physical components of stress for the y_i-coordinate system.
(E) In an integration along the hole centerline, the variable of integration can be changed from y_2 to p_{12}.
(F) The y_3-surface through the centerline is plane and is a plane of reflectional symmetry for the speed field and stream surfaces.
(G) The hole is so deep that $p_{12} = N_1 = N_2 = 0$ on its base.
(H) The shear surface curvature is non-zero on the centerline, except possibly at a finite number of points.

The phrase *unidirectional shear flow* may be defined[16] as follows. A flow is a *shear flow* if the volume of no material element changes and there is a one-parameter family of material surfaces (called *shear surfaces*) each of which moves isometrically (i.e. the separation of each pair of neighboring particles in the surface is independent of time). A shear flow is *unidirectional* if, for each pair of neighboring shear surfaces, the direction of relative sliding is everywhere tangential to the same material line (a *line of shear*) at all time.

We refer the stress equations of motion to the orthogonal system of coordinates y_i (Fig. 11.6(a)) with certain coefficients expressed in terms of principal radii of curvature ρ_{ij} of the coordinate surfaces.[16] From (A) and (B), it follows[16] that this is a 'shear flow coordinate system' and that the y_3-surfaces are principal stress surfaces, i.e. that $p_{31} = p_{32} = 0$. From (F), it then follows that the No. 3 equation reduces to $\partial p_{33}/\partial y_3 = 0$, which is trivially satisfied. From (C) and (F), certain principal curvatures are zero. The No. 1 and No. 2 equations reduce to the following:

$$\frac{1}{h_1}\frac{\partial p_{11}}{\partial y_1} + \frac{1}{h_2}\frac{\partial p_{12}}{\partial y_2} + \frac{2p_{21}}{\rho_{23}} + \frac{p_{21}}{\rho_{21}} = \rho_{a_1} \qquad (11.11)$$

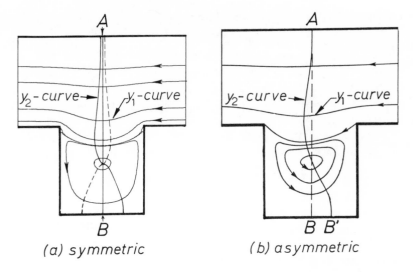

Fig. 11.6. Schematic diagrams of postulated orthogonal shear flow coordinate systems for flow past a liquid-filled hole with closed base. The diagrams show intersections with the plane $y_3 = 0$ which contains the hole centerline AB. Curves passing through the vortex center have been arbitrarily chosen to be smooth. Surfaces $y_2 = $ const. coincide with stream surfaces. In the symmetric case (a), the centerline AB is a (straight) y_2-curve ($y_1 = y_3 = 0$). In the asymmetric case (b), it is postulated that the y_2-curve through A meets the hole base (in a point B').

$$\frac{1}{h_1}\frac{\partial p_{21}}{\partial y_1} + \frac{1}{h_2}\frac{\partial p_{22}}{\partial y_2} - \frac{N_1}{\rho_{23}} + \frac{N_2}{\rho_{21}} = \rho_{a_2} \qquad (11.12)$$

where h_i^2 ($i = 1, 2, 3$) denote the diagonal components of the metric tensor, a_i denote the physical components of acceleration, and ρ_{23} and ρ_{21} denote the principal radii of curvature of the y_2-surface; by Dupin's theorem, the coordinate curves of an orthogonal system are lines of curvature on coordinate surfaces; ρ_{23} and ρ_{21} equal the radii of curvature of the y_1-curve and the y_3-curve, respectively, on a y_2-surface.

Let the centerline ($y_3 = y_1 = 0$) meet the upper wall at A and the base of the hole at B (Fig. 11.6(a)). Then, by integration along the centerline, we have

$$P^* := -p_{22}(A) + p_{22}(B) = -\int_B^A \frac{\partial p_{22}}{\partial y_2}\, dy_2 \qquad (11.13)$$

Using eqn (11.12), one may therefore write

$$P^* = P_e^* + P_i^* \tag{11.14}$$

where

$$P_e^* := -\int_B^A (N_1/\rho_{23} - N_2/\rho_{21})h_2 \, dy_2 \tag{11.15}$$

and

$$P_i^* := -\int_B^A (\rho a_2 - h_1^{-1} \partial p_{21}/\partial y_1)h_2 \, dy_2 \tag{11.16}$$

$N_1 = p_{11} - p_{22}$ and $N_2 = p_{22} - p_{33}$ denote the first and second normal stress differences[16] in unidirectional shear flow; $p_{21} = \sigma$, the shear stress. For a tensile normal stress i-component, $p_{ii} > 0$.

By hypothesis (E), the variable of integration in eqn (11.15) can be changed from y_2 to $\sigma = p_{21}$, and one can use the expression for $\partial p_{21}/\partial y_2$ given by eqn (11.11) to do this, provided that the range of integration can be divided into a finite number of subintervals throughout each of which p_{21} varies monotonically with y_2 and hence $\partial p_{21}/\partial y_2$ is non-zero; it is therefore necessary that, within each such subinterval, the expression

$$V := \rho a_1 - h_1^{-1} \partial p_{11}/\partial y_1 - (2/\rho_{23} + 1/\rho_{21})p_{21} \tag{11.17}$$

shall vanish nowhere. The integration limits become σ_A ($= p_{21}$ at A) and σ_B ($= 0$). The result may be written in the form

$$P_e^* = \int_0^{\sigma_A} \frac{N_1/\rho_{23} - N_2/\rho_{21}}{h_1^{-1} \partial p_{11}/\partial y_1 + (2/\rho_{23} + 1/\rho_{21})\sigma - \rho a_1} \, d\sigma \tag{11.18}$$

With $\rho a_1 = 0$ (creeping flow) and $\partial p_{11}/\partial y_1 = 0$ (assumption (D)), we thus obtain the Higashitani–Pritchard equation

$$P_e^* = \int_0^{\sigma_A} \frac{N_1/\rho_{23} - N_2/\rho_{21}}{2/\rho_{23} + 1/\rho_{21}} \frac{d\sigma}{\sigma} \tag{11.19}$$

Three particular cases are of special interest: the transverse slot, for which $\rho_{21} = \infty$; the parallel slot, for which $\rho_{23} = \infty$; and the circular or square hole, for which one may reasonably assume that $\rho_{21} = \rho_{23}$. In each case, the unknown non-zero curvature factor can be cancelled. We thus obtain the following remarkably simple results:

$$\text{Transverse slot: } P_e^* = \int_0^{\sigma_A} \frac{N_1}{2\sigma} \, d\sigma \qquad (11.20)$$

$$\text{Parallel slot: } P_e^* = \int_0^{\sigma_A} \frac{-N_2}{\sigma} \, d\sigma \qquad (11.21)$$

$$\text{Circular hole: } P_e^* = \int_0^{\sigma_A} \frac{N_1 - N_2}{3\sigma} \, d\sigma \qquad (11.22)$$

Baird[19] has noted that, by differentiating these integrals with respect to the upper limit variable σ_A, one may obtain the following alternative forms:

$$\text{Transverse slot: } N_1 = 2nP_e^* \qquad (11.23)$$

$$\text{Parallel slot: } N_2 = -nP_e^* \qquad (11.24)$$

$$\text{Circular hole: } N_1 - N_2 = 3nP_e^* \qquad (11.25)$$

Here,

$$n := \frac{d \log P_e^*}{d \log \sigma} \quad (\sigma = \sigma_A) \qquad (11.26)$$

For any liquid for which $N_i = c_i\sigma^2$ ($i = 1, 2$; $c_i = $ const.) over the range $(0, \sigma_A)$, it is easy to see that eqns (11.20), (11.21), and (11.22) reduce to eqns (11.6), (11.7), and (11.10), respectively, and also that $n = 2$. It follows, in particular, that the Higashitani–Pritchard equations agree with the Second Order Fluid equations. Do the former give a valid generalization of the latter? In attempting to answer this question by making comparisons with measured values of P_e^*, N_i, and σ, it is clear that liquids for which n differs significantly from 2 will be of special interest. For the comparisons made below, the differences between the two theories turn out to be mostly rather small in relation to the scatter of measurements.

In comparing measured quantities with predictions, abbreviations will be used for the equations, as explained in the accompanying table.

	Abbreviation	Transverse slot	Parallel slot	Circular hole	P_i^*
Second Order Fluid	SOF	(11.6)	(11.7)	(11.10)	0
Higashitani–Pritchard	HP	(11.20)	(11.21)	(11.22)	0
H–P–Baird	HPB	(11.23)	(11.24)	(11.25)	0
H–P–B–Lodge	HPBL	(11.23)	(11.24)	(11.25)	P_N^*

All the above equations agree on two important points: when inertia is negligible, there are monotonic relations between elastic hole pressures and normal stress differences; and, for a hole cross-section of given shape, *the hole cross-section dimension does not enter into these relations.* Tanner and Pipkin[10,13] suggest that such results are to be expected on grounds of dimensional analysis. Are they correct? For flows which are fully developed at the hole region and for sufficiently deep holes, dimensional analysis suggests that the relation should be expressible in the form

$$P^* = \sigma F(\text{Re}, b/h, N_1/\sigma, N_2/N_1, \tau\dot{\gamma}, N_1/G) \qquad (11.27)$$

where τ and G denote material constants having dimensions of time and modulus, respectively, and $F(\ )$ denotes a dimensionless function of unknown form. An important point is that, when $\text{Re} = 0$, b and h are the only two lengths involved: constitutive equations for polymeric liquids contain no material constants having the dimension of length, provided that we make the plausible assumption that these equations can be expressed in the form of relations between the body stress tensor at a typical particle P and the history of the body metric tensor at P and that no covariant derivatives of these tensor fields occur.[16] When $\text{Re} = 0$, eqn (11.27) shows that P^* is independent of hole size b to the extent that changes of b and h at constant b/h leave P^* unchanged. Experimental data support this, but also show[18,20] that, over a wide range of variables, P^* is independent of b/h. I cannot see how to explain this remarkable result by dimensional analysis alone. It is, however, predicted by the SOF and HP equations.

11.5. DISCUSSION OF THE HIGASHITANI–PRITCHARD ASSUMPTIONS

(A) This assumption means, in particular, that hole-induced stretching of the stream surfaces is negligible. For a rough estimate, let us consider the effect of hole-induced curvature of stream surfaces for flow past a transverse slot. For a small hole ($b \ll h$), we expect the principal curvature $\rho_{23}^{-1} = \varepsilon$, say, at any point to be small; hence $\partial p_{22}/\partial y_2 = \varepsilon h_2 N_1$ (the essential part of eqn (11.12)) is of first order in ε. The difference between the length of a curved segment of streamline and the corresponding straight line which would arise in the absence of the hole is, however, of second order in ε. This suggests (but does not prove) that an analysis of strain history near the hole would show that the departure from shear flow is of higher order than ε, and that, in consequence, the flow near the hole is approximately a shear flow, with the approximation improving for decreasing values of b/h.

(C) It is remarkable that the HP equations agree with data even under conditions in which photographs show that the stream surfaces are asymmetric.

(D) The assumption that $\partial p_{11}/\partial y_1 = 0$ on the hole centerline appears to be reasonable if the shear flow is torque-generated but questionable if it is pressure-generated. Let us suppose that we may write $p_{11} = p_{11,d} + p_{11,h}$, where $p_{11,d}$ denotes a contribution from the 'driven flow' (unperturbed by the hole) and $p_{11,h}$ denotes a hole-induced contribution. As an example of torque-generated shear flow, we may consider Couette flow between co-axial circular cylinders in relative rotation; then, because of the symmetry of the stress field with respect to arbitrary rotations about the common cylinder axis, we have $\partial p_{11,d}/\partial y_1 = 0$; it follows that $\partial p_{11}/\partial y_1 = \partial p_{11,h}/\partial y_1$, which may be assumed to be small for small holes; it would, however, need to be $O(\varepsilon^2)$ if it is to be negligible in the context of eqn (11.11) which contains a non-zero term $(2p_{21}/\rho_{23})$ of $O(\varepsilon)$, and I do not know whether this $O(\varepsilon^2)$ requirement can be justified. For pressure-driven shear flow, however, the situation appears to be worse, because $\partial p_{11,d}/\partial y_1$ is the pressure gradient which generates the main flow and is therefore large $(O(\varepsilon^0))$; I see no justification for neglecting it. These considerations suggest that different hole pressures might be found for torque-generated and for pressure-generated shear flows. Yet no such difference has been found experimentally or in the SOF analysis;[10] the latter does, however, show that, for a combined torque- and pressure-generated shear flow, a pressure gradient term (in $u\partial p^0/\partial x$ in equation (9) of reference 10) could become non-zero and might render inapplicable the SOF equation $P^* = N_1/4$.

(E) Possible difficulties in changing the variable of integration may arise in pressure-generated shear flow if the zeros in N_1 and σ occur at different locations on the centerline, so that the integrand N_1/σ becomes unbounded; if there are, in fact, singularities in the integrand, the question arises as to whether they are integrable. In addition, the sign of $\partial\sigma/\partial y_1$ can be expected to change along the centerline, so that separate integrations would be required, as noted above in connection with the requirement that eqn (11.17) vanish nowhere on the integration path in each zone.

(H) This assumption is introduced because, if the shear surface curvature were zero everywhere on the integration path, the numerator and denominator in the integrand of eqn (11.19) would vanish separately and so eqns (11.20)–(11.22) could not be derived.

In the evaluation of experimental data which follows, it will be seen that the differences between the HP and SOF predictions are mostly small, and that, where the difference appears to be significant (in comparison with the measurement scatter), the HP predictions are better than the SOF predictions. We consider data for high-viscosity (Re $<$ 0·1) and low-viscosity liquids separately.

11.6. HOLE PRESSURE DATA: HIGH VISCOSITY LIQUIDS

Figure 11.7 represents measured values of P^{**} for torque-driven flow past circular holes, for a 2% solution ('Z7') of polyisobutylene (Oppanol B200; $M_v = 4\,700\,000$) in an oligomer (Oppanol B1; $\eta_s = 0\cdot025$ Pa s at 25 °C). These values, and values for σ, N_1 and N_2, were obtained[21,22] from an extensive series of measurements made with cone–plate, plate–plate, and concentric cylinder rotational rheometers; flow birefringence data were found to be consistent with the N_1 data obtained from hole-free cone–plate data. Attempts to reconcile these data with data obtained using pressure holes led to the postulate[23] that polymeric liquids could generate large hole pressures having values independent of hole size. It is seen from Fig. 11.7 that changes in b/h do not affect P^{**}, and that cone–plate and concentric cylinder values are not very different; they are expected to be equal. Subsequent experiments with different concentric cylinder hole edges gave reason to believe that non-uniform concentric cylinder hole edges could have been responsible for the small differences shown in Fig. 11.7. For the data shown, Re $<$ 0·02; N_1/σ had values up to 12; $\eta_{rel} := \eta/\eta_s > 80$; η varied by a factor of 23; β varied in the range 0·040–0·097. These conditions are very far from the SOF conditions ($\eta =$ const.; $\beta = 0\cdot5$) for which (11.10) was derived; this is represented in Fig. 11.7 by the dashed curve ($P^* = (N_1 - N_2)/6$), which is seen to lie remarkably close to the measured values of P^{**}. It is reasonable to expect the difference $P^* - P^{**}$ to be small.[24] The agreement between the data and the SOF equation is remarkable. The values of $N_1/4$ and $- N_2/2$ are also shown (upper and lower dashed curves); the difference between them and $(N_1 - N_2)/6$ shows how far from the condition $\beta = 0\cdot5$ the data are (cf. eqn (11.9)). The values of the HP integral in eqn (11.22) also lie close to the data.

The agreement between data and the two theoretical curves shown in Fig. 11.7 suggests that, for some reason as yet unknown, the relation between hole pressure and normal stress differences is somewhat insensitive to changes made in the details of the derivations.

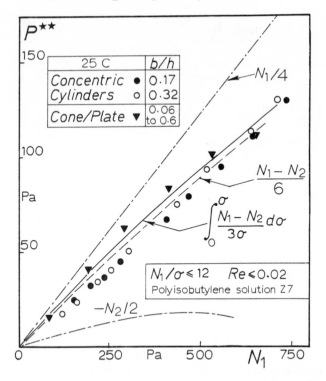

Fig. 11.7. Values of hole pressure P^{**} for a range of values of N_1 measured for circular holes by Kaye et al.[21] and Broadbent and Lodge[22] for a 2 wt% solution of polyisobutylene (Oppanol B200; $M_v = 4\,700\,000$) in an oligomer (Oppanol B1; viscosity 25 mPa s at 20 °C). Values obtained with cone–plate and concentric cylinder rheometers for different values of b/h are in fair agreement with each other and with values calculated from measured values of N_1, N_2, and σ by means of (i) the Higashitani–Pritchard integral (full curve) and (ii) one Second Order Fluid equation (11.10) (with an assumption $P^{**} = P^*$) for the case $\eta = $ constant and $\beta = 0.5$ (dashed curve, $(N_1 - N_2)/6)$; the agreement with (ii) is remarkable because, for the range of data shown, η varied by a factor of 23 and β varied from 0.04 to 0.097. If $\beta = 0.5$, the three dashed curves would coincide. Inertial contributions to P^{**} were negligible.

A second polyisobutylene solution batch (Z8) of composition nominally the same as that of 'Z7' was used by Pritchard[18,45] in a more extensive investigation of the effect of changing the hole diameters in the cone–plate pressure distribution apparatus used in the above experiments on 'Z7'. Figure 11.8 shows that the values of P^{**} measured for circular holes at a

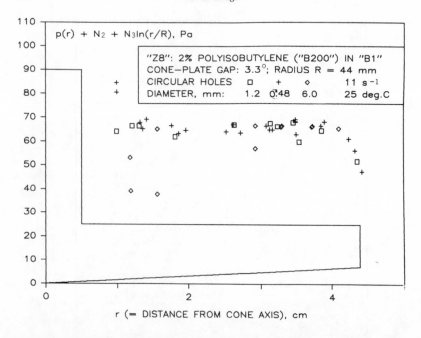

Fig. 11.8. Evidence that the hole pressure P^{**} is independent of hole diameter b for torque-driven shear flow when the inertial contribution to P^{**} is negligible. The data were obtained by Pritchard[18] for a polyisobutylene solution Z8 (having nominally the same composition as the solution Z7 featured in Fig. 11.7), using a cone–plate pressure distribution apparatus.[28] The ordinate represents values of $y = p(r) + N_2 + (N_1 + 2N_2)\ln(r/R)$, where $p(r)$ denotes the average, for two directions of cone rotation, of pressures recorded by a transducer connected to a circular hole in the horizontal plate; the hole center is at a distance r from the cone axis. The cone, of radius R, rotates in a sea of liquid on the horizontal plate which can be moved in its plane relative to the cone axis. The cone–plate gap profile is shown to scale. It is seen that, within the scatter, most points lie near a single horizontal line, showing that P^{**} ($= y$) is independent of b (in the range 0.5–6 mm) and of b/h (in the range 0·2–8). The deviation from the horizontal line of the four points at the right is attributed to a flow disturbance near the cone rim $r = R$. The other outlying points are subject to some uncertainty due to possible malfunctioning of a transducer.

given shear rate are substantially equal ($+3\%$ to -5% variation) for holes of diameter 0·48–6·02 mm and values of b/h in the range 0·2–8. These results are consistent with the SOF and HP predictions, made for $b/h \ll 1$. The observed constancy of P^{**} when the hole diameter b is changed by factors up to 12 and the ratio b/h is changed by factors up to 37 is remarkable and, as yet, unexplained. The Fig. 11.8 data are obtained from tabulated data supplied by Pritchard, from which I find that the numbers in columns 5 and 6 of reference 45 should be divided by $\log_e 10$.

The above data for 'Z7' and 'Z8' were obtained for torque-generated shear flow. For the rest of this chapter, we consider data obtained for pressure-generated shear flow. Schematic diagrams of the slit-die rheometers (called stressmeters) used are given in Fig. 11.9. The pressure gradient is determined either from pressures P_2, P_3 recorded with hole-mounted pressure transducers (Fig. 11.9(a)) or from pressures P_1, P_3 recorded with flush-mounted transducers (Fig. 11.9(b)). For brevity, we now use P_1 in place of $P_{1,\text{av}}$. The hole pressure $P^* = P_1 - P_2$ is determined from pressures P_1 and P_2 recorded with transducers which are flush- and hole-mounted, respectively. The three pressures are obtained at locations chosen to minimize the effects of die entrance and die exit disturbances to the assumed fully developed steady shear flow; when two identical holes are used (Fig. 11.9(a)), their hole pressure errors should be equal and hence one can determine the wall value σ of shear stress, unperturbed by hole errors, from the well known equation

$$\sigma = h(P_2 - P_3)/(2z) \tag{11.28}$$

where h and z denote the die height and the distance between hole center-lines measured along a line parallel to the main flow direction. The flow rate Q is measured either from the speed of rotation of a gear pump or

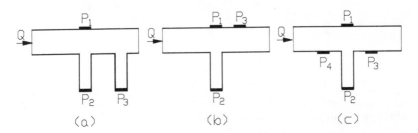

Fig. 11.9. Schematic diagrams of three transducer arrangements used to measure hole pressures $P^* = P_1 - P_2$ and $P^{**} = (P_3 + P_4)/2 - P_2$ for pressure-driven shear flow between fixed parallel walls of separation h. Values of wall shear stress σ, unperturbed by hole disturbances, are obtained from $P_2 - P_3$, $P_1 - P_3$, or $P_4 - P_3$, in cases (a), (b), (c), respectively, after multiplication by the factor $h/(2z)$, where z denotes the distance between the appropriate hole centers measured parallel to the main flow direction.

from the rate of rise of liquid flowing into an output cylinder; from the approximate wall shear rate

$$\dot{\gamma}_a := 6Q/(wh^2) \qquad (11.29)$$

where w ($\gg h$) denotes the width of the die cross-section, one can obtain the value of the wall shear rate $\dot{\gamma}$ (unperturbed by holes) from the well known slit-die analog of the Weissenberg–Rabinowitsch equation:[42]

$$\dot{\gamma} = (2 + m)\dot{\gamma}_a/3 \qquad (11.30)$$

where

$$m = \frac{d \log \dot{\gamma}_a}{d \log \sigma} \qquad (11.31)$$

Although the stressmeter design appears to be rather simple, measurement difficulties arise when the required pressure difference $P_1 - P_2$ is small in comparison with the local pressure P_1. One can either reduce P_1 (by using a positive drive pressure at the die entrance and negative pressure a the die exit,[24,25] or by having the measurement locations close to the die exit[26,27]) or use a system which measures the difference directly.[8,20] One must also check by direct measurement that leakage of liquid past the hole-mounted transducers is negligible.[9] It is also necessary to make corrections for systematic errors which can arise from small misalignment of the flush-mounted transducer effective center and the centerline of the opposite hole and from the use of a finite-width flush-mounted transducer[8] in a non-uniform pressure field; the effective center of such a transducer can move as the pressure gradient is increased.

Higashitani[24] measured P^* and P^{**} in a stressmeter with one hole-mounted and three flush-mounted transducers arranged as in Fig. 11.9(c). The extra flush transducer P_4 was used to evaluate $P^{**} = (P_3 + P_4)/2 - P_2$. For $b/h = 0.5$, the difference between P^* and P^{**} for a 0.6% aqueous solution of a polyacrylamide (Separan AP30), over a range of shear rates which gave values of N_1/σ up to 12, was at most 7% of P^*; this difference was hardly significant in relation to the scatter.[20] Although Re had values up to 8 (so that these experiments should not properly be included in the present section), the inertial contribution to hole pressure (estimated from (I), eqn (11.32), in Section 11.7) was at most only 1% of P^*, because of the high elasticity.

Figure 11.10 presents data obtained[26,29] with a molten low-density polyethylene (NPE952, melt flow index = 2, from Northern Petrochemicals) at 150 °C. A transverse slot stressmeter (Fig. 11.9(b)) was used with $b = h = 1$ mm; the pressures were measured at locations near the die exit. Stressmeter values for σ agreed with values obtained by H. M. Laun (BASF) using a Weissenberg 'rheogoniometer' modified by Meissner and by D.-K. Chang (RRC) using a similar rheogoniometer. Values of N_1 obtained from the two rheogoniometers were in reasonable agreement, and were used to determine the value of $n = \mathrm{d}\log N_1/\mathrm{d}\log\sigma = 1\cdot48$ for use in the HP equation (11.23); because n was constant, this procedure is equivalent to the use of eqn (11.26). The values of $P^*(\sigma)$ showed too much scatter for reliable use of eqn (11.26). It is seen from Fig. 11.10 that the HP prediction is consistent with the data, and that the SOF prediction is about 35% lower than the HP prediction.

Figure 11.11 shows similar results for a molten polystyrene (Styron 678)

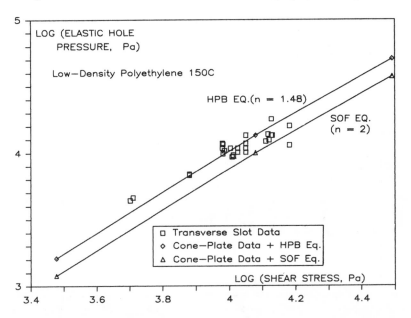

Fig. 11.10. Values of $\log P^*_e$ versus $\log\sigma$ measured by de Vargas[26,29] for molten low-density polyethylene flowing past the mouth of a transverse slot are consistent with values calculated by means of the Higashitani–Pritchard–Baird equations (11.23) and (11.26). Values of N_1 and σ were obtained from cone–plate measurements made by H. M. Laun and, independently, by D.-K. Chang. The Tanner–Pipkin[10] Second Order Fluid prediction (11.6) (lower straight line) lies about 35% lower than the HPB line; the viscosity varied by a factor of 2 over the range shown. Inertial contributions to hole pressure were negligible.

A. S. Lodge

at 190 °C obtained by Pike and Baird[27] with a somewhat similar stress-meter. Values of σ and N_1 were obtained with a Rheometrics cone–plate instrument. Viscosity values from the two instruments were fairly close. To evaluate the HP integral in eqn (11.20), I fitted a polynomial of the form $N_1/\sigma^2 = A + B\sigma + C\sigma^2$ to the cone–plate data. The HP curve in Fig. 11.11 is seen to be in reasonable agreement with the measured values of P^*. The SOF curve from eqn (11.6) is not very different from the HP curve, and is fairly close to the measured data points although the melt differs significantly from a Second Order Fluid because the viscosity varied by a factor of 2 over the range shown.

Figure 11.12 shows hole pressure data for a circular hole for a solution containing 28·5 g polystyrene (Pressure Chemicals 12a, $M_w = 670\,000 < 1·15\,M_n$) in 1 liter of Aroclors 1248 at 24 °C. The six highest points show

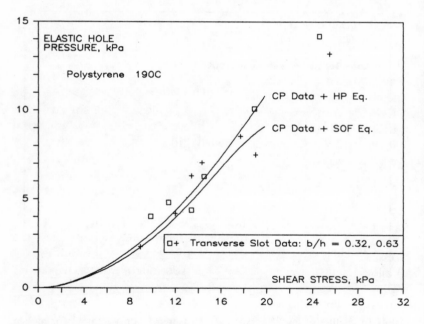

Fig. 11.11. Values of P_e^* versus σ measured by Pike and Baird[27] for molten polystyrene flowing past a transverse slot show no dependence on slot width b and, within the scatter, are consistent with the predictions (upper curve) of the Higashitani–Pritchard–Baird equations (11.23) and (11.26), evaluated with cone–plate data for N_1 and σ. The predictions (lower curve) of the Second Order Fluid equation (11.6) of Tanner and Pipkin[10] are also consistent with the measured points. Inertial contributions to P^* were negligible.

a small, systematic difference between values obtained for the two flow directions through the die, for unknown reasons. The averaged values, however, lie close to the HP curve obtained from eqn (11.25) with use of values for N_1 and N_2 which were obtained[30] from a truncated-cone and plate pressure-distribution rheometer[31] (the 'TCP' apparatus), in which values of $p(r)$, the pressure on the plate at distance r from the rotation axis, were obtained from hole-mounted pressure transducers. Since the N_1 and N_2 fields are uniform for the cone–plate geometry, hole pressure effects should be equal for each hole in the cone–plate zone, and hence one can use the familiar equation $N_1 + 2N_2 = -r\partial p_e/\partial r$ (where p_e denotes the value obtained from p after subtraction of the inertial contribution) to determine $N_3 := N_1 + 2N_2$. In order to obtain the value of N_2 from $p_e(R)$ (the value of $p_e(r)$ extrapolated to the rim $r = R$), it is necessary to make a correction for the hole pressure effect; the value of P^* obtained from an 'on-line stressmeter' with circular holes was used for this purpose, differences in the value of b/h for the two instruments being held to be unimportant in the light of data such as those shown in Figs 11.7 and 11.8. Figure 11.12 also shows that the SOF circular-hole prediction, eqn (11.10), is again close to the HP prediction, although the values of β (0·10–0·13) were significantly different from the value 0·5 used in the derivation of eqn (11.10); the viscosity showed little, if any, significant variation with shear rate. For other similar solutions, with polystyrene molecular weights of 390 000 and 860 000, agreement between measured values of P^* and HP predictions was also found.[8,32]

11.7. THE HPBL EQUATION: INERTIAL CORRECTION

In order to explore the possibility of attaining high shear rates in a stressmeter, it is necessary to attempt to extend the hole pressure analysis to allow for the effect of inertial forces, neglected in the SOF and HP treatments given above. In the first instance, one might attempt to take a step in this direction by hoping that, as Re is increased from zero, there would be a range of 'moderate' values of Re such that inertial forces make a significant contribution (represented by P_1^* defined in eqn (11.17)) to hole pressure while having negligible effect on the velocity field. The latter condition should be attainable if the inertial terms in the stress equations of motion could be equilibrated by a pressure field, either exactly or to a reasonable approximation.

If one could 'switch off' the N_1 and N_2 fields without changing the $\eta(\dot{\gamma})$

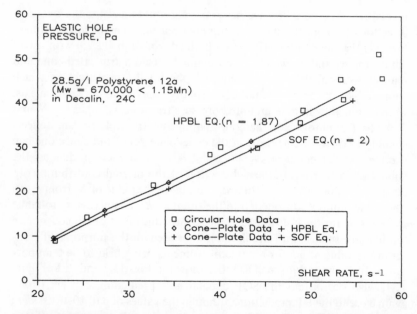

Fig. 11.12. Values of P_e^* versus $\dot{\gamma}$ measured by Tong[8] for a polystyrene solution flowing past the mouth of a circular hole of diameter 1 mm are, within the scatter, consistent with values (filled points) calculated by means of the HPBL equations (11.25) and (11.26) with use of values of N_1 and N_2 measured by Hou[30,31] with a cone–plate pressure-distribution apparatus. The predictions (lower curve) of the Second Order Fluid equation (11.10) for the case $\beta = 0.5$ are also close to the measured points (squares), although the actual values of β lay in the range of 0·10–0·13.

or velocity fields, the flow would be 'partially controllable' in the sense defined by Pipkin:[33] the velocity field is determined by the viscosity function $\eta(\dot{\gamma})$ alone and is unaffected by changes in the N_1 or N_2 fields. Pipkin has proved that the only such flows are flow between parallel plates and flow between concentric cylinders in relative rotation. There are, however, flows which are approximately partially controllable; shear flow between cone and plate in relative rotation is one important example: when $N_1 = N_2 = 0$ and $Re = 0$, the stress equations of motion are satisfied exactly by a unidirectional shear flow in which the shear surfaces are cones coaxial with the rotating cone, and the angular dependence of velocity and shear rate is governed by the viscosity function $\eta(\dot{\gamma})$ alone. The same statement is true even if N_1 and N_2 differ from zero provided that

$N_3 = 0$ (i.e. $\beta = 0 \cdot 5$); this is, incidentally, another example of Giesekus' theorem.[14] If N_3 is not zero, the stress equations of motion do not admit the foregoing unidirectional shear flow solution and there has to be a superposed 'secondary flow' velocity field. For gap angles of a few degrees, however, the secondary flow is extremely small[28] in comparison with the primary flow (the unidirectional shear flow), and one can still use the cone–plate system over a useful range of shear rates to obtain reliable values for N_1 and N_2. Under these conditions one may describe the cone–plate flow as 'approximately partially controllable'. Cone–plate data do, in fact, show that the pressure field for non-zero Re values can be expressed as a sum of an 'elastic' contribution (determined by N_1 and N_2) and an inertial contribution which is the same as that generated by a Newtonian liquid having density and viscosity values equal to those of the non-Newtonian liquid; remarkably enough, this is true even when the inertial contribution is greater than the elastic contribution.[20]

As noted above after eqn (11.16), $P_1^* = 0$ for creeping flow when $\partial p_{21}/\partial y_1 = 0$ on the hole centerline (assumption (C)); this is expected to be valid when the speed field and streamline surfaces have reflectional symmetry in the hole centerplane $y_1 = 0$, provided that the effects of the hole-induced perturbation to strain history can be neglected. When inertial effects are not negligible, the symmetry assumption (C) and the associated assumption (D) will be untenable in general; a possible exception could occur if the effect of elasticity just balanced the effect of inertia so that symmetry again prevailed. While there is evidence of a trend in this direction,[2] it would be too restrictive to rely on this possibility.

Accordingly, it is advisable to attempt to extend the HP analysis to accommodate speed field and streamline asymmetry. For this purpose, I retain all the HP assumptions (A)–(H) except for (C) and (D) which I replace by the following:

(C$_L$) The hole centerline is straight but the smooth y_2-curve of the orthogonal y_i-coordinate system which passes through the point A (the intersection of the hole centerline with the wall opposite the hole) meets the hole base, in some point B' (Fig. 11.6(b)).

(D$_L$) At all points of this curve AB', $\partial p_{11}/\partial y_1 = 0$.

These seem to me to be the simplest modifications to make to the HP analysis if it is to be extendable to asymmetric-stream-surface cases. An essential feature of the HP analysis is the use of an orthogonal (shear flow) coordinate system; if it exists, it allows one to simplify the stress equations of motion. The extension now proposed retains this feature by allowing the previously plane center surface $y_1 = 0$ to become curved. If the proposed assumptions (C_L) and (D_L) are valid, the rest of the HP analysis can be carried through without change except that P_i^* (defined by eqn (11.16)) need not be zero. Thus the effect of inertia is represented by the addition of a non-zero term P_i^* in eqn (11.14).

For a given liquid, P_i^*, defined by eqn (11.16), would presumably depend on the function $\eta(\dot\gamma)$ as well as on ρ. The evaluation of the integral in eqn (11.16) does not appear to be feasible, except by numerical methods for a given constitutive equation. Instead, I assume that an approximate evaluation is given by the equation

$$\text{(I)} \qquad\qquad\qquad P_i^* = P_N^* \qquad\qquad\qquad (11.32)$$

where P_N^* denotes the hole pressure for a Newtonian liquid of density ρ equal to that of the test liquid; the values of viscosity η_N and wall shear stress σ are chosen to be equal to the corresponding wall values (unperturbed by the hole) in the experiment with the test liquid. Let us refer to this as the *equivalent Newtonian liquid*. This assumption would be reasonable if the value of the inertial contribution P_i^* were insensitive to changes in the form of the viscosity function $\eta(\dot\gamma)$, and might not lead to significant error if $|P_i^*| \ll P_e^*$. For multigrade oils (such as BC30, considered below), this is not the case, but the shear rate dependence of η is small and the elasticity is small, so that eqn (11.32) again might not give much error.

According to the present assumptions for extending the HP analysis to accommodate flows with non-zero inertial effects, we thus have the final result that

$$P^* = P_e^* + P_N^* \qquad\qquad\qquad (11.33)$$

where the elastic contribution P_e^* is again given by eqns (11.20)–(11.22) or eqns (11.23)–(11.26), and P_N^* denotes the hole pressure for the 'equivalent Newtonian liquid'. A somewhat different treatment of the separation of inertial and elastic contributions to hole pressures has recently been given by Srinivasan,[41] who uses a different integration path.

11.8. HOLE PRESSURE DATA: LOW VISCOSITY LIQUIDS, HIGH SHEAR RATES

A commercial transverse-slot stressmeter has been developed[34] with the aim of measuring η and N_1 for multigrade oils at shear rates up to $10^6 \, s^{-1}$ and temperatures up to $150\,°C$, in order to approach running conditions in typical automotive journal bearings. Values of N_1 and η for 15 multi-grade oils obtained recently by Shell (UK) with one of these stressmeters have been compared[35] with values of the minimum oil film thickness H obtained by General Motors from direct measurements in an instrumented main bearing of a fired engine; a multiple linear regression analysis with $y = H$, $x_1 = \eta$, and $x_2 = N_1/(\dot{\gamma}\sigma)$ gave a correlation coefficient $R^2 = 0.70$; without x_2, it was found that $R^2 = 0.15$. These results suggest that gasoline mileage could be increased by the use of suitable multigrade oils with lowered viscosity and increased elasticity. If one wishes to use a stressmeter for rapid initial screening of new oil formulations, it would probably suffice if one could be sure that P_e^* is a monotonic increasing function of N_1 alone; a precise knowledge of the form of this function may not be essential for this, and perhaps for other, practical applications. Nevertheless, at this relatively early stage in stressmeter development, it is useful to investigate further the precise relation between P_e^* and N_1, by considering the validity of the SOF and HPB (or HPBL) equations, using data obtained from a Lodge Stressmeter® for High Shear Rates[34] (Model No. H301, on loan from Exxon Chemical Co.).

Typical die dimensions are as follows: length 6 mm; h 85 μm; b 45 μm; z 523 μm. Two transverse slots are used, as in Fig. 11.9(a). The three diaphragm-capacitance pressure transducers are used as null indicators, with servo-regulator-controlled air supplies on the electrode sides being used to restore the null positions. The three liquid pressures are thus converted to three air pressures which are led to two linear pressure-difference transducers at room temperature; their outputs give $P_1 - P_2$ and $P_2 - P_3$. A fourth transducer connected to the base of an output cylinder is used to measure the flow rate. Nitrogen or instrument air up to 500 psi is used to drive the liquid from an input cylinder through the die into the output cylinder. Small thermocouples up- and down-stream from the die are used to monitor the temperature rise (usually less than 1 degree C) due to viscous heating. A detailed description of the instrument[35] and the methods used to evaluate P_e^* and P_f^* has been published elsewhere.[7]

Some recent developments[7,8] in flush-transducer technique are of particular importance when hole pressure measurements in pressure-driven shear flow are used to determine N_1 for low-elasticity liquids such as multi-grade oils and molten undiluted polymers. When a flush-mounted transducer (of finite width) is used to measure pressure in a non-uniform pressure field, where is the effective center of the transducer, and does this center move as the pressure gradient is increased? For diaphragm-capacitance transducers, measurements and calculations[8] have shown that the center does move, and that the effect can be expressed in terms of a 'finite-width contribution' P_f^* to P^*. Because the diaphragm deflections are extremely small, it is safe to assume additivity in the sense that

$$P^* = P_e^* + P_N^* + P_f^* \tag{11.34}$$

when inertial and elastic contributions are not zero. P_f^* depends on the transducer diaphragm tension, diameter, and distance from the electrode, as well as on the pressure gradient $\partial p_{22}/\partial y_1$; for a given transducer and given die height, therefore, we may express P_f^* in the form

$$P_f^* = \sigma G(T, \sigma) \tag{11.35}$$

for some function G; the diaphragm tension may vary with temperature T. From values of P^* measured for a range of shear stresses for two Newtonian liquids (for which $P_e^* = 0$) having viscosities of about 10 and 20 mPa s at the working temperature, one can evaluate P_f^* and P_N^* separately[7] on the basis of eqn (11.12) and an assumption that two polynomials in σ can be used to represent the functions f and G in eqns (11.2) and (11.35) for given values of T, b, and h. The values of P_N^* shown in Fig. 11.4 were obtained in this way.

Values of the elastic hole pressure P_e^* for a range of values of shear stress σ are shown in Fig. 11.13 for a 10·3 wt% solution (D2) of polyisobutylene (Oppanol B50, $M_v = 400\,000$) in decalin. The points represent complete sets of single readings for two runs over the range shown. The figure also includes values of P_e^* calculated by means of the HPBL equations (11.23), (11.26), and (11.34) in which values of N_1 and σ were obtained from measurements[36] made with Walters' torsional balance rheometer (TBR) —a parallel plate rotational rheometer which can be used at shear rates up to 20 700 s^{-1}. The TBR thrust gives values for $N_1 - N_2$, from which values of N_1 were calculated using a value $\beta = 0·1$ which had been obtained for low shear rates in another cooperative measurement program[37] for a similar solution (D1) with PIB of higher molecular weight. The difference between N_1 and $N_1 - N_2$ is hardly significant in comparison with the scatter of data shown in Fig. 11.13. Corresponding values for P_e^*, obtained with the SOF equation (11.6) and (11.34) are also shown in Fig. 11.13. The range of measurement common to both instruments extends up to $\dot{\gamma} = 20\,700$, $N_1/\sigma = 4$, Re = 0·1; viscosity varied from 2 to 0·2 Pa s, with consistent values from the two instruments. The smallest value of η_{rel} was 70.

It is seen that the TBR measurements confirm the validity of the HPBL equations used with the transverse-slot stressmeter data as a method for

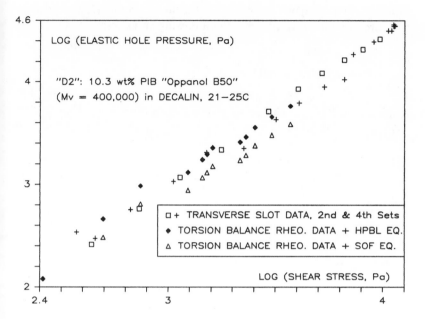

Fig. 11.13. Values of $\log P^{*}_{e}$ versus $\log \sigma$ (squares and crosses) measured by Lodge[7] for a polyisobutylene/decalin solution D2 flowing past the mouth of a transverse slot are consistent with values (filled diamonds) calculated from the HPBL equations (11.23), (11.26), (11.32), and (11.33) combined with values of $N_1 - N_2$ calculated by Lodge *et al.*[36] from values of thrust measured in a narrow-gap parallel-plate rheometer (the 'torsion balance rheometer'). A value $\beta = 0.1$ was assumed. The predictions (open triangles) of the Tanner–Pipkin[10] Second Order Fluid equation (11.6), modified by means of eqn (11.32), are about 60% lower than the measured points. The viscosity varied by a factor of 10 over the range of measurement shown. The results support the use of transverse-slot hole pressure measurement and the HPBL equations as a means of measuring N_1 up to shear rates of $20\,700\,\mathrm{s}^{-1}$ (the highest value in the common range of measurement).

measuring N_1 at shear rates up to $20\,700\,\mathrm{s}^{-1}$. It is also seen that the SOF equation gives values which are about 60% lower than the measured values.

Because there is no established method for measuring N_1 at shear rates above $20\,700\,\mathrm{s}^{-1}$, some assumption must be made in order to test the validity of stressmeter measurements (and the HPBL equations) at higher shear rates. For this purpose, it is natural to use the familiar 'time–temperature superposition' properties[44] commonly exhibited by solutions of flexible homopolymer molecules. In the present context, partial derivatives are to be interpreted using the following variables:

Dependent variables: $\quad \sigma,\ \sigma_p,\ \sigma_r,\ \sigma_{pr},\ N_1,\ N_{1r},\ P_e^*,\ P_{er}^*$

Independent variables: $\quad T,\ \dot{\gamma}_r$

Here, $\sigma_p := \sigma - \eta_s \dot{\gamma}$; $\dot{\gamma}_r := \dot{\gamma} a(T)$, where $a(T)$ is a function of the absolute temperature T alone, chosen to give 'superposition'; and $X_r := \rho_o T_o X / (\rho T)$ where X denotes any stress or pressure variable and ρ_o denotes the value of density ρ at some chosen temperature T_o.

Liquids are said to satisfy a *time–temperature superposition principle* in a temperature range $T_1 < T < T_2$ and a 'reduced shear rate' range $\dot{\gamma}_{r1} < \dot{\gamma}_r < \dot{\gamma}_{r2}$ if a function $a(T)$ can be found such that

$$\partial \sigma_{pr} / \partial T = 0 \tag{11.36}$$

and

$$\partial N_{1r} / \partial T = 0 \tag{11.37}$$

Such equations are satisfied by the Rouse–Zimm bead–spring theory for dilute polymer solutions,[43] provided that certain model parameters h^*, N are independent of T, and also by Oettinger's recent development[38] of these theories which predicts a shear-rate-dependent viscosity and a non-zero N_2.

Stressmeter data given below are in approximate agreement with the equations

$$\partial P_{er}^* / \partial T = 0 \tag{11.38}$$

$$\partial L^* / \partial T = 0 \tag{11.39}$$

where

$$L^* := \frac{\partial \log \sigma_{pr}}{\partial \log \dot{\gamma}_r} \bigg/ \frac{\partial \log \sigma_r}{\partial \log \dot{\gamma}_r} \tag{11.40}$$

It follows from eqns (11.36)–(11.40) that

$$\partial (N_1 - 2n P_{er}^*) / \partial T = 0 \tag{11.41}$$

where

$$n = \frac{\partial \log P_{er}^*}{\partial \log \dot{\gamma}_r} \bigg/ \frac{\partial \log \sigma_r}{\partial \log \dot{\gamma}_r} \tag{11.42}$$

in agreement with eqn (11.26). Hence, if independent measurements show that $N_1 = 2nP_e^*$ at T_1 and the above properties hold for $T_1 < T < T_2$ and $\dot{\gamma}_0 < \dot{\gamma} < \dot{\gamma}_1$, it follows that $N_1 = 2nP_e^*$ at T_2, and that the HPBL equation (11.23) is valid up to a higher shear rate $\dot{\gamma}_2 = \dot{\gamma}_1 a(T_1)/a(T_2)$. The only assumption involved here is that eqn (11.37) is valid, because the range of validity of the remaining equations (11.36), (11.38), and (11.39) can be established by direct stressmeter measurements. For most liquids tested to date, the relative viscosity is high (> 10) and so one might expect eqn (11.39) to be approximately valid; for one oil BC30, however, η_{rel} varies from 1·6 to 1·2, and the approximate validity of eqn (11.39) found by measurement is somewhat surprising.

The stressmeter data in Fig. 11.14 show that $P_{er}^*(\dot{\gamma}_r)$ and $\sigma_r(\dot{\gamma}_r)$ are independent of T in the range 21–111 °C; the σ range extends to 11 kPa (at 21 °C). At 21 °C for σ up to 3·5 kPa, the N_1 data are consistent with those from the TBR (Fig. 11.13). If eqn (11.37) is valid up to 111 °C, it follows that the HPBL equations (11.23), (11.26), and (11.34) are valid (for these data) up to $\sigma = 3·5$ kPa at 111 °C, i.e. up to $\dot{\gamma} = 112\,000\,\text{s}^{-1}$; here, $\text{Re} = 3$, $-P_N^*/P_e^* = 0·06$, and $\eta_{rel} > 50$. Although the TBR test does not go above $\sigma = 3·5$ kPa for this liquid, the fact that the stressmeter data (P_{er}^* and σ_r) exhibit the superposition properties over the whole range shown gives some reason for confidence in the view that these data should give valid N_1 measurements over this range, which extends the shear rate range up to $\dot{\gamma} = 290\,000\,\text{s}^{-1}$ and the reduced shear rate range up to $\dot{\gamma}_r = 390\,000\,\text{s}^{-1}$ (with $a(T) = 1$ at 111 °C). For D2, there was no significant difference between σ and σ_p.

In an attempt to extend the shear rate range up to $\dot{\gamma} = 10^6\,\text{s}^{-1}$, a sample of D2 was diluted with decalin, giving an 8·7 wt% solution labelled D2b. Stressmeter data satisfied eqns (11.36), (11.38), and (11.39) over the whole range of measurement, namely: 60–99 °C; $\dot{\gamma}$ up to $1·2 \times 10^6\,\text{s}^{-1}$, Re up to 96, and $-P_N^*/P_e^*$ up to 0·16. If eqn (11.37) is valid and if TBR data (now being obtained) confirm the HSRSM data over common ranges of T and σ, it will follow that the stressmeter can be used to give values of N_1 at shear rates up to $1·2 \times 10^6\,\text{s}^{-1}$. For these data, $12 < \eta_{rel} < 61$.

For an experimental multigrade oil BC30, the solvent contribution $\eta_s\dot{\gamma}$ was a much larger fraction of shear stress than in the case of the other liquids considered above; it was found that $1·2 < \eta_{rel} < 1·6$, and that eqns (11.36), (11.38), and (11.39) were satisfied for most data within the scatter of measurements. It was also found that $\sigma_r(\dot{\gamma}_r, T)$ varied with T to a significant extent, represented by the non-zero values of $K(T)$ used in Fig. 11.15. The superposition of data shown in Fig. 11.15 (except at the highest temperature and shear rates, where errors in σ measurement due

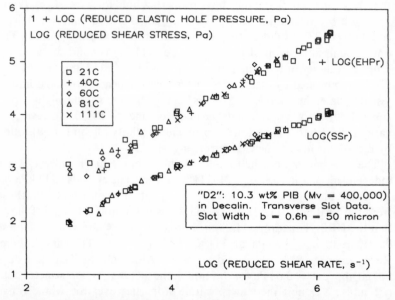

Fig. 11.14. Values of $\log P^*_{er}$ (upper points) and $\log \sigma_r$ (lower points) measured by Lodge[7] for the polyisobutylene solution D2 featured in Fig. 11.13 flowing past the mouth of a transverse slot satisfy a time–temperature superposition principle over the range of temperatures (21–111 °C) investigated. For this solution, $\sigma_p = \sigma$ within 1%. The results suggest that transverse slot hole pressure measurements coupled with the HPBL equations can give values of N_1 up to shear rates of 290 000 s^{-1} (the highest value for the data shown).

to the use of non-degassed liquid are thought to have arisen) establishes the validity of eqn (11.39). No TBR data are available for this oil, whose elasticity is probably too small for TBR measurements to be made. The validity of eqn (11.36) is shown by the superposition of data in the lower curve of Fig. 11.16; at high $\dot{\gamma}$, 74 °C data are anomalous. The anomalous values are believed to be influenced by errors in the shear stress measurement arising from the presence of microbubbles of sizes comparable with the die height. In other experiments made with an ultra-high-shear-rate-viscometer[7] having a die height of 25 μm, it has recently been found that measurements made with decalin at shear rates up to 5×10^6 s^{-1} have anomalously high shear stress values and that the anomaly can be removed by thorough degassing prior to measurement; this viscometer is similar to the stressmeter but has a rigid wall in place of the flush-mounted

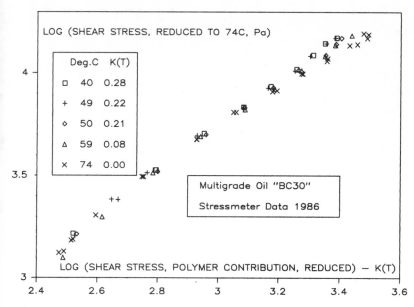

Fig. 11.15. Data points representing values of $\log \sigma_r$ versus $\log \sigma_{pr}$ obtained at different temperatures for a multigrade oil BC30 are seen to be superposable by horizontal shifts $K(T)$, except for the highest 74 °C points, which may be in error due to microbubble effects. The superposition shown establishes the approximate validity of eqn (11.39).

transducer. The anomaly attributed to bubble trouble tends to become more evident at low viscosities and high shear rates.

In evaluating n by means of eqn (11.42), the anomalous 74 °C data were omitted. The HPBL equations (11.23), (11.34), and (11.42) have been used to evaluate N_1 at each temperature; the results are plotted in reduced form in Fig. 11.16 (upper points). It is seen that there is reasonable time–temperature superposition of the form (11.37), within the scatter of measurement, which evidently increases as the reduced shear rate decreases. The greatest shear rate is $1.2 \times 10^6 \text{s}^{-1}$, which was obtained at 74 °C; the greatest value of reduced shear rate $\dot{\gamma} a_T$ is $2.7 \times 10^6 \text{s}^{-1}$; for these data, $N_1 / \sigma < 1$. These results afford some confidence for the view that the stressmeter can give values of N_1 to a reasonable approximation up to shear rates of 10^6s^{-1}.

For these data, the greatest value of Re was 83 and, for the D2b data, 96. In 1983, data taken with BC30 were interpreted[20] to mean that elastic and inertial contributions to P^* were additive (as assumed) up to but not

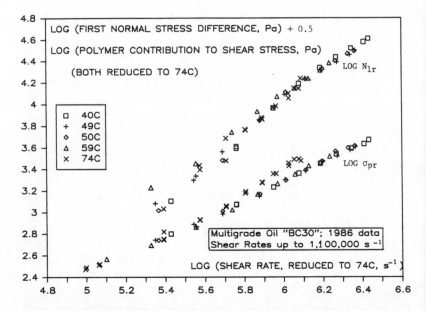

Fig. 11.16. Values of $\log N_{1r}$ (upper points) and $\log \sigma_{pr}$ (lower points) versus $\log \dot{\gamma}_r$ for the multigrade oil BC30 satisfy a time–temperature superposition principle, except for the highest 74 °C σ_{pr} points, which may be in error due to microbubble effects. The values of N_1 were obtained by means of the HPBL equations (11.23), (11.26), (11.34), and (11.42), together with (11.39), applied to values of hole pressure P^* measured by Lodge[7] for flow past the mouth of a transverse slot. The near superposition shown suggests that the method gives approximate values of N_1 up to shear rates of $1\,100\,000\,\mathrm{s}^{-1}$ (the highest value used, at 74 °C) and up to reduced shear rates of $2\,700\,000\,\mathrm{s}^{-1}$.

above Re = 15; now, however, we see no such restriction. The present method of evaluating P_f^* is believed to be more reliable than the 1983 method whose validity depends on an unsupported assumption that the elasticity of 'Bright Stock' was negligible.

The fact that, for BC30, $P_{er}^*(\dot{\gamma}_r)$ and $\sigma_{pr}(\dot{\gamma}_r)$ are independent of T while $\sigma_r(\dot{\gamma}_r, T)$ depends on T is of interest in another important connection. In spite of published counter examples,[20] it is sometimes argued that $N_1(\dot{\gamma})$ can be calculated from $\sigma(\dot{\gamma})$. The different time–temperature superposition behavior of P_e^* and σ found for BC30 suggests that BC30 furnishes another counter example. Another very important counter example has recently been published[37] for D1: a 2% solution of polyisobutylene (Oppanol B200, $M_v = 4\,700\,000$) in decalin. The solution was degraded by passage through a gear pump for various periods at increasing pump speeds. Periodically, the pump speed was lowered to a fixed value and the viscosity η and hole pressure P^* were measured. It was found that there was negligible change in the viscosity and that P^* decreased by about 30%. It is well known that η and $N_1/\dot{\gamma}^2$, at low shear rates, depend on very different moments of the molecular weight distribution; presumably, the very high molecular weight molecules break first, with a noticeable effect on N_1 but not on η. These data, obtained with an On-Line Stressmeter which can be used in a sample-testing or in an on-line mode, suggest that such an instrument could usefully be used to monitor polymerization reactions with the hope of obtaining better quality control than that attainable by measurement of viscosity alone.

11.9. DISCUSSION AND CONCLUSIONS

Space limitations prevent me from doing justice to the important work of Baird[27] and coworkers who have made extensive flow birefringence studies of the detailed stress distribution in flow of polymer melts past transverse slots, or to the increasing number of computations of hole pressures made with various constitutive equations.[40] Some other published measurements of hole pressures have given results which seem to be very different from mine; I have discussed these measurements elsewhere.[20,25,26] I believe that the apparent discrepancies can be attributed in each case to one or more experimental difficulties: use of insufficiently sensitive transducers; attempts to mount a flat transducer flush with a cylindrical wall; small leakage of test liquid through holes; and failure to investigate the flush transducer finite-width effect.

The results presented above are encouraging: they suggest that hole pressure measurements can be used to determine values of N_1 for molten polymers up to moderate shear rates, and for multigrade oils and other low-viscosity liquids up to shear rates as high as $1\,000\,000\,\text{s}^{-1}$. Moreover, the measuring techniques developed for this purpose have also led recently to very small slit die viscometer experiments which suggest that multigrade oil viscosities in the few mPa s range can be measured up to shear rates as high as $5\,000\,000\,\text{s}^{-1}$. These results have been published elsewhere.[7]

In regard to the SOF and HPBL equations relating hole pressures and normal stress differences, all reliable available experimental data show that the equations have a range of approximate validity (usually within a scatter band of about $\pm 10\%$) which extends far outside the range of validity of assumptions used in deriving the equations. This paradox is as yet unresolved.

With the aim of illuminating the physical principles underlying the use of hole pressure data for determining N_1 and N_2, I have here presented data for only a few polymeric liquids. Results for a greater variety of liquids have been given elsewhere.[20] Possible limitations of the method could arise if the test liquid has a yield stress: it could not then be used in the holes, because large errors in pressure transmission could occur; this is of importance for many liquids of industrial interest, e.g. molten ABS, molten filled polymers, and other polymeric liquids containing rigid particle additives. Limited experiments have, however, suggested that one can use a different liquid to fill the holes without invalidating the method: in one example, glycerine was used to fill the holes when mayonnaise was measured in the On-Line Stressmeter.[20] It would also be desirable to use stable (nearly incompressible) molten polymer in the holes with the possibility of making periodic bleeds to fill the holes with fresh, undegraded polymer. This would clearly be essential if the melt Stressmeter is to be successfully used with molten polymers such as PVC. These possibilities have, however, not yet been adequately investigated.

ACKNOWLEDGEMENTS

For financial support, I am grateful to Exxon Chemical Co.; the US Army Research Office (grant No. DAAG29-84-K-0046, and grant No. DAAL-03-86-K-0174 to the Engine Research Center); and E. I. Du Pont de Nemours & Co. (for polymer science and engineering grants to the Rheology Research Center). I gratefully acknowledge technical assistance from R. Williams and D. H. Hutchins. Professors W. G. Pritchard, B. A. Finlayson and D. G. Baird kindly furnished tabulated data, and Dr R. B. Rhodes (Shell Development Co.) provided base stock viscosity data. I have had many helpful discussions with Professors W. G. Pritchard and D. S. Malkus.

REFERENCES

1. S. A. Trogdon and D. D. Joseph, *J. Non-Newtonian Fluid Mech.*, 1982, **10**, 185.
2. T. -H. Hou, P. P. Tong and L. de Vargas, *Rheol. Acta*, 1977, **16**, 544.

3. T. Cochrane, K. Walters and M. F. Webster, *Phil. Trans. Roy. Soc.,* 1981, **A301**, 163.
4. A. S. Lodge, *Elastic Liquids*, Academic Press, New York, 1964.
5. N. R. Jackson and B. A. Finlayson, *J. Non-Newtonian Fluid Mech.,* 1982, **10**, 55.
6. M. J. Crochet, S. DuPont and J. M. Marchal, *Trans. Soc. Rheol.,* 1986, **30**, S91.
7. A. S. Lodge, SAE Paper No. 870243, 1987.
8. P. P. Tong, PhD thesis, University of Wisconsin–Madison, 1980.
9. A. S. Lodge, *J. Rheol.,* 1983, **27**(5), 497.
10. R. I. Tanner and A. C. Pipkin, *Trans. Soc. Rheol.,* 1979, **13**, 471.
11. E. A. Kearsley, *Trans. Soc. Rheol.,* 1970, **14**(3), 419.
12. R. I. Tanner, *Phys. Fluids,* 1968, **9**, 1246.
13. A. C. Pipkin and R. I. Tanner, *Mechanics Today,* 1972, **1**, 262.
14. H. Giesekus, *Rheol. Acta,* 1963, **3**, 59.
15. W. O. Criminale, J. L. Ericksen and G. L. Filbey, *Arch. Rat. Mech. Anal.,* 1958, **1**, 410.
16. A. S. Lodge, *Body Tensor Fields in Continuum Mechanics*, Academic Press, New York, 1974.
17. K. Higashitani and W. G. Pritchard, *Trans. Soc. Rheol.,* 1972, **16**, 687.
18. W. G. Pritchard, *Phil. Trans. Roy. Soc.,* 1971, **A270**, 508.
19. D. G. Baird, *Trans. Soc. Rheol.,* 1975, **19**, 147.
20. A. S. Lodge, *Chem. Eng. Commun.,* 1985, **32**, 1.
21. A. Kaye, A. S. Lodge and D. G. Vale, *Rheol. Acta,* 1968, **7**, 368.
22. J. M. Broadbent and A. S. Lodge, *Rheol. Acta,* 1971, **10**, 557.
23. J. M. Broadbent, A. Kaye, A. S. Lodge and D. G. Vale, *Nature,* 1968, **217**, 55.
24. K. Higashitani, PhD thesis, University of Wisconsin–Madison, 1973.
25. K. Higashitani and A. S. Lodge, *Trans. Soc. Rheol.,* 1975, **19**, 307.
26. A. S. Lodge and L. de Vargas, *Rheol. Acta,* 1983, **22**, 151.
27. R. D. Pike and D. G. Baird, *J. Rheol.,* 1984, **28**(4), 439.
28. N. Adams and A. S. Lodge, *Phil. Trans. Roy. Soc.,* 1964, **A256**, 149.
29. L. de Vargas, PhD thesis, University of Wisconsin–Madison, 1979.
30. T.-H. Hou, PhD thesis, University of Wisconsin–Madison, 1980.
31. A. S. Lodge and T.-H. Hou, *Rheol. Acta,* 1981, **20**, 247.
32. A. S. Lodge, *IUPAC Proc. 28th Macromol. Symp.,* 1982, p. 774.
33. A. C. Pipkin, *Quart. Appl. Math.,* 1968, **26**, 87.
34. The Bannatek Co., Inc., PO Box 5472, Madison, Wisconsin 53705-0472.
35. T. W. Bates, B. Williamson, J. A. Spearot and C. K. Murphy, S.A.E. Paper No. 860376, 1986.
36. A. S. Lodge, T. S. R. Al-Hadithi and K. Walters, *Rheol. Acta,* 1987, **26**, 516.
37. G. A. Alvarez, A. S. Lodge and H.-J. Cantow, *Rheol. Acta,* 1985, **24**, 368.
38. H. C. Oettinger, *J. Chem. Phys.,* 1986, **84**, 4068; University of Wisconsin–Madison Rheology Research Center Report RRC109, 1986.
39. J. Meissner, *Rheol. Acta,* 1975, **14**, 471.
40. D. S. Malkus and M. F. Webster, 1986, *J. Non-Newtonian Fluid Mech.,* 1987, **25**, 93.
41. R. Srinivasan, *Rheol. Acta,* 1987, **26**, 107.
42. K. Walters, *Rheometry*, Chapman and Hall, London, 1975, eqn (5.27).

43. A. S. Lodge and Yeen-jing Wu, *Rheol. Acta,* 1971, **10,** 539.
44. H. Markovitz, *J. Polym. Sci., Symposium No. 50*, 1975, p. 431.
45. W. G. Pritchard, *Rheol. Acta,* 1970, **9,** 200.

Chapter 12

Sliding Plate and Sliding Cylinder Rheometers

J. M. DEALY

Department of Chemical Engineering, McGill University, Montreal,
Canada

and

A. J. GIACOMIN

Department of Mechanical Engineering, Texas A & M University,
College Station, Texas, USA

12.1. INTRODUCTION

The present review is concerned with rheometers that are particularly advantageous for the generation of large, rapid transient shear deformations in highly viscous, non-Newtonian fluids, viz. sliding plate and sliding cylinder rheometers. Large, rapid deformations are particularly useful for the study of time dependent structural changes and nonlinear viscoelasticity, and a number of material functions have been defined to facilitate the interpretation and presentation of nonlinear viscoelastic data.[1] The rheometers described here are thus of particular value in the evaluation of

383

rheologically complex materials that are processed using industrial machinery. Included in this category of materials are molten plastics, elastomers, concentrated polymer solutions, asphalts, bread doughs, and other concentrated suspensions.

The instruments most commonly used to measure the response of such materials to shearing deformations, i.e. pressure flow rheometers and rotational rheometers, are unsuitable for the study of responses to large transient deformations. For this type of deformation, 'sliding surface' rheometers have been found advantageous, i.e. instruments in which a more or less uniform shear is generated by the rectilinear motion of one surface relative to a second surface parallel to it. Both sliding plate ('plane Couette') flow and sliding cylinder ('telescopic shear') flow have been used to advantage.

The purpose of this review is to summarize the advantages and limitations of sliding plate and sliding cylinder rheometers and to survey the various ways they have been used.

12.1.1. Limitations of Rotational and Pressure Flow Rheometers

The measurement of the pressure drop associated with the flow of a fluid in a straight channel, either a capillary or a slit, is the oldest and most popular single rheological technique. However, the only well defined rheological property that can be reliably measured in such an instrument is viscosity.[2] Since the flow field is not homogeneous, pressure flow rheometers cannot be used to study time dependent phenomena such as viscoelasticity and thixotropy. In particular, the shear rate varies across the channel, and at the entrance it varies in the flow direction. Furthermore, at the entrance there is a strong extensional mode of deformation superposed on the shear flow.

In rotational rheometers, the shear rate is nearly constant for a fluid element, and the response to transient deformations can be studied. The cone and plate geometry is popular, because the shear rate is approximately uniform, only a small sample is required, and sample insertion is simple. However, deviations from the ideal uniform shear rate distribution are present at all rotational speeds[3] and can cause significant errors for large cone angles, low viscosities or high speeds.[4] For materials having large values of the first normal stress difference, instrument compliance is a serious problem. For highly elastic materials, anomalous flow at the free surface is the most serious problem that arises in the use of cone–plate rheometers, and for such instruments this phenomenon often limits the shear rate at which reliable results can be obtained to values below $1 \, \mathrm{s}^{-1}$.[5,6]

For small amplitude oscillatory shear, the parallel disk geometry has several advantages over the cone–plate.[7] However, the shear rate is not uniform, and the study of nonlinear effects requires complex methods of data reduction[8,9] and in most cases the assumption of a constitutive equation.[10-12] The problem of shear rate nonuniformity can be circumvented to some extent by the use of a shear stress transducer.[13] Such an arrangement is especially well suited to use as an in-line process rheometer,[14] but it is not suitable for precise scientific measurements.

The eccentric rotating disk rheometer has been used to determine linear viscoelastic properties,[15-18] but it has not been found to be generally useful for the study of nonlinear effects. Only one deformation pattern can be generated, and the results cannot be related quantitatively to other nonlinear material functions.[19]

Concentric cylinders are, theoretically, the best geometry for a rotational rheometer, as the ideal flow is an exact solution of the entire equations of motion.[20] Furthermore, when the gap is small, the shear rate becomes practically uniform.[21] In fact, such rheometers have been used for the study of nonlinear viscoelasticity in polymeric liquids.[22-25] However, the Weissenberg (rod climbing) effect tends to draw fluid out of the gap.[26] In addition, loading and cleaning are inconvenient, and maintaining concentricity is difficult when small gaps are used, especially if the rheometer is operated at elevated temperature.

12.2. SLIDING PLATE RHEOMETERS

12.2.1. Advantages and Disadvantages

The generation of shear deformations by the linear motion of one flat plate relative to another has certain advantages over the use of rotational flows. Edge failure is a much less severe problem, so higher shear rates can be reached for elastic liquids. Anisotropic materials can be studied by variation of the angle between the sample orientation and the direction of motion. Widely available and versatile tensile testing frames and actuators can be used to support and drive the rheometer for high-force, large-displacement applications. In addition, birefringence studies are facilitated.

There are also some disadvantages in comparison with rotational rheometers. The total strain is limited by the rheometer length and end effects, and the normal stress differences cannot be measured except by means of birefringence techniques.

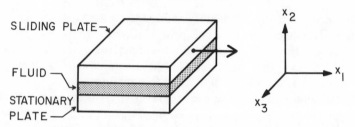

Fig. 12.1. Basic features of sliding plate geometry.

12.2.2. Basic Equations

The basic features of the sliding plate geometry are shown in Fig. 12.1. Sliding plate rheometers are either strain-controlled or stress-controlled. Most generate a controlled rate of deformation and use a load cell to measure the total shearing force. The deformation can be generated by the crosshead of a tensile testing machine, or by some other electromechanical or servohydraulic linear actuator. Conversely, the force can be controlled by a weight suspended by a pulley or by a feedback loop containing a servohydraulic actuator, and the resulting strain can then be measured.

The shear stress, σ, is determined by measuring the force, F, required to drive the motion of the moving plate (or the force required to hold the stationary plate in place) and dividing it by the wetted area, A, of the plates:

$$\sigma = F/A \qquad (12.1)$$

The shear strain, γ, is the displacement, X, of the moving plate divided by the distance, h, between the plates:

$$\gamma = X/h \qquad (12.2)$$

The shear rate, $\dot{\gamma}$, is the velocity, V, of the moving plate divided by the gap:

$$\dot{\gamma} = V/h \qquad (12.3)$$

12.2.3. Sources of Error

The principal sources of error associated with the use of sliding plate rheometers are listed in Table 12.1. Nearly all these are most severe for large deformations of viscoelastic materials. In order to minimize errors due to shear wave propagation and viscous heating, and to provide the maximum shear strain for a given plate displacement, it is desirable to make the gap, h, as small as possible. This means that the flatness and

TABLE 12.1
Sources of Error for Sliding Plate Rheometers

A. Nonideal rheometer geometry
  1. Plates not flat
  2. Plates not parallel
  3. Fluctuations in h due to play

B. Instrument friction contribution to F

C. End and edge effects
  1. Due to surface tension
  2. Due to stress mismatch at free surfaces

D. Shear wave propagation due to sample inertia

E. Secondary flow due to normal stress differences

F. Uncertainty as to wetted area, A
  1. Due to imperfect sample loading
  2. Due to loss of adhesion during shearing

G. Nonuniform material properties
  1. Due to temperature nonuniformity
  2. Due to loss or absorption of water or solvent
  3. Due to chemical degradation

H. Cohesive failure (fracture) of the sample

---

parallelism of the plates must be maintained to very close tolerances. Also, any fluctuation in the gap spacing during operation must be kept very small. Thus the machining and alignment of the plates must be carried out with great care. Furthermore, the mechanism used to support and guide the moving plate must have minimal play, i.e. it is necessary to have a very tight fit of the sliding or rolling components of the support mechanism for the moving plate. However, any friction arising from the motion of these components will contribute to the measured force, F, and will result in an error in the calculation of the shear stress.

For this reason, many of the sliding plate rheometers that have been used have been of the 'sandwich' type illustrated in Fig. 12.2. There are two sample layers and two outer plates, with a central plate. Here there are no net lateral forces on the central plate, and gap uniformity is maintained by the samples themselves. However, this requires that the moving and stationary plates be precisely aligned and that the distance between the

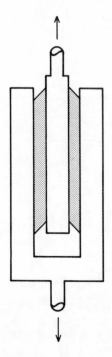

Fig. 12.2. Basic elements of 'sandwich' rheometer.

outer plates be uniform and unaffected by forces arising from the test. Furthermore, both samples must have the same size and shape and must be positioned precisely opposite each other on either side of the central plate. In order to avoid asymmetrical gravitational forces on the central plate, the rheometer is usually mounted vertically.

12.2.3.1. End and Edge Effects

When elastic materials are to be studied at large shear strains, the most serious limitation of sliding plate rheometers is the inhomogeneity of the deformation due to edge and end effects. By 'edge' we mean the free surface parallel to the direction of motion, while an 'end' is a free surface that is initially normal to the direction of motion. These surfaces are indicated in Fig. 12.3. End effects arise from two causes; one of these is surface tension, and the other is the mismatch between the state of stress associated with ideal simple shear and the hydrostatic stress that acts on a free surface by the surrounding atmosphere.

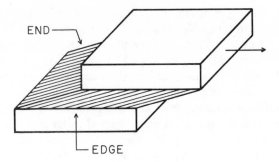

Fig. 12.3. End and edge effects in sliding plate rheometer.

Laun and Meissner[27] have estimated the error due to surface tension in the shear stress calculated using eqn (12.1). They assumed that the sample deforms in such a way that the free surfaces are always flat, i.e. that the sample is always a parallelepiped. From the definition of the static surface tension, α, they showed that, when a sample of initial length L undergoes an amount of shear strain γ, the contribution, σ_α, to the apparent shear stress is given by

$$\sigma_\alpha = \frac{2\alpha\gamma}{L\sqrt{1 + \gamma^2}} \tag{12.4}$$

In their low shear rate studies of molten plastics, Laun and Meissner found that this contribution was negligible. However, surface tension did pose a problem in creep recovery (recoil) experiments where the intention is to reduce the actual shear stress to zero. As is explained below, the free surfaces cannot behave in the simple way assumed by Laun and Meissner, because this would require an imbalance of the forces acting at the free surfaces. However, it is likely that these effects themselves contribute larger errors to the calculated shear stress than the surface tension.

We turn now to the question of the mismatch of the stresses at the free surfaces. What we mean by this is that the stress field in a material whose ends behave in the ideal way shown in Fig. 12.1 cannot possibly balance that which exists in the surrounding medium. This medium is usually air, but the mismatch problem persists as long as it has rheological properties different from those of the sample, even if the only difference is that the sample and the surrounding medium are Newtonian fluids with different viscosities. This problem was first pointed out by Philippoff.[28]

In order to maintain a balance between the stresses in the sample and in the surrounding medium, the free surfaces must behave differently from the ideal situation in which they are flat. The result can be a secondary, circulatory flow, a distortion of the shape of the surface, a tearing of the sample (cohesive failure) or a pulling away from the wall (adhesive failure). In fact, these will occur in various combinations depending on the rheological nature of the sample.

The problems resulting from end effects in sliding plate flow are most severe when elastic materials are subjected to large strains. Theoretical treatments of end effects in elastic materials have been presented by Read[29] and by Rivlin and Saunders.[30] These theories predict that the apparent shear stress calculated on the basis of eqn (12.1), with the sample assumed to be a parallelepiped, is below the true shear stress and decreases as the length to thickness ratio, L/h, increases.

Andrade[31] observed dramatic edge irregularities in viscous gels, and Gent et al.[32] observed the shear stress distribution across a square rubber sheet. The latter authors made their observation by measuring the surface shear stress locally at different positions in a sample under static strain, and the shear stress was found to be highly nonuniform, even for very small shear strains.

Toki and White[33] found that end effects in a sliding plate rheometer posed a serious problem in the measurement of the nonlinear viscoelastic properties of elastomers. To correct the data, an empirical formula was derived based on the arbitrary subtraction of the exposed area of the shearing plates from the original sample area. Giacomin and Dealy[34,35] found that significant spurious phase shifts resulted from the use of a load cell to determine the shear stress in their studies of the response of molten plastics to large amplitude oscillatory shear. On the other hand, Liu et al.[36] concluded that end effects were not a problem in their studies of concentrated polymer solutions at shear rates up to $4 \cdot 8 \, \text{s}^{-1}$ and total strains up to 48. Clearly, the importance of end effects is strongly dependent on the nature of the material being studied and the maximum strain and strain rate involved.

12.2.3.2. Shear Wave Propagation

Another source of inhomogeneous deformation is shear wave propagation. This is only a factor in nonsteady test modes, but it is precisely this type of test that is necessary to study viscoelasticity. Shear wave propagation is a potential problem in any rheometer when transient tests are to be performed. However, because sliding plate rheometers can be used at larger strains and strain rates than rotational rheometers, special care must be taken to ensure that inertial effects do not compromise the validity of the results.

Because of inertia in the sample material, a change in the velocity of the moving surface cannot instantaneously cause the acceleration of every material element that would be necessary to keep the strain and strain rate independent of x_2. In a Newtonian fluid subjected to the sudden start-up of motion by the moving surface at constant velocity, the velocity distribution is given by a Fourier series.[37] At longer times, the series is dominated by the first term, and the asymptotic approach to steady state becomes exponential, with a 'half life' of $h^2\rho/\pi^2\eta$. We note that the approach to steady state is asymptotic and is most rapid when the gap is small and the viscosity is large. This phenomenon is thus only a serious problem for liquids of rather low viscosity, in which case it is necessary to use the smallest possible gap.

The behavior of elastic liquids at the inception of steady shear flow has been analyzed theoretically[38,39] and observed experimentally.[40] In some cases, the theories predict a reflection of the shear wave from the stationary surface, and this has been observed in collagen solutions.[40] One possible effect of sample inertia is an overshoot in the measured stress. Since stress overshoot is a common feature of the stress growth function in viscoelastic fluids, care must be taken to ensure that an observed overshoot is a rheological effect rather than an inertial effect.

It is also of interest to consider the case of oscillatory shear, which is widely used to study both linear and nonlinear viscoelasticity. The strain is given by

$$\gamma = \gamma_0[\sin(\omega t)] \tag{12.5}$$

For a Newtonian fluid, the criterion for neglecting the effect of inertia on the strain field is

$$\frac{h^2\omega\rho}{2\eta} \ll 1 \tag{12.6}$$

Analyses have also been presented for the 'second order fluid'[41] and for a material exhibiting linear viscoelastic behavior.[42,43] MacDonald *et al.*[42] considered the case of small deviations from a linear velocity profile in deriving a criterion for neglect of inertial effects. In order for the storage modulus to be reasonably free of errors due to acceleration, the criterion is

$$\frac{h^2\omega\rho\eta''}{6|\eta^*|^2}\left[2 + \left(\frac{\eta'}{\eta''}\right)^2\right] \ll 1 \tag{12.7}$$

while for negligible error in the loss modulus the criterion is

$$\frac{h^2\omega\rho\eta''}{6|\eta^*|^2} \ll 1 \qquad (12.8)$$

Schrag[43] has carried out a more thorough analysis, and his general criterion for neglecting the nonlinearity of the displacement profile is

$$h/\lambda_s \ll 1 \qquad (12.9)$$

where λ_s is the shear wavelength, which is related to the complex modulus and the loss angle as follows:

$$\lambda_s = \frac{2\pi}{\omega\sqrt{\rho/|G^*|}\,\cos^2(\delta/2)} \qquad (12.10)$$

For the case of a fluid having a density of $10^3\,\text{kg}\,\text{m}^{-3}$ and a complex viscosity of $1\,\text{Pa}\,\text{s}$, Schrag concludes that, in order to permit the use of frequencies up to several Hz, it is necessary that h/λ_s be less that $1/30$.

12.2.3.3. Other Sources of Error

It is clearly advantageous to make the gap as small as possible to minimize shear wave problems. However, Burton *et al.*[44] found, in their steady shear study of high molecular weight polystyrene melts using a parallel disk rotational rheometer, that at sufficiently small gaps the apparent shear stress decreased as the gap was further decreased at a fixed shear rate. They attributed this to the atypical behavior of the polymer molecules in contact with the disk surface. This suggests that there is a lower limit to h for very high molecular weight polymeric materials.

Another possible cause of nonlinearity in the velocity distribution is secondary flow. It has already been mentioned that secondary flow can occur as an end effect. Another cause is as a result of a positive first normal stress difference, which would have the effect of drawing material in from the ends of the sample and 'pumping' it out at the edges, as shown in Fig.

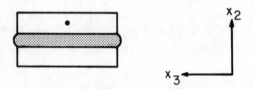

Fig. 12.4. Effect of first normal stress difference on edges.

12.4. This effect is thought to be small, but no theoretical analysis of the phenomenon seems to have been made.

We have considered above only the role of end effects and secondary flows in shear stress measurement. However, these same phenomena also have the effect of making it impossible to make a direct measurement of normal stress differences. If a pressure transducer is mounted with its diaphragm flush with the face of one of the plates, it is possible to measure σ_{22}, if the transducer is not vented, or $\sigma_{22} - P$ if it is vented, where P is the hydrostatic pressure in the surrounding atmosphere. However, there is no way to make a direct measurement of σ_{11} or σ_{33}, and neither of these is equal to P, because of uncertainty as to the details of the stress distribution near the ends and edges. However, information about normal stress differences can be inferred from birefringence measurements.

Equations (12.1) and (12.2) assume that the sample wets the plates over the entire area of nominal contact. This means that any zones of noncontact will contribute to an error in the calculated stress. Moreover, the presence of such zones will cause deviations from the desired, homogeneous shear deformation. Zones of noncontact can result from gas bubbles trapped at the sample–plate interface or a loss of adhesion in response to the stresses generated by the deformation. A related phenomenon is the cohesive failure of the sample in response to these stresses. At sufficiently high stress levels, adhesive and/or cohesive failure is bound to occur, but little is known as yet about the fundamentals of the fracture of elastic liquids.

In presenting the results of rheological measurements, it is almost always assumed that the sample is at a uniform, known temperature. However, this can never be precisely the case because of viscous dissipation. Whenever a viscous material is deformed, some of the work of deformation is converted into internal, thermal energy by means of viscous dissipation. This increase in thermal energy will result in a temperature increase, unless it is removed by the flow of heat. However, heat only flows when there is a temperature gradient. Thus a temperature gradient in the sample is inevitable. To illustrate this point, consider the steady state sliding plate shear of a Newtonian fluid with a constant viscosity. If both plates are at a fixed temperature, T_0, the steady state temperature distribution is

$$T(x_2) \;=\; T_0 + \frac{\eta \dot{\gamma}^2 h^2}{2k}\left[\frac{x_2}{h} - \left(\frac{x_2}{h}\right)^2\right] \tag{12.11}$$

The maximum temperature rise occurs at the midplane:

$$T_{\max} - T_0 = \frac{\eta \dot{\gamma}^2 h^2}{8k} \qquad (12.12)$$

Clearly, viscous heating will be a problem when η, $\dot{\gamma}$ and h are large and k is small. However, the use of the steady state analysis provides a worst case estimate of the maximum temperature rise, and in practice we can often make our rheological measurement before sufficient viscous heat has been generated for the temperature to approach its steady state distribution.

The presence of many of the sources of error mentioned above can be detected by varying the gap, h. If the values of the material function are not affected, the errors are under control.

12.2.4. Use of Shear Stress Transducers

Many of the possible sources of error associated with the use of sliding plate rheometers can be eliminated or dramatically reduced if the shear stress is measured locally, at the center of the sample, rather than inferred from the total driving force, F. This would be especially advantageous in the study of the response of viscoelastic materials to large strains.

First, such a technique is immune to the effects of instrument friction. Thus the support/guide mechanism for the moving plate can be adjusted to have minimum play without regard to the introduction of significant sliding friction. It is thus unnecessary to use a 'sandwich' configuration, and sample preparation and insertion are much simplified. Knowledge of the exact wetted area is no longer required, as only the area of the shear sensitive surface of the transducer needs to be known to determine the shear stress.

A related advantage is that changes in the sample occurring at its free surfaces due to oxidation and loss or absorption of water or solvent have a minimal effect on the stress and strain in the neighborhood of the shear stress transducer for an extended period of time. By contrast, in cone–plate and parallel disk rheometers, the free surface at which degradation and composition changes first occur is at the maximum radius where it has the maximum effect on the measured torque. Another important advantage of local shear stress measurement, especially at very high strains, is the elimination of end effects so that the true shear stress response to very large deformations can be determined.

Devices for the local measurement of shear stress exerted on a flat or cylindrical surface have been developed to measure skin friction associated with the flow of air.[45,46] Shear stress detectors have also been used to study the behavior of soils,[47] granular materials[48–53] and rubbers.[32] A shear stress transducer suitable for use in the study of the viscoelastic behavior of highly viscous liquids is a more recent invention.[13] Such a transducer has been used successfully in sliding plate rheometers to study the behavior of polymeric liquids at room temperature[54] and of molten plastics.[55,34]

12.2.5. Applications of Sliding Plate Rheometers

Sliding plate rheometers have been used for studying nonlinear viscoelasticity in soaps,[56] asphalt,[57] concentrated polymer solutions,[58–60] bulk liquid polymers,[61–67] molten plastics,[68–72] filled polymers,[73] filled elastomers,[74,75] and rubbers.[76] Sliding plate rheometers of the sandwich type have also been used for measuring the nonlinear viscoelastic properties of foods.[77,78] Hibberd and Parker[79,81] and Faubion *et al.*[82] concluded that a sliding plate rheometer of the single sample variety was best suited to the measurement of nonlinear viscoelastic properties of bread doughs.

Commercial instruments designed to measure the linear viscoelastic properties of solid materials, such as the Rheovibron, the Metravib Viscoelasticimeter and the Dynastat, can be modified for use with viscoelastic liquids by use of sandwich or sliding cylinder fixtures.[83,84]

12.2.5.1. Studies of Polymeric Liquids

Weight-driven sandwich rheometers have been used to determine the low shear rate viscosity and steady state compliance of thermoplastics.[27,66] Laun[69] has developed another sandwich rheometer in which the middle plate is fixed and the outer plates are rigidly connected to a moving cage which is driven by a pneumatic cylinder. This instrument is thus basically a creepmeter; it was specifically designed to study molten plastics at shear stresses approaching those occurring in actual processing operations.

Meissner and coworkers have extended the use of sliding plates to include shearing in two directions.[62,67] This was done by using two electromechanical linear actuators perpendicular to each other. The two relevant components of the shear stress were measured independently using two load cells.

Sliding plate rheometers have been used to measure birefringence in bulk polymers[61,71] and in polymer solutions.[58,85] In this way, information about normal stress differences can be obtained by use of the stress optical law.[86] By the use of glass windows or entire plates made of glass, the measurement of birefringence in the 1,3-plane is straightforward. Haghtalab[85] used glass windows, and mounted a shear stress transducer in the stationary plate so that the 1,3 birefringence and the shear stress could be measured simultaneously.

Kimura et al.[61] concluded that sliding plate geometry was better suited to birefringence measurements than cone–plate geometry. They devised an elaborate technique to ensure that the edges were flat so that birefringence measurements in the 1,2-plane could be made. The moving plate was coupled to the crosshead of a tensile testing machine. This instrument has been used for studies of nonlinear viscoelasticity in polybutadiene[61] and in polystyrene solutions.[58]

Soong and his coworkers[36,59] used a sandwich type sliding plate rheometer for the study of nonlinear viscoelasticity in concentrated polymer solutions. In order to maintain alignment, it was found necessary to use guide rods for the outer plates. Friction in the bearings resulted in a noisy stress signal from the load cell, and the studies were limited to shear rates less than $5 \, s^{-1}$. Deformations studied included stress growth, stress relaxation after cessation of steady shear, interrupted shear, large amplitude oscillatory shear, small amplitude oscillatory shear superposed on stress growth, and exponential shearing. This versatility in the choice of deformation histories was made possible by the use of a programmable servohydraulic drive system.

Giacomin and Dealy[34,55] have developed a sliding plate rheometer for the study of nonlinear viscoelasticity in molten plastics. This instrument employs a shear stress transducer so that the results are unaffected by edge and end effects, by degradation at the free surface or by lack of knowledge of the exact sample size. A precision linear bearing table is used to support the moving plate. Only about 4 ml of sample material are needed, and they prepared samples of commercial thermoplastics in the form of rectangular plaques in a heated press. The moving plate is driven by an MTS Systems servohydraulic linear actuator with computer control, so that any type of strain history can be programmed. This rheometer can generate total strains up to 400 and shear rates up to $200 \, s^{-1}$. This instrument can be used to measure the complex modulus over several decades of frequency, the viscosity over several decades of shear rate, as well as a wide range of nonlinear viscoelastic properties.

12.2.5.2. High Shear Rate Techniques

For studies involving very high shear rates, sliding plate rheometers are at a disadvantage because the total strain is limited by the maximum displacement of the movable plate. However, this problem can be overcome by the use of a sandwich geometry with a very long, flexible band or film acting as the central plate. In the 'band viscometer' developed for use with printing inks,[87,88] a weight attached to the end of the long band, preferably made of polyester film, draws ink from a reservoir into the gap between two metal blocks that form the outer plate walls. The 'sliding film rheometer', designed for use with molten plastics, also makes use of a long flexible tape, made of steel in this case. The tape moves at high speed from a feed reel to a motor-driven take-up reel.[89,90] The reservoir is continuously supplied with melt by an extruder, and the shear stress is inferred from the shear force on one of the side walls.

12.2.5.3. Strong Shear Flow

Doshi and Dealy[91] have suggested that sliding plate rheometers can be used to generate 'strong' shear flows in polymeric liquids, i.e. ones that induce a high degree of molecular stretching and alignment. Shear flow is commonly thought of as a 'weak' flow, in contrast to uniaxial extension which is the most common example of a strong flow. However, this distinction arises from the comparison of 'steady simple shear', in which the shear rate, $\dot{\gamma}$, is constant, with 'steady simple extension', in which the Hencky strain rate, $\dot{\varepsilon}$, is constant. Doshi and Dealy show that it is possible to generate a strong shear flow by use of a shear strain that increases exponentially with time:

$$\gamma(t) = A[\exp(\alpha t) - 1] \tag{12.13}$$

Cone–plate rheometers are unsuitable for such experiments, because the shear rate increases exponentially, and edge effects would begin to interfere with the measurement very early in the test. Zülle *et al.*[92] used a sliding plate rheometer to study the response of polyisobutylene to exponential shear.

12.2.6. A Commercial Sliding Plate Rheometer

A sliding plate rheometer is now commercially available from MTS Systems Corporation.[93] This rheometer was developed for use with molten plastics but can be used to study other viscoelastic materials such as elastomers and bread dough. A shear stress transducer[13] is used to avoid end and edge effects and other errors associated with the use of a total load cell to determine shear stress. Studies can be carried out at temperatures up to 250 °C. Only a few grams of sample are required, and the rheometer is easily opened for cleaning and sample insertion.

A servohydraulic actuator generates the motion of the moving plate. The position control loop is under computer control and a version of the BASIC programming language, developed especially for materials testing, is used to set up strain patterns. The rheometer can be used to determine

the storage and loss moduli and the viscosity at shear rates from 0·1 to
200 s^{-1}. In addition, a wide variety of nonlinear viscoelastic properties can
be measured by programming the computer to generate multiple, bidirec-
tional step strains, start-up and cessation of steady shear, interrupted
shear, large amplitude oscillatory shear, and exponential shear.

12.3. SLIDING CYLINDER RHEOMETERS

12.3.1. Introduction

Sliding cylinder rheometers have no edge effects and require no bearings
or bushings to maintain the gap spacing. They were first used at the
beginning of the century and have continued to find application from time
to time.[94–96] More recently they have been used to study molten plastics,[97,98]
polymer solutions[99] and bread dough.[100–104] A falling rod viscometer widely
used to estimate the high shear rate viscosity of printing inks is also based
on the sliding cylinder principle.[105]

The basic features of the sliding cylinder rheometer are shown in Fig.
12.5. The material under test is contained in the annular gap between a

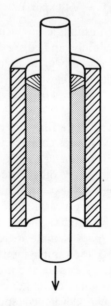

Fig. 12.5. Basic features of sliding cylinder geometry.

solid inner cylinder or rod with radius r_i and a hollow cylinder with wall radius r_o. The length of the sample is L, the driving force is F, and the relative displacement is X.

12.3.2. Basic Equations

The shear stress at the wall of the inner cylinder is related to F, which we take to be positive, as follows:

$$\tau_w \equiv -\tau_{rz}(r_i) = \frac{F}{(2\pi r_i L)} \tag{12.14}$$

If the relative cylinder velocity is V, the velocity distribution for a Newtonian fluid is given by

$$v(r) = V\left[\frac{\ln(r/r_o)}{\ln(r_i/r_o)}\right] \tag{12.15}$$

The shear rate at the wall of the inner cylinder is

$$\dot{\gamma}_w \equiv -\left(\frac{\partial x}{\partial r}\right)_{r_i} = \frac{V}{r_i \ln(r_o/r_i)} \tag{12.16}$$

The velocity has been taken as positive in the direction of motion so that the shear rate and the shear stress have negative values, and the quantities γ_w and τ_w are defined, for convenience, so that they have positive values. The viscosity of a Newtonian fluid can then be calculated as follows:

$$\eta = \frac{\tau_w}{\dot{\gamma}_w} = \frac{F\ln(r_o/r_i)}{2\pi LV} \tag{12.17}$$

For a power law fluid with $\sigma = K|\dot{\gamma}|^n$, the velocity profile is given by

$$v(r) = V\left[\frac{(r/r_o)^{1-1/n} - 1}{(r_i/r_o)^{1-1/n} - 1}\right] \tag{12.18}$$

This equation can be used to derive relationships for calculating the power law parameters K and n from experimental data.

If a sliding cylinder rheometer is designed so that the relative gap width, $(r_o - r_i)/r_o$, is very small, then the shear strain becomes nearly uniform and is given approximately by the simple expression

$$\gamma = X/(r_o - r_i) \tag{12.19}$$

where X is the axial displacement of one cylinder relative to the other. Since $(r_o - r_i)$ is simply the gap spacing, this equation is equivalent to eqn

(12.2) for the sliding plate geometry. Thus, when the gap is small, shear strain and shear rate can be calculated without knowledge of the constitutive equation of the material. For larger gaps, however, there is no straightforward method for determining the local shear strain when the constitutive equation is unknown.

In his studies of the complex modulus of bread doughs, Hibberd[101–104] carried out oscillatory shear experiments with several gap spacings and extrapolated curves of the logarithm of G' and G'' versus $(r_o - r_i)$ to zero to obtain values of the moduli assumed to correspond to the small-gap shear expression (eqn (12.19)). The data were found to fall on a straight line for small values of the gap.

The sources of error for sliding cylinder rheometers are the same as for sliding plate rheometers, except that edge effects are absent, and there is no bearing friction. End effects, however, are still present.

12.3.3. Applications of Sliding Cylinder Rheometers

Myers and Faucher[97] used a sliding cylinder rheometer to measure the viscosity of molten polymers at low shear rates. An Instron testing machine was used to drive the piston at various speeds, and F was measured by means of a compressive load cell.

McCarthy[106] studied the dynamic mechanical properties of molten polymers by forcing the inner cylinder to oscillate in the axial direction. His rheometer incorporated a unique sample loading technique that avoided the preparation of a molded preform. A ring-shaped melting chamber surrounding the outer cylinder is charged with resin and, after being melted, it is extruded into the rheometer gap by means of a second ring which is forced down by the manual application of a torque. The oscillation of the inner cylinder is driven by an MTS Systems servohydraulic linear actuator. The oscillating cylinder is hollow and made from magnesium to minimize its mass. Its temperature is controlled by means of a ribbon heater next to its inner wall.

In their studies of nonlinear viscoelasticity in concentrated polymer solutions, Tsai and Soong[99] found the sliding cylinder geometry to be preferable to sliding plates. Signal noise in the load cell output was found to be lower for the sliding cylinder rheometer than for their sliding plate rheometer. (The noise in the sliding plate rheometer was due to friction in the precision guide rods used to maintain parallelism.) A novel sample loading technique was used. Designed for use with materials that can be poured, it is a convenient method to ensure that the material in the gap is bubble free. The instrument was equipped with a programmable MTS servohydraulic drive system permitting great flexibility in flow pattern selection.

Maxwell[98] has developed a very simple sliding cylinder rheometer for the study of stress relaxation after cessation of steady shear in molten plastics. In Maxwell's rheometer, the outer cylinder is driven at constant speed, while the central rod is held in place by a force transducer. Samples are premolded in two halves. Maxwell notes that this rheometer is limited to use at small strains; in his own work the maximum strain was 1. This instrument has been used to determine the liquid–liquid transition temperature, T_{ll}, in several polymers.[107]

Finally we mention a concentric cylinder rheometer in which the inner cylinder can both translate and rotate so that shear in two orthogonal directions can be studied.[108]

REFERENCES

1. J. M. Dealy, *J. Rheol.*, 1984, **28**, 181.
2. J. M. Dealy, *Rheometers for Molten Plastics*, Van Nostrand Reinhold, New York, 1982.
3. G. Heuser and E. Krause, *Rheol. Acta*, 1979, **18**, 553.
4. J. G. Savins and A. B. Metzner, *Rheol. Acta*, 1970, **9**, 365.
5. P. T. Gavin and R. W. Whorlow, *J. Appl. Polym. Sci.*, 1975, **19**, 567.
6. D. S. Pearson and W. E. Rochefort, *J. Polym. Sci., Polym. Phys. Ed.*, 1982, **20**, 83.
7. K. Walters and R. A. Kemp, *Rheol. Acta*, 1968, **7**, 1.
8. W. C. MacSporran and R. P. Spiers, *Rheol. Acta*, 1982, **21**, 193.
9. W. C. MacSporran and R. P. Spiers, *Rheol. Acta*, 1984, **23**, 90.
10. R. L. Powell and W. H. Schwartz, *J. Polym. Sci., Polym. Phys. Ed.*, 1979, **17**, 969.
11. R. L. Powell and W. H. Schwartz, *J. Rheol.*, 1979, **23**, 323.
12. E. Ganani and R. L. Powell, *J. Rheol.*, 1985, **29**, 931.
13. J. M. Dealy, US Patent 4 463 928, 1984.
14. J. M. Dealy, US Patent 4 571 989, 1986.
15. B. Maxwell, *Polym. Eng. Sci.*, 1967, **7**, 145.
16. R. J. J. Jonpschaap, K. M. Knapper and J. S. Lopulissa, *Polym. Eng. Sci.*, 1978, **18**, 788.
17. T. N. G. Abbott and K. Walters, *J. Fluid Mech.*, 1970, **40**, 205.
18. P. Payvar and R. I. Tanner, *Trans. Soc. Rheol.*, 1973, **17**, 449.
19. L. H. Gross and B. Maxwell, *Trans. Soc. Rheol.*, 1972, **16**, 577.
20. J. S. Dodge and I. M. Krieger, *Rheol. Acta*, 1969, **8**, 480.
21. T. M. T. Yang and I. M. Krieger, *J. Rheol.*, 1978, **22**, 413.
22. T. T. Tee and J. M. Dealy, *Trans. Soc. Rheol.*, 1975, **19**, 595.
23. S. Onogi, T. Masuda and T. Matsumoto, *Trans. Soc. Rheol.*, 1970, **14**, 275.

24. T. Matsumoto, Y. Segawa, Y. Waroshina and S. Onogi, *Trans. Soc. Rheol.*, 1973, **17**, 47.

25. S. Onogi and T. Matsumoto, *Polym. Eng. Rev.*, 1981, **1**, 45.

26. J. M. Dealy and T. K. P. Vu, *J. Non-Newt. Fluid Mech.*, 1977/78, **3**, 127.

27. H. M. Laun and J. Meissner, *Rheol. Acta*, 1980, **19**, 60.

28. W. Philippoff, in *Physical Acoustics*, Vol. II-B, W. P. Mason (Ed.), Academic Press, New York, 1965.

29. W. T. Read, *J. Appl. Mech.*, 1950, **17**, 349.

30. R. S. Rivlin and D. W. Saunders, *Trans. Inst. Rubber ind.*, 1949, **24**, 296.

31. E. N. da C. Andrade, *Proc. Roy. Soc.* (Lond.), 1911, **85**, 448.

32. A. N. Gent, R. L. Henry and M. L. Roxbury, *J. Appl. Mech.*, 1974, **41**, 855.

33. S. Toki and J. L. White, *J. Appl. Polym. Sci.*, 1982, **27**, 3171.

34. A. J. Giacomin, PhD thesis, Chem. Eng., McGill University, Montreal, 1987.

35. A. J. Giacomin and J. M. Dealy, The effect of free boundaries in melt rheometers, Paper G3, 58th Annual Meeting Soc. Rheol., Tulsa, Oklahoma, Oct. 1986.

36. T. Y. Liu, D. W. Mead, D. S. Soong and M. C. Williams, *Rheol. Acta*, 1983, **22**, 81.

37. G. K. Batchleor, *An Introduction to Fluid Mechanics*, Cambridge University Press, Cambridge, 1967, p. 191.

38. Y. Mochimaru, *J. Non-Newt. Fluid Mech.*, 1983, **12**, 135.

39. A. Narain and D. D. Joseph, *Rheol. Acta*, 1982, **21**, 228.

40. A. W. Chow and G. G. Fuller, *J Non-Newt. Fluid Mech.*, 1983, **12**, 135.

41. H. Markovitz and B. D. Coleman, *Adv. Appl. Mech.*, 1964, **8**, 69.

42. I. F. MacDonald, B. C. Marsh and E. Ashare, *Chem. Eng. Sci.*, 1969, **24**, 1615.

43. J. L. Schrag, *Trans. Soc. Rheol.*, 1977, **21**, 399.

44. R. H. Burton, M. J. Folkes, K. A. Narh and A. Keller, *J. Mater. Sci.*, 1983, **18**, 315.

45. J. Dickenson and N. D. Vinh, *Proc. 5th Canad. Congr. Appl. Mech.*, 1975, p. 515.

46. K. C. Brown and P. N. Joubert, *J. Fluid Mech.*, 1969, **35**, 737.

47. J. R. F. Arthur and K. H. Roscoe, *Civ. Eng. Public Wks Eng. Rev.*, 1961, **56**, 659.

48. S. L. Agarwal and S. Venkatesan, in *ASTM STP* No. 392, 1965, p. 152.

49. P. M. Blair-Fish and P. L. Bransby, *J. Eng. Ind., Trans. ASME*, **17**, Feb. 1973.

50. U. Tüzün and R. M. Nedderman, *Chem. Eng. Sci.*, 1985, **40**, 337.

51. J. W. Delaplaine, *A.I.Ch.E.J.*, 1956, **2**, 127, 371.

52. G. Broersma, *Behavior of Granular Materials*, Stam Tech. Publ., Culemborg, The Netherlands, 1972, p. 49.

53. J. Smid and J. Novosad, *Powder Technol.*, 1970/71, **4**, 322.

54. J. M. Dealy and S. S. Soong, *J. Rheol.*, 1984, **28**, 355.

55. A. J. Giacomin and J. M. Dealy, *J. Rheol.* (SPE ANTEC Tech. Papers), 1986, **32**, 711.

56. J. E. Bujake, *J. Colloid Interface Sci.*, 1968, **27**, 229.

57. T. D. Khong, S. L. Malhotra and L.-P. Blanchard, *Rheol. Acta*, 1979, **18**, 382.

58. K. Osaki, S. Kimura and M. Kurata, *J. Rheol.*, 1981, **25**, 549.
59. N. Sivashinsky, A. T. Tsai, T. J. Moon and D. S. Soong, *J. Rheol.*, 1984, **28**, 287.
60. T. Y. Liu, D. S. Soong and M. C. Williams, *J. Polym. Sci., Polym. Phys. Ed.*, 1984, **22**, 1561.
61. S. K. Kimura, K. Osaki and M. Kurata, *J. Polym. Sci., Polym. Phys. Ed.*, 1981, **19**, 151.
62. J. Meissner, *Chemie*, 1984, **38**, 35.
63. S. Middleman, *Trans. Soc. Rheol.*, 1969, **13**, 123.
64. F. P. LaMantia, B. de Cindio, E. Sorta and D. Acierno, *Rheol. Acta*, 1979, **18**, 369.
65. D. Acierno *et al.*, *Trans. Soc. Rheol.*, 1977, **21**, 261.
66. S. M. Fruh and F. Rodriguez, *A.I.Ch.E.J.*, 1970, **16**, 907.
67. H. P. Huerlimann and J. Meissner, Multidirectional shear rheometer for polymer melt, Int. Conf. Viscoelasticity of Polymeric Liquids, Grenoble, Jan. 1986.
68. M. Fujiyama and M. Takayanagi, *Kogyo Kagaku Zasshi*, 1969, **72**, 1163.
69. H. M. Laun, *Rheol. Acta*, 1982, **21**, 464.
70. J. Meissner, *Pure Appl. Chem.*, 1984, **56**, 369.
71. F. D. Dexter, J. C. Miller and W. Philippoff, *Trans. Soc. Rheol.*, 1961, **5**, 193.
72. M. Fleissner, *Angew. Makromol. Chem.*, 1981, **94**, 197.
73. F. Nazem and Y. Hill, *Trans. Soc. Rheol.*, 1974, **18**, 87.
74. S. Montes and J. L. White, *Rubber Chem. Technol.*, 1982, **55**, 1354.
75. I. Furuta, V. M. Lobe and J. L. White, *J. Non-Newt. Fluid Mech.*, 1976, **1**, 207.
76. C. Goldstein, *Trans. Soc. Rheol.*, 1984, **18**, 357.
77. F. Shama and P. Sherman, *J. Food Sci.*, 1966, **31**, 699.
78. M. Fukushima, S. Taneya and T. Sone, *J. Soc. Mater. Sci. Japan*, 1964, **13**, 331.
79. G. E. Hibberd and N. S. Parker, *Cereal Chem.*, 1978, **55**, 102.
80. G. E. Hibberd and N. S. Parker, *Cereal Chem.*, 1975, **52**, 3.
81. G. E. Hibberd and N. S. Parker, *Cereal Chem.*, 1979, **56**, 232.
82. J. M. Faubion, P. C. Dreese and K. C. Diehl, in *Rheology of Wheat Products*, Amer. Assoc. Cereal Chemists, St. Paul, Minnesota, 1985, p. 91.
83. B. H. Shah and R. Darby, *Polym. Eng. Sci.*, 1976, **16**, 46.
84. T. Murayama, *J. Appl. Polym. Sci.*, 1982, **27**, 80.
85. A. Haghtalab, M.Eng. thesis, Chem. Eng., McGill University, Montreal, 1985.
86. J. Janeschitz-Kriegl, *Polymer Melt Rheology and Flow Birefringence*, Springer Verlag, Berlin/New York, 1983.
87. H. H. Hull, *J. Colloid Sci.*, 1952, **7**, 316.
88. A. C. Zettlemoyer, *Offic. Dig. Fed. Paint Varnish Prod. Club*, 1960, **32** (424), 615.
89. F. C. Starr, US Patent 4 466 274, 1984.
90. Slocumb Corp., Wilmington, Delaware, USA.
91. S. R. Doshi and J. M. Dealy, *J. Rheol.*, 1987, **31**, 563.
92. D. Zülle, J. J. Linster, H. P. Hürlimann and J. Meissner, *J. Rheol.*, 1987, **31**, 583.
93. P. J. Cain, *Sliding Plate Rheometer for Viscoelastic Materials*, MTS Systems Corporation, Box 24012, Minneapolis, Minnesota 55424, USA.

94. M. Segel, *Physik. Z.*, 1903, **4**, 493.
95. A. Pochettino, *Nuovo Cimento*, 1914, **8**, 77.
96. D. Tollenaar and M. C. Bisschop, *J. Colloid Sci.*, 1955, **10**, 151.
97. A. W. Myers and J. A. Faucher, *Trans. Soc. Rheol.*, 1968, **12**, 183.
98. B. Maxwell, in *Order in the Amorphous State of Polymers*, S. E. Keinath, R. L. Miller and J. K. Rieke (Eds), Plenum, New York, 1986.
99. A. T. Tsai and D. S. Soong, *J. Rheol.*, 1985, **29**, 1.
100. G. E. Hibberd, W. J. Wallace and K. A. Wyatt, *J. Sci. Instr.*, 1966, **43**, 84.
101. G. E. Hibberd and W. J. Wallace, *Rheol. Acta*, 1966, **5**, 193.
102. G. E. Hibberd, *Rheol. Acta*, 1970, **9**, 497.
103. G. E. Hibberd, *Rheol. Acta*, 1970, **9**, 501.
104. G. E. Hibberd, *Rheol. Acta*, 1975, **14**, 151.
105. G. Pangalos and J. M. Dealy, *J. Oil Col. Chemists Assoc.*, 1985, **68**(3), 59.
106. R. V. McCarthy, *J. Rheol.*, 1978, **22**, 623.
107. B. Maxwell and K. S. Cook, *J. Polym. Sci., Polym. Symp.*, 1985, **72**, 343.
108. A. Gotsis, MS thesis, Virginia Polytechnic Institute and State University, Blacksburg, 1983.

Chapter 13

Commercial Rotational Instruments

G. J. BROWNSEY

ARFC Institute of Food Research, Norwich, UK

13.1. INTRODUCTION

Materials generally show a broad spectrum of behaviour, the rheological properties lying between the extremes of a truly elastic and an ideally viscous response. The rheological testing procedures involve measuring the response of a material to an applied deformation but, given that ideality in response is rarely encountered, a straightforward rheological test is not usually sufficient for a complete material characterisation. Also, materials often show considerable time dependent changes as well as markedly non-linear responses to an applied stress or strain, so that the rheological tests need to be chosen carefully. The deformation, or strain, can be applied in a variety of ways but the aim of any study, in establishing a relationship between material properties and the stress–strain–time conditions, means that only relatively simple and well characterisable shear conditions are used. Understandably, the most usual approach is to shear the material between two surfaces. Now, since it is only the relative movement within the material that is important, the approach used does not require that any one surface be stationary. However, from a practical point of view, a simple arrangement is to move the surfaces in contact with

405

the material rather than move the material itself. Here it is important that there be good coupling between the material and the boundary surfaces so that 'slip' does not occur since it is vital that the material in contact with the boundary surfaces be undergoing an identical motion to that of the surfaces themselves. By satisfying this requirement any measure will be a reflection of the properties of the bulk material and not those of an indeterminate part.

One of the drawbacks of a quasi-stationary material approach is that of maintaining stable material conditions during a test. This stability cannot always be guaranteed; indeed, under normal conditions of extrusion, it is never attained. A distinct advantage of a rotational rheometer/viscometer is that all of the material is undergoing shear, but this may not necessarily be uniform throughout the material volume. With such rotational instruments, the materials are predominantly viscous or capable of flow, rather than the more structured, elastic semi-solids. Also, the sample volumes can vary considerably, the minimum being less than 1 ml. Effects of continuous shear can also be monitored: the structural degradation and the more general time dependent processes that occur are readily observed.

In the past, many rotational devices have been used merely as viscometers in what was essentially a quality control environment. Their advantages have been that they could be precalibrated and were easy to use, an example of this being the Brookfield viscometer which has enjoyed widespread use whilst retaining a degree of portability. Generally, most instruments share a common feature, that of the rotation of one surface about a common axis while the other remains stationary. Modifications to this basic arrangement do occur, such as when the rotational axis is displaced, giving rise to an eccentric type of motion, or where both surfaces are rotating, possibly about misaligned axes. Such axial rotations are usually unidirectional, though they can be restricted to a small angular displacement thereby giving the possibility of an oscillatory motion. The surfaces between which the material is confined are either plane or cylindrical, though others are possible. In at least one instrument, the Balance Rheometer, the surfaces are spherical, this being a prerequisite for its mode of operation.

It is perhaps advantageous to consider briefly the basic design of a rotational device and highlight many of the important features. Assume that one surface is stationary whilst the other is moving at a fixed distance from it. With the absence of any material within the gap, any rotational displacement of the movable component will not influence the stationary surface. However, due to both the mass and shape of the rotatable component, its motion will be influenced by its inertia, this being especially noticeable during non-steady state periods of motion. Once a constant rotational state has been established, the only energy required to sustain this uniform motion will be that required to overcome the frictional drag in any bearings. Such resistance to motion can be regarded as negligible only when extreme care has been taken in instrumental design and manufacture or when the material response is significant by comparison. By resorting to air bearings or electromagnetic devices, such frictional losses can be minimized but their use often conflicts with other requirements. Whatever the arrangement used, the bearings must be axially stiff.

If a material is now introduced into the gap, a viscous drag and/or elastic response will result. Such a response should not be observed for air alone. This extreme end of the measurement regime, that of very low torques, is often very important, especially when measuring yield values directly. However, whatever the material, be it a fluid or a concentrated dispersion, it must provide a reaction to the imposed strain and so couple both the stationary and mobile surfaces. Attachment to only the mobile surface will merely increase the moment of inertia of the rotating assembly which, though detectable and measurable, would not provide any information on material properties. The material must therefore bridge the gap, both completely and uniformly. Usually this gap dimension is predetermined by instrumental design or measurement configuration, though it may be determined by the material itself and can vary from a few microns to a very large value indeed. Ideally, if a Couette geometry is chosen, the gap should be as narrow as possible with the radius as large as possible, thereby providing an approximately uniform shear rate distribution within the material. Such an arrangement would be preferential when studying markedly shear thinning fluids.

It is often easier to confine a material in a horizontal rather than a vertical manner and, if the gap is very narrow, capillary action may by usefully employed. Unfortunately, narrow gaps require that machine tolerances and alignment be very precise. Tests on well characterised material standards should be undertaken and will usually highlight any instrumental imperfections.

It should also be appreciated that, apart from the usual torque reaction to an imposed shear, there is also a normal force component (Weissenberg effect) which can become significant at high shear rates or with polymeric fluids of high molecular weight that are markedly shear thinning. This component does provide another means of determining material constants and it has been used as the basis of a purpose built viscometer,[1] though it

G. J. Brownsey

has not been developed commercially. In a parallel plate instrument, the presence of a normal force will, if possible, alter the plate separation. Only very high stiffness will alleviate this effect but this stiffness in itself imposes severe conditions on the driven and stationary assemblies since the usual measurement of force requires a compliant transducer. However, a feedback mechanism can be used to maintain the gap dimensions.

Care should be taken to achieve isothermal conditions; to maintain both boundary surfaces at constant temperature is often very difficult. Metal is the preferred material owing to its good thermal conductivity. Also, it is useful to be able to observe the sheared material directly. This provides confidence in the results obtained and helps avoid misinterpretation, such as could occur if shear fracture were suddenly to appear.

The measurement geometry chosen for any study is not of major significance here, as far as the performance of the rheometer itself is concerned. More important is the means of detection, be it through a measured displacement or by a reaction to an imposed force. Basically, two different procedures are used. The first is where the device indicates the reactive couple that arises in rotating one surface. Necessarily, both the mobile component and the reaction to its rotation/displacement are measured on the same drive shaft. Another procedure requires measuring the reactive torque or displacement at the quasi-stationary surface. This approach is, from a design aspect, somewhat easier to achieve since the motor and measuring assemblies are now separated and there is greater freedom in design.

The underlying strategy of these rotational instruments is that the driven surface is controlled by a feedback mechanism so that its angular velocity, angular displacement or resultant torque is maintained at a constant value. This feedback can be either electrical or mechanical; with a little ingenuity, almost any desired condition is achievable in either a static or a dynamic state. The drive assembly must, however, be capable of maintaining precise control, under a wide range of operating conditions, in both rotational speed and torque. Stepper motors have often been used, replacing the more usual servo-motors since they have the advantage of very high holding torques and precisely controlled speeds coupled with high positional rigidity and accuracy. However, it should be remembered that stepper motors have only a limited achievable angular resolution (say 200 steps/rev) so that smooth operation is not possible except at the higher stepping rates. At very low stepping rates, this erratic motion may be problematical since the angular velocity is no longer constant. Therefore, to overcome this, higher motor speeds, coupled to a gearbox, may be considered a suitable alternative.

It would not be appropriate to give a detailed account of the many commercial instruments that are in use at the present time. Many have been in use for a very long time and excellent articles exist on both their design concept and handling.[2-4] Consequently, it is better to concentrate on recently introduced rheometers and, where appropriate, outline their basic features. For ease of description, the range of instruments is best classified into two groups: the bench devices, which are predominantly controlled strain devices, and the larger research machines which offer a far wider range of facilities.

13.2. BASIC ROTATIONAL INSTRUMENTS

Ravenfield provide a range of viscometers that utilise the same basic frame where the motor is vertically mounted above the sample position. It is housed in an inner frame which is restrained axially by springs, these torque springs being readily exchanged using a 'cartridge' system approach. The complete assembly is moved to set the gap, a dial micrometer allowing a positional resolution of $2 \cdot 5 \, \mu m$ vertically. The model BS Wide Range Viscometer is a recently introduced instrument (October 1984) and incorporates a thermally controlled servo-mechanism to maintain a constant gap when operating in cone–plate mode. A temperature controlled facility is available (-50 to $+210\,°C$) using an externally regulated bath, and the complete mechanical unit stands on its electronic console, thereby making it a quite compact system. The viscometer uses a drum unit for torque calibration and provides basic rotational speeds from 8 to $420 \, rad \, s^{-1}$, though this range is expandable. Under programmable control, a variety of speed ramp and time programs are available, with a minimum ramp time of 5 s. The maximum operational torque is dependent on the rotational speed chosen and varies from $0 \cdot 176$ to $0 \cdot 785 \, N \, m$; with the torque assembly of $0 \cdot 02 \, N \, m$ fsd, resolution is typically $10^{-5} \, N \, m$. Both the rotor and stator are protected by a torque limiting clutch, the measurement itself relying on a non-contacting inductive transducer. For manual operation, a digital display provides a direct readout of torque or rotational speed. An analogue output is also available to permit rheograms to be drawn, with an option of an RS232 interface to allow computer control. The standard measurement heads provide a shear rate range from 20 to $> 10^6 \, s^{-1}$, though the basic device does not include temperature control.

Viscometers (UK) Ltd provide four basic instruments, the LV8, RV8, RV4 and HV8, covering a low to high viscosity range. It is a modular approach whereby one can purchase the required items, such as a temperature control unit, analogue drive, spindles and remote sensing head. The measuring head unit is itself quite small and can be attached to a small laboratory stand. A direct visual indication of viscosity is provided, with rotational speed manually selected from a predetermined set of four or eight speeds. These speeds are machine dependent and cover the range 0.03–$10 \, \mathrm{rad \, s^{-1}}$. The viscometer is usually operated in 'dip' bob mode, a switch allowing internal calibration of the instrument with respect to the measuring assembly used. By using the options available, temperature can be controlled from ambient to $260 \, ^\circ\mathrm{C}$ with an accuracy of $0.2 \, ^\circ$, and viscosities from 20 to $10^8 \, \mathrm{mPa \, s}$ can be determined to within 1%.

All Brookfield viscometers employ the basic principle of sensing the torque, using a calibrated spring, required to maintain a constant angular velocity of an immersed spindle. They are very well known devices, marketed over 45 years, which have now been updated to take account of the advances in electronics, the viscometers having a digital display that is continually refreshed. They have analogue output, multiple speeds and interchangeable spindles (threaded coupling) so they can handle a wide range of fluids. It is very convenient that the accessories from earlier models also fit the latest viscometers. Both the digital and dial reading viscometers have four maximum torque ranges available of 67×10^{-6}, 0.7×10^{-3}, 1.4×10^{-3} and $5.7 \times 10^{-3} \, \mathrm{N \, m}$, together with a limited number of switch selectable speeds (4 or 8) from 0.03 to $10 \, \mathrm{rad \, s^{-1}}$. The digital viscometer cannot be hand-held during use, unlike the analogue dial equivalent type. With the available spindles the viscosity range covered is from $15 \, \mathrm{mPa \, s}$ to $64 \times 10^6 \, \mathrm{mPa \, s}$ with sample volumes typically several hundred ml. For lower viscosities an optional UL adaptor is provided.

The Wells-Brookfield Cone-Plate Viscometer has eight speeds and can handle sample volumes from 0.2 to $2 \, \mathrm{ml}$, with accessories such as temperature control permitting accuracies to $0.01 \, ^\circ$ from -30 to $+100 \, ^\circ\mathrm{C}$. A 'thermosel' system extends the temperature range to $300 \, ^\circ\mathrm{C}$, with larger volumes (8–$13 \, \mathrm{ml}$) measurable by coaxial cylinder geometry (shear rate range of 0.08–$93 \, \mathrm{s^{-1}}$).

The Brookfield Digital Viscometer DV-II is called a new generation viscometer and has a membrane sensitive display panel on the front of the motor housing to allow intermediate display of shear stress, viscosity or $\%$ viscosity scale on the digital readout. An RVDT is used to measure the relative position of the pivot shaft, this being a measure of torque. The eight-speed motor can be switched on/off, the display can be auto-zeroed and the device has an analogue output and an RS232 (1200 baud) interface for the serial output of data to a micro for data storage or calculation.

The Brookfield Rheoset is classed as a new programmable viscometer having a torque range from 6.7×10^{-5} to $28.7 \times 10^{-3}\,\mathrm{N\,m}$. The microprocessor that is attached, by a ribbon cable, to the measuring head has a 40-digit LCD display and integral strip printer. The keyboard allows BASIC programming of the 32k RAM with additional features to provide specific rheological tasks to be undertaken easily if required. The rotational speeds are fully programmable from 0.01 to $26\,\mathrm{rad\,s^{-1}}$ in steps of as little as 0.01 if required. With the available torque ranges, viscosities from 0.5 to $10^9\,\mathrm{mPa\,s}$ can be measured, even as a function of temperature or elapsed time. The unit has a program backup, power supply and a cassette interface for program storage.

The Haake Rotovisco system is a firmly established range of instruments where both the torque measurement system and the motor drive are normally integrated into one unit. The usual viscometer configuration is that of Couette mode. The measuring head has an electronically controlled d.c. motor whose speed is switch selectable and maintained to within 0.1% of the preassigned value. Temperature control is typically to $0.1\,^\circ$ with torque linearity to 0.3%. The basic units are the RV12, RV2/3 and RV100. The RV12 is of modular design, offers 30 fixed speeds within the range $0.1\text{--}53\,\mathrm{rad\,s^{-1}}$, and this can be further reduced by a gear option by $\times 10$ or $\times 100$. Three measuring units are available with maximum torques of 0.015, 0.05 and $0.15\,\mathrm{N\,m}$. In association with a speed programmer PG142 and x–y recorder, flow curves can be automatically recorded.

The RV2 is designed for the higher shear rates, having 40 fixed speeds up to $100\,\mathrm{rad\,s^{-1}}$. The choice of measuring heads is also extended, with four covering the range $0.005\text{--}0.5\,\mathrm{N\,m}$ fsd.

The universal instrument in the Haake range is the RV100 which incorporates a shear rate programmer and x–y–t recorder. Maximum rotational speed is $52\,\mathrm{rad\,s^{-1}}$ with programmable speeds preset in 1% steps, the torque being measured by the deflection of a low compliance spring (max. deflection $\sim 8.7\,\mathrm{mrad}$). The rheometer is designed for routine quality control measurements and has the option of three measuring heads.

If a Couette system is required for measuring very small sample volumes at low shear rates then the instrument most suitable is the RV100/CV100 system. Air is now required to supply the air bearing in the CV100. This instrument operates in a slightly different manner in that the outer cylinder is the driven surface with the inner cylinder connected to the torque measuring head via the air bearing. The inner cylinder is set in its vertical position by a motor driven mechanism whose speed can be varied; this facility is considered useful when studying thixotropic materials. The upper torque limit is 0·001 N m, with rotational speeds from 0·02 to 21 rad s^{-1} at temperatures up to 95 °C. As an option the RV100/CV100 can oscillate at frequencies from 0·01 to 9·9 Hz and at amplitudes of 17 mrad to 0·68 rad. Analogue output is also provided so that, through the use of suitable interfaces, data and machine parameters can be processed under computer control to allow the determination of viscoelasticity. A Haake Rheocontroller is available, with standard IEEE-488 interface, to permit the connection of a computer to a Rotovisco with software available for Hewlett-Packard machines. Other options are an interface for an HP80 series micro which allows upgrading of the RV2/3, RV12 and RV100 systems.

The most recent addition to the Haake range, which is intended to replace many of the earlier instruments, is the Rotovisco RV20 (October 1986) (Fig. 13.1). The torque measuring systems (M series), with a maximum torque reading of 0·1 N m, have a resolution of 0·2% fsd and a maximum compliance of 8·7 mrad. With the RV20, ten different fixed rotational speeds can be preset with the capability of reducing the range by a factor of 10 and 100 giving a total of 30 speeds. The shear rate can be digitally displayed, as can temperature and shear stress (% fsd). This manually operated system can be ungraded to a semi-automatic mode by the addition of a speed programmer PG242 and chart recorder, thereby allowing such tests as ramping and cycling and even shear jump tests. For a fully computerised system an RV20 together with the RC20 Rheocontroller is required and provides the capability of dynamic measurements (on-line Fourier analysis of stress and strain) and thixotropic recovery tests. The RC20 has both serial and IEEE-488 interfaces. In dynamic mode, the RC20/CV100 directly controls the oscillating strain and is under full software control of a micro such as an IBM-XT. Oscillation is also possible with the M5-Osc option, which has a steady shear capability of 0·5–52 rad s^{-1} or with sinusoidal oscillation 0·05–5 Hz.

All these devices are essentially bench mounted and do not take up much space. However, peripherals such as chart recorders, computers, dry air supplies and thermocirculators can cause problems in this respect.

Contraves have developed a wide range of viscometers, for both process control and product development/research. Early instruments were the TV and STV viscometers, the Low Shear 100 and the Rheomat 30. This latter device has 30 preselectable speeds in a geometric progression from

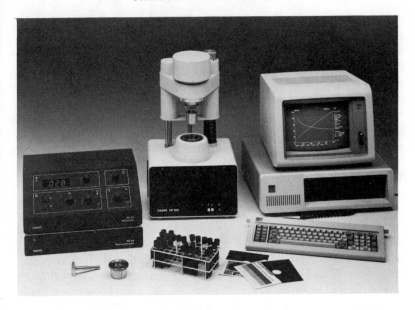

Fig. 13.1. Computerised package consisting of Rotovisco RV20, Rheocontroller RC20, measuring system CV100 and computer. (By courtesy of Haake.)

5×10^{-3} to $36 \, \text{rad s}^{-1}$, and torques are available from as low as 4.9×10^{-3} to $0.049 \, \text{N m fsd}$. Both the torque measurement and drive assemblies are in the same drive unit, the compliance for measurement being from 3.5 to 35 mrad for the ranges indicated. The drive is also provided with an electromagnetic brake, enabling relaxation studies. By using a programmer, the Rheoscan 30, far greater instrument control is possible. A wide range of measuring geometries are available. In the cone–plate mode, the gap is preset by the use of a spherical bearing that is attached to the apex of the cone. However, when using extremely viscous and adhesive materials, it is possible to remove this fixture whilst cleaning the platen, so care is required. This instrument was phased out during 1986, with other rheometers such as the Rheomat 115 superseding it.

The Contraves Rheomat 115 is a standardised viscometer, bench mounted and quite sturdy, with both measuring components on the driven axis. In standard Couette mode, sample loading is certainly an acquired technique, the sample generally having to be introduced into the cup before offering the assembly (with bob) up into the instrument. The sample is also not easy to see during a test since the temperature controlled jacket and stand obscure a clear view. The viscometer is microprocessor controlled and has a torque range from 5×10^{-4} to 50×10^{-3} N m, which corresponds to an internal reading of 0–1000 (max. compliance 0·034 rad). Fifteen speeds are selectable by using one plug-in module, giving a range of 5×10^{-3} to 80 rad s^{-1}. Gear options of $\times 10$ and $\times 100$ reduce this rotational speed range. To achieve a measure of automation, a combined programmer/chart recorder, the Rheoscan 115, can be fitted, which allows control at up to 779 speeds instead of the usual 15. Additionally, shear rate programs can be set up, but stress recovery following the cessation of shear is not easy to perform. This is not helped by the inbuilt delay between the command and speed operation, but it is primarily due to the machine's dependence on the integral chart recorder. However, it is possible to circumvent this to some extent, and use a micro as a data-logger. Contraves also support a Rheoanalyser option which is an inter-face that permits the viscometer's parameters to be set up and data captured. The computer (HP) merely interrogates the interface at uniform time intervals and at the end of a test the data can be analysed by the appropriately chosen software.

The Contraves Low Shear 30 is another instrument that can be used with the Rheoanalyser if required. It is essentially a rheometer system for the determination of viscoelastic properties within the low shear regime. Here the outer cup rotates or oscillates and the torque is sensed on the inner cylinder. In pure rotation, thirty speeds from 1·2 m rad s^{-1} to 10 rad s^{-1} are possible. There is an option to add the oscillatory drive system which covers the range $0·2 \times 10^{-3}$ to 1·63 Hz and the drive has an electromagnetic clutch. The torque assembly consists of a torsion wire support for the bob and an optical device to sense the very low twist. A restoring force is then used, via a coil, to hold the zero (null) position. The torque range is selectable in five steps from $9·5 \times 10^{-10}$ to 6×10^{-6} N m. The sinusoidal oscillation is usually preset to give a maximum angular deflection of 0·52 rad, although other values of 0·26 or 0·13 rad are per-mitted and are produced by an exchangeable eccentric cam drive. The rotational speed can also be externally controlled by a d.c. voltage (0–6 V). This instrument is best suited to biological materials where the viscosity is low and available sample volumes are small.

Other instruments in the range include the Rheomat 135 and Rheomat 145, which are modular rheometer systems. The Rheomat 135 has a maximum torque of 0·2 N m with rotational speeds from 20×10^{-6} to 82 rad s^{-1}. The cone–plate system has a separate controller with integral microprocessor and keyboard, and can perform both shear jump and angle jump tests. Of the recently introduced Rheomat 100 series, the Rheomat 108 is the simplest viscometer, with eight speeds, mains adaptor, rechargeable batteries and a concentric cylinder assembly. The viscometer is of the 'dip-in' type and can display viscosity, shear stress/rate, torque or temperature on a digital display. The eight speeds cover the range 5–104 rad s^{-1} with torque values up to $7 \cdot 5 \times 10^{-3}$ N m. There is also an analogue output of torque. Other units are the Rheoscan 100, a programmable unit for rotational speed and temperature, using plug-in modules to operate for up to 10 hours. The Contraves CP400 is a cone–plate measuring system for temperatures up to 400 °C.

The Physica range of instruments includes the viscometer Viscolab LC1 and the rheometer Viscolab LC10. The LC1 uses concentric cylinders with 27 speeds (9 × 3 ranges) from 0·1 to 84 rad s^{-1}, selected in sequence by thumbwheel switches. The torque range is up to 50×10^{-3} N m with a standard temperature range from -10 to $+90$ °C. The measurement of torque is said to be achieved without relying on deflection. The LC10 is a similar instrument except that it can be used with a flow curve programmer FP10 or with the Viscolab computer system. Sample volumes depend on the geometry and vary from 0·5 to 100 ml, with shear rates from 1·3 to 3979 s^{-1}.

The Bohlin Visco 88 (Fig. 13.2) is a portable viscometer, battery powered for up to 8 hours of use in the field or laboratory. It employs the concentric cylinder geometry with the inner cylinder rotating with or without an outer cylinder attached. The drive and torque measurement are via this inner cylinder drive unit with the rotational speeds fixed in eight steps from 2 to 100 rad s^{-1}. The speeds are set in geometric progression and the viscometer has a built in temperature sensor and liquid crystal display of all measured and calculated functions such as viscosity, shear rate, torque, temperature, stress and rotational speed (Hz). In use, the viscometer must be calibrated at each switch-on by using water, which can be particularly troublesome if oil based fluids are being studied. However, this is being changed so that the calibration is achieved internally when desired. The bobs are also easier to connect, being altered to push fits. There are eight different measuring geometries based on two outer cylinders and three bobs and only these can be used if the display is to provide correct readings. External output of torque to a chart recorder is also provided and there is an RS232 series interface to allow the control of all functions on a micro and also collect data. The shear rate range is from 4 to 1208 s^{-1} with a torque range up to 10×10^{-3} N m. The shear stress and viscosity indication has both a low and high reading warning

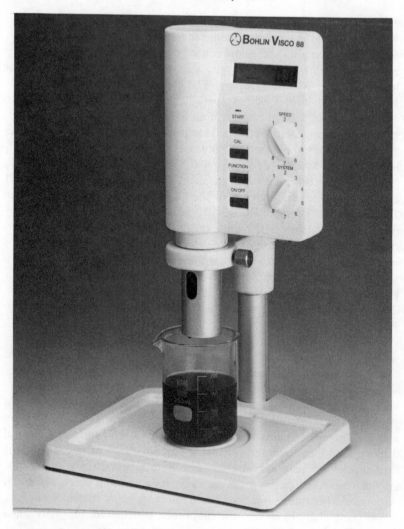

Fig. 13.2. Bohlin Visco 88. (By courtesy of Bohlin Reologi UK Ltd).

that indicates that the measurement is out of range, even though a torque value is provided. It would be very useful if such viscometers had memory facilities to hold previous readings.

Only a few of the many bench devices have been mentioned, most of these controlled strain viscometers being rotational only, though some of the latest machines do provide the capability of oscillatory strain control. As such, this allows a more detailed investigation of the fluid, but equally important are the tests performed under conditions of controlled stress. Probably one of the best known controlled stress instruments is the Deer Variable Stress Rheometer, whose development can be traced from the early articles which discussed the use of air turbines both to support and to apply a constant stress to an inner cylinder of a Couette arrangement.[5,6] The Deer rheometers, PDR81 series II and III, were essentially all from the same family, closely following the original design. The latter devices were marketed by Rheometer Marketing UK, but following their demise it is not known whether the instrument is still in production, so maintenance may prove more difficult than in the past. The rheometer is well constructed and quite compact. The associated electronic console and optional sweep programmer are separate units with an x–y or y–t chart recorder being necessary. Air is also required, which should be of instrument quality. Many of the difficulties encountered with this rheometer can be associated with a faulty air bearing usually arising from poor handling. The induction drive motor assembly is vertically mounted above the air bearing, the lower drive shaft being available to attach both tachometer and an angular displacement scroll as well as the couplings for the measuring assemblies. The angular displacement is monitored by a non-contacting proximity transducer coupled with an eccentric scroll having two working regions of some 1·7 rad diametrically opposite each other, though linearity is restricted to only 1 rad. A fixing pin is used to lock the scroll assembly, this effectively defining a zero position datum from which all displacements can be subsequently measured.

There is a range of platens, cups and cones, but not all are marked for ease of identification, so they should be checked before use. The method of attachment of these assemblies to the drive shaft is neither robust nor adequate for precision work. The complete rheometer can be levelled and the freewheeling of the air bearing can be reduced by adjusting the bias voltage to the motor. On some instruments this can be a particularly frustrating task, with balance (when achieved) often being displaced from the datum. The maximum torque capacity is 5×10^{-3} N m with a displayed resolution of typically 1×10^{-7} N m. Analogue output of angular displacement and angular velocity are available but not the applied torque. Typical angular resolution is 1 m rad. Though a bench device, the rheometer is quite sensitive and should be isolated from the majority of structurally borne vibrations if it is to be used at the lower end of its range. In operation, gap settings are easy with the complete motor assembly being lowered. The integral fluid circulating jacket is transparent, making it easy to check for trapped air that often results in poor temperature control. Temperatures from 5 to 85 °C are standard, any lower temperatures not being advisable because of the problems of condensation on the rheometer. Measurements are straightforward and, by inspection of the supplied manual giving the instrumental constants, viscosities, stresses and strains can be calculated from the raw data. The stress is applied through a switch selection so that transient tests are easy to perform. A semi-automatic operating mode can be achieved by using a programmer, but shear is always unidirectional though there appears to be no reason why oscillation could not be implemented. With the programmer attached, there is also an analogue signal proportional to the applied torque available. J. Deer was originally involved with this rheometer but has since participated in the design of a similar device that is sold by Carri-med.

This new and improved controlled stress instrument is the Controlled Stress (CS) Rheometer by Carri-med. At a prototype stage it has been referred to as a Rheodeer,[7] but it is essentially a new rheometer that enjoys many of the advantages that computer control provides both in machine control and data acquisition. Like many new instruments, performance of the earlier models was not without limitations, but these have been identified and corrected, mainly through the user feedback that the company encourages. This feature has helped both the manufacturer and the user; it is a policy that another company, Bohlin Reologi, promote quite actively.

The main external features of the instrument (Fig. 13.3) are its electronic console, onto which is directly attached the motor drive assembly. It is conveniently placed, leaving a large flat area as a workspace. A wide torque range is possible through three different versions of the motor drive. These are the CS50, CS100 and CS500 with full scale torque values of 5×10^{-3}, 10×10^{-3} and 50×10^{-3} N m respectively. Thumbwheel switches select the applied torque with a resolution of either 1×10^{-7} or 5×10^{-7} N m. Temperature is similarly selected, with resolution of 0.1 °, and there is a digital display of angular velocity for speeds up to 50 rad s^{-1}. Unlike the Deer rheometer, the CS machines have no visible bias control, since this operation, though necessary, is performed automatically by hardware. There is a visual indication when stability has been achieved but this can take up to 40 s. Measurement of angular velocity uses an optical encoder disc whilst the proximity displacement transducer operates by measuring the distance between itself and the surface of a specially machined disc. The transducer position is itself adjustable over a full 360 ° which is extremely useful when setting up the instrument. Unfortunately

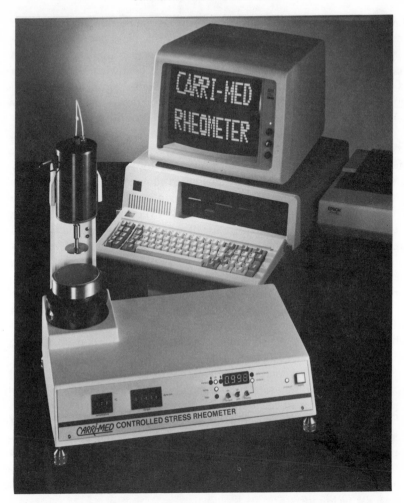

Fig. 13.3. Carri-Med Controlled Stress Rheometer. (By courtesy of Carri-Med).

the measurement region is still limited to ~ 1 rad. A novel feature of operation is the automatic setting of the predetermined gap (cone–plate, parallel plate). The lower platen assembly and Peltier heating/cooling block moves upwards, under pneumatic control, taking approximately 5 s to advance the 20 mm though the speed is said to be adjustable. The gap can be preset by a micrometer adjustment to within 5 μm and is quite reproducible except when very viscous materials are being studied. With low viscosity fluids, problems of trapped air in the sample (cone–plate mode) frequently occur, so the ram loading principle is not always beneficial. Apart from power and air, a low volume water circulation supply is required for the Peltier block, to remove excess heat when the rheometer is being used below room temperature. A stable air pressure is also considered advantageous, with pressure fluctuations being kept below $34 \, kN \, m^{-2}$.

The instrument can be manually operated but this restricts its use, so the computer control system should really be regarded as essential. Earlier models used an Apple IIe microcomputer but this has been superseded by an IBM with IEEE-488 interface. A limited range of creep, flow analysis and oscillatory software is available and is continually being updated. The creep software is quite good and that for flow (both stress and shear rate flow modes) makes quite extensive use of models such as Casson, Bingham and Herschel–Bulkley for data analysis. For oscillation, the frequency range is from 0·001 to 10 Hz, this being set by the software which both generates the waveform and calculates the phase angle. Though the programs available are menu driven, familarity makes their operation somewhat easier to follow. They are certainly adequate as a basis from which to start a rheological study; since the IBM version was only available in 1986, the suite of programs does not yet reflect the capability of the rheometer.

With the degree of computer control that this instrument has, it is easy to allow oneself to rely totally on the automated nature, both in performance and subsequent calculation. Certainly, for the oscillation regime, a visual indication of the materials' responses in real time, such as a chart recorder could provide, would be beneficial. This would avoid misinterpretation of many non-linear effects and provide a check on the performance of the rheometer. Understandably, this rheometer brings the characterisation of viscoelastic materials into the laboratory, as a nonspecialist technique.

The Sangamo Visco-Elastic Analyser (Integrated Petronics) is another controlled stress device that has been around for many years. The torque can be applied in a continuous, stepwise or oscillatory mode, and in appearance the instrument is very similar to the Deer. Angular displacement is either 0·5 or 0·02 rad with a resolution of better than 10^{-4} rad. Optional is an IEEE interface to allow control and data acquisition, and it has the facility to realign (twist) the lower platen assembly in order that the displacement transducer can record within its linear range. Unfortunately this rheometer is no longer marketed but Rheo-Tech International now provide a new version stress instrument called the Rheo-Tech VER (viscoelastic rheometer). The pushbutton console is replaced by a pressure sensitive membrane panel and there is a high temperature option that replaces the usual water jacket for temperatures up to 300 °C. Apart from controlled stress, a preset shear rate can be selected and the shear stress monitored, this mode permitting the simulation of fixed shear rate processes. Software is available for IBM micros and the machine has a specification of: torque 9.8×10^{-7} to 5.8×10^{-3} N m; angular velocity up to 100 rad s^{-1}; oscillatory frequencies from 1×10^{-5} to 10 Hz with a gap setting accuracy to 10^{-6} m. A portable steady shear rate viscometer (Visco-Tech 8) was also released in 1986, being a quality control device, with speeds from 0·5 to 105 rad s^{-1}.

13.3. RESEARCH RHEOMETERS

This group of rheometers are most easily identified by their size, cost and flexibility in use. Certainly they are not cheap, and the majority are floor standing. Their flexibility means that they are ideal for research rather than the more routine type of work. The most widely known rheometer in past years for the study of viscoelasticity has been the Weissenberg Rheogoniometer. This is a widely distributed machine, the prototype of many new instruments, which has undergone various modifications over the years. The R-20 has retained its drive mechanism of synchronous motor and multistage gearbox, providing rotational speeds of the lower platen from 3.6×10^{-6} to 78 rad s^{-1}. It has an electromagnetic clutch-brake assembly to facilitate stress growth and relaxation tests, and for oscillatory work it has a second motor and drive to provide a selection of mechanically derived frequencies with amplitudes freely adjustable from 2 to 30 m rad. Here the lower platen is driven, with the upper, on an air bearing providing support for the torque measurement assembly. Normal forces and angular displacements are measured on the lower platen. A feedback servo-mechanism is incorporated to maintain a constant gap in the plate–plate mode. A problem here has been the overdamped nature of the normal force/torque measurement system

The flexibility of the Weissenberg is dictated by the model purchased (A, B, C or D). Model A provides for rotation only, whilst model D allows oscillatory (2.5×10^{-6} to 50 Hz) and normal force testing, as well as superposition of oscillation and constant rotation. A 10-piece set of calibrated torsion bars provide a torque capability from 0.55×10^{-11} to 1·4 N m, with normal force from 4.8×10^{-2} to 100 N. Each model is available manually operated or automated for computer control, with signal analysis using a transfer function analyser, but at the present time (September 1986) it is currently undergoing a complete upgrading by Carri-med, who recently acquired the instrument to add to their existing range. It is not expected that the new rheometer will be available until at least 1988.

In the early 1970s, quite sophisticated rheometers began to appear, one such device being that manufactured by the Instron Corporation.[8] The

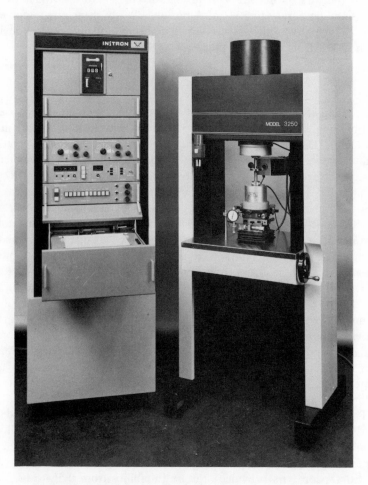

Fig. 13.4. The Instron 3250. (By courtesy of Instron.)

Instron 3250 Rotary Rheometer (Figs 13.4 and 13.5) is a floor standing machine with the capability of measuring both torque and normal forces; with suitable options, it can function in the eccentric rotating disc (ERD) mode. The mechanical aspects comprise of a direct drive (no clutches) digitally controlled motor which, together with an optical encoder, provide the equivalent of 128 000 steps/rev. Axial runout of the air bearing is typically 5×10^{-8} m. In a typical parallel plate configuration, one platen is directly attached to the lower end of the driven shaft, precise machining being necessary for correct alignment since there is no provision to adjust this surface. The load cell is situated below, on a stage that is freely adjustable for both height, lateral displacement and rotation. The mechanical unit uses a closed frame very much like a figure '8' for

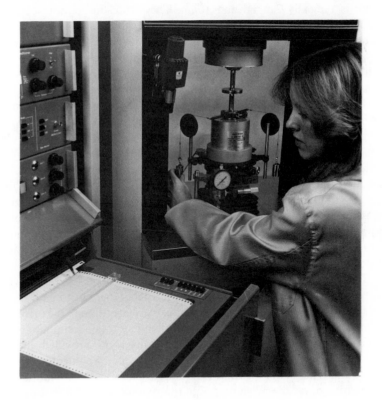

Fig. 13.5. The calibration technique for the Instron Rheometer. (By courtesy of Instron.)

increased stiffness, which is in excess of $10^9\,\mathrm{N\,m^{-1}}$ vertically and greater than $10^8\,\mathrm{N\,m^{-1}}$ transversely. However, like all structures, it has a characteristic resonance ($\sim 28\,\mathrm{Hz}$) whose amplitude has been kept as low as possible by the incorporation of friction dampers in the frame. The complete unit stands nearly 2 m high, all services of power and air being introduced at the base of the frame, together with a large umbilical that carries all command and response signals to another floor standing console unit. The console holds the temperature controller, drive control unit, analogue position control (optional but essential) and chart recorder, and can accommodate other peripherals that may be required.

In operation, the platen gap is very easily set by raising the lower load cell assembly. Two torque-normal force load cells are available with capacities of $20 \times 10^{-3}\,\mathrm{N\,m}$ (1 N) and $2\,\mathrm{N\,m}$ (100 N) respectively. Compliance is typically 2 m rad and $10\mu\mathrm{m}$. These transducers are not temperature controlled, a situation which should be remedied if studies over any reasonable length of time are required. Noise levels on the load cells are such that accuracies down to 1 in 20 000 fsd are easily attainable.

The drive unit is capable of rotation in either direction at speeds, in tenths of decade steps, from 1×10^{-6} to $260\,\mathrm{rad\,s^{-1}}$, selected by thumbwheel switches. Acceleration is typically $1200\,\mathrm{rad\,s^{-2}}$. Oscillation is provided through internally generated waveforms (0·01–100 Hz); sine, triangle and square in angular velocity as well as square in angular displacement can all be superimposed on a steady state rotation. The amplitude of oscillation can also be controlled and there is an LED indication when the motor is working outside its specification, such as high frequency at high amplitude. The frequencies and angular velocities can be updated at any time so that transient tests are easily performed. Analogue output of both torque and normal forces is available but that of angular position/velocity is only accessible if the angular position control facility is fitted. With this option, the rheometer can be driven from an external waveform generator, so the internal drive control unit becomes somewhat redundant. Since the motor is digitally controlled, there is no limit to the lower frequency attainable, except that the discrete motion of the drive will be apparent. The analogue position control allows total freedom to select frequency, amplitude ($+/-1$ rad) and even waveform, provided that the motor is driven within its operating range. Computer control is easy to achieve and is necessary if such calculations as phase angle and moduli are to be achieved. As the machine design is essentially modular and the raw data are easily available, it is up to the user to provide the necessary hardware or software for data analysis. A Solartron 1172 frequency response analyser is frequently used to determine amplitude and phase angles, using a correlation technique. It can also function as a frequency generator and provides a measure of phase angle to within $0.1°$; recent devices such as the Solartron 1250 are able to reduce this to $0.01°$. Hardware/software computer packages are available for signal analysis and these can easily be modified to suit the rheological field of study, but most users have developed their own support. The upper frequency limit is usually considered to be 100 Hz, but there is a load cell resonance in the region of 78 Hz, so the rheometer is generally restricted to lower frequencies. Overall, the instrument, which also has a radiant heating thermal chamber, is a good research instrument where emphasis has been placed on the mechanical aspects of the rheometer rather than on the software control or data analysis. Its flexibility is quite considerable and it can operate in both controlled strain and controlled stress modes, oscillatory or transient testing.

Also in the early 1970s, another general purpose rotational rheometer was designed by Rheometrics, who have since developed a specialised range of machines which are continually being updated. The Rheometrics Mechanical Spectrometer started as a bench standing device, an automated version being the RMS-605. This rheometer employed the criteria that rheological characterisation required tests to be taken over the variables of stress, strain, time and environment. Both torsion and compression testing were achievable with a built-in microprocessor undertaking signal averaging cross-correlation and all calculations. The d.c. torque motor was mounted above the sample position and, through the use of analogue control, could provide smooth angular rotation even at very low shear rates. Angular velocities were from 0.001 to $100 \, \text{rad s}^{-1}$, acceleration $> 900 \, \text{rad s}^{-2}$, and oscillation possible from 1.6×10^{-4} to 15.9 Hz at amplitudes of up to 0.5 rad. All waveforms were digitally generated internally with an integral chart recorder, printer and plotter providing hardcopy results. Operation of this rheometer was dependent on its integral controller. Torque transducers covered the range 9.8×10^{-5} to $0.19 \, \text{N m fsd}$ and were temperature compensated. A thermal chamber, forced convection, accommodates temperatures up to $400 \, °\text{C}$ with a nitrogen option to go down to $-150 \, °\text{C}$. This rheometer has since been superseded by the RMS-800. The new motor has extended performance and is capable of angular velocities from 1×10^{-6} to $100 \, \text{rad s}^{-1}$ and torque ranges from 9.8×10^{-6} to $0.9 \, \text{N m}$ with normal forces from 0.001 to $2 \, \text{N fsd}$. Axial runout in the motor has been reduced to less than $1.5 \times 10^{-6} \, \text{m}$ and, in the quest for extremely low compliance that is

necessary for accurate transient and normal force measures, a new transducer has been designed. It is a force rebalance transducer having two
servos to maintain zero steady state displacement of the platens. The
instrument can also perform creep and recovery tests. Data analysis uses
a correlation technique for sinusoidal oscillatory testing and an IBM
micro can be attached.

The Rheometrics System-4 is a relatively recent introduction that arose
from the desire to undertake a more complete material characterisation
than would be possible using any single rheometer. This is principally
because, in designing a specific instrument, conflicting requirements such
as torque capability, inertia and axial runout are usually encountered and
cannot be overcome for best performance. Consequently, the System-4
was designed, it being a modular concept with four different measuring
heads that can be positioned, as required, over the test area. The test
systems included are steady shear, transient shear, fluids and tensile
testing.[9] Specialised devices are still available, such as the Rheometrics
Dynamic Analyser (RDA-700), which is similar to the earlier dynamic
spectrometer in its main operation, being one of forced sinusoidal shear
oscillation. Frequency ranges are from 1.59×10^{-3} to 79 Hz at temperatures from -150 to $+500\,°C$. It has an automatic compensation to
maintain material expansion/contraction by keeping the normal force
constant. Complete computer control is possible, software being available
for strain sweeps, frequency sweeps and stress relaxation and temperature
sweeps.

The Rheometrics Dynamic Spectrometer (RDS-7700 Series II) is the
latest design in dynamic spectrometers which provides, as an option, a
continuous shear capability. It can also be upgraded to the RMS-800, can
operate in either manual or automatic modes, and uses a dedicated microcomputer. It also is equipped with a stepped motor to control axial
servo-positioning.

Specifically for fluids, there are the Rheometrics Fluids Rheometer
(RFR-7800) and the Rheometrics Fluids Spectrometer (RFS-8400 and
RFS-8500); these are designed for low to medium viscosity fluids. The
RFR has both steady and dynamic shear modes at angular velocities from
1×10^{-4} to 100 rad s^{-1} with oscillation from 1.59×10^{-5} to 79 Hz. It has
a humidity controlled environmental chamber with the drive motor
housed in the lower part of the frame. Thus, in Couette flow, it is only the
outer cylinder that rotates. Torque range is typically 0.01 N m fsd with
normal force of 1 N; calibration is by dead weights. For signal analysis, it
uses a built-up signal generator to act as a reference for cross-correlation.

The measurement period is $1\cdot5 \times$ (frequency period) in oscillation, with a phase resolution of $0\cdot1°$. For constant rotation, it measures 2000 points over $1\cdot6$ s and provides an average, though the capability exists to average over longer time periods. Stress relaxation and creep studies can easily be undertaken.

The Viscoelastic Testers RVE-M and RVE-S are specifically designed for melts (M) and viscoelastic solids (S) and are ideal for repetitive studies. The RVE-M, in auto mode, has a frequency range of $1\cdot59 \times 10^{-2}$ to $15\cdot9$ Hz and is usually used in cone–plate or parallel plate mode. The RVE-S is specifically designed for torsional testing of solid samples and can measure the shear moduli over the range 10^5–10^{11} Pa. Both devices are similar, except that the RVE-S has a torque capacity of $0\cdot9$ N m as against $0\cdot19$ N m for the RVE-M.

The Rheometrics Stress Rheometer allows materials to be tested under conditions of controlled stress by creep and relaxation studies. The machine has a very high angular resolution ($\sim 20 \times 10^{-6}$ rad) and can record at very low shear rates. All phases of the instrument are controlled by a built-in processor. The RSR has a drag cup motor and a very stiff air bearing. It is described by Franck[10] as having a torque capability of $4\cdot9 \times 10^{-6}$ to $9\cdot1 \times 10^{-3}$ N m, and with 25 mm parallel plates has a stress range of $1\cdot6$–3200 Pa. Temperature can be varied from ambient to 350 °C, and both the creep and recovery are monitored at a sampling rate of $0\cdot02$ Hz. An optional CRT is available for graphics display of the data.

The Rheometrics series of machines are probably the most widely used of the new rheometers, in spite of their very high cost. However, the market is certainly not at capacity, as has been shown over the past few years by Bohlin Reologi (Sweden) who have developed a range of rheometers and viscometers. At present, their principal rheometer is the Bohlin Rheometer System whose top of the range machine is the Model VOR (viscosity–oscillation–relaxation test) (Figs. 13.6 and 13.7). This rheometer was introduced in 1983; the prototype has since been modified and upgraded. It is a surprisingly compact unit and very robustly manufactured. Originally its computer control was by a Facit but this has since been changed to an IBM compatible microcomputer with special interface. Two motors are used, one for the constant rotation and another for the oscillation, a clutch choosing the desired drive. In Couette mode the outer cylinder is driven from below with the torque sensed by the inner cylinder attached to a torsion spring (or bar) via an air bearing. Integral temperature control is provided and the gap setting is achieved by lowering the complete inner cylinder/air bearing/torsion bar. Rotational

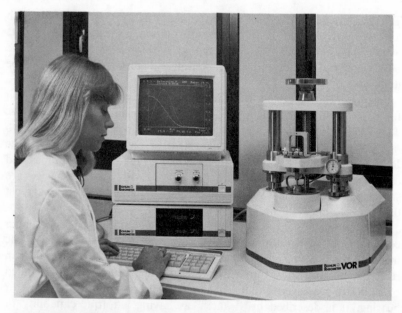

Fig. 13.6. Bohlin VOR Rheometer. (By courtesy of Bohlin Reologi UK Ltd.)

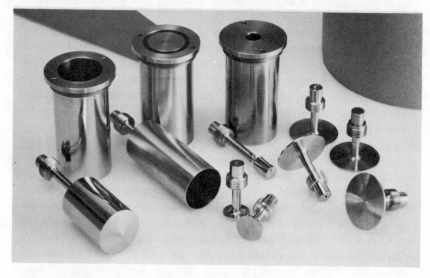

Fig. 13.7. The measuring assemblies for the Bohlin VOR. (By courtesy of Bohlin
Reologi UK Ltd.)

speeds are from 135×10^{-6} to $135 \, \text{rad s}^{-1}$ and torsion bars are available for the range $19 \cdot 6 \times 10^{-6}$ to $24 \cdot 4 \times 10^{-3} \, \text{N m}$. The frequency range is $0 \cdot 001$–$20 \, \text{Hz}$ (14 points), the waveform being generated through software with signal analysis also performed automatically using fast Fourier transformations. The software is impressive and is menu driven with much disc access, so a hard disc system is to be preferred. Rotational speeds and frequencies are preset in the software and the strain and torque signals are now accessible as analogue levels. The maximum angular deflection of the drive system is $0 \cdot 02 \, \text{rad}$.

Stress relaxation can also be performed, with the measurement period chosen within the range 1–$22\,000 \, \text{s}$; a ramp rise time is adjustable from $20 \, \text{ms}$ to $20 \, \text{s}$. For the slower rotational speeds a gearbox is used and both directions of rotation are possible with some 60 speeds being accessible. Originally the rheometer used torsion springs as the sensing elements but these were found to be quite difficult to secure if frequently changed; torsion bars are now used. The design of the device, especially the bridge arrangement that secures the torque sensing elements, does restrict the rheometer to the lower torque values but is well within the machine design.

The Bohlin Controlled Stress Rheometer (BCS) (Fig. 13.8) was introduced in 1986. The sample is contained in a stationary lower compartment. Temperature control is provided (5–$95\,^{\circ}\text{C}$) and the controlled torque applied on the rotatable upper geometry using a drag-cup motor principle. The angular deflection is monitored as a function of time with high resolution ($10^{-5} \, \text{rad}$) and a full $360\,^{\circ}$ linear range. The maximum continuous torque that can be applied is $0 \cdot 001 \, \text{N m}$ with a resolution of $2 \times 10^{-7} \, \text{N m}$. The sample can also be preconditioned with a short duration torque of $0 \cdot 1 \, \text{N.m}$. Rotational speeds from 10^{-5} to $50 \, \text{rad s}^{-1}$ are measurable and the machine has optional software for oscillatory stress measurements via the microcomputer. At the present time, the instrument is undergoing user trials by those research groups who have used the earlier VOR machine.

Gottfert Werkstoff-Prufmaschinen have a rheometer for measuring the viscosity and thermosetting of polymers as well as an Elastograph 76.85 which is a microprocessor controlled rotorless shear vulcameter. It has a fixed oscillation frequency of $0 \cdot 83 \, \text{Hz}$ with amplitudes variable from 17×10^{-4} to $14 \times 10^{-3} \, \text{rad}$. Torque is measured on the lower oscillating surface from $0 \cdot 5$ to $10 \, \text{N m}$ with normal forces from $0 \cdot 5$ to $10 \, \text{kN fsd}$.

The Toyoseiki (Japan) Rheolograph series provide quick and precise measurements of dynamic viscoelasticity of a wide range of materials. The Rheolograph Liquid (654) is a double concentric cylinder type of instrument, undertaking measurement at a constant shear rate on volumes of

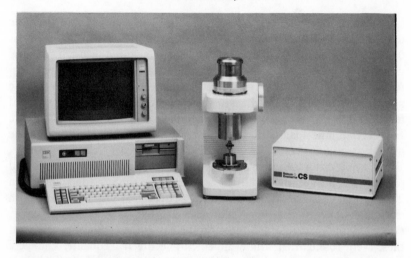

Fig. 13.8. Bohlin CS Rheometer. (By courtesy of Bohlin Reologi UK Ltd.)

less than 1 ml. The outer lower assembly rotates, via a clutch mechanism, with a shear rate range of 1–$99\,\mathrm{s}^{-1}$ and shear stresses from 0.01 to $5\,\mathrm{N\,m}^{-2}$. Oscillation is also possible at a fixed amplitude of $17 \times 10^{-3}\,\mathrm{rad}$ at frequencies of either 0.5 or $1.0\,\mathrm{Hz}$. Temperature control is provided from 10 to 60 °C, with a digital indication of the measured and calculated results. The other instruments in the range (651–653) do not use rotational shear.

Iwamoto Seisakusho (Japan) no longer produce the Autoviscometer III but have an improved version, the IR-200. This is a conventional coaxial type rheometer; measurements can be made in both cone–plate and Couette geometries. It has a d.c. servo-motor rotating the outer/lower member via a reduction gear system allowing steady state or dynamic oscillatory measures as well as transient phenomena. Constant rotational speed is from 5.2×10^{-3} to $0.52\,\mathrm{rad\,s}^{-1}$ or from 0.52 to $52\,\mathrm{rad\,s}^{-1}$. Oscillation amplitude is to $0.03\,\mathrm{rad}$ at frequencies from 0.8×10^{-3} to $83 \times 10^{-3}\,\mathrm{Hz}$ or 83×10^{-3} to $8.3\,\mathrm{Hz}$. Torque is measured via a torsion wire or pipe, capable of measuring from 5.6×10^{-5} to $10.18\,\mathrm{N\,m\,deg}^{-1}$. With the fixtures applied (1 ° cone, 3 ° cone and Couette assembly) shear rates from 0.06 to $2000\,\mathrm{s}^{-1}$ are possible, with shear stresses from 7.4×10^{-2} to $6.3 \times 10^{3}\,\mathrm{N\,m}^{-2}$. Normal forces can be measured by using an optical device to a maximum value of $4.9\,\mathrm{N}$, and another option allows the rotational speeds (and frequencies) to be extended down to $5.2 \times 10^{-5}\,\mathrm{rad\,s}^{-1}$.

All the latest rheological instrumentation provides far greater information than the earlier, single point devices. For routine work, there is much in favour of the use of a precalibrated viscometer; the use of instrumental constants can save much time if applied intelligently. However, as in many other fields of instrumentation, the computerised approach has been seen as an aid to the widespread application and use of a rheology/material science approach. Interpretation of results is relatively straightforward, so much so that great faith is often placed on the manufacturer providing a suitable instrument. It is easy to use such rheometers beyond their design specifications unless there is an understanding of rheology. Nevertheless, all this computational support, though making it easier for the technician, should not detract from the use of other instruments such as chart recorders and oscilloscopes to check and obtain hard-copy evidence of the machines' performance. A manual override is often useful on an auto- mated device, and calibration, using well characterised fluids, can be used both to check performance and to establish the operating criteria for any other fabricated measuring assemblies that may be considered suitable. Steady state conditions or those of dynamic equilibrium are now well established techniques at the medium to low frequencies, but emphasis is now being placed on the start/stop or transient response approach. These require more stringent instrumental conditions, the quality of results depending a great deal on the rheometer's manufacture, this having improved greatly in recent years. Whatever the technique chosen, it should be but one of the many used. In supporting a successful material charac- terisation, the greater one's knowledge of rheology the more likely one is to succeed.

REFERENCES

1. G. S. Beavers and D. D. Joseph, *J. Fluid Mechanics,* 1975, **69,** 475.
2. J. R. Van Wazer, J. W. Lyons, K. Y. Kim and R. E. Colwell, *Viscosity and Flow Measurement*, Interscience, New York, 1963.
3. R. W. Whorlow, *Rheological Techniques*, Ellis-Horwood, Chichester, 1980.
4. D. C. Cheng, Warren Spring Lab. Report LR282(MH), 1979.
5. S. S. Davis, J. J. Deer and B. Warburton, *J. Phys. (E),* 1968, **1,** 933.
6. S. S. Davis, *J. Phys. (E),* 1969, **2,** 102.
7. E. Ernst, *Arztl. Lab.,* 1982, **28,** 21.
8. C. J. Drislane, J. P. DeNicola, W. M. Wareham and R. I. Tanner, *Rheol. Acta,* 1974, **13,** 4.
9. J. M. Starita, in *Rheology*, Vol. 2, G. Astarita, G. Marrucci and L. Nicolais (Eds), Plenum Press, New York, 1980, pp. 229–34.
10. A. J. P. Franck, *J. Rheol.,* 1985, **29,** 833.

Chapter 14

Flow Visualisation in Rheometry

M. E. MACKAY* AND D. V. BOGER

*Department of Chemical Engineering, University of Melbourne,
Parkville, Victoria, Australia*

INTRODUCTION

Figure 14.1 illustrates the place of rheometry in the process for solving a non-Newtonian fluid mechanics problem for an incompressible fluid. Given that the flow problem and boundary conditions can be specified, the basic and established tools to effect a solution for the problem are the Cauchy momentum equations (conservation of momentum) and the continuity equation (conservation of mass). However, these equations can only be solved when the stresses are related to the velocity field via a constitutive equation. With the exception of Newtonian fluids and some

* Present address: Department of Chemical Engineering, University of Queensland, St Lucia, Queensland 4067, Australia.

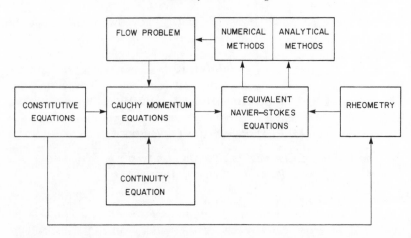

Fig. 14.1. Illustration of the function of rheometry in the scheme of solving a non-Newtonian fluid mechanics problem.

simple non-Newtonian fluids, e.g. power-law fluids, where fluid elasticity is of no importance, the relevant constitutive equation is not known and must be chosen from a range of available possibilities. It is the parameters in the constitutive equation, such as viscosity, relaxation time and retardation time, in the Oldroyd B model, for example, which must be measured in rheometry in order to define the flow problem completely so that it can be solved by numerical and rarely by analytical methods. Having solved the fluid mechanics problem for the stress and velocity field, the solution must be checked because of the assumed constitutive equation. At this stage, flow visualisation techniques can be used to observe the velocity and/or stress field for comparison with prediction. If the comparison is good, the constitutive equation is adequate and the problem is solved. Unfortunately this process has only been successful for relatively simple elastic liquids[1] in squeeze film flows,[2] Stokes flow around a sphere,[3,4] isothermal spinning,[5] and drop breakup in filament extension.[6]

Thus flow visualisation for observation of the velocity and stress field and rheometry for measurement of the basic material parameters are both essential in the development of non-Newtonian fluid mechanics for viscoelastic fluids. However, flow visualisation techniques in rheometers where the flow field is well understood, such as torsion and Couette flows, are of importance only for the purposes of establishing parameters required, such as the stress-optic coefficient in birefringence, for quantitative observation in more complex flow fields. In the latter category of flow field are the so-called strong inlet and exit flows, which are important in rheometry (capillary and slit rheometry) and in relatively simple flow fields for testing constitutive equations in non-Newtonian fluid mechanics.

This chapter first examines birefringence as a technique for stress measurement in flowing viscoelastic fluids. The technique is discussed in some detail particularly in regard to determination of the stress-optic coefficient where well understood viscometric flows need to be used. Emphasis is then placed on the use of the technique in non-viscometric entry and exit flows, which are both important in rheometry, but where difficulties still remain in interpretation of the observations in terms of the basic stress field.

Flow visualisation techniques for streak-line observation and point velocity measurement are then briefly discussed. Unlike birefringence, these techniques require no calibration in terms of a flow field of known kinematics or stress field. Hence there is no discussion on the use of these techniques for well understood viscometric flows such as torsion and Couette flows, but the treatment concentrates on a detailed examination of tubular entry flows, where the importance of streak-line observation and point velocity measurement in terms of the ultimate solution of this important flow field is emphasised.

14.2. BIREFRINGENCE MEASUREMENTS

Flow birefringence is a non-destructive optical technique which is used to measure the stresses within a flowing fluid. It is hoped that birefringence can be used in conjunction with velocity measurements to map both the stress and velocity (and hence the velocity gradient) fields on a point by point basis to test the predictions of a rheological equation of state (constitutive equation) in complex flow geometries. This being the case, the most suitable equation of state could then be identified and confidently used to predict the flow field in another geometry. The method, although extremely tempting, is not exact and without assumptions. It is concluded at the end of this section that, while birefringence measurements are certainly accurate in predicting stresses in simple shear flows for flexible molecules, they are only qualitative or semi-quantitative in flows where moderate to large elongational elements exist, i.e. the flows of most interest to the rheologist.

Birefringence (optical double refraction) is due to a difference between the principal refractive indices within a material. Birefringence is easily observed by twisting a piece of perspex (plexiglass) between crossed polarisers. Bands of colours will appear which represent different levels of the principal refractive indices.* By using what is termed the stress-optic relation the bands are related to the stresses within the material. Briefly, the stress-optic relation may be stated as follows: the stress and refractive index ellipses are coaxial and the differences in the principal refractive indices are directly proportional to those of the stresses.

Birefringence also occurs with particle suspensions and polymer solutions and melts during flow and, just as in static systems such as perspex, the stress-optic relation is postulated to be valid. Flow birefringence was observed independently by Mach[7] and Maxwell[8] in 1873; it is due to orientation of the particles or macromolecules which results in optical anisotropy. Since then, flow birefringence has gained much popularity as a method for direct measurement of fluid stresses in complex geometries.

A complete survey of the recent literature can be found in references 9 and 10. Here a discussion on the stress-optic relation is first presented, followed by sections on measurement techniques and experimental studies in various geometries.

14.2.1. Stress-Optic Relation

Before looking at more complicated fields, we consider first a two-dimensional stress or refractive index field. When monochromatic, linearly polarised light enters an optically active medium it is resolved into two waves, called the ordinary and the extraordinary, which move with different velocities. The velocity (v) is related to the refractive index (n) by

$$n = \frac{c}{v} \tag{14.1}$$

where c is the speed of light in vacuum. Thus one can see that the medium will have two principal refractive indices owing to the ordinary and extraordinary light waves. The relative phase difference, δ, is

$$\delta = \frac{2\pi L}{\lambda_1} (n_{P1} - n_{P2}) \tag{14.2}$$

where L is the propagation length of the light, λ_1 the light wavelength, and

---

* A principal coordinate system is one that rotates a given tensor, e.g. the refractive index, so that it has only diagonal elements. These diagonal values are the eigenvalues of the original tensor, and their direction is given by the eigenvectors. The eigenvalues can be visualised as scaling the axes of an ellipse at an inclination given by the eigenvectors.

the subscripts P1 and P2 stand for principal directions ($\mathbf{n}$ is a tensor). Birefringence is usually given the symbol Δ and is equal to $(n_{P1} - n_{P2})$; note that Δ is dimensionless.

Light travelling within the medium is elliptically polarised and the inclination angle of the major axis of the light or optic ellipse makes an angle χ_O with the polarisation axis (see Hecht and Zajac[11] for an excellent discussion on elementary optics). The stress-optic relation can be written in mathematical terms as

$$\Delta = C(\sigma_{P1} - \sigma_{P2}) \tag{14.3a}$$

and

$$\chi_O = \chi_M \tag{14.3b}$$

with σ representing the stress tensor, χ_M the inclination angle of the mechanical or stress ellipse, and C the stress-optic coefficient which is a function of the material and temperature.

From a theoretical viewpoint the stress-optic relation is found to be valid for flexible macromolecules at low extensions and rigid particles where Brownian motion dominates. Leal and Hinch[12] as well as Talbott[10] have shown that the stress and optic ellipses are not coaxial for rigid particles undergoing weak Brownian motion. The reader is referred to some reviews[13–20] for comprehensive surveys of the literature.

Before leaving this discussion on the stress-optic relation, a frequently encountered stress field needs to be discussed to elucidate the behaviour of χ_M and hence χ_O. Consider

$$\sigma_{ij} = \begin{pmatrix} \sigma_{11} & \sigma_{12} & 0 \\ \sigma_{12} & \sigma_{22} & 0 \\ 0 & 0 & \sigma_{33} \end{pmatrix} \tag{14.4}$$

where the usual rheological convention is used with 1 being the flow direction, 2 the shear and 3 the neutral. The three principal stresses (eigenvalues) are

$$\sigma_{P1} = \tfrac{1}{2}(\sigma_{11} + \sigma_{22}) + \sqrt{\tfrac{1}{4}N_1^2 + \sigma_{12}^2} \tag{14.5a}$$

$$\sigma_{P2} = \tfrac{1}{2}(\sigma_{11} + \sigma_{22}) - \sqrt{\tfrac{1}{4}N_1^2 + \sigma_{12}^2} \tag{14.5b}$$

$$\sigma_{P3} = \sigma_{33} \tag{14.5c}$$

where N_1 is the first normal stress difference, equal to $(\sigma_{11} - \sigma_{22})$. The principal directions corresponding to σ_{P1} and σ_{P2} are orthogonal and the first makes an angle $\chi_M^{(1)}$ with the 1-axis:

$$\tan_2 \chi_M^{(1)} = \frac{2\sigma_{12}}{N_1} \qquad (14.6)$$

The third principal direction is incident with the 3-axis and is orthogonal to the first and second.

For steady Poiseuille flow of a Newtonian fluid between plane walls, N_1 is zero and we find $\chi_M^{(1)}$ is always 45°. $\chi_M^{(1)}$ can deviate from 45° for a fluid which has σ_{12} and N_1 non-zero. In particular, near the wall, where the shear rate is greatest, the largest deviation is expected to occur. The principal directions are incident with the flow coordinates when σ_{12} is zero, as is the case with elongational flows.

14.2.2. Measurement of Birefringence

There are many optical instruments (polariscopes) which may be used to measure birefringence. For the practical rheologist using highly birefringent materials, a plane or circular polariscope consisting of polarisers and quarter-wave plates is adequate (Δ should be greater than 10^{-5}–10^{-4}). A more sensitive method employs compensators such as the Ehringhaus or the de Sénarmont (see references 20 and 21) which are capable of measuring birefringences of order 10^{-7} and greater. The phase-modulated technique of Koeman and Janeschitz-Kriegl[22] and Frattini and Fuller[23] is more sophisticated and capable of measuring smaller birefringences on the order of 10^{-8}. Most birefringence research in flow fields of interest to the rheologist has dealt with highly birefringent polymer melts and solutions, so equations for the polariscope necessary to analyse these data are developed.

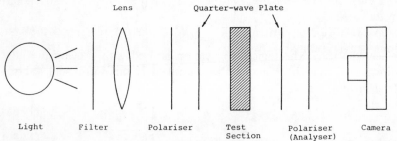

Fig. 14.2. Polariscope to measure the birefringence of highly birefringent materials. The light source consists of the light, monochromatic filter, and lens. The arrangement shown is for a circular polariscope; removal of the quarter-wave plates produces a plane polariscope. The wave normal direction is from left to right.

A polariscope is shown schematically in Fig. 14.2. A plane polariscope consists of a light source with two polarisers on either side of the test section; the polariser nearest the camera is termed the analyser. A dark-field polariscope has the polarisation axis of the analyser orthogonal to that of the polariser; a light-field instrument has the axes parallel. Bands representing various values of retardation would result for either method and are best analysed by the Walker[24] matrix method. Walker developed matrices based on Stokes parameters specifying the state of polarisation of an optical component which are multiplied in series. The column matrix for the Stokes parameters leaving a polariser (or 'ingoing' to the polariscope) whose axis lies along the x-axis (arbitrary) is

$$\mathbf{I}_i = E_x^2 \begin{pmatrix} 1 \\ 1 \\ 0 \\ 0 \end{pmatrix} \tag{14.7}$$

where E_x is the x-component of the electric vector. The first component is of interest as it specifies the intensity. Using the nomenclature of Walker (see also reference 20) the 'outgoing' column matrix for a plane polariscope is given by

$$\mathbf{I}_o = \mathbf{P}(\alpha)\mathbf{R}(\beta, \delta)\mathbf{I}_i \tag{14.8}$$

where $\mathbf{R}(\beta, \delta)$ represents a matrix for an optical component (in this case the test section) with a relative retardation δ at an angle β to the x-axis, and $\mathbf{P}(\alpha)$ represents the matrix for a polariser whose axis is at an angle α to the x-axis.

The relative transmittance ($T = I_{o,1}/I_{i,1}$, where 1 represents the first component) is found to be

$$T = \tfrac{1}{2} + \tfrac{1}{2}\cos 2\alpha(1 - 2\sin^2 2\beta \sin^2 \delta/2) \tag{14.9}$$

For the dark-field case ($\alpha = \pi/2$)

$$T = \sin^2 2\beta \sin^2 \delta/2 \text{ (dark field)} \tag{14.10}$$

and the relative transmittance is zero when

$$\delta = 2n\pi \qquad (n = 0, 1, 2, \ldots) \tag{14.11a}$$

$$\beta = \frac{n\pi}{2} \qquad (n = 0, 1, 2, \ldots) \tag{14.11b}$$

The birefringence is determined by combining eqns (14.2) and (14.11a):

$$\Delta = n\frac{\lambda_1}{L} \quad (n = 0, 1, 2, \ldots) \tag{14.12a}$$

Bands of equal δ will be black in monochromatic light. They are coloured in white light, with the exception of the zeroth order band which is black. For this reason they are termed isochromatics and are related to the magnitude of the principal refractive indices. Bands of equal β are always black and move if the polariser and analyser are rotated together in the crossed position. These bands are related to the direction of the principal refractive indices and are termed isoclinics (χ_0 is defined to be less than 45°). Clearly

$$\chi_0 = \beta \tag{14.12b}$$

The properties of the birefringence and the isoclinic angle make their determination simple. The polariser and analyser are rotated together using white light, and the black zeroth order isochromatic is determined since it will appear stationary. The isochromatics are more distinct in monochromatic light and are determined by 'counting out' from the zeroth order with the filter in place. The isoclinic angle is found by rotating the polariser and analyser to known angles and noting the position of the dark band.

A circular polariscope has

$$\mathbf{I}_o = \mathbf{P}(\pi/2)\mathbf{R}(3\pi/4, \pi/2)\mathbf{R}(\beta, \delta)\mathbf{R}(\pi/4, \pi/2)\mathbf{I}_i \tag{14.13}$$

where $R(\pi/4, \pi/2)$ and $\mathbf{R}(3\pi/4, \pi/2)$ represent quarter-wave plates whose 'fast axes' are at the given angles to the incident radiation. From this one obtains

$$T = \sin^2 \delta/2 \tag{14.14}$$

Thus a circular polariscope eliminates the isoclinic angle and the isochromatics are immediately determined.

The birefringence and isoclinic angle may be readily determined using the above methods. However, the rheologist usually desires the stresses; to obtain these the stress-optic relation must be applied (eqns (14.3) and (14.12)). In the following section the determination of C, the stress-optic coefficient, and the validity of the stress-optic relation are critically examined.

14.2.3. Experimental Studies in Various Geometries

The experimental studies of many research teams throughout the world are summarised below. The sections are divided to examine each

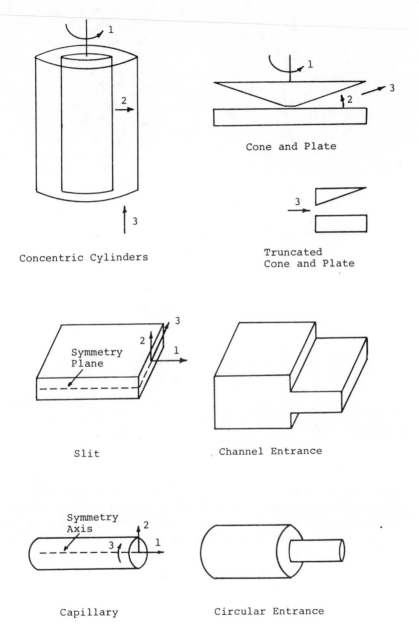

Fig. 14.3a. Flow geometries of interest.

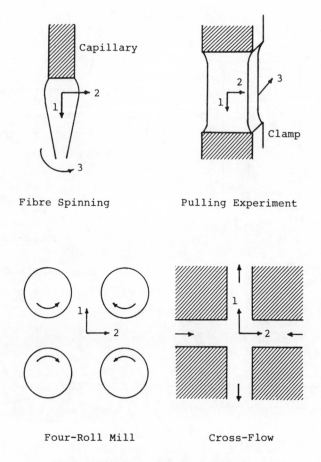

Fig. 14.3b. Flow geometries of interest.

particular geometry (see Figs 14.3a and 14.3b): concentric cylinders (Couette flow), cone and plate (torsion flow), slit and capillary, elongational and tubular and planar entrances. Where applicable the results are examined to determine the validity of the stress-optic relation as well as further information which may be extracted from the measurement. Rather than reference all the papers within the text, Table 14.1 was prepared with comments to indicate the nature of the work.

14.2.3.1. Concentric Cylinders Torsion Flow

The concentric cylinders geometry (see Fig. 14.3a) was the first to be used in flow birefringence.[7,8] Because of this, and its simplicity, it is frequently

TABLE 14.1
Birefringence Literature Review Arranged by Geometry and Year of
Publication

Flow geometry	Reference	Comments[1]
Concentric cylinders	Backus and Scheraga[25]	Concludes detergent micelles are rod-like.
	Wayland[26]	Colloidal suspension and pure liquid system; measured transition shear rate.
	Philippoff[27]	Stress-optic relation valid for 15% PIB/decalin.
	Frishman and Tsvetkov[28]	Solvent and high velocity gradient effects with PS (polystyrene).
	Peebles et al.[29]	MY suspensions' viscosity and birefringence properties of suspensions.
	Janeschitz-Kriegl and Papenhuijzen[30]	Concentration, temperature effects of viscosity and birefringence.
	Peterlin and Munk[18]	Data for numerous systems presented and interpreted.
	Tsvetkov et al.[31]	Rigidity of PPBA calculated.
	Tsvetkov et al.[32]	Rigidity and rotary diffusion coefficient of PPPhTPhA calculated.
	Vinogradov et al.[33]	Oscillatory deformation of various polymers.
	Tsvetkov et al.[34]	Flexibility of PPPhTPhA (poly-p-phenylene terephthalamide) and other polymers calculated.
	Vinogradov and Malkin[35]	Textbook on rheology with a multitude of data.
Cone and plate	Dexter et al.[36]	Viewed perpendicular to 1–3 plane of PE in parallel plates.

(continued)

TABLE 14.1—*contd.*

Flow geometry	Reference	Comments[1]
Cone and plate (contd.)	Gortemaker[21]	Birefringence and stress time variation experiments with melts. S-OR confirmed at low shear rates ($< 1\,s^{-1}$). Also used concentric cylinders.
	Gortemaker *et al.*[37]	See Gortemaker[21]
	Gortemaker *et al.*[38]	See Gortemaker[21]
	Laun *et al.*[39]	See Gortemaker[21]
Capillary or slit	Philippoff[40]	Rigid and flexible molecule systems investigated by viewing along the 1-axis of capillary and found $n_{22} - n_{33}$ non-zero for rigid systems. Other planes studied.
	Philippoff[41]	Theory to accompany 40
	Whitehead[42]	Birefringence of PS solution in slit. Calculated wall shear stress within 10% of homogeneous flow shear stress.
	Wales and Philippoff[43]	Viewed along 1-axis of capillary using various melts and $n_{22} - n_{33}$ non-zero.
	Wales[44]	Viewed along 2 and 3 axis in slit using various melts and $n_{11} - n_{33}$ non-zero. S-OR valid up to $\sim 10^4$ Pa. (used cone and plate geometry).
	Mackay[9]	Various melts investigated in slit and interpretation of birefringence measurements found to be involved.
	McHugh *et al.*[45]	Isoclinic band spreading explained in slit flow.

(*continued*)

TABLE 14.1—*contd.*

Flow geometry	Reference	Comments[1]
Elongation	Gurnee et al.[46]	Birefringence and stress measurements of a PS sheet and S-OC found to be non-constant under creep and relaxation.
	Saunders[47-49]	Birefringence and stress measurements of various polymers. S-OR found valid with non-Gaussian interpretation.
	Ziabicki and Kedzierska[50,51]	Classic papers on fibre spinning. Relation between birefringence and spinning stress complex.
	Frank and Mackley[52]	Birefringence measured in two roll mill, molecular orientation localised.
	Crowley et al.[53]	Birefringence measured in four roll mill, molecular orientation localised.
	Matsumoto and Bogue[54]	Birefringence and stress measured of PS film under transient conditions of time and temperature, S-OR found invalid at high stress.
	Talbott[10]	Birefringence and stress measured for polymer solution, S-OR found invalid at moderate stresses.
	Talbott and Goddard[55]	See Talbott[10]
	van Aken and Janeschitz-Kriegl[56]	Birefringence and stress measured in planar elongational flow for PS, S-OR found valid up to moderate stresses, polymer is elongation thinning.
	Cressely and Hocquart[57]	Birefringence of PEO (polyethylene oxide measured in cross flow cell, molecules stretched most in centre.

(*continued*)

TABLE 14.1—contd.

Flow geometry	Reference	Comments[1]
Elongation (contd.)	Fuller and Leal[58]	Birefringence measured in four roll mill; compared to molecular theories.
	Onogi et al.[59]	Birefringence and stress measured (in separate apparatus) in shear flow of liquid crystal solutions, S-OR not valid. Residual stresses from capillary found important in fibre spinning.
	Kimora et al.[60]	Birefringence and stress measured in shear and elongation of solid PB, S-OR confirmed.
	Gardner et al.[61]	Birefringence and velocity measured of PS solutions in cross flow cell, molecules extended in centre, entanglement layer at wall postulated, velocity measurements taken (see also papers cited within).
	Macosko et al.[62]	Birefringence measured in planar elongation shaped die of PS melt, birefringence near centre the same regardless of lubrication.
	Muller and Froelich[63]	Birefringence and stress measured in uniaxial elongation for PS melt, S-OR found invalid at high stresses.
Entrance (including converging flow)	Prados and Peebles[64]	Birefringence measured in slit, converging, diverging and flow around a cylinder of MY, velocity profiles calculated and diverging flow different from converging.
	Tordella[65]	Birefringence and pressure drop measured in circular entrance for polymer melts, birefringence patterns differ between linear and branched PE.

(continued)

TABLE 14.1—*contd.*

Flow geometry	Reference	Comments[1]
	Fields and Bogue[66]	Birefringence measured in channel entrance for PS solution, compared to BKZ theory predictions.
	Tordella[67]	See Tordella;[65] melt fracture discussed.
	Boles *et al.*[68]	Birefringence measured in channel entrance for PIB solution, stresses concentrate along the centre line.
	Han and Drexler[69,70]	Birefringence and velocity measured in channel entrance for various melts, compared to modified second-order theory.
	Brizitsky *et al.*[71]	Birefringence measured in channel entrance for various melts, elongational stresses extend to downstream channel and are a function of MWD.
	Yoo and Han[72]	Birefringence and wall pressures measured in converging channel for PE and PP melts, wall normal stress behaves differently from centre line.
	Horsman and Merzkirch[73]	Scattered light birefringence used for MY solutions.
	Eisenbrand and Goddard[74]	Birefringence and velocity measured in circular entrance for a polymer solution, unsteadiness in birefringence noted near entrance.
	Checker *et al.*[75]	Birefringence and velocity measured in channel entrance of PE and PP melts, ordering of polymer chain considered.
	Crater and Cuculo[76]	Birefringence and velocity measured in circular entrance of PET, various entrance geometries investigated.

(*continued*)

TABLE 14.1—contd.

Flow geometry	Reference	Comments[1]
Entrance (including converging flow) (contd.)	Aldhouse et al.[77]	Birefringence measured in entrance flow of high density PE, multiple relaxation times necessary to describe stresses.

[1] Abbreviations: PIB = Polyisobutylene, PS = Polystyrene, MY = Milling Yellow Solution, PPBA = Poly-p-Benzamide, PPPhTPhA = Poly-p-Phenylene Terephthalamide, PE = Polyethylene, S-OR = Stress-Optic Relation, S-OC = Stress-Optic Constant, PEO = Polyethylene Oxide, PB = Polybutadiene, MWD = Molecular Weight Distribution, PP = Polypropylene, PET = Poly(Ethylene Terephthalate).

employed. However, it is well known that the shear field is inhomogeneous within the gap (see reference 78 and papers cited therein), thus somewhat limiting the apparatus. One desires the gap to be as small as possible to eliminate this effect; however, the limitations of a very small gap are alignment difficulties and the ability to view through the gap for birefringence measurements.

A rigorous check of the stress-optic relation in this geometry was carried out by Philippoff[27] for a polyisobutylene solution. He viewed along the 3-axis while rotating the inner cylinder. The isoclinic angle and birefringence were measured using Sénarmont compensation at each shear rate. Using a similar apparatus the shear stress was measured whilst the first normal stress difference was determined in a cone and plate geometry (Fig. 14.3a).

The interpretation of these data was carried out by noting that (see eqns (14.4) and (14.5))

$$\sigma_{12} = \tfrac{1}{2}(\sigma_{P1} - \sigma_{P2})\sin 2\chi_M^{(1)} \qquad (14.15)$$

or using the stress-optic relation (14.3)

$$\Delta \sin 2\chi_O^{(1)} = 2C\,\sigma_{12} \qquad (14.16)$$

Philippoff plotted the optic and shearing stress data from the two instruments according to eqn (14.16) and obtained a linear relation indicating a constant stress-optic coefficient. He also used the normal stress data to calculate $\chi_M^{(1)}$ (see eqn (14.6)), compared this to the measured $\chi_O^{(1)}$ and found the two equal at equivalent shear rates. Therefore the stress-optic relation was confirmed, at least for this system and level of principal stresses ($\sigma_{P1} - \sigma_{P2} \approx 2 \times 10^3\,$Pa).

Besides being used as a calibration device, concentric cylinders can be used to find the first normal stress difference and to investigate orientation effects in shearing and oscillatory flow. The use of the measurements for the calculation of the stresses, both shearing and normal, for rigid particles and micelles is *not* recommended since Leal and Hinch[12] have shown that the stress-optic relation is *not valid* at moderate to large deformation gradients for these systems. On the other hand, stresses of the order $10^4\,$Pa can be calculated for flexible molecules in the melt (Section 14.2.3.2). However, the stress-optic coefficient, C, must be known and the *use of literature values is not recommended* since deviations of 10–20% or more are common. The measurements provide shear orientation information for both systems (rigid and flexible) and allow for the testing of models provided that the various types of anisotropy (shape, intrinsic, macro-form, microform)[18] are considered.

In summary, this geometry is a useful calibration device to find the stress-optic coefficient (eqn (14.16)) as long as the above remarks are considered. The inhomogeneity of the shear field should be noted, as well as the appearance of secondary flows if the inner cylinder is rotated. The design is simple, and viewing is fairly easy, making it attractive as a birefringence measurement instrument, so it is a valuable device to view flow orientation effects in a variety of systems.

14.2.3.2. Cone and Plate Torsion Flow

To overcome the problem of shear field inhomogeneity, a small angle cone and plate geometry is used (Fig. 14.3a). Only one research group has used this geometry,[20,21,37-39,44] albeit a truncated cone and plate viewed in the 3-direction. The stress-optic relation was found to be valid for polymer melts in both transient and steady shear conditions up to shear stresses on the order of 10^4–$10^5\,$Pa (some deviation that occurred in the transient measurement was attributed to mechanical delay of the apparatus). It should be noted that high density polyethylene yielded the best results and validity of the stress-optic relation, perhaps indicating that chain branching significantly alters the physics of the flow and applicability of the stress-optic relation.

The design of the apparatus is very involved, certainly more so than that with the concentric cylinders. There are also difficulties with 'parasitic' velocity gradients in the apparatus;[21] this will be discussed in the next sub-section. Thus the concentric cylinder device is recommended despite its inherent limitations.

14.2.3.3. Capillary and Slit Flows

For pressure driven or Poiseuille flow in these geometries the shear field is inhomogeneous. The shear rate is zero at the symmetry axis and increases to a maximum at the wall for the capillary whilst the infinitely wide slit has a zero shear rate along its symmetry plane and a maximum at the wall (Fig. 14.3a). It is straightforward to verify for well developed flow that

$$\sigma_{rz} = \frac{1}{2} \left| \frac{\partial p}{\partial z} \right| r \quad \text{(capillary)} \tag{14.17}$$

$$\sigma_{xy} = \left| \frac{\partial p}{\partial x} \right| y \quad \text{(slit)} \tag{14.18}$$

where p is pressure, z and x the flow directions (1-direction) and r and y the shear directions (2-direction). Thus, by measuring the pressure drop, the shear stress field is easily calculated.

Although the shear stress is linear with shear direction for both geometries, there is a fundamental difference between the two regarding birefringence measurements. One can view parallel to the z or r direction in the capillary.[40,41,43,65,67] Viewing along the z-axis gives information about $(n_{P2} - n_{P3})$, and along the r-axis about $(n_{P1} - n_{P2})$. However, interpretation of these data, especially in the r-axis experiment, is difficult[65,79-81] as the stresses vary in the r-direction. The infinitely wide slit overcomes this problem as the stresses change only in the y-direction and can be viewed along z. Thus one can determine $(n_{P1} - n_{P2})$ by placing the slit in the polariscope with the neutral axis parallel to the wave normal direction. However, no slit can be infinitely wide, and side walls must be installed which influence the flow and stress fields. Wales[44] has recommended a slit width to depth ratio of at least 10/1 to minimise the influence of side walls. His recommendation comes from birefringence measurements viewing along the 2-axis (i.e. $n_{P1} - n_{P3}$).

Even for a large width to depth ratio, a parasitic effect is evident and greatly influences the isoclinic angle rather than the isochromatics. The isoclinic angle is determined by rotating the crossed polars counter-clockwise from the original orientation of zero degrees (analyser polarisation direction parallel to x-axis). Theoretically a *thin* dark band should descend from the top wall and reach the symmetry plane at 45° rotation. Mackay[9]

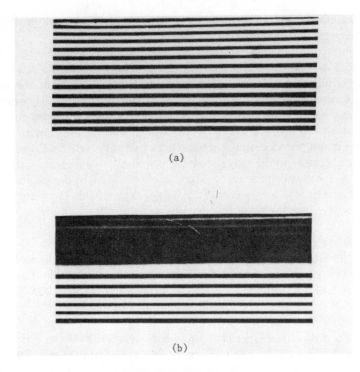

(a)

(b)

Fig. 14.4. Birefringence patterns for high density polyethylene in slit flow: (a) isochromatic pattern; (b) 40° isoclinic pattern for the same flow rate as in (a) (note the width of the dark band).

and Wales[44] have shown that for polymer melts a *thick* dark band, which sometimes covers the entire upper half, descends from the top wall (Fig. 14.4). The problem, of course, is what position within this band corresponds to the isoclinic angle. McHugh *et al.*[45] explained that it is the variation of σ_{12} and N_1 along the wave normal that produces the spreading. The explanation was based on the experimental evidence of Fröcht[82] that normal and shear stresses parallel to the wave normal produce no birefringence in static systems (i.e. σ_{13}, σ_{23}, σ_{33} when viewed along the 3-axis).

Gortemaker[21] and Wales[44] have shown that χ_O equals χ_M in the cone and plate geometry. However, Mackay[9] found χ_O (slit) difficult to determine, and a comparison to χ_M (cone and plate) was inconclusive. Mackay also noticed a peculiar double banded zero-degree isoclinic with a polystyrene melt at high shear rates and low temperatures. This may have been a parasitic effect or a changeover from positive to negative birefringence as has been observed for polystyrene fibres.[83]

The interpretation of birefringence measurements in these geometries is complicated. The axial symmetry of the capillary makes the analysis difficult whilst the side walls influence the isoclinic angle in the slit (applying a lubricant on the side walls may eliminate this effect). However, the slit is a useful calibration device as C found by Mackay[9] agrees within 5–10% with the values given by Wales[44] which were obtained in a truncated cone and plate for similar melts. This is due to the relative insensitivity of $\sin 2\chi_0$ to χ_0 in the range 35–45° which most polymer melts assume at low to moderate shear rates. More work needs to be done with the capillary geometry. With a proper analysis of the data this geometry may be attractive since there are no apparent parasitic effects.

14.2.3.4. Elongational Flows

Elongational flows have been generated by using many techniques such as: fibre spinning, pulling experiments, four-roll mill and cross-flow cells (Fig. 14.3b). What is immediately obvious from Table 14.1 is that the stress-optic relation appears to be invalid in a number of instances[10,46–51,54,55,59,63] for elongational flows.

There are two cases where the stress-optic relation has been reported to be valid in elongational flow.[56,60] In the first investigation van Aken and Janeschitz-Kriegl[56] measured the stress and birefringence of two impinging streams for a polystyrene melt. The elongational viscosity of the polystyrene apparently was elongation thinning, suggesting that the physics for this particular polymer is different from that for others used where the relation failed and where the polymers apparently all undergo elongation thickening. This particular polystyrene may exhibit similar rheological properties to the high density polyethylene noted in Section 14.2.3.2 which is suspected to incur elongation thinning also.[84] Thus, elongation thinning polymer melts appear to adhere to the stress-optic relation at higher stress levels. The other study[60] does not discuss the stresses obtained in a pulling experiment; they are thought to be low and not a crucial test of the relation.

Matsumoto and Bogue[54] and Muller and Froelich[63] showed that the stress-optic relation is not valid for a polystyrene melt at principal stress differences in excess of approximately 5×10^5 Pa, while Talbott[10] and Talbott and Goddard[55] reached the same conclusion for polymer solutions for stresses in excess of 10^3 Pa. The melts and solutions were not fully characterised in shearing flow, so it is not possible to interpret these data to understand the dynamics and deformation of the molecules. However, it appears that the stress-optic relation is not usable at a principal stress difference of order 5×10^5 Pa for polymer melts (note the difficulty in obtaining stresses of this order in shearing experiments). This deviation may be due to the finite length of the macromolecule and will be discussed below. The velocity was not measured in any of the above cited references.

The two-roll[52] or four-roll[53,58] mill and cross-flow geometries[57,61] have significant elongational gradients near the centre (Fig. 14.3b). Using a four-roll mill, Fuller and Leal[58] determined that the birefringence reaches a saturation value indicative of the finite extensibility of the macromolecule.[17] Their birefringence–elongation rate data were fitted well by taking this factor into account and may explain the deviation from the stress-optic relation as noted above. The effect of elongation on the birefringence–stress relation may be stated (this formalism was developed

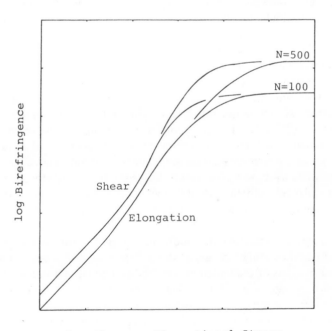

Fig. 14.5. Birefringence versus stress in both shear and elongational flow for a dumb-bell with an inverse Langevin spring of 100 and 500 statistical segments; the units are arbitrary.

by Kuhn and Grün;[85] see also Phan-Thien and Tanner[86] and Fuller and Leal[87]) as follows:

'Consider a macromolecule made of a number of cylindrical rods (statistical segments) joined at the end on universal joints with the polarisability (proportional to the refractive index[16,18]) greater in one direction within each rod. The macromolecule is suspended in a Newtonian fluid and the hydrodynamic friction confined to spheres attached to the two end rods. As the deformation gradient is increased the two spheres separate until they are at the maximum allowed by the contour length. By increasing the gradient further the stress will continue increasing due to the finite viscosity of the carrier fluid; however, the birefringence will not increase as the polarisability and hence the refractive index difference remain constant or saturate since the macromolecule is fully extended.'

This effect is shown in Fig. 14.5 in arbitrary units for a polymer molecule with 100 and 500 statistical segments (note that by taking into account finite extensibility the elongational viscosity *does not* increase without bound[86,88]). The deviation from the stress-optic relation occurs at small deformations in simple elongational flow. For example, the dimensionless shear rate (shear rate times relaxation time) where the relation fails is about 0·316 and saturation occurs at 100, whilst in simple elongation the dimensionless elongation rate where deviation arises is 0·0316 and saturation is at 3·16. Clearly, deviations would be much more obtainable in elongational flow than in shear, and this may explain the observation of a non-linear stress-optic relation in the former but not in the later. Similar observations to those by Fuller and Leal have been made by the research group at Bristol (reference 61 and papers cited therein) in a cross-flow cell. They have also observed a birefringent 'entanglement layer' attached to the wall.

In conclusion, experimental studies have shown the stress-optic relation to be invalid at higher principal stress differences. This deviation is explained in terms of the finite extensibility of the macromolecule. Thus, in flows where significant elongational gradients exist, as discussed in the next section, the calculated stresses may be in error, except possibly for the case where the polymer or solution undergoes elongation thinning.

14.2.3.5. Tubular and Planar Entry Flows
Entrance flows from a large to small pipe or duct (Fig. 14.3a) are important in polymer processing, understanding flow property measurement in

capillary rheometry, and more recently as a test problem for numerical methods (see reference 89 for a recent review on this problem). For viscoelastic fluids a large vortex forms in the corner and the streak-lines form a 'wine glass' shape entering the smaller pipe or duct. Mackay *et al.*[90] have demonstrated for a circular entrance that the wine-glass shape of the central core is readily predicted by neglecting the influence of the vortex and treating the core as a fibre. The prediction of the core shape is accurate; however, the major assumption is that the stresses within the core dominate and are due to elongation. This will be shown to be true by birefringence measurements.

As shown in Table 14.1, numerous research groups have used birefringence to investigate entrance flows. Tordella[65,67] was the first to demonstrate that the birefringence patterns are different between low and high density polyethylene. White[84] surveyed the literature and determined that the former polymer undergoes elongation thickening whilst elongation thinning occurs in the latter. Thus, at equivalent flow conditions in a circular entrance, one would expect the stress levels as well as the birefringence to be much greater for low density polyethylene. This is demonstrated in Fig. 14.6. Note the qualitative difference between the patterns, the greater stress values for low density polyethylene, and the concentration near the centre line. Recently White and Baird[91] demonstrated differences in the flow patterns and correlated them with separate elongational measurements. Birefringence therefore gives an indication of the stresses developed, and clearly shows the large stresses developed in the core (note the dark area in the corners, indicative of low stress levels, in Fig. 14.6), in agreement with the assumption of Mackay *et al.*[90]

In addition to birefringence measurements of polymer melts in a planar entrance, Han and Drexler[69,70,92] measured the velocity using streak photography. They analysed the data with a modified second-order theory and found qualitative agreement. Streak photography is not generally accurate for calculating velocity gradients; thus, despite the high quality of the work, a study should be completed using more accurate means. They did find that significant normal stresses developed in the central core region, in agreement with Tordella. These stresses were in some cases greater than 10^5 Pa and may have been in error (Section 14.2.3.4).

Eisenbrand and Goddard[74] measured the superficial birefringence of a polymer solution in circular entrance flow and found the birefringence to increase with flow rate and to become unstable in certain cases after 3–4 min, which may be similar to the instabilities shown by Nguyen and Boger[93] using streak photography. Checker *et al.*[75] and Aldhouse *et al.*[77]

(a)

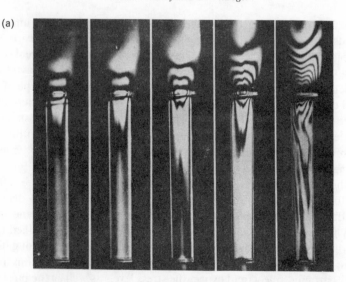

(b)

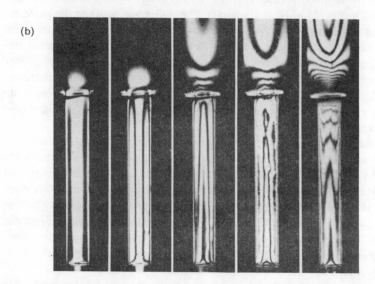

Fig. 14.6. Isochromatic patterns for entry flow of (a) low density polyethylene and (b) high density polyethylene. The number of isochromatics increases faster with shear stress for low density polyethylene than for high density polyethylene. Reprinted from reference 65 with permission of John Wiley and Sons, New York.

measured the birefringence of a high density polyethylene melt in a uniquely shaped planar-type entrance. The width to depth ratio is very small though, at best being 7·6/1 and at worst approximately 2/1, and the results may be influenced by the side walls. They discuss chain ordering effects and find the maximum birefringence to increase with flow rate[75] and that the stresses need to be modelled by multiple relaxation times.[77]

Summarising, the studies all indicate high stresses near the centre line or plane which increase with flow rate and appear to increase more rapidly with elongation thickening materials than those that undergo elongation thinning. There is a great need to complete a study which calibrates the birefringence in shearing and elongational flows and subsequently relates these to the entrance flow measurement. This, combined with accurate velocity measurements and a well characterised fluid (both steady and dynamic properties measured), would elucidate exactly the stress and deformation within a material and allow for comparison with prediction using constitutive equations. Thus far, the closest any research team has come is the study by Han and Drexler[69,70,92] where the fluid was characterised with a slit rheometer (i.e. found viscosity and C from pressure drop measurements) and this was related to velocity using streak photography and birefringence measurements in a plane entrance with a modified second-order theory. The results are inconclusive as the stresses measured by birefringence may be incorrect due to the non-linearity in the stress-optic relation.

14.3. STREAK-LINE OBSERVATION AND POINT VELOCITY MEASUREMENT

An extensive variety of flow visualisation techniques exist,[94-96] ranging from streamline flow field images to velocity measurements and, as already discussed, stress field imaging using birefringence. By far the most active area of flow visualisation in non-Newtonian fluid mechanics has been the observation of streamline images for both polymer melts and solutions in entry flows—a flow field of importance as a test problem for numerical simulation in viscoelastic fluid mechanics. Tables 14.2 and 14.3 summarise these observations (excluding birefringence) for polymer melts and solutions in both slit and tubular entries. Even a casual glance at these tables indicates that most of the effort has been directed towards the observation of streamline images using tracer particles in the flow. Until recently little attention had been directed towards point velocity measurement both in this flow field and in others of interest in rheometry.

TABLE 14.2

Flow Visualisation Studies for Polymer Melts in Entry Flows

Investigator	Year	Material[1]	Entry Geometry[2]	Flow Visualisation Method
Tordella[97]	1957	LDPE	Flat entry, $\beta \approx 32$	Carbon black tracer, cine film
Clegg[98]	1958	LDPE, HDPE	Flat and conical entries	Coloured core, cine film
Schott and Kagham[99]	1959	LDPE	Flat entry, $\beta = 5\cdot3$	Coloured layers, cine film
Bagley and Birks[100]	1960	LDPE, HDPE	Flat entry, $\beta = 20$	Carbon black threads, cine film
Bagley and Schreiber[101]	1961	LDPE	Conical entry, 20°–180°	Carbon black threads, cine film
Ballenger and White[102]	1970	LDPE, HDPE, PMMA, polystyrene, polypropylene	Flat entry	Coloured threads, cine film
den Otter[103]	1970	Linear and branched PDMS	Flat slit entry	Carborundum, still photo
*Ballenger et al.[104]	1971	LDPE, HDPE, polystyrene, polyproplyene	Flat entry $\beta \approx 7$	Coloured threads, cine film
Vinogradov et al.[105]	1972	Polybutadiene	Flat slit entry	Stained glass particles, flow birefringence
Han and Drexler[70]	1973	HDPE, polystyrene, polypropylene	Flat, 60° tapered	Streak photography
Oyanagi[106]	1973	HDPE	Flat entry, $\beta = 11 - 26$	Section solidified plug, or flow birefringence
*White and Kondo[107]	1977	Polystyrene, LDPE, HDPE	Flat entry, $\beta = 5\cdot75$ 35°, 65°, 63°, 80°, 90° and 128° slit entry	Coloured threads, cine film
Mackley and Moore[122]	1986	HDPE	Unique shape in slit entry, $\beta = 15$	Laser dopplermeter
*White and Baird[91]	1986	Polystyrene, LDPE	Slit entry, $\beta = 5\cdot9$	Tracer particles, videotape.

* Observations accompanied by independent viscosity and normal stress measurement.

[1] Abbreviations: LDPE = Low Density Polyethylene, HDPE = High Density Polyethylene, PDMS = Poly(Dimethyl Siloxane)

[2] β is the contraction ratio.

TABLE 14.3
Flow Visualisation Studies for Polymer Solutions in Entry Flows

Investigator	Year	Material[1]	Entry Geometry[2]	Flow Visualisation Method
Vinogradov and Manin[108]	1964	Al naphthenate/gasoline	60°, 180° slit entry	Polarised light, still photo
Giesekus[109]	1968	PAA/H_2O, 1·6–4% PIB/decalin, 4%	Flat die entry 60–180° slit entry	Streak photography
*Metzner *et al.*[110]	1969	PAA/H_2O, 0·5%	Re-entrant tube	Streak photography
Ballenger and White[102]	1970	PIB/mineral oil, 2·5%	Flat die entry, $\beta = 21$	Carbon black tracers
*Ballenger *et al.*[104]	1971	PIB/mineral oil, 2·5%	Flat die entry, $\beta = 21$	Carbon black tracers
*Boger and Ramamurthy[111]	1972	$Methocel/H_2O$, PAA/H_2O	Flat die entry, $\beta = 2$	Streak photography
Oliver and Bragg[112]	1973	PAA/H_2O	Flat die entries	Dye tracers, still photo
*Pearson and Pickup[113]	1973	$PAA/glycerin - H_2O$	Flat die entry flat tapered slit entries	Streak photography
*Tomita and Shimbo[114]	1973	PEO solutions, 2·5–5%	Flat die entry	Not specified
Ramamurthy[115]	1974	$PAA/glycerine - H_2O$, 1·5%	Flat die entry	Streak photography
Strauss and Kinast[116]	1974	PAA/H_2O, 0·12%	Tapered slit entry	Streak photography
Busby and Macsporran[117]	1976	PAA/H_2O	Re-entrant tube	Laser dopplermeter
*Cable and Boger[118]	1978	PAA/H_2O	Flat die entry, $\beta = 2·4$	Streak photography and cine film
*Nguyen and Boger[93]	1979	PAA/corn syrup	Flat die entry, $\beta = 4·08, 7·68, 12·3, 14·6$	Streak photography and cine film
*Ramamurthy and McAdam[119]	1980	PAA/H_2O	Flat die entry, $\beta = 13·2$	Laser dopplermeter
*Cochrane *et al.*[120]	1981	PAA/corn syrup	Various geometries	Streak photography
*Walters and Rawlinson[121]	1982	PAA/corn syrup	Flat slit entry, $\beta = 13·3$	Streak photography
Dembek[123]	1982	PIB/Low MW PIB	Flat die entry, $\beta = 5·33, 10·7$	Streak photography
*Boger *et al.*[124]	1986	PAA/corn syrup, PIB/PB	Flat die entry, $\beta = 4·4, 6·8, 16·5$	Streak photography

(continued)

TABLE 14.3—contd.

Investigator	Year	Material[1]	Entry Geometry[2]	Flow Visualisation Method
*Evans and Walters[125]	1986	PAA/corn syrup	Flat slit entry, $\beta = 4$, 16, 80, various corners used	Streak photography
*Lawler et al.[126]	1986	PIB/PB, PAA/glycerine — H_2O	Flat die entry, $\beta = 4$	Laser dopplermeter

* Observations accompanied by independent viscosity and normal stress measurement.
[1] Abbreviations: PAA = Polyacrylamide, PIB = Polyisobutylene, PEO = Poly(Ethylene Oxide), PB = Poly(1-Butene)
[2] β is the contraction ratio.

14.3.1. Techniques for Streak-line Observation and Point Velocity Measurement

Streak photography has been the most common technique used for the recording of flow patterns in non-Newtonian fluid mechanics. In this technique, where the fluid under investigation needs to be optically clear, a cross-section of the flow is illuminated with a thin planar light source, thus enabling the visualisation of flow patterns when small, highly reflective tracer particles are suspended in the fluid. When a photograph is taken of the flow field, perpendicular to the plane of illumination, the lines produced on the photographic negative as tracer path images are called streak-lines. Streak-lines approximate fluid particle path lines when small, neutrally buoyant tracer particles are used in the fluid. A wide variety of tracer particles can be employed, depending on the density of the fluids to be investigated, the intensity of the light source employed, and the speed and characteristics of the photographic film. In our work for highly viscous polymer solutions we have used a pigment sold under the trade

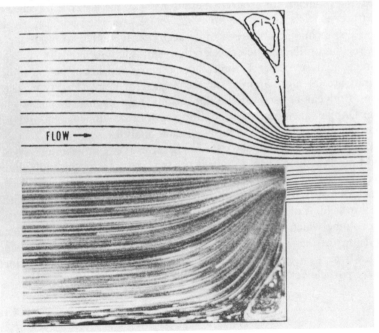

Fig. 14.7. Comparison of the streamlines predicted by Viriyayuthakorn and Caswell[127] with the experimental observations of Nguyen and Boger[93] for a Newtonian fluid in creeping flow in a 4 to 1 circular contraction.

name Timica Sparkle (titanium dioxide coated mica flakes with a size range of 15–40 μm and a density of 200 kg m^{-3}). For accurate observation of the flow patterns, optical distortion due to the presence of curved surfaces and differences in the index of refraction of the fluid under investigation and its containing conduit should be minimised.

Figure 14.7 illustrates the type of result that can be obtained with the technique. Here the streak-lines predicted by Viriyayuthakorn and Caswell[127] with finite element numerical methods are compared to the streak-line observations of Nguyen and Boger[93] for an inelastic Newtonian fluid in creeping flow in a circular 4 to 1 contraction. Note the excellent agreement between theoretical prediction and experimental observation.

Streak-line photographic techniques can also be used for velocity measurement (see e.g. Cable and Boger[118]). For point velocity measurement the light source is flashed at known time intervals with the camera shutter open during the flash triggering period, which produces two comet-like images on the photograph. The clearly defined head of each image can be used as a reference for accurate measurement of the distance travelled by the tracer particle during the time interval between the two flash triggerings. The technique, although quite accurate, is limited to moderate to low regions of fluid particle acceleration, and is labour intensive in regard to data analysis. Laser Doppler anemometry and laser speckle photography are far more appropriate techniques for point velocity measurement. Both can be used for two-dimensional velocity measurements while laser Doppler anemometry can be adopted for three dimensions, and both can be highly automated in terms of data analysis.

Laser Doppler anemometry (LDA) involves the pointwise analysis of a real-time flow field. The flow field needs to be translucent and suitably seeded to scatter laser light. The incident laser beam is split into two beams which intersect at the point of measurement (measuring volume) within the flow field. A photomultiplier receives the light signals from the measuring volume which are analysed continuously for the Doppler frequency shift (f_D) of the scattered light (f_s) compared to the incident frequency (f_i), where $f_D = f_s - f_i$. The Doppler frequency is directly proportional to the particle velocity according to the equation

$$f_D = \frac{1}{\lambda_l} \bar{v}(\mathbf{e}_s - \mathbf{e}_i) \tag{14.19}$$

where λ_l is the laser light wavelength, $\bar{v}$ is the velocity component parallel to $(\mathbf{e}_s - \mathbf{e}_i)$, and $\mathbf{e}_s$ and $\mathbf{e}_i$ are unit vectors in the scattered and incident light directions respectively. A basic LDA system measures only one component of velocity, predetermined by the optical setup. More elaborate systems are available which use multicolour laser sources to provide complete velocity vector information. Costs of such systems can be very high.

Although the technique has been available for a considerable time, few results have been published in the non-Newtonian fluid mechanics literature. An excellent paper by Lawler *et al.*[126] describes an automated two-colour LDA velocimeter which was used to examine two velocity components in transient and steady flows of Newtonian and constant viscosity elastic fluids. Point velocity observations were compared with finite element predictions for flow between eccentric cylinders and for flow through an axisymmetric sudden contraction. Other more general references on the subject are listed.[128-131]

Laser-speckle interferometry is an inexpensive technique (compared with LDA) which can provide two-component velocity data in transparent fluid systems. The technique involves illuminating a two-dimensional plane of a suitably seeded flow field with a pulsing light source (of known pulse frequency) and recording two or more successive speckle images on photographic film. Analysis of this full field speckle image is performed by pointwise scanning of the image with a low power laser and recording the resultant fringe characteristics of the transmitted interference pattern. Basically the velocity at each point of the flow field is determined using the equation

$$v = \frac{\lambda_1 D_s}{mt\Delta X} \tag{14.20}$$

where D_s is the distance between image and analysis screen, t is the time between individual exposures, ΔX is the fringe spacing, λ_1 is the low power laser wavelength, and m is the magnification (image size/actual size). The directional components of the velocity can also be determined from the orientation of the interference fringes which are normal to the velocity vector direction. Although the technique is very accurate, simple to set up and use, inexpensive, and can provide data on two velocity components, it has received almost no attention in the non-Newtonian fluid mechanics literature with the exception of our own paper published in 1983[132] which describes the technique and illustrates its use in tubular entry flows.

Figure 14.8 demonstrates the effectiveness of laser-speckle interferometry in providing pointwise axial and radial velocity data across an accelerating flow field. The analysis, conducted for an inelastic Newtonian fluid, was performed 0·27 tube diameters upstream of the contraction

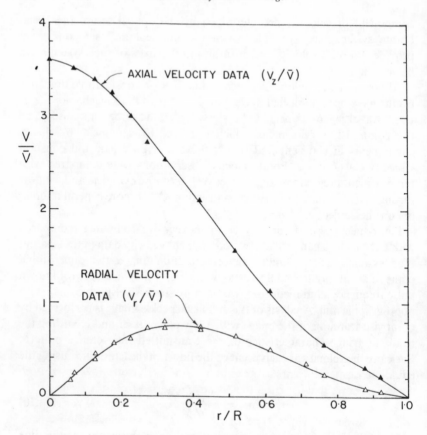

Fig. 14.8. Dimensionless velocity data obtained with laser speckle photography 0·27 diameter upstream of the contraction plane for a Newtonian fluid flowing in an abrupt circular contraction.

plane in a circular 4 to 1 contraction, where the velocity profile is accelerating from the upstream Poiseuille distribution as the fluid approaches the contraction. The reader who is interested in speckle photography and its use for velocity measurement in flowing fluids should consult the papers by Meynart.[133–135]

14.3.2. Tubular Entry Flows of Viscoelastic Fluids

The basic elements for laminar flow through an abrupt circular contraction are illustrated in Fig. 14.9. The flow progresses from being fully

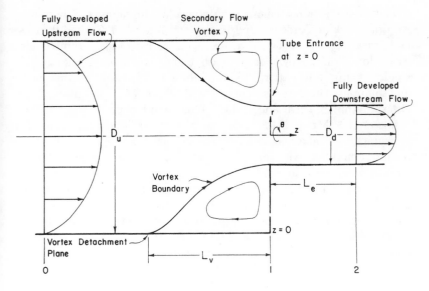

Fig. 14.9. Basic elements of an entry flow, for flow from a large tube through an abrupt entry into a smaller tube.

developed at a plane some distance upstream from the contraction to fully developed in the downstream tube at a distance L_e from the contraction plane. The entry length, L_e, is the distance required from the contraction plane ($z = 0$) for the centre-line velocity to become 98 or 99 per cent of its fully developed value. The behaviour of Newtonian and inelastic non-Newtonian fluids in terms of the pressure drop both with and without inertia in the flow is now well understood.[89] Flow visualisation (streak-line observation and point velocity measurement) has played an important role in gaining this understanding. The low Reynolds number (Re < 0·1) entry flow problem for viscoelastic fluids remains of considerable interest, as already stated, because of its importance in rheometry, in polymer processing, and now as a test problem for finite element simulation. The problem for viscoelastic fluids remains largely unsolved, i.e. the observations made with flow visualisation particularly in regard to the size and shape of the secondary flow vortex have not yet been predicted for any real fluid with any constitutive equation. The flow visualisation observations in this flow field are briefly reviewed in order to emphasise the important role that flow visualisation is playing in the development of non-Newtonian fluid mechanics.

Flow visualisation studies, using streak photography and beginning with the work of Tordella[97] and Bagley and Birks,[100] illustrated the existence of a large recirculating vortex in the corner of an abrupt circular entry flow at low Reynolds number. Extensive but largely qualitative studies of entry flow patterns followed for a wide range of polymer melts and solutions. These works were reviewed by Tordella,[67] Dennison,[136] den Otter,[137] White,[138] Petrie and Denn,[139] White and Kondo,[107] Boger[89,140] and White *et al.*[141] Many of the early works were for limited flow rates, for uncharacterised materials, and were more concerned with flow instabilities (melt fracture) than with stable flow patterns. However, it is clear that the large vortices are associated with excess entry pressure drops which are significantly higher than those expected and now predicted for Newtonian or inelastic shear thinning fluids. Also it was observed that some viscoelastic molten polymers exhibit large vortices while others do not (Ballenger and White[102]). Giesekus[109] and Ramamurthy[115] (for polymer solutions) and Ballenger and White[102] (for some polymer melts) demonstrated that these vortices grow with increasing flow rate, whilst in the same paper Ballenger and White showed results for other molten polymers where the vortices are small and do not grow with flow rate. All the workers suggested that fluid elasticity was responsible for the vortex growth, but the question as to why the vortex grows for some materials and is either not present or does not grow for others remained unresolved until the work of Cogswell[142] and White and Kondo.[107] Both authors suggested that materials with an elongational viscosity that increases with elongational rate exhibit vortex enhancement (growth), while no (or only small) vortices are present for materials where the elongational viscosity decreases or remains constant with elongation rate. White and Baird[91] confirmed this conclusion in a definitive paper where streak-line flow visualisation was combined with good flow property measurement. Steady shear properties (η and N_1), dynamic properties (G' and G''), and elongational stress growth data were measured for two different molten polymers. One (low density polyethylene) exhibited large vortices and vortex growth, and the other (polystyrene) exhibited almost no secondary flows in a planar 5·9 to 1 contraction. At the conditions of observation, both flows were characterised by about the same Weissenberg number, yet the flow fields were quite different. The difference was in the elongational flow properties of the polymers. Vortex growth was clearly associated with unbounded elongational stress growth with time at fixed elongational strain rates, while the absence of the vortex was associated with bounded elongational stress growth. The observation was consistent with the White and Kondo premise that large vortices and vortex growth constitute a stress relief mechanism. Thus all viscoelastic fluids do not exhibit large vortices and vortex growth in entry flows. The presence and characteristics of the vortex are strongly dependent on elongational flow properties.

Constitutive equations that might be useful to characterise shear thinning and elastic fluids, such as the molten polymers used in the experiments of White and Baird,[91] are at this stage normally too complex for use with the equations of motion for a numerical solution of the entry flow problem. This presupposes, of course, that all material constants are available from the basic flow property measurement, which is hardly ever the case. Thus the choice of a constitutive equation for examination of the entry flow of viscoelastic fluids has been a compromise between simplicity and practical reality. Although attempted solutions for creeping flow in a circular contraction for other constitutive equations are available, the most common choice of constitutive equation has been the convected Maxwell or the Oldroyd B model. Important papers that should be consulted are those of Mendelson *et al.*[143] and Keunings and Crochet,[144] while numerical solution techniques and results for viscoelastic fluids in entry flows have been reviewed by Crochet and Walters[145] and Crochet and Davies.[146]

In order to link flow visualisation more directly to numerical simulation, emphasis is now being placed on flow visualisation using constant viscosity elastic fluids (the so-called Boger fluid) in entry flows.[1] The series of streak photographs reproduced in Fig. 14.10 is typical of the vortex growth behaviour observed in contracting flows for constant viscosity elastic liquids.[93,120,121,124,125] Although there have been many attempts, the vortex growth illustrated in Fig 14.10 has not been predicted (even qualitatively) for these ideal elastic liquids, or for any viscoelastic fluid. Since even the qualitative aspects of the entry flow field have not been predicted, detailed velocity field observations are not yet required, which may explain why there has been so little effort directed towards point velocity measurement in this flow field.

Recent streak-line observations in tubular entry flows do establish at least one reason why numerical simulation for this flow field has been unsuccessful. Further examination of the streak photographs in Fig. 14.10 shows that, at low values of $\lambda\dot{\gamma}$, the vortex is virtually identical in shape and size to that observed and predicted for an inelastic Newtonian fluid (see Fig. 14.7); λ is a shear rate dependent relaxation time based on the downstream shear rate, $\dot{\gamma}$, equal to $N_1/2\eta\dot{\gamma}^2$. Here the vortex boundary is concave with its centre of rotation near the corner of the upstream tube.

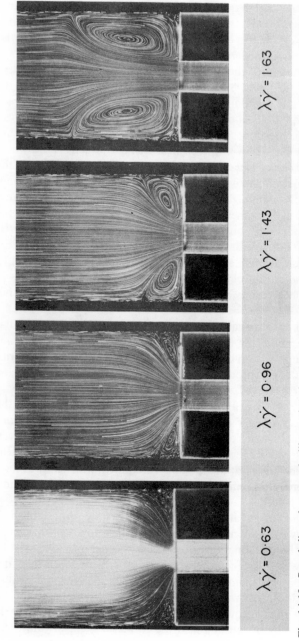

Fig. 14.10. Streak-line photographs illustrating the changing vortex growth as a function of $\lambda\dot{\gamma}$ for a constant viscosity elastic liquid flowing in a 4·08 to 1 circular contraction.[124] The fluid used for the observations (a dilute solution of high molecular weight polyacrylamide dissolved in water and corn syrup) is characterised by a constant viscosity, $\eta = 9·75\,\mathrm{N\,s\,m^{-2}}$, and by $\lambda_0 = 0·308\,\mathrm{s}$ and/or $\lambda_1 = 1·132\,\mathrm{s}$ and $\alpha = 0·373$, where λ_0 is the limiting or low shear rate Maxwell relaxation time whilst λ_1 and α are the Oldroyd B relaxation time and retardation parameter respectively.

$\lambda\dot{\gamma} = 0·63$ $\lambda\dot{\gamma} = 0·96$ $\lambda\dot{\gamma} = 1·43$ $\lambda\dot{\gamma} = 1·63$

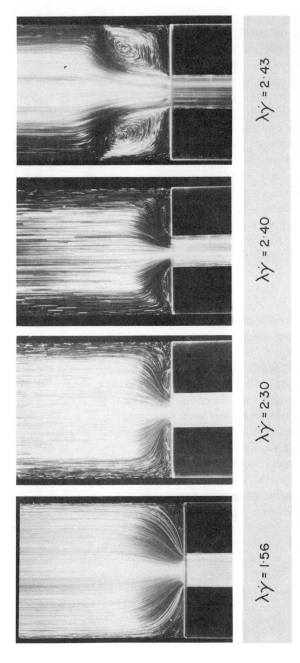

$\lambda\dot{\gamma} = 1.56$ $\lambda\dot{\gamma} = 2.30$ $\lambda\dot{\gamma} = 2.40$ $\lambda\dot{\gamma} = 2.43$

Fig. 14.11. Streak-line photographs illustrating the changing vortex shape and growth as a function of $\lambda\dot{\gamma}$ for a constant viscosity elastic liquid flowing in a 4·08 to 1 circular contraction. The fluid is characterised by $\eta = 25.1\,\mathrm{N\,s\,m^{-2}}$, and by $\lambda_0 = 0.149\,\mathrm{s}$ and/or $\lambda_1 = 1.19\,\mathrm{s}$ and $\alpha = 0.143$. Complete steady and dynamic shear properties for the fluid are available.[124]

As $\lambda\dot{\gamma}$ increases, the centre of rotation of the cell shifts towards the tube entrance and the cell boundary straightens until, at higher $\lambda\dot{\gamma}$, the cell boundary is convex with the centre of rotation of the vortex positioned close to the tube entrance or *lip*. This lip vortex now grows and the re-attachment length of the cell increases for $\lambda\dot{\gamma} \geqslant 1$. Such behaviour has been consistently observed for the constant viscosity polyacrylamide in corn syrup solutions for the contraction ratio $\beta \geqslant 4$ when the vortex growth is not a significant function of β. The change in shape of the vortex boundary without a change in the re-attachment length of the cell has not been predicted by any numerical simulation. A lip vortex like that illustrated in Fig. 14.10 was first observed using streak photography in entry flows for viscoelastic fluids by Giesekus,[109] more recently by Dembek[123] and consistently by Walters and co-workers in circular entry flows and in other entry flow geometries.[120,121,125]

The transition in flow from a corner to a lip vortex and a mechanism for the change in shape of the vortex boundary is not apparent from the streak photographs shown in Fig. 14.10, nor was it apparent from experiments conducted with the polyacrylamide in corn syrup solutions conducted in contraction ratios up to 15. However, the transition and a mechanism becomes apparent from the streak photographs shown in Fig. 14.11 for another constant viscosity elastic liquid with steady and dynamic flow properties similar to those of the fluid used for the observations shown in Fig. 14.10 for flow in a 4 to 1 circular contraction.* Here the re-attachment length and shape of the cell remain similar to those for the Newtonian cell with increasing $\lambda\dot{\gamma}$ to a value of about 1·6. At this stage the re-attachment length of the secondary flow vortex *decreases* as $\lambda\dot{\gamma}$ increases, effectively reaching a zero value at $\lambda\dot{\gamma} = 2\cdot37$. The decrease in the size of the corner vortex is not an inertial effect as expected for Newtonian fluids when $N_{Re} > 1$ since the downstream Reynolds number never exceeds 0·0192 for the streak photographs shown in Fig. 14.11. The decrease in the dimensionless re-attachment length, $X(= L_v/D_u$; Fig. 14.9), with increasing $\lambda\dot{\gamma}$ occurs at the same time as the formation of an independent vortex (at $\lambda\dot{\gamma} = 2$) which emanates from the tube entrance lip. The lip vortex ultimately destroys the corner vortex, and vortex growth occurs for $\lambda\dot{\gamma} > 2\cdot40$. Thus two distinctly different flow pattern developments for two constant viscosity elastic fluids with essentially the same time constants are observed for creeping flow in the same circular 4 to 1

---

*A polyisobutylene–polybutene fluid characterised by a constant viscosity, $\eta = 25\cdot1\,\mathrm{N\,s\,m^{-2}}$, and by $\lambda_0 = 0\cdot149\,\mathrm{s}$ and/or $\lambda_1 = 1\cdot19\,\mathrm{s}$ and $\alpha = 0\cdot143$ was used for the observations shown in Fig. 14.11;[124] the material parameters are described in reference 124 and the caption of Fig. 14.10.

contraction. Clearly, the two materials are not similar and differ in some unmeasured flow property, most likely the elongational viscosity, and clearly the flow visualisation results identify this difference.

Lawler et al.[126] provided a better understanding of the differences in the flow patterns illustrated in Figs 14.10 and 14.11. Using an automated two-colour laser Doppler velocimeter they were able to make very accurate axial and radial velocity measurements in a circular 4 to 1 contraction for both Newtonian and elastic liquids. The experimental techniques were demonstrated by comparison of the two-component velocity measurements for a Newtonian fluid with the results obtained using the finite element code developed by Kim-E et al.[147] The agreement between the velocity observations and numerical prediction is very impressive. For the ideal elastic fluid the authors established that, at a lower critical value of Weissenberg number (or Deborah number), the flow changed from a steady two-dimensional motion, nearly identical to the Newtonian kinematics, to a time periodic flow with a tangential velocity component which fluctuated about zero. Multiple time period (three-dimensional) motions were observed for an increasing range of Weissenberg numbers until, at a second critical Weissenberg number, the flow suddenly reverted back to a two-dimensional, time independent motion. The observations of Lawler et al.[126] and our own (Boger et al.[124]) are indeed identical: an elastic liquid in tubular entry flow can experience two transitions to a time dependent three-dimensional flow—one transition at low Weissenberg numbers and another transition at significantly higher values of Weissenberg number. In between the two critical Weissenberg number regions, vortex growth in a steady two-dimensional flow is observed. All attempts at numerical simulation fall at approximately the lower critical conditions observed for the unsteady three-dimensional flow. Although far more experimentation is required to characterise the multiple unsteady flows observed at the lower critical Weissenberg number, it is clear that any numerical simulation aimed at predicting the observed stable vortex growth flow must be generalised to three dimensions and time dependence, even at low Weissenberg number. Thus flow visualisation, both in terms of streak-line photography and point velocity observation, has now defined the complexity of the tubular entry flow problem. It remains to be seen if these complexities can be predicted.

14.4. CONCLUSION

Flow visualisation in rheometry has been reviewed with regard to a major challenge in non-Newtonian fluid mechanics—the solution of non-viscometric flow problems for viscoelastic fluids. To meet this challenge it is essential that the stress field and/or the velocity field and streak-lines be observed and quantified in non-viscometric flow fields so that the tools available (constitutive equations) for solution of such problems can be validated and established. Optical birefringence as a technique for stress measurement has been discussed in some detail particularly in regard to determining the stress-optic coefficient where well understood viscometric flows need to be used to establish the value of this coefficient. Having established the stress-optic coefficient, the use of the technique for flows with a significant elongational component has been examined. For such important flows it is concluded that the technique must be used with great care since its validity is in question.

Flow visualisation techniques for streak-line observation and point velocity measurement were then described. The chapter concluded with a summary review on the influence streak photography and point velocity measurements have had in gaining an understanding of the flow phenomena observed in tubular entry flows for viscoelastic fluids. Although the flow phenomena observed, particularly in regard to the secondary flow vortex, have not yet been predicted, the flow visualisation with well characterised ideal elastic fluids has delineated the complexity of the entry flow for the numerical analyst. Clearly, the challenge remains to predict even the qualitative aspects of this flow. Multidimensional point velocity measurements in this flow and others of interest in rheometry are indeed rare and will be required for well characterised fluids to provide firm validation of a theoretical solution for the problem. Once such a solution is available, with the associated stress field prediction, the validity of the birefringence technique for stress measurement in this elongational flow can be assessed. Many challenges remain for the experimentalist to obtain good qualitative flow visualisation observations, using well characterised viscoelastic fluids, in flow fields, with a significant elongational component.

ACKNOWLEDGEMENTS

Research in non-Newtonian fluid mechanics in Chemical Engineering at the University of Melbourne is supported by the Australian Research Grants Scheme. The help of Rod Binnington in the organisation of the review is gratefully acknowledged. Dr M. E. Mackay is grateful for a

University of Melbourne Postdoctoral Research Fellowship which allowed the completion of this work.

REFERENCES

1. R. J. Binnington and D. V. Boger, *J. Rheol.*, 1985, **29**, 887.
2. N. Phan-Thien, N. Dudek, D. V. Boger and V. Tirtaatmadja, *J. Non-Newtonian Fluid Mech.*, 1985, **18**, 227.
3. R. P. Chhabra, P. H. T. Uhlherr and D. V. Boger, *J. Non-Newtonian Fluid Mech.*, 1980, **6**, 187.
4. F. Sugeng and R. I. Tanner, *J. Non-Newtonian Fluid Mech.*, 1986, **20**, 281.
5. T. Sridhar, R. K. Gupta, D. V. Boger and R. J. Binnington, *J. Non-Newtonian Fluid Mech.*, 1986, **21**, 115.
6. D. W. Bousfield, R. Keunings, G. Marrucci and M. M. Denn, *J. Non-Newtonian Fluid Mech.*, 1986, **21**, 79.
7. M. E. Mach, *Optisch-Akutische Versuche*, Calve, Prague, 1873.
8. J. C. Maxwell, *Collected Papers*, Vol. III, Cambridge University Press, London, 1890.
9. M. E. Mackay, Behaviour of polymer solutions and melts in shearing and elongational flow using streak photography and birefringence, PhD thesis, University of Illinois, Urbana, 1985.
10. W. Talbott, Streaming birefringence in extensional flow of polymer solutions, PhD thesis, University of Michigan, Ann Arbor, 1978.
11. E. Hecht and A. Zajac, *Optics*, Addison-Wesley, Reading, Massachusetts, 1979.
12. L. G. Leal and E. J. Hinch, *Rheol. Acta*, 1972, **11**, 190.
13. H. G. Jerrard, *Chem. Rev.*, 1959, **59**, 345.
14. H. A. Scheraga and R. Signer, in *Technique of Organic Chemistry*, 3rd edn, Vol. 1, Part III, A. Weissberger (Ed.), 1960, p. 2387.
15. R. E. Harrington, in *Encyclopedia of Polymer Science and Technology*, Vol. 7, Wiley, New York, 1967, p. 100.
16. H. Janeschitz-Kriegl, *Adv. Polym. Sci.*, 1969, **6**, 170.
17. A. Peterlin, *Pure Appl. Chem.*, 1966, **12**, 563.
18. A. Peterlin and P. Munk, in *Physical Methods of Chemistry*, Vol. I., Part IIIc, A. Weissberger and B. Rossitter (Eds), Wiley, New York, 1972, p. 271.
19. A. Peterlin, *Ann. Rev. Fluid Mech.*, 1976, **8**, 35.
20. H. Janeschitz-Kriegl, *Polymer Melt Rheology and Flow Birefringence*, Springer-Verlag, New York, 1983.
21. F. H. Gortemaker, A flow birefringence study of stresses in sheared polymer melts, PhD thesis, Delft, 1976.
22. B. Koeman and H. Janeschitz-Kriegl, *J. Phys. (E)*, 1979, **12**, 625.
23. P. L. Frattini and G. G. Fuller, *J. Rheol.*, 1984, **28**, 61.
24. M. J. Walker, *Am. J. Phys.*, 1954, **22**, 170.
25. J. K. Backus and H. A. Scheraga, *J. Colloid Sci.*, 1951, **6**, 508.

26. H. Wayland, *J. Appl. Phys.*, 1955, **26**, 1197.
27. W. Philippoff, *J. Appl. Phys.*, 1956, **27**, 984.
28. E. V. Frishman and V. N. Tsvetkov, *J. Polym. Sci.*, 1958, **30**, 297.
29. F. N. Peebles, J. E Prados and E. H. Honeycutt Jr, *J. Polym. Sci.*, 1963, **C5**, 37.
30. H. Janeschitz-Kriegl and J. M. P. Papenhuijzen, *Rheol. Acta*, 1971, **10**, 461.
31. V. N. Tsvetkov, G. I. Kudryavtsev, I. N. Shtennikov, T. V. Peker, E. N. Zakharova, V. D. Kalmykova and A. V. Voldkhina, *Eur. Polym. J.*, 1976, **12**, 517.
32. V. N. Tsvetkov, I. N. Shtennikova, T. V. Peker, G. I. Kudryavtsev, A. V. Voldkhina and V. D. Kalmykova, *Eur. Polym. J.*, 1977, **13**, 455.
33. G. V. Vinogradov, A. I. Isayen, D. A. Mustafaev and Y. Y. Podolsky, *J. Appl. Sci., Polym. Sci.*, 1978, **22**, 665.
34. V. N. Tsvetkov, N. V. Pogodina and L. V. Starchenko, *Eur. Polym. J.*, 1981, **17**, 397.
35. G. V. Vinogradov and A. Ya. Malkin, *Rheology of Polymers*, Springer-Verlag, New York, 1980.
36. F. D. Dexter, J. C. Miller and W. Philippoff, *Trans. Soc. Rheol.*, 1961, **5**, 193.
37. F. H. Gortemaker, M. G. Hansen, B. de Cindio and H. Janeschitz-Kriegl, *Rheol. Acta*, 1976, **15**, 242.
38. F. H. Gortemaker, M. G. Hansen, B. de Cindio, H. M. Laun and H. Janeschitz-Kriegl, *Rheol. Acta*, 1976, **15**, 256.
39. H. M. Laun, M. H. Wagner and H. Janeschitz-Kriegl, *Rheol. Acta*, 1979, **18**, 615.
40. W. Philippoff, *Trans. Soc. Rheol.*, 1961, **5**, 149.
41. W. Philippoff, *Trans. Soc. Rheol.*, 1961, **5**, 163.
42. J. C. Whitehead, Birefringent studies of a viscoelastic fluid in channel flow, MS thesis, University of Tennessee, Knoxville, 1964.
43. J. L. S. Wales and W. Philippoff, *Rheol. Acta*, 1973, **12**, 25.
44. J. L. S. Wales, The application of flow birefringence to rheological studies of polymer melts, PhD thesis, Delft, 1976.
45. A. J. McHugh, M. E. Mackay and B. Khomami, *J. Rheol.*, 1987, **31**, 619.
46. E. F. Gurnee, L. T. Patterson and R. D. Andrews, *J. Appl. Phys.*, 1955, **26**, 1106.
47. D. W. Saunders, *Trans. Faraday Soc.*, 1956, **52**, 1414.
48. D. W. Saunders, *Trans. Faraday Soc.*, 1956, **52**, 1425.
49. D. W. Saunders, *Trans. Faraday Soc.*, 1957, **53**, 860.
50. A. Ziabicki and K. Kedzierska, *J. Appl. Polym. Sci.*, 1962, **6**, 111.
51. A. Ziabicki and K. Kedzierska, *J. Appl. Polym. Sci*, 1962, **6**, 361.
52. F. C. Frank and M. R. Mackley, *J. Polym. Sci, Polym. Phys. Ed.*, 1976, **14**, 1121.
53. D. G. Crowley, F. C. Frank, M. R. Mackley and R. G. Stephenson, *J. Polym. Sci., Polym. Phys. Ed.*, 1976, **14**, 1111.
54. T. Matsumoto and D. C. Bogue, *J. Polym. Sci., Polym. Phys. Ed.*, 1977, **15**, 1663.
55. W. Talbott and J. D. Goddard, *Rheol. Acta*, 1979, **18**, 505.
56. J. A. van Aken and H. Janeschitz-Kriegl, *Rheol. Acta*, 1980, **19**, 744.
57. R. Cressely and R. Hocquart, *Proc. Int. Congr. Rheol.*, 1980, p. 377.

58. G. G. Fuller and L. G. Leal, *Proc. Int. Congr. Rheol.*, 1980, p. 393.
59. Y. Onogi, J. L. White and J. F. Fellers, *J. Non-Newtonian Fluid Mech.*, 1980, **7**, 221.
60. S. Kimora, K. Osaki and M. Kurata, *J. Polym. Sci., Polym. Phys. Ed.*, 1981, **19**, 151.
61. E. Gardner, E. R. Pike, M. J. Miles, A. Keller and K. Tanaka, *Polymer*, 1982, **23**, 1435.
62. C. W. Macosko, M. A. Ocansey and H. H. Winter, *J. Non-Newtonian Fluid Mech.*, 1982, **11**, 301.
63. R. Muller and D. Froelich, *Polymer*, 1985, **26**, 1477.
64. J. W. Prados and F. N Peebles, *A.I.Ch.E.J.*, 1959, **5**, 225.
65. J. P. Tordella, *J. Appl. Polym. Sci.*, 1963, **7**, 215.
66. T. R. Fields Jr and D. C. Bogue, *Trans. Soc. Rheol.*, 1968, **12**, 39.
67. J. P. Tordella, in *Rheology*, Vol. 5, F. E. Eirich, (Ed.), Academic Press, New York, 1969, p. 57.
68. R. L. Boles, H. L. Davis and D. C. Bogue, *Polym. Eng. Sci.*, 1970, **10**, 24.
69. C. D. Han and L. H. Drexler, *J. Appl. Polym. Sci.*, 1973, **17**, 2329.
70. C. D. Han and L. H. Drexler, *J. Appl. Polym. Sci.*, 1973, **17**, 2369.
71. V. I. Brizitsky, G. V. Vinogradov, A. I. Isayev and Y. Y. Podolsky, *J. Appl. Polym. Sci.*, 1978, **22**, 751.
72. H. J. Yoo and C. D. Han, *J. Rheol.*, 1981, **25**, 115.
73. M. Horsman and W. Merzkirch, *Rheol. Acta*, 1981, **20**, 501.
74. G. D. Eisenbrand and J. D. Goddard, *J. Non-Newtonian Fluid Mech.*, 1982, **11**, 37.
75. N. Checker, M. R. Mackley and D. W. Mead, *Phil. Trans. Roy. Soc.* (London), 1983, **A308**, 451.
76. D. H. Crater and J. A. Cuculo, *J. Polym. Sci.,. Polym. Phys. Ed.*, 1983, **21**, 2219.
77. S. T. E. Aldhouse, M. R. Mackley and I. P. T. Moore, *J. Non-Newtonian Fluid Mech.*, 1986, **21**, 359.
78. T. M. T. Yang and I. M. Krieger, *J. Rheol.*, 1978, **22**, 413.
79. H. Aben, *Exp. Mech.*, 1966, **6**, 13.
80. H. Aben, in *Optical Methods in Mechanics of Solids*, A. Legarde (Ed.), Noordhoff, Rockville, Maryland, 1981, p. 41.
81. D. C. Drucker and W. B. Woodward, *J. Appl. Phys.*, 1954, **25**, 510.
82. M. M. Frӧcht, *Photoelasticity*, Vol. II, Wiley, New York, 1948.
83. J. F. Rudd and R. D. Andrews, *J. Appl. Phys.*, 1956, **27**, 996.
84. J. L. White, *J. Appl. Polym. Sci., Appl. Polym. Symp.*, 1978, **33**, 31.
85. W. Kuhn and F. Grün, *Kolloid-Z.*, 1942, **101**, 248.
86. N. Phan-Thien and R. I. Tanner, *Rheol. Acta*, 1978, **17**, 568.
87. G. G. Fuller and L. G. Leal, *J. Non-Newtonian Fluid Mech.*, 1981, **8**, 271.
88. J. F. Stevenson and R. B. Bird, *Trans. Soc. Rheol.*, 1971, **15**, 135.
89. D. V. Boger, *Ann. Rev. Fluid Mech.*, 1987, **19**, 157.
90. M. E. Mackay, D. U. Hur, R. J. Binnington and D. V. Boger, in preparation for *Polym. Eng. Sci.*
91. S. A. White and D. G. Baird, *J. Non-Newtonian Fluid Mech.*, 1986, **20**, 93.
92. L. H. Drexler and C. D. Han, *J. Appl. Polym. Sci.*, 1973, **17**, 2355.
93. H. Nguyen and D. V. Boger, *J. Non-Newtonian Fluid Mech.*, 1979, **5**, 353.

94. W. Lauterborn and A. Vogel, *Ann. Rev. Fluid Mech.*, 1984, **16**, 223.
95. W. J. Yang (Ed.), *Flow Visualisation*, Vol. III (Proc. 3rd Int. Symp. Flow Visualization), Hemisphere Publishing Corp., Washington, 1983.
96. M. Van Dyke, *An Album of Fluid Motion*, Parabolic Press, Stanford, California, 1983.
97. J. P. Tordella, *Trans. Soc. Rheol.*, 1957, **1**, 203.
98. P. L. Clegg, *Trans. J. Plast Inst.*, 1958, **26**, 151.
99. H. Schott and W. S. Kagham, *Ind. Eng. Chem.*, 1959, **51**, 844.
100. E. B. Bagley and A. M. Birks, *J. Appl. Phys.*, 1960, **31**, 556.
101. E. B. Bagley and H. P. Schreiber, *Trans. Soc. Rheol.*, 1961, **5**, 341.
102. T. F. Ballenger and J. L. White, *Chem. Eng. Sci.*, 1970, **25**, 1191; *J. Appl. Polym. Sci.*, 1971, **15**, 1949.
103. J. L. den Otter, *Plastics and Polymers*, 1970, **38**, 155.
104. T. F. Ballenger, I. J. Chen, J. W. Crowder, G. E. Hager, D. C. Bogue and J. L. White, *Trans. Soc. Rheol.*, 1971, **15**, 195.
105. G. V. Vinogradov, N. I. Insarova, B. B. Bviko and E. K. Bortsenkova, *Polym. Eng. Sci.*, 1972, **12**, 323.
106. Y. Oyanagi, *Appl. Polym. Symp. No. 20*, 1973, p. 123.
107. J. L. White and A. Kondo, *J. Non-Newtonian Fluid Mech.*, 1977/78, **3**, 41.
108. G. V. Vinogradov and V. N. Manin, *Kolloid Z., Z. Polym.*, 1964, **201**, 93.
109. H. Giesekus, *Rheol. Acta*, 1968, **7**, 127.
110. A. B. Metzner, E. A. Uebler and C. F. Chan Man Fong, *A.I.Ch.E.J.*, 1969, **15**, 750.
111. D. V. Boger and A. V. Ramamurthy, *Rheol. Acta*, 1972, **11**, 61.
112. D. R. Oliver and R. Bragg, *Can. J. Chem. Eng.*, 1973, **51**, 287.
113. J. R. A. Pearson and T. J. F. Pickup, *Polymer*, 1973, **14**, 209.
114. Y. Tomita and T. Shimbo, *Appl. Polym. Symp. No. 20*, 1973, p. 137.
115. A. V. Ramamurthy, Laminar flow of viscous and viscoelastic fluids in the entrance region of a pipe, PhD thesis, Monash University, Clayton, Victoria, Australia, 1970; *Trans. Soc. Rheol.*, 1974, **18**, 431.
116. K. Strauss and R. Kinast, *Colloid Polym. Sci.* 1974, **252**, 753.
117. E. T. Busby and W. C. Macsporran, *J. Non-Newtonian Fluid Mech.*, 1976, **1**, 71.
118. P. J. Cable and D. V. Boger, *A.I.Ch.E.J.*, 1978, **24**, 896, 992; 1979, **25**, 152.
119. A. V. Ramamurthy and J. C. H. McAdam, *J. Rheol.*, 1980, **24**, 167.
120. T. Cochrane, K. Walters and M. F. Webster, *Phil. Trans. Roy. Soc. (London)*, 1981, **A301**, 163.
121. K. Walters and D. M. Rawlinson, *Rheol. Acta*, 1982, **21**, 547.
122. M. R. Mackley and I. P. T. Moore, *J. Non-Newtonian Fluid Mech.*, 1986, **21**, 337.
123. G. Dembek, *Rheol. Acta*, 1982, **21**, 553.
124. D. V. Boger, D. U. Hur and R. J. Binnington, *J. Non-Newtonian Fluid Mech.*, 1986, **20**, 31.
125. R. E. Evans and K. Walters, *J. Non-Newtonian Fluid Mech.*, 1986, **20**, 11.
126. J. V. Lawler, S. J. Muller, R. A. Brown and R. C. Armstrong, *J. Non-Newtonian Fluid Mech.*, 1986, **20**, 51.
127. M. Viriyayuthakorn and B. Caswell, *J. Non-Newtonian Fluid Mech.*, 1980, **6**, 245.

128. F. Durst, A. Melling and J. H. Whitelow, *Principles and Practice of Laser Doppler Anemometry*, Academic Press, New York, 1976.
129. T. S. Durrani and C. A. Greated, *Laser Systems and Flow Measurement*, Plenum Press, New York, 1977.
130. I. E. Drain, *The Laser Doppler Technique*, Wiley, New York, 1980.
131. E. O. Schulz-Du Bois (Ed.), *Photo Correlation Techniques in Fluid Mechanics*, Springer, Berlin, 1983.
132. R. J. Binnington, G. J. Troupe and D. V. Boger, *J. Non-Newtonian Fluid Mech.*, 1983, **12**, 255.
133. R. Meynart, *Rev. Phys. Appl.*, 1982, **17**, 301.
134. R. Meynart, *Appl. Opt.*, 1983, **22**, 535.
135. R. Meynart, *Phys. Fluids*, 1983, **26**, 2074.
136. M. T. Dennison, *Trans. J. Plast. Inst.*, 1967, **35**, 803.
137. J. L. den Otter, *Plastics and Polymers*, 1970, **38**, 155.
138. J. L. White, *Appl. Polym. Symp. No. 20*, 1973, p. 155.
139. J. S. Petrie and M. M. Denn, *A.I.Ch.E.J.*, 1976, **22**, 209.
140. D. V. Boger, *Advances in Transport Processes*, A. S. Mujundar and R. A. Mashelker (Eds), Wiley Eastern, New York, 1982, p. 43.
141. S. A. White, A. D. Gotsis and D. G. Baird, *J. Non-Newtonian Fluid Mech.*, 1987, **24**, 121.
142. F. N. Cogswell, *Polym. Eng. Sci.*, 1972, **12**, 64.
143. M. A. Mendelson, P. W. Yeh, R. A. Brown and R. C. Armstrong, *J. Non-Newtonian Fluid Mech.*, 1982, **10**, 31.
144. R. Keunings and M. J. Crochet, *J. Non-Newtonian Fluid Mech.*, 1984, **14**, 279.
145. M. J. Crochet and K. Walters, *Ann. Rev. Fluid Mech.*, 1983, **15**, 241.
146. M. J. Crochet and A. R. Davies, *Numerical Simulation of Non-Newtonian Flow*, Rheology Series, Vol. 1, Elsevier, Amsterdam, 1984.
147. M. E. Kim-E, R. A. Brown and R. C. Armstrong, *J. Non-Newtonian Fluid Mech.*, 1983, **13**, 341.

Chapter 15

The Rheology of Two-Phase Flows

L. A. UTRACKI

*National Research Council Canada, Industrial Materials Research
Institute, Boucherville, Quebec, Canada*

NOTATION

A_i	equation constants
A_0, A	initial and final flow channel cross-section in convergent flow; eqn (15.84)
a_i	semiaxis in eqns (15.22), (15.23); parameters
a_c, a_T	concentration and temperature shift factor
B, B_0	extrudate swell and its value for Newtonian liquid, respectively
C_{ij}	elastic constants in eqn (15.86)
D	droplet deformability defined in eqn (15.101); characteristic diameter defined in eqn (15.118)

D_c, D_e	capillary and extrudate diameter, respectively
D_r	rotational Brownian diffusion coefficient, eqn (15.18)
d, d_i	diameter, diameter of ith generation of particles in polydisperse suspensions; eqns (15.15) and (15.16)
$d_{v/s}$	volume-to-surface average particle diameter, eqn (15.120)
$\bar{d}$	average value of d
E	elasticity of interphase in eqn (15.114)
E	(subscript) uniaxial extension; (superscript) excess value
E_{sep}	energy required to separate two particles; eqn (15.36)
e	shape factor in eqn (15.56)
F, F_y, F_m	function, its yield value and that of a matrix, eqn (15.43)
$\mathbf{F}_{ij}$	interparticle interaction force in eqn (15.65)
$\tilde{F}_{max}$	dimensionless stress at yield per drop in eqn (15.116)
f	free volume fraction
f_i	orientation function in eqns (15.86)–(15.95)
$f(x)$	function of a parameter x
G, G', G''	shear modulus, and storage and loss dynamic shear moduli, respectively
G'_y, G''_y	yield values for G' and G''
$\tilde{G}$	dimensionless shear rate defined in eqn (15.111)
g	acceleration due to gravity
g_i	orientation function in eqns (15.86)–(15.94)
H	enthalpy
$\bar{H}_G$	reduced gross relaxation spectrum in eqns (15.156) and (15.157)
J, J_0, J_e^0	creep compliance, its value at $t = 0$ and steady state J; eqn (15.48)
$k_i \simeq 1/\phi_{mi}$	constants in eqn (15.14)
k_i	equation constants in eqn (15.42)
k_H, k_M	Huggins, Martin constants
L	length of a dispersed particle
$L(\tau)$	retardation spectrum
M, M_w, M_n	molecular weight and its weight and number averages, respectively

M	parameter in eqn (15.35)
M_e	entanglement molecular weight
m_i	parameters of eqns (15.33) and (15.46)
N_1, N_2	first and second normal stress difference
N_1^+, N_2^+	normal stress growth functions
n	power law exponent; eqn (15.74)
n_i	number of particles
n_e	entanglement degree of polymerization; eqn (15.147)
P	pressure
Pe	Peclet number; eqn (15.18)
P_e	entrance–exit pressure drop in capillary flow
p, p^*	aspect ratio and its generalized value
$\mathbf{r}_{ij}$	center-to-center distance between particles; eqn (15.65)
r, r_c	radial position of a particle and its critical value
R^*	gas constant
R	hard spheres diameter ratio; eqn (15.10)
R_c	particle diameter-to-capillary diameter ratio; eqn (15.27)
Re	Reynolds number; eqn (15.31)
R_0	distance from center of a particle
R_T, R_T^0	Trouton ratio and its limit at small deformation rates
r_h	parameter in eqn (15.158)
$\langle \mathbf{S} \rangle$	elastic stress component of spherical suspension; eqn (15.65)
S_i	initial slope of stress growth function in uniaxial extension
s	subscript indicating suspension
s_i	specific surface area of ith particle
T	temperature
T_m, T_g	melting point; glass transition temperature
T_s	separation temperature; eqn (15.146)
t, t_p	time, period of rotation for anisometric particles; eqn (15.17) and (15.30)
U	particle velocity; eqn (15.31)
U_i	functions defined in eqns (15.75)–(15.79)
V, V_i	volume, volume of ith fraction of particles; eqn (15.13)

w_i	weight fraction of specimen i
X_{ij}	energetic interaction parameter; eqn (15.125)
x	variable
x_i	mole fraction
Y	packing function; in eqn (15.2)
α, α_i	equation parameters; eqns (15.4), (15.22), (15.23) etc.
α_i	polarizabilities; eqn (15.95)
2α	convergence angle; eqn (15.152)
β	Onsager parameter in eqn (15.147)
β_1, β_{12}	slip factor in Lin's equations (15.154), (15.155)
Γ_0	critical parameter for droplet breakup
$\gamma, \dot{\gamma}$	strain, rate of strain in shearing
$\dot{\gamma}_c, \dot{\gamma}_y$	critical value of $\dot{\gamma}$ for onset of dilatancy or yield
γ_R	recoverable shear strain
γ_r	strain recovery
ΔE_η	activation energy of flow
$\Delta G_m, \Delta G_{el}$	Gibbs free energy of mixing and an elastic contribution
ΔH_m	heat of mixing
ΔV	overlapping volume; eqn (15.36)
δ	segmental density; eqn (15.147)
$\varepsilon, \dot{\varepsilon}$	Hencky strain in extension and rate of straining, respectively
ε^*	Lennard-Jones characteristic constant
ε_{max}	maximum filament shrinkage; eqn (15.156)
ε_b	maximum strain at break
$\eta, \eta_0, \eta_\infty$	shear viscosity and its upper and lower Newtonian plateau value
η', η'', η^*	dynamic, loss and complex viscosity, respectively
η_E, η_E^+	elongational viscosity, stress growth function in extension at $\dot{\varepsilon} = const$
η_r, η_{sp}	relative, specific viscosity
$\eta_r^0, \eta_{E,r}$	zero-shear relative viscosity, relative viscosity in elongation
$[\eta], [\eta]_s, [\eta]_a$	intrinsic viscosity, intrinsic viscosity of suspensions and that for anisometric particle suspensions
$[\eta]_E, [\eta]_{E,d}$	emulsion and deformable droplet emulsion intrinsic viscosity, respectively

η_p, η_m	viscosity of dispersed liquid and matrix liquid of emulsion; eqn (15.96)
η_i, η_{si}, η_{ei}	interface viscosity and its shear and extensional components respectively
$\eta_{r,i}$	relative viscosity of ith generation of particles in polydisperse suspension
η^+, η_E^+	time dependent viscosity (or the stress growth function) in shear and uniaxial extension
η_{app}	apparent viscosity
θ	anisometry factor; eqns (15.84), (15.85)
θ_h	parameter; eqn (15.158)
κ	parameter defined in eqn (15.100)
Λ, λ	viscosity ratios defined in eqns (15.98) and (15.99), respectively
v, v_0	dynamic interfacial tension coefficient and its equilibrium value
v_{ij}	kinematic viscosity coefficient; eqn (15.131)
Ξ	function defined in eqn (15.63)
ρ	density
σ, σ^*	shape constant in eqns (15.20) and (15.21), and Lennard-Jones constant, respectively
σ_{ij}	i,j component of the stress tensor
$\sigma_{crit}(t)$	critical value of shear stress to break bonds in a thixotropic system; eqn (15.38)
σ_y, $\sigma_{y,c}$, $\sigma_{y,E}$	yield shear stress, its value in compression and extension, respectively
σ_{ij}^+	stress growth function in shear ($ij = 12$) or elongation ($ij = 11$)
σ_c	critical shear stress for droplet breakup
σ_m	critical shear stress for melt fracture
τ	retardation time; eqn (15.49)
τ^*	relaxation time
τ^2	free volume contribution; eqn (15.125)
Φ	Farris volume fraction as defined in eqn (15.12)
ϕ, ϕ_m	volume fraction; maximum packing ϕ
$\phi_{m,N}$	ϕ_m for N generations of spheres; eqns (15.8), (15.9)
ϕ_{m0}, $\phi_{m\infty}$	maximum volume packing fraction at shear stress $\sigma = 0$ and $\sigma \rightarrow \infty$, respectively
ϕ_F	effective volume of a flock; eqn (15.37)
ϕ_1	angle of orientation of a spheroid; eqn (15.30)

χ_{ij}	thermodynamic interaction coefficient between species i and j; eqn (15.123)
$\Psi(t)$	retardation function; eqns (15.48), (15.49)
ψ, ψ_0	first normal stress difference coefficient and its value at $\dot{\gamma} \to 0$
ψ, ψ_0	fiber orientation angle in convergent flow; eqns (15.84), (15.85)
ω	frequency
~	indicates reduced variables
*	(superscript) reducing variables

15.1. INTRODUCTION

There is renewed interest in multiphase flows. This has arisen from the need for information by diverse industries, as well as from intellectual curiosity within the scientific community, now armed with new mathematical and physical tools. In the polymer industry, future developments in the area of polymer alloys, blends and composites (PABC) will depend, to a great degree, on the ability of suppliers and processors to control the morphology of the finished product. In the petroleum industry the behavior of drilling mud and high pressure flow of liquids through porous media is crucial for secondary and tertiary oil recovery. There is a growing trend in developing technology for slurry transporation of coal, ore and other large volume particulate materials. Here again the role of multiphase flow is important.

The rheological behavior of PABC is decidedly most complex and interesting. This complexity makes it difficult to understand and control PABC behavior without reference to simpler systems. This chapter presents a historical sequence of increasing difficulty, starting with suspensions of monomodal hard spheres in Newtonian liquids and ending with polymer blends.

The feature common to all multiphase systems is of course the presence of distinguishable phases. For the simplest case of a dilute dispersion of one phase in another, one may ask (i) how the presence of the dispersed phase affects the continuous phase, (ii) how stress and deformation rate gradients affect the distribution, shape and orientation of the dispersed phase, (iii) what is the effect of the interface, and (iv) what is the combined effect of the influences (i)–(iii) on the measured response of the material. Only the simplest cases may be able to provide answers to these questions.

However, to understand what the measured quantity of a function means, an attempt must be made to postulate a reasonable answer to all four.

Most of the rheological equations of state were derived assuming the material to be (1) a continuum, with no discontinuity from one point to another, (2) homogeneous, i.e. without a concentration gradient, and (3) isotropic, i.e. having properties not dependent on an orientation direction. There is an obvious dichotomy between the theoretical assumptions for continuum theories and the observed behaviors of most multiphase systems. In some cases the assumptions do not seem critical i.e. dispersion of small spherical particles flowing through a large conduit can be analyzed in terms of continuum theories, but this is seldom so for fiber suspensions.

Rheological properties are most frequently measured[1-5] for (I) steady state shearing, (II) dynamic shearing, and (III) stretching. These can be classified according to strain (γ), vorticity (Ω), uniformity of stress and uniformity of strain rate. A summary is given in Table 15.1, referring mainly to steady state performance, which is easily achieved for large strain measurements. For small strain testing in dynamic fields, steady state is limited to the linear viscoelastic zone of low strain and frequency. However, for multiphase systems large and small strain measurements cause two distinctly different morphologies. So, for multiphase systems (by contrast with rheometry of homogeneous, single phase liquids) selection of the deformation mode according to the four classification criteria in Table 15.1 usually provides different information: when information for e.g. die flow modeling is required, the steady state shear data should be used; when the rheological properties of specimens are of interest, small strain dynamic testing provides better results.

Stretching flow, with its moderate strains, is a special case; here it is assumed that steady state can be achieved at relatively low strains, so the properties are measured under homogeneous, irrotational conditions. However, this situation exists only for low molecular weight simple liquids. For high molecular weight polymeric fluids, strain hardening is the rule and steady state conditions can seldom be achieved with commercial instruments. The situation is further complicated for multiphase systems. During flow start-up, anisometric particles rapidly align with principal stress direction; that is, just as for large strain shear flow, steady state extension does not provide information on rheological behavior of the original specimen but rather on its oriented version.

It thereby follows that only steady state dynamic testing can be used to characterize multiphase materials. In principle, the information on the

TABLE 15.1
Classification of Rheological Methods of Measurements

No.	Method	Strain	Vorticity	Uniformity of Stress	Uniformity of Strain rate	Comment
I.	Steady State Shear	Large	Yes			
I.1	Sliding plate (drag)			Homogeneous	Homogeneous	Small gap, h
I.2	Poiseuille (capillary or slit)			Variable with radius and length	Not uniform	Large L/d
I.3	Rotational Couette			Linear with gap	Not uniform	Small gap, Δr
I.4	Rotational cone-and-plate			Homogeneous	Homogeneous	Cone angle $< 4°$
I.5	Rotational parallel plates			Linear with radius	Linear with radius	Small gap and shear rates
II.	Dynamic Shear	Small	Yes			
II.1	Couette			Variable	Variable	
II.2	Cone-and-plate			Uniform	Uniform	
II.3	Parallel plates			Linear	Linear	
III.	Extensional Flows	Moderate	Irrotational			
III.1	Uniaxial			Homogeneous	Homogeneous	
III.2	Biaxial			Homogeneous	Homogeneous	

original specimen as well as its modification by shear or extension is part of the start-up or transitory flows. It is hoped that theoretical developments will soon allow these deformations to be more thoroughly explored.

15.2. SUSPENSIONS OF SOLID PARTICLES IN A LIQUID

15.2.1. Suspensions in Newtonian Liquids
These frequently behave like non-Newtonian fluids. Deviation increases with the volume fraction of dispersed particles, ϕ. For anisometric particles or particle aggregates the non-zero first normal stress function, N_1, is observed. Shear fields are known to change morphology even in the simplest case of uniform, hard spheres. Section 15.2.1 considers only Newtonian flows; non-Newtonian effects are discussed in Section 15.2.2.

15.2.1.1. Uniform, Hard Spheres Suspensions
For Newtonian liquids these have been the subject of ongoing theoretical and experimental attention. Early works have been reviewed by Frish and Simha,[6] Rutgers[7] and Thomas,[8] with more recent contributions by Utracki,[9-11] Mewis,[12] Metzner[13] and others. Quite unique in depth and scope is the review of microrheology of dispersions by Goldsmith and Mason.[14]

Theories derive from three assumptions:

(i) The diameter of rigid particles is large compared with that of the suspending medium molecules, but small compared with the smallest dimension of the rheometer.
(ii) The flow is at steady state, without inertial, concentration gradients or wall slip effects.
(iii) The liquid medium adheres perfectly to the particles.

There may be a fourth assumption for inter-particle interaction, depending on the theory.

Of the many relations between relative viscosity and ϕ:

$$\eta_r = \eta/\eta_0 = f(\phi) \tag{15.1}$$

(where η and η_0 are, respectively, the viscosity of the suspension and of the medium) recent research[9] suggests two:

$$\left. \begin{array}{c} \eta_r^0 = 1 + [\eta]_s \tilde{\eta}_0 \phi \\ \tilde{\eta}_0 = 4(1 - Y^7)/[4(1 + Y^{10}) - 25Y^3(1 + Y^4) + 42Y^5] \\ Y = [2(\phi_m/\phi)^{1/3} - 1]^{-1} \end{array} \right\} \tag{15.2}$$

$$\ln \eta_r^0 = [\eta]_s \phi / (1 - \phi / \phi_m) \tag{15.3}$$

In eqns (15.2) and (15.3), the superscript 0 indicates zero rate of shear, $[\eta]_s$ is the intrinsic viscosity, and ϕ_m is the maximum packing volume fraction. Equation (15.2) was rigorously derived by Simha.[15] The author used a cell model of the hard sphere suspension, placing the particles in the center of the spherical shells, with radius, inversely proportional to ϕ, dependent on the hydrodynamic interactions. Equation (15.3) was first proposed by Mooney[16] by considering successive additions of rigid, uniform spheres to the liquid. The relation can also be derived from the free volume theory.[17,18]

Both (15.2) and (15.3) are two-parameter equations; for uniform hard spheres in random packing $[\eta]_s = 2.5$ and $\phi_m = 0.62$. For non-uniform particles the relations were found to be valid provided the parameters were approximately selected (by independent experiments or curve fitting).

The third relation

$$\eta_r^0 = (1 + \alpha\phi)^\beta \tag{15.4}$$

with α and β parameters, was originally proposed by Einstein[19,20] for very dilute suspensions ($\alpha = 2.5$, $\beta = 1$). If $\beta < 0$ then eqn (15.4) becomes any of the 'relative fluidity' equations discussed in the literature since 1920. Hess[21] and later Vand[22] proposed eqn (15.4) with $\alpha = -2.5$ and $\beta = -1$ for concentrations in excess of 50 vol%. De Bruyn[23] obtained better results using $\alpha = -1.73$ and $\beta = -2$. Equation (15.4) with the latter value of β was re-derived several times e.g. by Maron and Pierce[24] and by Quemada.[25] In spite of 'wrong' limits (note that for $\beta < 0$, $\phi_m = -1/\alpha$, but then for $\phi \to 0$, $\eta_r^0 \simeq 1 + (2/\phi_m)\phi$, which reduces the Einstein's equation only if $\phi_m = 0.8$!), equation (15.4) with $\beta = -2$ continuously finds its advocates.[13] There is almost as much support for eqn (15.4) with $\beta = -2.5$.[26-28] An interesting approach to this problem was taken by Krieger and Dougherty[29] who proposed eqn (15.4) with $\alpha = -1/\phi_m$ and $\beta = -[\eta]_s \phi_m$. Note that these constants give eqn (15.4) not only the correct low and high values but also sufficient flexibility to accommodate systems with different numerical values of $[\eta]_s$ and ϕ_m.

There are several ways to pack even monodispersed, hard spheres resulting in a large variation of ϕ_m (Table 15.2).

Equations (15.2)–(15.4) predict that η_r^0 should be independent of diameter, d. However, it was recognized early on that properties of suspensions of small particles with $d \ll 1 \mu m$ should show higher η_r^0 than theoretically predicted by a simple hydrodynamic argument. There are three reasons to expect this effect: (i) the low mobility of liquid molecules

TABLE 15.2
Maximum Packing Volume Fraction in Suspensions of Uniform Hard Spheres

No.	Arrangement	$\phi_m \times 10^3$	Ref.	Comments
I.1	Cubical	523·6	30	Theoretical
I.2	Single-staggered (cubical tetrahedral)	604·5	30	Theoretical
I.3	Double-staggered	698·0	30	Theoretical
I.4	Pyramidal (face-centered cubical)	740·5	30	Theoretical
I.5	Hexagonal close-packed	740·5	30	Theoretical
I.6	Random-loose	601	31	Experimental limits
I.7	Random-dense	637	31	for steel spheres
I.8	Random-loose	596	32	Experimental limits
I.9	Random-dense	641	32	for nylon spheres
I.10	Average random-loose	589 ± 14	33	Average of published
I.11	Average random-dense	639 ± 32	33	experimental data
I.12	Most probable random	620	–	Experimental average

adsorbed on the particle surface;[34] (ii) the contribution due to thermal (Brownian) motion; and (iii) effects of colloidal aggregation of particles.[35] The data from 16 laboratories were examined by Thomas.[8] After correcting for diameter effects the author obtained good superposition of data onto one single dependence, empirically expressed as

$$\eta_r^0 = 1 + 2 \cdot 5\phi + 10 \cdot 05\phi^2 + 0 \cdot 00273 \exp(16 \cdot 6\phi) \qquad (15.5)$$

The correlation among eqns (15.2)–(15.5) can be found elsewhere.[9] Another set of complicating effects in uniform hard sphere suspensions is due to orientation or structure formation under flow conditions.[36] These will be discussed later.

15.2.1.2. Particle Size Distribution Effects
In the limiting region of dilute suspensions where the linear relation derived by Einstein[19,20] holds, the only shape dependent parameter $[\eta]_s = 2 \cdot 5$ is independent of polydispersity. The effect becomes important only at $\phi \geqslant 0 \cdot 2$;[7] below this limit, blending two generations of spheres with the diameter ratio

$$R = d_1/d_2 \qquad (15.6)$$

resulted in a small depression of η_r^0.[37,38]

The importance of particle size distribution on rheological behavior is most conveniently discussed in terms of the maximum packing volume fraction. Most of the relations between η_r^0 and ϕ can be conveniently cast in terms of reduced variables:

$$\tilde{\eta}_0 = \tilde{\eta}_0(\tilde{\phi}) \qquad (15.7)$$

$$\tilde{\eta}_0 \equiv (\eta_r^0 - 1)/\phi[\eta]_s \quad \text{and} \quad \tilde{\phi} = \phi/\phi_m$$

Accordingly, any increase in ϕ_m reduces $\tilde{\phi}$ and effectively lowers η_r^0 at a constant value of ϕ.

Equation (15.2), for example, predicts that η_r^0 for 60 vol% of loading of spherical particles decreases from 21,142·0 to 18·6 with increase of ϕ_m from its reasonable value for random packing of uniform spheres (0·620) to $\phi_m = 0·945$. The latter value, as will be shown, is a reasonable maximum which may be obtained for tailored distributions of spherical particles. Reduction of η_r^0 by a factor of 1138 can generate substantial savings for the manufacturer.

The problem of maximization of ϕ_m by designing appropriate mixtures of particles with specific diameter ratios and specific concentrations has been critical to numerous industries. The need to maximize ϕ_m originates not only in its ability to reduce η_r^0 but also in generating higher modulus organic or inorganic composites, improving hiding power of paint, obtaining high power propellents and explosives, etc. Several approaches have been used to increase ϕ_m.

(1) McGeary[39] data for maximum values of $\phi_{m,2}$ (subscript 2 indicates binary mixture) obtained by blending two generations of uniform diameter hard spheres with diameter ratio R are shown in Fig. 15.1. There is a simple relation between $\phi_{m,2}(R = 1) = \phi_m$ and $\phi_{m,2}(R \to \infty) = \phi_{m,2}(\infty)$:

$$\phi_{m,2}(\infty) = \phi_m + (1 - \phi_m)\phi_m \qquad (15.8)$$

Experimentally, $\phi_m = 0·625$ and $\phi_m(R > 80) = 0·845 - 0·860$. From eqn (15.8) (assuming $\phi_m = 0·625$), $\phi_{m,2}(\infty) = 0·859$. Equation (15.8) can easily be generalized for N generations of spheres, each with $R^N \to \infty$:

$$\phi_{m,N}(\infty) = \phi_{m,N-1}(\infty) + [1 - \phi_{m,N-1}(\infty)]\phi_{m,N-1}(\infty) \qquad (15.9)$$

From eqn (15.9), assuming $\phi_m = 0·625$, one finds $\phi_{m,2} = 0·859$, $\phi_{m,3} = 0·980, \phi_{m,4} = 1·000$. In practical terms, since only at $R^N > 100$ are the conditions for $R \to \infty$ approached, and since the smallest diameter should not be below $0·1\,\mu m$, this method can generate binary or ternary mixtures with expected $\phi_m \leqslant 0·980$.

For random packing of binary spheres the dependence $\phi_{m,2} = \phi_{m,2}(R)$

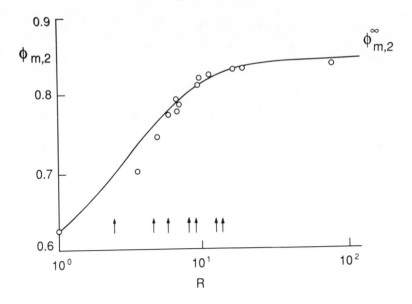

Fig. 15.1. Maximum packing volume fraction as a function of particle diameter ratio.

can be expressed in the form of the nested growth function:

$$\phi_{m,2} = \phi_{m,2}(\infty)\{1 - \exp[a_0 + a_1\exp(-a_2 R)]\} \qquad (15.10)$$

where the a_i are parameters. Taking $\phi_{m,2}(\infty) = 0.859$, $a_0 = -4.2$, $a_1 = 3.2$ and $a_2 = 0.1$, the curve in Fig. 15.1 was generated. In spite of the approximate nature of selected parameters, a reasonable fit to McGeary's data is obtained.

(2) Another method of designing multimodal suspensions of spheres with high ϕ_m starts by assuming a crystal-like arrangement of uniform spheres, then calculating the maximum diameter of the second generation of spheres to go into spaces left between the first generation spheres, then the third generation to go into new spaces, etc. These calculations have been carried out several times[30,40,41] assuming either hexagonal or cubic structure. An example is shown in Table 15.3. The arrows in Fig. 15.1 indicate the space filling values of R. Note that the addition of the second generation spheres with $R < 2.42$ has a deleterious effect—it disrupts the close packing that decreases ϕ_m.

(3) Still another method uses the log-normal distribution as the desired

TABLE 15.3
Calculated Space Filling Distribution for Hexagonal Hard Sphere Arrays

Sphere generation number	R	N	$\phi_i \times 10^3$	$\phi_m \times 10^3$
1	1·0	1	740·5	740·5
2	2·42	1	52·6	790·3
3	4·44	2	16·8	809·9
4	5·65	8	32·6	842·5
5	8·06	8	11·3	853·8
6	9·01	4	4·0	857·8
7	12·4	12	4·7	862·5
8	12·5	12	4·5	867·0
9	13·9	24	6·6	873·6

final result. This method has been applied to both uniform and random packing of nearly spherical particles. Setting R_N and ϕ_N as the diameter and the volume fraction of Nth generation particles, the method requires that

$$R_N = A^{1-N}$$

$$\phi_N = \phi_m / R_N \qquad (15.11)$$

$$\sum_1^\infty V_N = 1$$

where A is a parameter. For five generations of particles with $R_N = 100$, $\phi_m \simeq 0.94$ was obtained.

(4) In some applications not only high ϕ_m but also uniform porosity and ease of handling are important. For such applications Ritter's method for non-segregating mixtures seems to be most suitable.[42,43] Four generations of particles are required with the diameter ratios 1:3 $\pm$ 0·4:9 $\pm$ 2:17 $\pm$ 3 at respective volume fractions of 0·4, 0·1, 0·1 and 0·4. Experimentally, $\phi_m = 0.78$ and uniform porosity were obtained. Higher ϕ_m were reported for other compositions, but the small particles tended to settle at the bottom and the porosities were not as good.

(5) Farris[44] derived the following relation for polydisperse systems:

$$\eta_r = \Pi \eta_{r,i}(\Phi_i) \qquad (15.12)$$

In order to achieve the lowest η_r in systems containing the same total volume fraction of solids, Farris' calculations require that

$$\Phi_i = V_i/\Sigma_i V_i = \text{const} \tag{15.13}$$

In eqn (15.13), V_i is the volume of the ith generation of spheres. It is customary to assign the subscript $i = 0$ to the liquid and $i = 1$ to either the smallest or the largest particles. Parkinson *et al.*[45] combined eqns (15.3), (15.12) and (15.13), writing

$$\eta_r^0 = \Pi_i \exp[2 \cdot 5\, \phi_i/(1 - k_i \phi_i)] \tag{15.14}$$

where the ϕ_i are the volume fractions of each generation of (spherical) particles and the k_i depend on the particle diameter, d_i, according to the empirical relation (valid for both emulsions and suspensions)

$$k_i = 1 \cdot 079 \exp(0 \cdot 01008\, d_i^{-1} + 0 \cdot 0029\, d_i^{-2}) \tag{15.15}$$

where d_i is in μm. The data[45] can also be represented by a simpler dependence:

$$k_i = 0 \cdot 168\, d_i^{-1 \cdot 0072} \tag{15.16}$$

For monodisperse suspensions $k = 1/\phi_m = 1 \cdot 3506$.

To illustrate the η_r^0 dependence on ϕ_m, the data for suspensions of binary spheres[46] are shown in Fig. 15.2 as η_r^0 versus $1/R$. It can be seen that for low $\phi < 0 \cdot 55$ the effect is small, not exceeding a factor of 4, but for $\phi > 0 \cdot 59$ blending two generations of spheres can reduce η_r^0 by at least two decades.

15.2.1.3. Suspensions Containing Anisometric Particles

The flow properties of non-spherical particle suspensions are less well known. At the onset of shearing, the particles begin to rotate with the period

$$t_p = 2\pi(p + p^{-1})/\dot{\gamma} \tag{15.17}$$

where p is the aspect ratio ($p \equiv a_{max}/a_{min}$, where a_{max} and a_{min} are respectively the maximum and minimum particle dimension) and $\dot{\gamma}$ is the rate of shear. The rate of rotation goes through a periodic acceleration for rods, at times $t = 0$, $t_p/2$ and t_p, and for discs at $t = t_p/4$ and $3t_p/4$. Due to these orientational effects the $[\eta]$ is a periodic function of time, gradually damped to reach a steady state value.[47] Under steady state shearing, the particles continue to rotate. For small ones the rotary Brownian motion becomes important at Peclet numbers

$$\text{Pe} = \dot{\gamma}/D_r \tag{15.18}$$

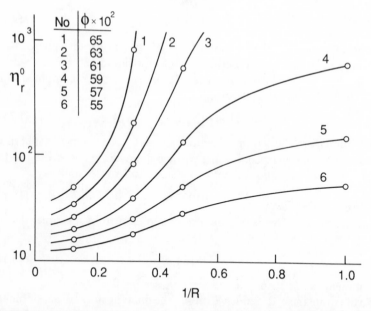

Fig. 15.2. Zero shear relative viscosity versus ratio of particle diameter at volume fraction $\phi = 0.55-0.65$.

Pe < 1 (D_r is the rotary diffusion coefficient). Thus the flow depends on p and Pe resulting in non-Newtonian behavior. These aspects will be discussed later in this chapter.

Since rheological effects are related to particle orientation, the theoretical description must combine the kinetics of motion with rheology. Furthermore, since orientation is determined by the deformation tensor (Table 15.1), there is no direct, general correlation between rheological responses of these suspensions tested under different modes of deformation.

For hard sphere suspensions, eqn (15.2) or (15.3) provided a single smooth dependence from infinitely dilute to concentrated systems. This is no longer true for suspensions of anisometric particles, where crowding and mode of deformation affects the orientation. In the infinitely dilute region, one may define the intrinsic viscosity of anisometric particles, $[\eta]_a$, either in steady-state or time-dependent form. For rigid dumb-bells[48]

$$[\eta]_a = 3(L/d)^2/2 \tag{15.19}$$

where L is the sphere separation and d their diameter. For ellipsoids of rotation and rigid rods[49]

$$[\eta]_a = \frac{14}{15} + \frac{p^2}{5}\left[\frac{1}{3(\ln 2p - \sigma)} + \frac{1}{\ln 2p - \sigma + 1}\right] \quad (15.20)$$

where σ is the numerical constant. For ellipsoids of rotation $\sigma = 1\cdot5$, and for rigid rods $\sigma = 1\cdot8$. Equation (15.20) holds for $p > 20$. It provides the upper bounds for freely rotating particles. For time averaged optimum orientation, Goldsmith and Mason[14] wrote

$$[\eta]_a = p^3/[3(\ln 2p - \sigma)(p + 1)^2] \quad (15.21)$$

Haber and Brenner[50] derived a general relation for $[\eta]_a$ of triaxially anisometric ellipsoids:

$$[\eta]_a = \frac{4}{15}\frac{\alpha''_1 + \alpha''_2 + \alpha''_3}{\alpha''_1\alpha''_2 + \alpha''_2\alpha''_3 + \alpha''_3\alpha''_1} + \frac{1}{5}\left[\frac{a_2a_3(\alpha_2 + \alpha_3)}{\alpha'_1(a_2^2\alpha_2 + a_3^2\alpha_3)}\right.$$

$$+ \frac{a_3a_1(\alpha_3 + \alpha_1)}{\alpha'_2(a_3^2\alpha_3 + a_1^2\alpha_1)} + \frac{a_1a_2(\alpha_1 + \alpha_2)}{\alpha'_3(a_1^2\alpha_1 + a_2^2\alpha_2)}\right]$$

$$- \left[\frac{a_1^2 - a_2^2}{a_1^2\alpha_1 + a_2^2\alpha_2} + \frac{a_2^2 - a_3^2}{a_2^2\alpha_2 + a_3^2\alpha_3} + \frac{a_3^2 - a_1^2}{a_3^2\alpha_3 + a_1^2\alpha_1}\right]^2 \Big/ 5$$

$$\times \left[\frac{a_1^2 + a_2^2}{a_1^2\alpha_1 + a_2^2\alpha_2} + \frac{a_2^2 + a_3^2}{a_2^2\alpha_2 + a_3^2\alpha_3} + \frac{a_3^2 + a_1^2}{a_3^2\alpha_3 + a_1^2\alpha_1}\right]$$

$$(15.22)$$

where the a_i are lengths of semi-axes

$$\alpha_i = (\Pi_i a_i)\int_0^\infty dx/(a_i^2 + x)\Delta x \quad (15.23)$$

with

$$\Delta x = [\Pi_i(a_i^2 + x)]^{1/2}$$
$$\alpha'_i = a_ja_k(\alpha_j - \alpha_k)/(a_j^2 - a_k^2)$$
$$\alpha''_i = (a_j^2\alpha_i - a_k^2\alpha_k)/(a_j^2 - a_k^2)$$

For $a_1 = a_2 = a_3$, $\alpha = 2/3$, $\alpha' = 2/5$ and $\alpha'' = 4/15$, which leads to the Einstein value $[\eta]_a = 5/2$. For ellipsoids of revolution, eqn (15.23) can be expressed in terms of p and integrated analytically.

In the region of infinite dilution the particle rotates freely without being affected by the presence of others. Accordingly, $[\eta]_a$ is a measure of particle hydrodynamic volume defined by its geometry. The customary definition of the dilute region is that where particles are not restricted in their motion, i.e. to $\phi < p^{-2}$. Outside this region the two-body interactions have to be taken into account. One can postulate that this can be done using a power series expression:

$$\tilde{\eta}_0 = 1 + k_H[\eta]_a\phi + \ldots \qquad (15.24)$$

where, by analogy with polymer solutions, the Huggins constant, k_H, expresses the particle–particle interactions. Its value is theoretically known for hard sphere suspensions; eqn (15.2) gives $k_H = 5/16\,\phi_m$. For aniso-metric particles k_H depends on the type of flow, on shape and on orienta-tion. For rigid rods or dumb-bells flowing through pipes experimentally $k_H = 0\cdot7 + 0\cdot2$. Within the dilute region the period of rotation, given by eqn (15.17), increases with ϕ. At the limit, due to crowding, no free rotation is possible.

In the semi-concentrated region, $p^{-2} < \phi < p^{-1}$, movement takes place in two dimensions. Rheologically this results in a decrease of the apparent hydrodynamic volume of the particles, observed as a decrease in the rate with which η_r increases with ϕ.[51]

It has been proposed[52] that the effect by crowding on $[\eta]_a$ be considered as similar in its limit to that induced by high strain rates. For rods[53]

$$[\eta]_0/[\eta]_\infty = p/1\cdot17 \qquad (15.25)$$

where subscripts 0 and ∞ indicate limits $\dot{\gamma} \to 0$ and $\dot{\gamma} \to \infty$, respectively. For discs the numerical factor of $1\cdot17$ ought to be changed to $3\cdot31$. Doi and Edwards predicted that for rods $\eta_r^0 \propto \phi^3$.[54]

Within the concentrated region, $\phi > 1/p$, as ϕ approaches the maximum packing value, theoretically η_r should rapidly increase toward infinity. Experimentally, a series of complicating factors (to be discussed in later sections) are observed. Invariably, all these lead to highly non-Newtonian behavior and the zero-shear viscosity can be extracted only after a series of correcting procedures.

Alternatively, one can use a pragmatic approach and describe η versus ϕ dependence in a wide range of concentration by a hard sphere equation (15.2) or (15.3) taking $[\eta]_s$ and ϕ_m as adjustable. Owing to the aforemen-tioned orientational effects, usually the dilute region of freely tumbling particles has to be treated separately from semi-concentrated and con-centrated ones. The limiting concentration is easy to calculate from the encompassed volume of freely rotating rods or plates. The relation between $[\eta]_a$ and ϕ_m on the aspect ratio p for discs and rods can be approximated by

$$[\eta]_a, \phi_m = a_0 + a_1 p^{a_2} \tag{15.26}$$

with the a_i being parameters. An example of their values is given in Table 15.4.

To sum up, experimentally there are numerous difficulties in obtaining the results which obey basic continuum theory assumptions. By simple geometrical argument, a concentration difference must exist between the bulk of the sample and the layer near the wall. For fiber suspensions these effects have been reviewed by Maschmeyer and Hill.[57,58] The old rule-of-thumb in chemical engineering requires that the smallest dimension of the measuring device (e.g. capillary diameter) should be at least 10 times larger than the largest dimension of the flowing particle. For dilute suspensions of hard spheres, Brenner[59] showed that the measured value of η_r is

$$\eta_{r,exp} = 1 + (5\phi/2)(1 + 61 R_c^2/75) \tag{15.27}$$

where $R_c = d/D_c$ is a ratio of particle diameter to capillary diameter. For $D_c \simeq 10d$ the error is about 1%.

The other problem is generation of well dispersed suspensions. Theory requires that particles be separated and randomly oriented, but due to strong solid–solid interactions, and low limit of the dilute, free-tumbling region ($\phi < p^{-2}$) this requirement is seldom attained. The presence of aggregates and/or orientation invariably leads to non-Newtonian behavior.

Finally, the particles are assumed to be non-deformable under the test condition, i.e. rigid and non-breakable. The latter requirement is particularly difficult to observe when measuring suspensions of rigid fibers in viscous media.

TABLE 15.4
Experimental Values of Parameters a_i of Eqn (15.26)

No.	Particle	Y	$p_m{}^a$	a_0	a_1	a_2	Ref.
1.	Discs	$[\eta]$	50	2·51	0·1127	1	55
2.	Discs	$1/\phi_m$	50	1·29	0·0598	1	11
3.	Rods	$[\eta]$	50	2·34	0·1636	1	11
4.	Rods	$1/\phi_m$	150	1·38	0·0376	1·4	56

^{a} Maximum value of aspect ratio used to determine the parameters a_i.

15.2.1.4. Troutonian Viscosity of Suspensions

When the extensional field is irrotational and under steady state flow conditions the particles remain oriented in the direction of stress. In uniaxial flow they align with the main axis in the flow direction; in biaxial they lie on the stretch plane.

Batchelor derived the following relation for dilute suspensions of rods with aspect ratio p in a Newtonian liquid:[60]

$$\eta^0_{E,r} = 3 + 4\phi p^2 / 3 \ln (\pi/\phi) \tag{15.28}$$

where $\eta^0_{E,r} = \eta^0_E/\eta_0$ is the relative extensional viscosity within the Troutonian range of extensional rates, $\dot{\varepsilon} \to 0$. For $\phi \to 0$ the Trouton ratio

$$R^0_T = \lim_{\dot{\gamma},\dot{\varepsilon} \to 0} \eta_E/3\eta \tag{15.29}$$

is unity.

As illustrated in Fig. 15.3, R^0_T depends strongly on p. For hard spheres ($p = 1$) even at high concentration, $\phi = 0.7$, only a modest increase is predicted: $R^0_T = 1.21$. This may explain why in the rheology of rigid sphere suspensions the entrance–exit pressure drop correction in capillary flow can be neglected.[61]

The experimental data[62-64] confirm the theoretical predictions. Even for concentrated supensions with $\phi > 1/p$ the agreement is reasonable. One may expect this result since fibers do not rotate in uniaxial flow and the maximum packing of fiber cross-sectional areas defines the concentration limits. As the Fig. 15.3 comparison shows, experimental errors tend to be higher than predicted. Owing to difficulties in measuring extensional viscosity the discrepancy may not originate in theory.

15.2.2. Suspensions in Newtonian Liquids; Non-Newtonian Flows

As indicated in Section 15.2.1, the Newtonian behavior of suspensions is limited to low concentrations. An exception seems to be the irrotational flow of anisometric particles where the rate of strain independent region extends to concentrations where strong non-Newtonian behavior would be expected in shear. These rate of deformation dependent phenomena will be summarized below.

15.2.2.1. Orientation

The orientation of particles in flow is of particular interest for microrheology. To be able to predict the macroscopic rheological properties, a detailed description of phase behavior is required. In this field, contributions from the Pulp and Paper Research Institute of Canada by Mason and later by van de Ven and their co-authors are of exceptional value. The

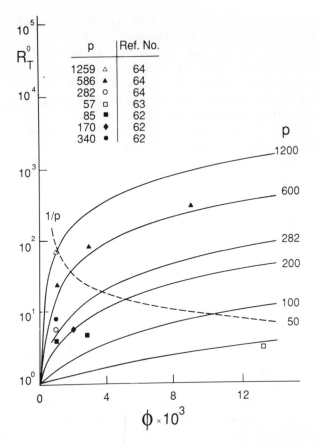

Fig. 15.3. Zero deformation rate Trouton ratio versus volume fraction of fibers with aspect ratio p; the limit of the dilute region, $1/p$, is also indicated.

earlier results were brilliantly summarized by Goldsmith and Mason.[14] The theoretical and experimental work allowed the establishment of the angle of orientation of a spheroid:

$$\phi_1 = \arctan[p^* \tan(2\pi t/t_p)] \qquad (15.30)$$

where for cylinders and discs $p^* = p$ and $1/p$, respectively. Accordingly, for rods the maximum velocity of rotation occurs at $t/t_p = 0$, 1/2, 3/4, 5/4,... For $p^* = 1$, $\phi_1 = 2\pi t/t_p$, i.e. the spheres rotate with constant velocity. In non-uniform shear fields (Poiseuille flow) the particles rotate with velocity predicted by eqns (15.17) and (15.30) in accordance with the value of $\dot{\gamma}$ appropriate to the radial location of the sphere in the capillary. Near the wall, for finite diameter spheres, the immobile layer of the suspending medium causes a reduction of rotational and translational velocity. The effect scales with the square of the diameter. The wall also causes a geometric exclusion effect, i.e. had the axial migration of particles been absent, there would be lower than average concentration of particles near the wall, and retardation of their motion. However, axial migration does exist at a rate increasing nearly linearly with Reynolds number:

$$\text{Re} = \rho U d / \eta_0 \qquad (15.31)$$

where U is the particle velocity; $U = \dot{\gamma}d$. At a higher concentration the difference in velocities of particles located at different radial positions results in the formation of transient multiplets behaving similarly to rods. Under these circumstances the rate of axial migration is accelerated, and the flow profile flattens. Experimentally, for $\phi = 1/3$, $R_c = 0.056$ and 0.112, partial and complete plug flows were observed, respectively.[65,66] Similarly, plug flow of discs or rod suspensions was observed with non-rotating particles (note that $\dot{\gamma} = 0$ in the plug flow region), with the major axis aligned in the direction of flow.

Hoffman,[67,68] Strivens,[69] Krieger and Choi[70] and van de Ven and co-workers[47,71,72] reported on the dilatant flow of concentrated suspensions of uniform and polydispersed spheres ($\phi > 1/2$). A dramatic change in light diffraction pattern was systematically observed[67,68] at $\dot{\gamma} > \dot{\gamma}_C$ where $\dot{\gamma}_C$ is the value of $\dot{\gamma}$ for the onset of dilatancy. van de Ven and his collabora-tors[72,72] demonstrated that the distance between sliding layers of uniform spheres in a parallel plate rheometer depends on ϕ and $\dot{\gamma}$; changes of up to 10% were measured. Strivens provided a detailed study of the instrument dependence of the phenomenon. The effect was found to be related to the acceleration of particle motion, 'joining' in the gap and compression of the particle stabilizing layer.

The dilatant behavior of binary sphere suspensions in capillary flow was recently reported by Goto and Kuno.[38] The fascinating part of the story is that at constant loading, $\phi \simeq 0.2$, dilatancy was observed only within a relatively narrow range of composition, $0.714 < x \leqslant 0.976$, where x represents the fraction of larger spheres. Furthermore, the magnitude of the effect was found to be related to R; at $\phi \simeq 0.2$, $x = 0.945$, the sharpest increase of η_r with $\dot{\gamma}$ was observed for particle diameter ratio $R = 4.74$. After high speed filming of the flow the authors calculated the number of particles, n, near the capillary wall (defined as an annular volume with thickness equal to diameter of larger sphere). The results are illustrated in Fig. 15.4. The authors concluded that (i) η_r primarily depends on the number of larger particles near the wall, (ii) at low $\dot{\gamma}$ smaller particles cause migration of the larger away from the wall, resulting in a decrease of η_r for binary mixture, and (iii) at high $\dot{\gamma}$ the small particles nearly completely vacate the wall area, forcing the larger ones away from the centre toward the wall, which in turn causes the dilatant behavior.

In Couette flow spheres migrate toward the outer cylinder.[73-75] In shearing, a 'shear fractionation' of spherical particles has been observed by Giesekus[76] and more recently by Prieve et al.[77,78] The observations are not identical. Giesekus observed that, during torsional shearing of binary

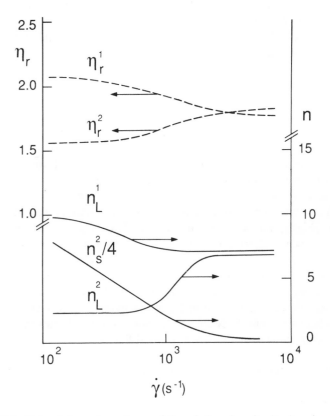

Fig. 15.4. Rate of shear dependence of the relative viscosity (top) and number of particles near the wall.

sphere suspensions, the larger and the smaller spheres separated into two different annular volumes, i.e. for each sphere size a critical equilibrium radial distance had to be postulated. On the other hand, Prieve et al. reported that for each sphere diameter and speed of rotation there is a critical radius; in the parallel plate rheometer, a particle located at $r < r_c$ was observed to migrate inward, whereas that placed at $r > r_c$ migrated outward. There is no theoretical explanation for either observation.

Recently Matsumoto et al.[79] reported that in the cone-and-plate geometry the storage, G', and loss, G'', shear moduli of non-rigid, uniform, spheres decrease monotonically with test time (or number of cycles). G' and G'' were observed to decrease by 4 decades, but steady state shearing for 15 s returned G' and G'' to the initial values. Since the phenomenon depended on the rigidity as well as on the uniformity of shape and size, development of a structure during the dynamic test must be postulated.

The data of Hoffman[67,68] are also interesting for another reason. At $\phi \geqslant 0.53$ and low values of $\dot{\gamma}$ the power law index

$$n = d \ln \sigma_{12} / d \ln \dot{\gamma} \qquad (15.32)$$

approaches zero. For the system styrene–acrylonitryle (SAN) latex in ethylene glycol, addition of salt decreased n to zero. The experiment was performed in order to demonstrate that increased interparticle interaction causes the onset of dilatation to move to higher $\dot{\gamma}$. However, it also demonstrated that at these relatively high concentrations, $\phi = 0.54$, there is a yield stress, σ_y, in shear flow for small ($d = 324$ nm) sphere suspensions. Years later, on the basis of experiments with polystyrene (PS) latices without charge, and with anionic or cationic charge, $d = 175$ nm, $\phi \leqslant 0.2$, Onogi and Matsumoto[80] wrote: 'suspensions of particles having strong attractive forces show yield value, while suspensions of particles having repulsive forces behave like Newtonian liquids, because particles cannot aggregate to form special structures'. Yield stress is associated with a three-dimensional structure of liquid behaving like an elastic solid at stresses below σ_y. The evidence accumulated so far indicates that there is a full spectrum of structures, from liquid-like, i.e. $\sigma_y = 0$, to solid-like with large σ_y (e.g. hydrated gelatin). For anisometric particles at $\phi > 1/p$, yield may be due to mechanical interlocking of particles. For spheres it mainly originates from interparticle interactions. When these interactions are weak $\sigma_y \to 0$ is observed, with the arrow indicating the time effect; had the experiment been conducted at $\dot{\gamma} < \dot{\gamma}_y$ no yield behavior would be noted. The value of $\dot{\gamma}_y$ depends on the strength of interparticle interactions as well as on ϕ; e.g. for $\phi = 0.1$ and 0.2 of neutral PS particles,[80] $\dot{\gamma}_y = 0.35$ and $2.4\,(s^{-1})$, respectively.

In uniaxial extensional (convergent) flow there is evidence of spherical particles moving toward the center of the stream.[38] Convergent flow of glass fibers, $p = 200–800$, in Newtonian media at $\phi \leqslant 10^{-4}$ was studied by Murty and Modlen.[81] The fiber orientation angle ψ (derived as an average angle between the fiber axis and flow direction) changed from 45° (random) to about 15°. The orientation started upstream from the convergence. For a low viscosity medium, jamming at the entrance region was responsible for as much as 60% of fibers being left out.

Owing to the accelerated rotation of fibers in a shear field (see eqn (15.28)) alignment of fibers in Couette flow should take place. The theoretical and experimental results[82] are shown in Fig. 15.5. The theory indicates that the shear field is about half as efficient at causing fiber alignment as planar extension. However, the shear field is rarely homogeneous, and during the flow fibers undergo breaking, bending or coiling,[83] causing a further reduction of alignment efficiency.[84] Further details on various modes of orientational behavior of flowing suspensions can be found in

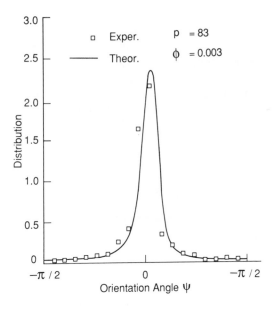

Fig. 15.5. Distribution of fibers with aspect ratio $p = 83$ at concentration $\phi = 0.003$ versus the orientation angle in Couette flow.

excellent reviews by Cox and Mason,[85] Batchelor[86] and Leal.[87] It is recognized that at higher fiber loading, $\phi p > 1$, the rheological response of aligned fibers resembles that of liquid crystals.

15.2.2.2. Aggregation, Agglomeration and Flocculation

One fundamental assumption of continuum theories is structure stability (Newtonian flows) or, alternatively, a well defined process of its changes (non-Newtonian behavior). As indicated in Section 15.2.2.1, orientational effects in layered concentrated suspensions of spheres are responsible for either dilatant or pseudoplastic behavior. Strong interparticle interaction may lead to yield stress or strong transient behavior. In short, there is an intimate relation between the liquid structure and its rheological response; change in one causes a corresponding change in the other.

Aggregation, agglomeration and flocculation are structural phenomena[88] ranging from transient rotating doublets[29] to pseudo-solid-like behavior of flocculated suspensions with yielding.[79,88-93] The aggregation can be due to interparticle thermodynamic interactions, chemical bonding or crowding in simple geometric terms. The latter type prevails in shear flows of suspensions of anisometric particles.

There are numerous theories based on structural models of suspensions briefly reviewed by Mikami.[94,95] More recent derivations can also be found.[92-95] Wildemuth and Williams[92] considered the effect of shear stress dependent maximum packing volume fraction, ϕ_m, on η_r. The mechanism responsible for variation of ϕ_m is stress dependent flocculation; defining $\phi_{m,0}$ and $\phi_{m,\infty}$ as the values of ϕ_m at normalized shear stress $\tilde{\sigma}_{12} \to 0$ and $\tilde{\sigma}_{12} \to \infty$, respectively, the authors derived the relation

$$\phi_m = (\phi_{m,0} + \phi_{m,\infty}\tilde{\sigma}_{12}^m)/(1 + \tilde{\sigma}_{12}^m) \qquad (15.33)$$

where m is an experimental constant with reported values of $1\cdot00-1\cdot17$. The interesting facet of eqn (15.33) is that it can be used to predict values of yield stress, $\tilde{\sigma}_y$, if m, $\phi_{m,0}$ and $\phi_{m,\infty}$ are known:

$$\tilde{\sigma}_y = (\phi - \phi_{m,0})/(\phi_{m,\infty} - \phi) \qquad (15.34)$$

The shear stress normalization

$$\tilde{\sigma}_{12} = \sigma_{12}/M \qquad (15.35)$$

where M, the fourth parameter of the theory, normalizes the flocculation process in terms of the stress sensitivity; the larger the value of M, the less sensitive the system. A more complex form of σ_y was proposed by Lin et al.:[93]

$$\sigma_y = C[(8/\pi)(E_{sep}/\Delta V_{ave}) + kC] \qquad (15.36)$$

where $C = \phi_F(C^{\circ}_{fp}\phi - \phi_F)$, E_{sep} is the energy required to separate two particles, ΔV_{ave} the overlapping volume, k an empirical constant to improve fit of the equation (the first term in the square brackets is theoretical), ϕ_F is an effective flock volume fraction and

$$C^{\circ}_{fp} = \lim_{\phi \to 0} \phi_F/\phi \qquad (15.37)$$

Denisov et al.[96] as well as Brady and Bossis[97] reported on numerical simulation of suspension rheology. In the first case the authors used the 6–12 Lennard–Jones potential with the usual meaning of ε^* and σ^* as characteristic constants (with dimensions of energy and length, respectively) of the interacting species. If R_0 is a measure of distance from the center of the particle at which action of the potential begins, then the necessary condition for dilatant behavior is $R_0 \geqslant \sigma^*$ and particle concentration exceeding a critical value dependent on the system.

The Stokesian dynamics method was used by the other authors.[97] The simulation provided valuable information on the influence of various microstructural elements on the macroscopic viscosity. The relative velocity of two particles in suspension provides the most important contribution to energy loss. As ϕ increases, correlation of interparticle motion also increases. The hydrodynamic lubrication results in an increased number of particles acting as a single agglomerate. The maximum packing volume fraction, ϕ_m, takes on a meaning as a percolation-like threshold for η to increase to infinity due to the formation of infinite clusters.

Microstructural theories of suspensions have frequently been reviewed.[98–101] The aspects which these theories appear to solve with ease are the 'intractable'[102] phenomena of thixotropy and rheopexy or anti-thixotropy.

The term thixotropy refers to a continuous decrease of stress with time under steady state deformation rate, and subsequent recovery when the flow stops. There are several books[103–106] and reviews[99,107,108] dealing with the subject. The phenomenon is related to molecular or macroscopic changes in associations. Bonding must be weak enough to be broken by flow-induced hydrodynamic forces. If dispersion is very fine, even slight interactions will be sufficient to produce a thixotropic effect. On the other hand, as the dispersion gets coarser, larger (but reversible) forces are required. In the case of suspensions of anisometric particles, the effect is particularly strong. For spheres, the effect can be modified by changes in type and concentration of ionic groups at the surface.

Time dependency enters into the consideration of the rheological response of any viscoelastic system, viz. polymer solutions or melts. In the steady-state testing of viscoelastic materials, the selected time scale is usually chosen to allow the system to reach an equilibrium value. Depending on the system and the deformation rate, the stress may reach equilibrium at $t > 10^4$ s, i.e. on a time scale comparable to the thixotropic experiments. More direct distinctions between these two systems are the usual lack of elastic effects and larger strain values at equilibrium observed for the thixotropic materials. There is a correlation between these two phenomena, and theories of viscoelasticity based on thixotropic models have been formulated.[109,110]

Inherent in the concept of thixotropy is the yield stress. Both the microstructural and continuum theories postulate that the material behaves as a Bingham body at stresses below a critical value, i.e. in constant stress experiments

$$\dot{\gamma}(t) = 0 \quad \text{for} \quad \sigma_{12} < \sigma_{crit}(t) \tag{15.38}$$

The definition of σ_{crit} given by the inequality (15.38) is very similar to that of the yield stress:

$$\dot{\gamma} = 0 \quad \text{for} \quad \sigma_{12} < \sigma_y \tag{15.39}$$

where the time scale is not important. This, however, has a profound effect on the shape of the flow curves. The presence of σ_y causes the apparent viscosity, η_{app}, to increase to infinity upon reduction of $\dot{\gamma}$ to zero:

$$\eta_{app} = (\sigma_y + \sigma_{12})/\dot{\gamma} \tag{15.40}$$

with the slope

$$\partial \ln\eta_{app}/\partial \ln\dot{\gamma}|_{\dot{\gamma}\to0} = -1 \tag{15.41}$$

By contrast, in thixotropic systems, experimentally η 'at rest' has a finite value and the rate of shear dependence of the equilibrium viscosity does not necessarily follow eqn (15.41).

15.2.2.3. Steady State Flows

The classification recognizes three types: dilatant, D (shear thickening); Newtonian, N (within any range of $\dot{\gamma}$ or σ_{12}); and pseudoplastic, P (shear thinning). Similarly, in extensional flow the liquids may be stress hardening (SH), Troutonian (T) and stress softening (SS). By definition, the responses considered here are taken at sufficiently long times to ensure equilibrium, and the yield effect, Y, is subtracted. Since, within the experimental range of stress or rate of deformation, several types can be observed, there exist a variety of flow curves. Four of the more common ones are shown in Fig. 15.6.

To understand the flow, the yield effect should first be subtracted. There are several methods for determining σ_y. Among these is the modified Casson equation[111]

$$\sigma_{12}^{1/2} = k_0 + k_1(\eta_a\dot{\gamma}/\eta_0)^{1/2} \tag{15.42}$$

where k_0 and k_1 are constants, η_0 and η_a are the zero shear and apparent viscosities of the dispersing liquid, respectively. Equation (15.42) was rewritten by Utracki[10] as

$$F^{1/2} = F_y^{1/2} + aF_m^{1/2} \tag{15.43}$$

where F may be shear stress, σ_{12}, elongational stress, σ_E, shear loss modulus, G'', etc., F_y indicates the yield value of F, F_m is the F-value of pure

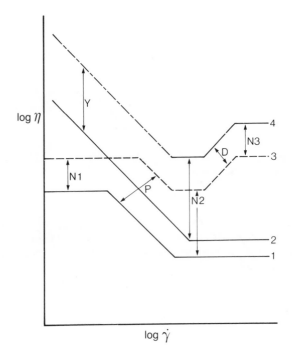

Fig. 15.6. Schematic flow curves, $\log \eta$ versus $\log \dot{\gamma}$, for four types of dispersion; N, Y, P and D indicate Newtonian, yield, pseudoplastic and dilatant flows.

matrix liquid at the same deformation rate as F, and a is a measure of the relative value of F. For instance, if $F = \sigma_{12}$ then F_y is the yield stress in shear, σ_y, and $a^2 = \eta_r$, i.e. eqn (15.43) predicts a straight line dependence for Newtonian liquids with yield value of F_y. In Fig. 15.7 the results of dynamic shear testing for polypropylene (PP) filled with mica are presented.[55] The concentration dependence of σ_y can be expressed either as[10]

$$\sigma_y = K(\phi - \phi_0)^n \qquad (15.44)$$

or as[55]

$$\sigma_y = A_1 \exp(A_2\phi) \qquad (15.45)$$

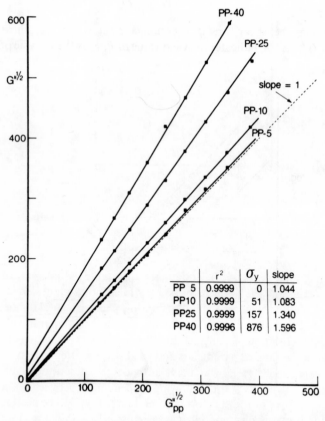

	r^2	σ_y	slope
PP 5	0.9999	0	1.044
PP10	0.9999	51	1.083
PP25	0.9999	157	1.340
PP40	0.9996	876	1.596

Fig. 15.7. Modified Casson plot for polypropylene/mica at 180 °C; $\phi = 0, 0.0342,$ 0.0961 and 0.175.[55]

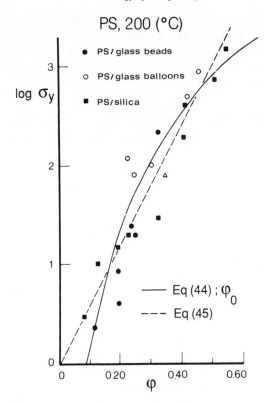

Fig. 15.8. Apparent yield stress σ_y versus ϕ for polystyrene filled with glass beads and balloons: solid line, eqn (15.44) with $\phi_0 = 0$; broken line, eqn (15.45); points, data of Kataoka *et al.*[112]

In these relations, K, ϕ_0, n, A_1 and A_2 are adjustable parameters. In Fig. 15.8 these relations are applied to data for filled polystyrenes.[112]

Another method requires a simultaneous fit of experimental data to one or other constitutive equation in which a parameter or parameters are related to σ_y.[11] In principle, any combination of models providing correlation between rheological parameters and yield stress written in terms of the same independent variables may provide a description of the phenomenon. Recently[10] the following dependence between viscosity, $\eta = \eta(\dot\gamma)$ or $\eta' = \eta'(\omega)$, and deformation rate was found to be particularly suitable for Newtonian/pseudoplastic systems, N1 + P in Fig. 15.6:

$$\eta = \eta_0[1 + (\dot\gamma\tau^*)^{m_1}]^{-m_2} \qquad (15.46)$$

with η_0 the Newtonian viscosity, τ^* an average relaxation time, m_1 and m_2 parameters of the equation dependent on the breadth of the relaxation time spectrum.[113]

Similarly the relation

$$\sigma_y = a_1 \omega^{1-a_2} \qquad (15.47)$$

with a_i being parameters, was found[114] to be particularly suitable for describing the frequency dependent apparent yield stress in rigid polyvinylchloride formulations.

Measurements of creep and elastic recovery also provide a sensitive, direct means of detecting σ_{crit} and σ_y. The methods require a simultaneous fit of time dependent strain, $\gamma(t)$, at a constant stress, σ_{12}, to the compliance equation

$$J(t) \equiv \gamma_{12}(t)/\sigma_{12} = J_0 + J_e^0 \Psi(t) + t/\eta \qquad (15.48)$$

where the retardation function, $\Psi(t)$, depends on the retardation spectrum

$$\Psi(t) = \left[\int_{-\infty}^{+\infty} L(\tau^*)(1 - \exp^{-t/\tau}) d\ln\tau \right] \Big/ J_e^0 \qquad (15.49)$$

For $\sigma_{12} < \sigma_y$ the parameters J_0, J_e^0, $L(\tau^*)$ and η are independent of σ_{12}. Alternatively, plotting the recoverable strain versus stress allows detection of σ_y as the maximum value of stress below which the Hookean behavior is obtained. Polymer latices and suspensions of carbon black in linseed oil and clay or calcium carbonate in aqueous media analyzed by Amari and Watanabe[115] provide examples. The values of σ_y determined from creep and those from shear viscosity were found to be in good agreement.

There are several direct methods of measurement of σ_y. Dzuy and Boger[116] used a rotational vane viscometer. Yield stresses in compression and elongation have been directly measured for PP/mica and polyethylene/mica systems using standard rheological instruments. In the first case[55] $\sigma_{y,c}$ was calculated from unrelaxed stress values in parallel plate geometry, using the Rheometrics Mechanical Spectrometer. In the second case[52] $\sigma_{y,E}$ was taken as the critical stress value below which no sample deformation was observed during 30 minutes of straining in the Rheometrics Extensional Rheometer. Good agreement between $\sigma_{y,c}$ and σ_y (calculated from eqn (15.43) was obtained. For unoriented particles the von Mises criterion for plastic flow of solids should be obeyed, i.e. $\sigma_{y,c} = 3^{1/2}\sigma_y$. Indeed, for the low concentration systems, $\sigma_{y,c} > \sigma_y$. However, for highly concentrated ($\phi > \phi_m$) samples $\sigma_{y,c} \simeq \sigma_y$, indicating that the compressive yielding occurs via the shear mode, i.e. the flakes are oriented at these loadings.

Two semi-empirical equations frequently used to describe η versus $\dot{\gamma}$ dependence for dispersions are the four-parameter Cross dependence[117]

$$(\eta - \eta_\infty)/(\eta_0 - \eta_\infty) = 1/(1 + a_0\dot{\gamma}^{a_1}) \qquad (15.50)$$

and the Williamson relation[118]

$$(\eta - \eta_0)/(\eta_0 - \eta_\infty) = 1/(1 + a_2\sigma_{12}) \qquad (15.51)$$

where η_0 and η_∞ are Newtonian viscosities at $\dot{\gamma} \to 0$ and $\dot{\gamma} \to \infty$ respectively and the a_i are parameters. Equation (15.51) was formally derived by Krieger and Dougherty[29] based on the model of doublet formation and break. Theoretically, a_2 is proportional to the ratio of the particle volume to thermal energy:

$$a_2 \propto d^3/R^*T$$

with the proportionality factor being empirical. Equations (15.50) and (15.51) are frequently written in terms of η_r.[119-121]

Recently[120] a new four-parameter relation was proposed:

$$\eta/\eta_\infty = \{[1 + (\dot{\gamma}\tau)^{a_1}]/[(\eta_\infty/\eta_0)^{1/2} + (\dot{\gamma}\tau)^{a_1}]\}^2 \qquad (15.52)$$

The source of the relation is eqn (15.4) with $\beta = -2$ and the structural parameter α expressed in terms of ϕ and $\dot{\gamma}$.

There is obviously less flexibility in the 3- than in the 4-parameter equation. Nevertheless eqn (15.51) has been found to describe many systems well. All these relations (15.50)–(15.52) are valid for Newtonian–pseudoplastic–Newtonian cases. The work of Krieger and Choi[70,121] is particularly informative. The authors measured the shear viscosity of sterically stabilized polymethylmethacrylate (PMMA) spheres in silicone fluid (SF) whose viscosity varied from $\eta_0 = 8$ to $450\,\text{mPa s}$. In high viscosity fluids the thixotropy and yield stress were observed. The yielding was well described by the Casson equation (15.42). The magnitude of σ_y was found to depend on ϕ, the viscosity of the SF and the temperature. Dispersions in low viscosity SF, $\eta_0 = 10\,\text{mPa s}$, followed eqn (15.51) expressed in terms of the reduced variables, $\eta_r = \eta_r(\sigma_r)$, with $\sigma_r = d^3\sigma_{12}/R^*T$. For most systems at $\sigma_r \simeq 3$ the lower Newtonian plateau was observed. However, when shear stress was further increased, dilatant behavior was observed. Dilatancy was found to depend on particle size, SF viscosity and temperature.[70] The authors reported small and erratic normal stresses.

It should be stressed that eqns (15.50)–(15.52) were derived to describe the pseudoplastic behavior of fluids with the upper, η_0, and lower, η_∞, Newtonian plateau. They should not be used to describe shear variation of viscosity for systems showing yield or dilatancy.

Hinch and Leal[122] derived the following set of relations expressing the particle stresses in dilute suspensions with small Pe $\ll$ 1:

$$\sigma_{12,p} = \phi\sigma_{12}^0[f_0(p^*) + 0(\text{Pe}^2)] \tag{15.53}$$

$$N_{1,p} = \phi\sigma_{12}^0[\text{Pe}\,f_1(p^*) + 0(\text{Pe}^3)] \tag{15.54}$$

$$N_{2,p} = \phi\sigma_{12}^0[\text{Pe}\,f_2(p^*) + 0(\text{Pe}^3)] \tag{15.55}$$

where σ_{12}^0 is the shear stress in the medium and $f_i(p^*)$ are the three shape factors illustrated in Fig. 15.9. For small aspect ratio $p^* \to 1$, p^* can be written in terms of excentricity, e:

$$p^* = 1 + e \tag{15.56}$$

Introducing eqn (15.56) into eqns (15.53)–(15.55) one obtains

$$\sigma_{12,p} = \phi\sigma_{12}^0\{5/2 + e^2[78/441 + 109/(180 + 5\text{Pe}^2)] + 0(e^3)\} \tag{15.57}$$

$$N_{1,p} = \phi\sigma_{12}^0[216e^2\text{Pe}/35(36 + \text{Pe}^2) + 0(e^3)] \tag{15.58}$$

$$N_{2,p} = \phi\sigma_{12}^0[-36e^2\text{Pe}/35(36 + \text{Pe}^2) + 0(e^3)] \tag{15.59}$$

There are two important observations: (i) for $e \to 0$ particle shear stress reverts to the Einstein value and both $N_{1,p}$ and $N_{2,p}$ vanish; (ii) $N_{2,p} = -N_{1,p}/6$.

Similar analysis provided the following estimates for infinite rods $(p^* \to \infty)$:

$$\sigma_{12,p}/\Xi \propto 0\cdot5p^{*2}\ln p^* \tag{15.60}$$

$$N_{1,p}/\Xi \propto 0\cdot2p^{*2}\ln p^* \tag{15.61}$$

$$N_{2,p}/\Xi \propto 0(1)p^{*2}\ln p^* \tag{15.62}$$

where

$$\Xi \equiv \phi\sigma_{12}^0\text{Pe}^{-1/3} \tag{15.63}$$

For infinite discs $(p^* \to 0)$ the right-hand side of eqns (15.60)–(15.62) should read $3/p^*$, $0\cdot3p^*$ and $-0\cdot08/p^*$, respectively. It is evident that in the presence of Brownian motion the rate of shear dependence for $\sigma_{12,p}$, $N_{1,p}$ and $N_{2,p}$ for rods and for discs is expected to be the same, a cube root of

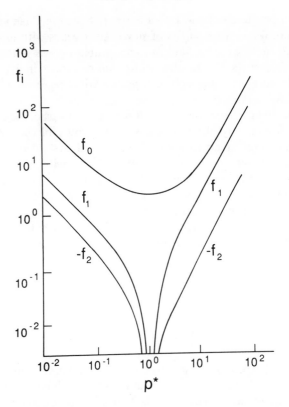

Fig. 15.9. Functionals f_i versus particle aspect ratio p^*; $p^* < 1$ for discs, $p^* > 1$ for fibers.

the strain rate, $\dot{\gamma}^{1/3}$. Newer theoretical developments in suspension rheology can also be found.[123–127]

As evidenced by eqns (15.54) and (15.55), the origin of suspension elasticity lies in anisometry of particles; rotation of asymmetric particles provides a mechanism for energy storage, Brownian motion for its recovery. For suspensions of spheres this mechanism does not exist and N_1 is expected to vanish, although owing to inertial effects within a wide range of Reynolds numbers, Re $\leqslant 21\cdot6$, negative values of N_1 were predicted:[127]

$$N_1 = \rho\phi(d\dot{\gamma})^2(0\cdot287\mathrm{Re}^{1/2} - 4/3) \qquad (15.64)$$

where ρ and d are respectively particle density and average diameter.

There is very little experimental information on N_1 for suspensions of spheres in Newtonian liquids. In a recent publication Chan and Powell[128] stated that, for up to $\phi = 0.3$ of sieved glass beads with $d = 25\text{--}28\,\mu\text{m}$ suspended in Newtonian fluid, no measurable N_1 was found in the full range of $\dot{\gamma} \leqslant 10^2\,(\text{s}^{-1})$. The observation was confirmed in dynamic testing where the storage modulus $G' \simeq 0$ was found. Krieger and Choi[70,121] also reported $N_1 \simeq 0$.

Lem and Han[129] reported $N_1 \simeq 0$ for calcium carbonate and for clay suspensions in nearly-Newtonian unsaturated low molecular weight polyester at loadings of up to about $30\,\text{vol}\%$ and $\dot{\gamma} \leqslant 10^2\,(\text{s}^{-1})$. However, suspension of high density polyethylene particles with $d = 20$ and $40\,\mu\text{m}$ showed positive values of N_1 at low loadings and negative at high loading. For $20\,\mu\text{m}$ particles the change of sign occurred at $\phi = 0.2\text{--}0.25$ and $\dot{\gamma} = 30\,(\text{s}^{-1})$, and for $40\,\mu\text{m}$ particles at $\phi \simeq 0.26$ and $\dot{\gamma} \simeq 10\,(\text{s}^{-1})$.

Theoretically[130] the interparticle interactions contribute directly and via modification of microstructure to the elastic stress component of spherical suspensions:

$$\langle \mathbf{S}^{\text{P}} \rangle N = \sum_{i=2}^{N} \sum_{j<i} \mathbf{r}_{ij} \mathbf{F}_{ij} \tag{15.65}$$

where N is the number of particles, $\mathbf{r}_{ij}$ center-to-center separation of i and j particles with pairwise interparticle interaction force $\mathbf{F}_{ij}$.

One would expect the elastic stress contribution in suspension of spheres in Newtonian liquids to be observed either at high concentrations or in strongly interacting systems. Gadala-Maria[131,132] reported that, for suspensions of polystyrene spheres ($d = 40\text{--}50\,\mu\text{m}$) in silicone oil at $\phi \leqslant 0.55$, N_1 increased linearly with $\dot{\gamma}$. The same result was obtained by Brady and Bossis in their numerical simulation experiment.[97] In lieu of a summary, the N_1 results for suspensions of spheres in Newtonian liquid are schematically illustrated in Fig. 15.10.

The suspensions of anisometric particles in Newtonian liquids are expected to show elastic effects. Indeed, for large N_1,[133-136] Weissenberg rod-climbing effects[57,64,137-139] and large capillary entrance–exit pressure drops (or Bagley correction)[57,58,136] were reported. On the other hand, not unexpectedly, no increase in extrudate swell was observed in the presence of anisometric particles.[137]

The report by Goto et al.[136] provides the most detailed insight into the N_1 behavior of fiber suspensions in Newtonian liquids:

$$N_1 = \phi A_0 \dot{\gamma}^{A_1} \tag{15.66}$$

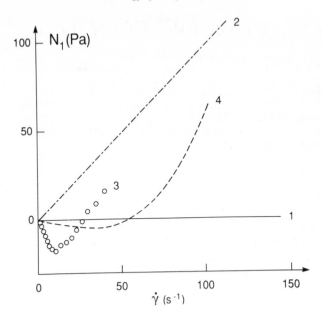

Fig. 15.10. Schematic of N_1 versus $\dot{\gamma}$ dependence for suspension of spheres in Newtonian liquids. 1. Theory and experiments for $\phi \leqslant 0\cdot3$.[122,128] 2. Theory and experiments for $\phi > 0\cdot4$.[130-132] 3. PE powder, $\phi = 0\cdot258$.[129] 4. Theory for non-interacting spheres suspensions[127] (not to scale).

with

$$A_0 = a_0 + a_1 \phi \tag{15.67}$$

and

$$A_1 = a_2 - a_3 \phi^2 \tag{15.68}$$

The values of a_i are listed in Table 15.5. The exponent A_1 for spheres = 1, while for fibers, depending on their flexibility, aspect ratio and concentration, $A_1 \simeq 0\cdot5$–$1\cdot5$. Note that for most suspensions $\phi p > 1$, i.e. the systems are concentrated without the possibility of free rotation of rigid fibers. As the concentration increases, A_1 decreases toward fractional values. There appears to be no correlation between A_1 and p. On the other hand A_0, which is an intensity factor, increases with p. However, interestingly enough for flexible Nylon and Vinylon fibers, A_0 is one order of magnitude larger than would be expected on the basis of the rigid fiber aspect ratio.

TABLE 15.5

Empirical Constants in Eqns (15.67) and (15.68) for Fiber Suspensions in Glycerin[136]

No.	Fiber	p	$\phi \times 10^3$	a_0	$a_1 \times 10^{-2}$	a_2	$a_3 \times 10^{-2}$
1.	Glass	150	5, 10, 15	0	90·6	1·24	26
2.		300	2·5, 5, 7·5, 10	236	270	1·02	26
3.	Carbon	143	2·5, 5, 10	10	36	1·53	38
4.		429	2·5, 5, 10	40	434	1·31	54
5.	Nylon	200	2·5, 5, 10	232	960	0·89	23
6.		300	2·5, 5, 10	2640	2720	0·78	23
7.	Vinylon	286	2·5, 5, 10	6900	0	0·78	23

The oscillatory (or dynamic-mechanical) testing of suspensions is gaining acceptance. The method is particularly suitable for studying suspensions of anisometric particles with well defined structures. One recent review included no reference whatsoever to dynamic testing in Newtonian liquids.[140] Ganani and Powell measured the dynamic behavior of spheres in Newtonian liquid, reporting that dynamic viscosity, η', behaves in a similar way to the steady state viscosity, and the storage modulus, G', in a similar way to N_1, i.e. for $\phi \leqslant 0.3$, $G' = N_1 \simeq 0$.

The rheological properties of pigment suspensions in dynamic fields were reviewed by Amari and Watanabe.[115] Owing to strong interparticle interactions in these colloidal dispersions, strongly non-Newtonian, as well as non-linear, viscoelastic behavior was observed.[141]

The dynamic measurements of suspensions of photosensitive PS spheres in diethyl phthalate at $\phi = 0.27-0.30$ allowed the authors[79] to demonstrate the effects of interactions on G', G'' and the relaxation spectrum H. They concluded that enhanced interactions and resulting aggregate formation shift the average relaxation time to higher values, in turn causing large increases in G' and G'' at low frequencies, ω. The dynamic tests were found to provide means for simple and detailed analysis of the aggregation process.

15.2.2.4. Transient Effects

In any system in which the structure changes with time upon imposition of stress, the transient effects should provide an important source of information. Doi's theoretical predictions of the stress growth in shear for semi-concentrated suspensions of fibers are schematically illustrated in Fig. 15.11.[142]

An ingenious experiment on dilute suspensions of rods ($\phi \leqslant 0.023$)

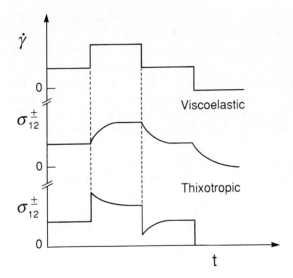

Fig. 15.11. Theoretical prediction of the shear rate variation effects on the stress growth and decay functions for viscoelastic and thixotropic liquids (after Doi[142]).

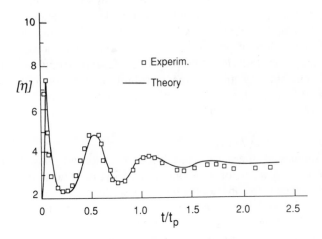

Fig. 15.12. Experimental (points) and theoretical (line) variation of intrinsic viscosity with reduced time; fibers with $p = 5.2$ were initially aligned normal to the shear direction, $\dot{\gamma} = 2.51\,\mathrm{s}^{-1}$.[143]

initially aligned (by application of an electrical field) normal to the direction of shear was described by Ivanov et al.[143,144] As shown in Fig. 15.12, there is excellent agreement with theory.[145,146] The shear stress varies in a periodic, damped fashion with t/t_p. The origin of the periodicity is the rotation of fibers in the shear field as predicted by eqn (15.17). The value of $[\eta]$ for aluminium coated Nylon fibers with $p = 5.05$ was observed to vary from 9.7 (perpendicular) to 2.3 (parallel orientation). This indicates that, due to Brownian motion, there is about 29° misalignment during one cycle.

Problems associated with start-up responses of semi-concentrated fiber suspensions in shear and extension were discussed by Dinh and Armstrong.[125] As shown in Fig. 15.13, the effects on N_1^+ and particularly on N_2^+ are predicted to be very large indeed. The theory for shear stress growth was tested in a later publication.[126] Unfortunately neither N_1^+ nor N_2^+ was measured. The authors concluded that, in good agreement with theory, η_r increased with ϕp^2, η^+ depended on total strain $\gamma = \dot{\gamma}t$, and η^+ versus γ showed a small local maximum.

The transient effects in suspensions of spheres have been discussed by Quemada et al.[120] and Chan and Powell.[128]

15.2.3. Suspensions in Non-Newtonian Liquids
The flow of polymer melts or solutions containing solid particles is discussed here. Earlier work in this field has been reviewed by Han,[147] and more recently by several other authors.[9,11,13,47,52,80,84,115,140,148–152] There is a growing interest in the flow of polymeric composites filled with anisometric, i.e. reinforcing, particles. Here, the properties depend strongly on the flow induced morphology and on the distribution of residual stresses. To optimize the processing and properties, it is important to know both the melt rheology and the orientation of the dispersed phase.

15.2.3.1. Newtonian Flows
In the absence of interlayer slip, addition of a second phase leads to an increase in zero-shear, or Newtonian viscosity, η_0. The simplest way to treat the system is to consider the relative viscosity as a function of volume loading, particle aspect ratio and orientation. There is no difference between the flow of suspensions in Newtonian liquids (see Section 15.3.2.1) and that of polymeric composites when the focus is on Newtonian flow. In order to observe Newtonian behavior of suspensions the flow of the medium must be Newtonian. This can be fairly well achieved for model systems based on polymer solutions, but rarely for commercial

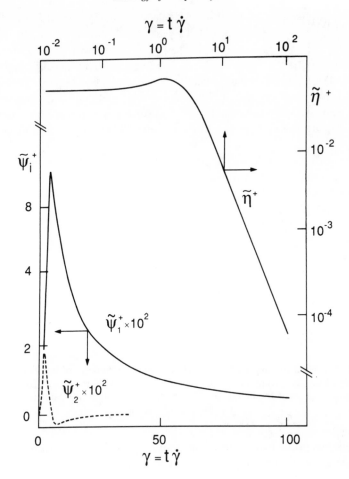

Fig. 15.13. The dimensionless stress growth coefficients for fiber suspensions versus shear strain; $\tilde{\eta}^+$ viscosity, $\tilde{\Psi}_1^+$ first normal stress difference, and $\tilde{\Psi}_2^+$ second normal stress difference.[125]

polymers. Frequently the dilemma is solved by using relative magnitude at the constant stress viscosity:

$$\eta_{rs} = \eta(\text{suspension})/\eta(\text{medium}) \text{ at } \sigma_{12} = \text{const} \qquad (15.69)$$

for relative viscosity of suspensions. An example of this treatment is shown in Fig. 15.14. The break in the dependence, indicating a sudden

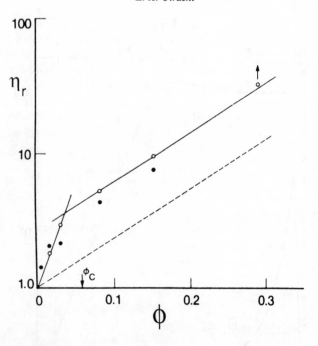

Fig. 15.14. Semi-log dependence of relative viscosity versus volume fraction for mica filled polyethylene; the broken line was calculated from eqn (15.70), and the solid lines represent the behavior below and above ϕ_c with intrinsic viscosities of 51·6 and 8·5, respectively.

decrease of $[\eta]$, coincides with the beginning of the concentrated region. The data are plotted in terms of the equation

$$\ln\eta_r = k[\eta]\phi \qquad (15.70)$$

Equation (15.70) is a simplified version of Martin's equation

$$\ln(\eta_{sp}/\phi[\eta]_s) = k_M[\eta]\phi \qquad (15.71)$$

k_M and $[\eta]_a$ were taken as adjustable parameters; with $\eta_{sp} = \eta_r - 1$, eqn (15.71) was proposed for suspensions by Bundenberg de Jong *et al.*[153] in 1932. Ten years later the relation was adopted for polymer solutions by Martin[154] and it has been known since as 'Martin's equation', valid for a wide range of concentrations in weakly interacting systems.

15.2.3.2. Non-Newtonian Flows

In Section 15.2.2 the non-Newtonian behavior of suspensions in New-tonian liquids was discussed. The effects observed for suspensions in polymeric fluids originate either from the non-Newtonian behavior of the medium or from the presence of filler particles. The problems associated with the first type have been discussed in the last two paragraphs of Section 15.2.3.1; those associated with the second type can best be discuss-ed under separate titles: yield, steady state; dynamic and extensional flows; and orientation and structure.

(a) Yield stress. As mentioned in Sections 15.2.2.1–15.2.2.3, yield occurs as a result of structure formation due to physical crowding of particles,[65,66] interparticle interactions[80] or steric-elastic effects of the medium.[70,121] Depending on the stability of the structure, the true or apparent yield stress can be obtained.

In Table 15.6 more recent examples of the polymer/filler systems with yield stress are listed. Similarly to suspensions in Newtonian liquids, the ones in molten polymer show yield stress due to crowding (highly con-centrated composite suspensions of large spheres,[112,166] fibers,[176-179] flakes[51,52,55,172,173] or interparticle interactions (carbon black, fumed silica, $CaCO_3$, etc.). So far, no σ_y has been reported due to steric-elastic effects. However, there is little doubt that the effect exists, even if not identified to date. In Fig. 15.15 an example of yield stress effect on G' in the PE/mica system is shown.[51] Determination of σ_y by means of the modified Casson equation (15.43) is illustrated in Fig. 15.7.

It is worth stressing that yield affects not only shear stress or loss behavior but also the normal stress or storage modulus.[11] Equation (15.43) has been successfully used substituting both G' as well as G'' for F. The magnitude of calculated yield values are not necessarily equal; for examined systems $G'_y > G''_y$ was obtained. Neglecting the yield stress (apparent or not) may have serious consequences on proper interpretation of elasticity.

(b) Elastic effects. There are several measures of the elastic effects: direct (e.g. N_1, N_2, G') or indirect (e.g. extrudate swell, B, entrance–exit pressure drop, P_e). It is customary to plot the measure of the elastic component versus that of the shear component: N_1 versus σ_{12}, G' versus G'', etc. For rheologically simple systems the dependencies are indepen-dent of temperature.[147]

White et al.[180] reported that, at constant $\phi = 0.2$ and σ_{12}, addition of

TABLE 15.6

Experimental Observation of Yield Stress in Filled Polymers

No.	Polymer	Filter	Concentration wt%	Concentration ϕ	Rheol. function	Range	Ref.
1.	Polypropylene (PP)	Talc	10–40		η	$\dot\gamma < 0.3$	155
2.	Polyisobutylene (PIB)	Carbon black	$w \leqslant 30$		η	$\dot\gamma < 10^{-3}$	156
3.	Solution of PIB in decalin	Glass beads, $d \simeq 30\,\mu m$		0.4	η	$\dot\gamma^* < 30$	157
4.	Polystyrene (PS)	Glass spheres, $d = 36$–$124\,\mu m$		0.51	η	$\dot\gamma < 0.1$	112
5.	Polyethylene (PE) Ionomer	Methyl methacrylate grafted Perlite, $d = 5.5\,\mu m$	$w < 30$	0.15	η	$\dot\gamma < 0.3$ $\dot\gamma < 1$	158
6.	PS	Carbon black		0.25	η, η', G'	$\dot\gamma, \omega < 0.3$	159
7.	PE	$CaCO_3$	40		η	$\dot\gamma < 10^{-2}$	160
8.	Aqueous solution of polyacrylamide (PAA)	Crosslinked PS particles, $d = 175\,\mu m$	$\leqslant 20$		G', G''	$\omega < 0.3$	161
9.	PS	$CaCO_3$, TiO_2, and Carbon black, $d \leqslant 500\,\mu m$	< 30		η_E^+	$\dot\gamma < 0.1$ $\dot\varepsilon < 0.5$	162,163
10.	PE, PS, PVC	$CaCO_3$	30, 40		G', G''	$\omega < 3$	164
11.	SBS, EPDM	Talc		0.17	η	$\sigma_{12} < 10^5\,Pa$	165
12.	PE	Steel spheres, $d = 15\,\mu m$		$\leqslant 0.7$	G', G''	$\omega < 10^2$	166
13.	Polydimethylsiloxane (PDMS)	Silica spheres, $d = 150\,nm$		$\leqslant 0.1$	η, N_1	$\dot\gamma < 1$	167
14.	PDMS	Fumed silica, $d \simeq 8\,nm$	$\leqslant 4.75$		η, N_1 η^-	variable	168 169

TABLE 15.6—*contd.*

No.	Polymer	Filler	Concentration wt%	φ	Rheol. function	Range	Ref.
15.	PVC	Glass beads, d = 38–44 μm			η', G'	$\omega < 0·1$	170
16.	Polyester elastomer, styrene–isoprene–styrene (SIS), PE, polyurethane (PU)	Ferrite, d ≃ 3 μm	≤85		η	$\dot{\gamma} < 200$	171
17.	PE	Mica, d ≃ 100 μm, p = 35	≤60	≤0·29	η', G'	$\omega < 1$	51, 172
					η_E^+		52, 173
18.	PP	Mica, d ≃ 100 μm, p = 35	≤60	≤0·29	η', G'	$\phi \geqslant 0·08$	55
19.	PE, PP	CaCO$_3$	≤56	≤0·34	η	$\sigma_{12} < 10^3$ Pa, $\dot{\gamma} < 0·1$	174, 175
20.	PE	Glass fibers, L = 430 μm, p = 14, and carbon fibers, L = 123 μm, p = 15	≤24	≤0·28, ≤0·11	η		176
21.	PE	Glass fibers, L = 434 μm, p = 31	30		η	$\dot{\gamma} < 1$	177
22.	PP	Glass fibers, L = 0·3–2 mm, d = 10 μm	≤40		G'	Strain dependence	178
23.	PP	Glass fibers, L ≤ 3 mm, d = 10 μm			η_E^+	$\dot{\varepsilon} < 0·1$	179

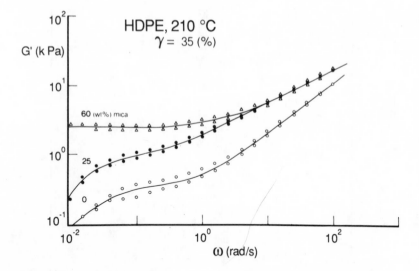

Fig. 15.15. Loss modulus versus frequency for high density polyethylene–mica at 210 °C.[51]

particulate fillers (glass beads, Franklin fibers, TiO_2, $CaCO_3$, carbon black or mica) to polystyrene (PS) lowers N_1. An opposite effect was observed for polycarbonate filled with glass fibers.[181,182] In the absence of a yield stress, as ϕ increased, the constant stress value of N_1 increased as well: $N_1(\sigma_{12} = \text{const}) \propto \phi$, in agreement with theoretical[122] and experimental[136] observations for fiber suspensions in Newtonian liquids. The difference in rheological behavior between fibers and flakes cannot be justified on theoretical grounds. Experimentally, the observations of White *et al.*[180] on the effects of mica additions to PS were confirmed by Utracki *et al.*[11,55] with data on polypropylene/mica systems. These results are illustrated in Fig. 15.16. At low deformation rates, the effects of yield on G' and G'' forced the curves to collapse into one. The effect was subtracted by plotting $(G' - G'_y)$ versus $(G'' - G''_y)$. It is evident that, as ϕ increases, the $(G' - G'_y)$ decreases at a constant value of $(G'' - G''_y)$.

When the elastic effects are compared at constant deformation rates a slightly different picture emerges. For fiber or flake filled polymer melts, an increase in ϕ results in an increase in N_1 or G', more pronounced for fibers, less so for flakes (see Fig. 15.15). For particulates the situation is less clear. Carbon black filled PS indicated[159] a strong increase of N_1 and G' with ϕ at constant rate of deformation. Similar effects were reported for suspensions of PS particles in aqueous solutions of polyacrylamide,[16] PS

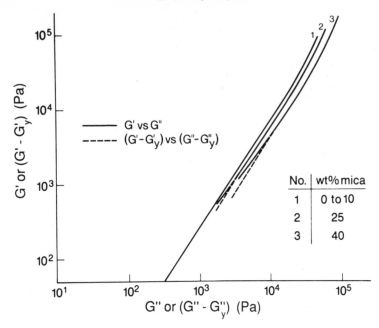

Fig. 15.16. G' versus G'' (solid lines) and $(G' - G'_y)$ versus $(G'' - G''_y)$ (broken lines) for polypropylene with mica at 180 °C.[11,55]

filled with TiO_2 or $CaCO_3$,[162] PE filled with steel spheres[166] or poly-dimethylsiloxane filled with silica spheres.[167] On the other hand, the N_1 (calculated from the slit rheometer pressure drop) of polypropylene filled with $CaCO_3$,[183] and that directly measured in a rotational rheometer for suspensions of uniform glass spheres in polyisobutylene solution[184] both decreased with ϕ at constant deformation rate.

There is little doubt that the addition of solids to polymer melts reduces the extrudate swell, B. In Fig. 15.17, B versus mica content in polypropylene at two shear rates is shown.[11,55] The phenomenon is well documented in the literature.[159,177,181,185–188] Crowson and Folkes[188] reported that B depends on the ratio $L/2D$, where L is fiber length and D capillary diameter. For $2D < L$, swelling was considerably larger ($B \simeq 5$) than when $2D > L$. Such an observation suggests that one reason for low swelling is the axial alignment of fibers. However, the situation is more complex since B is observed to decrease with ϕ for spherical particles or even for carbon black filled rubbers.[187] It seems that the low extrudate swell of composites originates in a flat flow profile related to yield stress.

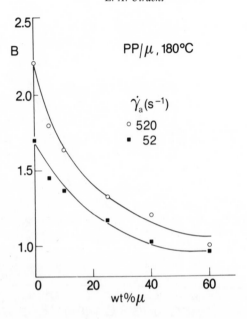

Fig. 15.17. Extrudate swell ratio, B, versus mica content in PP at 180 °C and at two apparent rates of shear, $\dot{\gamma}_a = 52$ and $520\,s^{-1}$.[11,55]

Plug flow at low filler content has frequently been reported.[14,189] If, during the flow, only a relatively thin annular layer of material undergoes deformation, the strain recovery can be expected to originate only in that layer. If, in addition, the material has a yield stress, then at the die exit only the shear $\sigma_{12} > \sigma_y$ can relax.

The entrance–exit pressure drop, P_e, in capillary or slit flow has been used as an indirect measure of elasticity.[190] However, recent computer simulations indicate[191–193] that increases of N_1 should lower, not augment, P_e. P_e appears to be linked to velocity rearrangements at the capillary entrance with not only σ_{12} and N_1 but also with the extensional properties playing an important role.[193] Cogswell[194] calculated the energy loss in free convergence due to the extensional field. It was recently demonstrated that these effects account for about 1/3 of total energy loss.[195]

Effects of particulate additions on P_e of polymer melts have seldom been reported. A sharp reduction of P_e at constant shear stress has been observed for the polypropylene/CaCO$_3$ system.[182] Addition of fibers[136,137] or flakes[55] to non-Newtonian fluids has an opposite effect. However, the latter publication showed that the effect depends on σ_{12}; at $\sigma_{12} > 10^5$ Pa, P_e seems to decrease with filler loading, although instabilities are suspected in this shear stress range.

(c) Extensional flows. The yield stress in extension, $\sigma_{11,y}$, has also been observed.[52,55,159,163,173,178,179,196] Yield stress is apparent in two related dependencies: (i) as a vertical displacement in the stress growth function at decreasing strain rates (see Fig. 15.18); and (ii) as a deviation from the theory at vanishing strain rates, $\dot{\varepsilon} \to 0$.[197] In agreement with the von Mises criterion, $\sigma_{11,y}/\sigma_y = 1 \cdot 3$–2 has been reported.[52]

For suspensions of uniform glass spheres in a 4% polyisobutylene solution the Trouton ratio decreased with ϕ.[184] At higher strains ($\varepsilon \simeq 4$) the decrease is by about a factor of 2. These results confirmed the early observation for the glass beads filled styrene–acrylonitryle (SAN) system[198] illustrated in Fig. 15.19. In the latter case the flow was Troutonian, with η_E independent of the rate of straining at $\dot{\varepsilon} \simeq 7 \times 10^{-6}$ to 7×10^{-4} (s^{-1}). Nicodemo *et al.*[199] argued that in extensional flow only the liquid undergoes deformation, and both η_E and ε should be corrected by

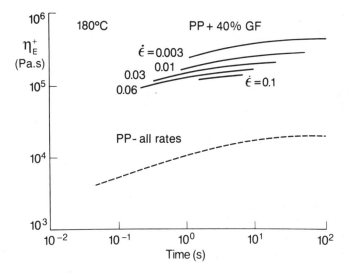

Fig. 15.18. Stress growth functions for PP (bottom curve) and for PP with 40 wt% of glass fiber (GF) (top five curves) at 180 °C; at different $\dot{\varepsilon}$ the functions superimpose for PP but not for PP/GF.[179]

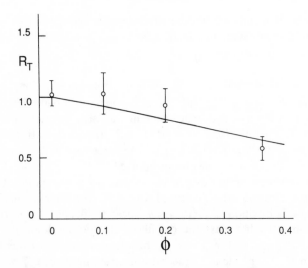

Fig. 15.19. Trouton ratio for glass spheres in SAN.[198]

dividing these quantities by a factor of $[1 - (\phi/\phi_m)^{2/3}]$. However, if the sample is strained volumetrically, as in the Nazem and Hill experiment, the correction should be $(1 - \phi/\phi_m)^{2/3}$. Using this factor $R_T = 1.05 \pm 0.11$ and the data in Fig. 15.19 were calculated.

The uniaxial elongational flow of polymer melts filled with small particles (carbon black, TiO_2, $CaCO_3$) has been a subject of investigation by White _et al._[159,162,163,200] Here the yield stress dominated the behavior. Experimental values of the ratio $\sigma_{11,y}/\sigma_y = 1.2$–$1.9$ were calculated in good agreement with the von Mises theoretical value of $\sqrt{3}$.

White and Tanaka[163] proposed a simple constitutive equation

$$\sigma_{11} - \sigma_{11,y} = 3\eta\dot{\varepsilon} \tag{15.72}$$

where η was taken as

$$\eta = G\tau^*/[(1 - 2\tau^*\dot{\varepsilon})(1 + \tau^*\dot{\varepsilon})] \tag{15.73}$$

with G and τ^* being respectively shear modulus and relaxation time. The theory is general, allowing for selection of a memory function $H(t)$ leading to expressions for η different from that in eqn (15.73).

For the power law model

$$\sigma_{12} = \sigma_1\dot{\gamma}^n \tag{15.74}$$

where $\sigma_1 = \sigma_{12}$ at $\dot\gamma = 1$ is the consistency index, Kawase and Ulbrecht[201] derived the expression

$$\sigma_1 = 2\sigma_{1,0}U[(6 + 4x^5)/(6 - 9x + 9x^5 - 6x^6)]^{n-1} \quad (15.75)$$

where $\sigma_{1,0}$ is the consistency index for the dispersing liquid:

$$U = [4n(2n - 1)(n + 1)U_1 - 12U_2 + 2U_3 + 3(n - 1)/2 - 9n(n - 1)$$
$$\times (6 + 4x^5)/2(2n + 1)(6 - 9x + 9x^5 - x^6)]$$
$$\times [3 (2 + 29n - 22n^2)/(2n + 1)] \quad (15.76)$$

$$U_1 = \{(1/2) + [(3 + 2x^5)n(n - 1)(2x^2 - 3/x + 7x - 6 - 6x\ln x)]/$$
$$[2(2 - 3x + 3x^5 - 2x^6)(2n + 1)]\}/[2(2n^2 + n)x^{-2n-3}/3$$
$$- (2n^2 + n)x^{-2n-2} + (2n^2/3 + n/3 - 1)x^{-2n}$$
$$- 2nx + (2n + 1)] \quad (15.77)$$

$$U_2 = -n(2n + 1)U_1x^{-2n-3}/3 + [(3 + 2x^5)n(n - 1)/$$
$$2x^2 (2 - 3x + 3x^5 - 2x^6)(2n + 1)] \quad (15.78)$$

$$U_3 = 2nU_1 - 3U_2 + 3n(n - 1)(3 + 2x^5)/$$
$$[(2 - 3x + 3x^5 - 2x^6)(2n + 1)] \quad (15.79)$$

where $1/x$ is the dimensionless radius of the model cell:

$$x = \phi/\phi_m \quad (15.80)$$

Equations (15.74)–(15.80) with $\phi_m = 0.605$ and $n \simeq 0.7$ provided excellent descriptions of the experimental data. It would be interesting to introduce into eqn (15.71) the expression

$$\eta = (\sigma_{12} + \sigma_y)/\dot\gamma \quad (15.81)$$

with $\sigma_{12} = \sigma_{12}(\phi, \dot\gamma, n)$ given by eqns (15.74) to (15.80).

A simpler dependence for suspensions in a power-law fluid (without the yield) was proposed by Goddard:[202]

$$\eta_{E,r} = \eta_E(\phi, \dot\varepsilon)/\eta_E(0, \dot\varepsilon) = 1 + 2\phi R_T p^{n+1}\{(1 - n)/n$$
$$\times [1 - (\pi/\phi)^{(n-1)/2n}]\}^n/(2 + n) \quad (15.82)$$

Equation (15.82) was found[173] to describe the η_E dependence of a PE/mica system well, provided the yield stress is first subtracted by means of Casson's equation (15.43).

Suetsugu and White[203] proposed a comprehensive constitutive equation for polymer melts containing small particles, which exhibit time dependent (thixotropic) responses combined with yield and non-linear viscoelastic behavior. For extensional steady state flow, eqn (15.73) was again applicable. However, to accommodate the non-linearity, the relaxation time was assumed to depend on the deformation rate:

$$\tau^* \; = \; \tau_0/(1 \; + \; \sqrt{3}a\tau_0\dot{\varepsilon}) \tag{15.83}$$

where a is a material constant. For PS with carbon black or $CaCO_3$, good agreement was obtained taking $a = 0.4$ and $\tau_0 = 5.4$ (s). The value of σ_y varied from 0.7 to 40 (kPa) depending on d and ϕ.

The recent constitutive equation proposed by Armstrong and coworkers[125,126] for semi-concentrated suspensions of anisometric particles in Newtonian liquids provides an elegant starting point for extension into non-Newtonian media. This may lead to a comprehensive and conceptually clear theory for polymeric composites.

Since elongational flow is irrotational, the particles should align with the stress. Composites with initially random orientation of fibers or flakes must have a period of rearrangement. At higher loading this results in a noisy stress signal observed for PE/mica[173] and PP/glass fiber[179] systems (see Fig. 15.20).

Efforts to study strain recovery and stress relaxation in systems containing flakes and fibers were unsuccessful. The phenomena seem to be complex, requiring multiple exponential decay functions and yield stresses.

(d) Final comments. To date, the systems considered have contained single types of particles: spheres, discs, fibers, etc. However, commercial materials are frequently more complex. Milewski[204] found synergistic performance effects when different filler types were combined. In general, the 'micro-packing' increased ϕ_m, enabling either use of less resin (i.e. high modulus product) or improvement of flowability at constant ϕ.[205] However, care must be taken to prevent undesirable behavior resulting from incorporation of fibers. As an example, in Fig. 15.21 the relative shear viscosity for suspensions containing $\phi = 0.15$ of glass fillers in silicone oil is shown. The composition of the filler changes from 100% spheres to 100% fibers. Yield stress in all compositions containing $\geq 20\%$ of fibers is evident.[206] Dilatant behavior for suspensions containing $\geq 60\%$ of spheres should be noted. When discussing suspensions of rigid anisometric particles, care must be taken in defining the aspect ratio. Flakes of

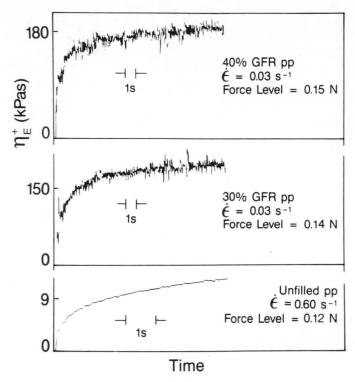

Fig. 15.20. Stress growth for PP filled with 0, 30 and 40 wt% of glass fiber at 180 °C; the elongational rates were selected in order to obtain a similar stress level.[179]

mica or glass, fibers of glass or carbon black, fibers of nylon, vinylon, cellulose etc. break or coil. These effects are well documented[6,51,55,172,207,208] but frequently ignored when interpreting results.

Other phenomena which complicate flow during rheological testing as well as in melt processing are related to flow instabilities. These may originate from filler coating or 'sizing' agents. Migration of the surface active ingredient to the die wall may cause a slip-stick flow instability, independently of whether the filler is present or not.[209] Similar types of behavior may be due to decreased maximum strain at break of the matrix on addition of fillers with poor affinity to it. During extensional flow in the convergent die region the flow lines break and reform.[210] This mechanism could provide an explanation for the oscillatory flow of the PP/glass fiber

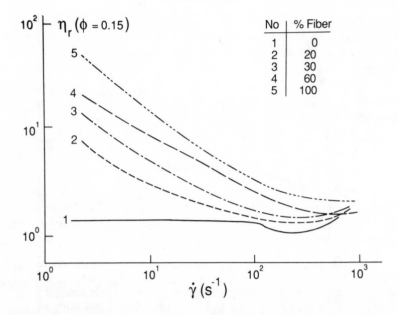

Fig. 15.21. Relative viscosity of glass spheres and fibers suspension in silicon oil at $\phi = 0.15$; composition of filler varies from 100% spheres to 100% fiber.[205]

system.[211] Still another type of instability, called 'order-disorder' transition, was presented by Wu.[212] The effect appears to be related to the orientation and packing of fibers in polyethyleneterephthalate (PET).

There are several reports indicating that additions of a small amount of filler may reduce the viscosity and improve stability in shear or extension.[52,173,178] The effects can sometimes be quite large: addition of $\phi \simeq 0.001$ of $2\,\mu$m diameter glass powder to PS melts resulted in reductions of η by 45%,[213] and addition of $\phi \simeq 0.05$–0.08 of mica to PE melts increased the values of the maximum strain at break from $\varepsilon_b \simeq 1$ to 2.7 at $\dot{\varepsilon} = 0.1\,\mathrm{s}^{-1}$.[173]

15.2.4. Orientation in Flow

Orientation of particles dispersed in Newtonian liquids was discussed in Sections 15.2.2.1 and 15.2.2.2. Overviews on rheology and structure development in polymeric liquid crystals have been published by Mansuripur[214] and White.[215]

The most powerful orientational fields are extensional. Using convergent and divergent flow channels it is possible to control orientation of anisometric particles. Most of the work in this area has been done with fiber-filled materials[151,152] but the effects are equally important for matrix polymers,[216] neat resins[217-220] or liquid crystals.[214,215]

According to Goettler,[151,152] plug flow may occur at $\phi \geqslant 0.05$ with the sheared layer less than 0·5 mm thick. The alignment is possible through the extensional flow in converging (or diverging) channels:

$$\frac{\tan \psi}{\tan \psi_0} = \left(\frac{A}{A_0}\right)^{3\theta/2} \tag{15.84}$$

where ψ is the angle between fiber axis and its local streamline, $\theta \equiv (p^2 - 1)/(p^2 + 1)$, A is the cross-sectional area of the channel, and subscript 0 indicates the initial position.

Vincent[221] derived the following dependence for convergent flow:

$$\tan \psi = C \exp(-3\varepsilon\theta/2) \tag{15.85}$$

where C is an integration constant dependent on the initial angle of the fiber, and ε is the extensional strain, $\varepsilon = \dot{\varepsilon}t$. The equivalence of these two equations is not accidental, since both are based on the same theoretical model.[222] Equation (15.84) or (15.85) approximates the experimental data quite well, except large strains (or convergence ratios) where the angle ψ tended toward a minimum value of 10–15°, instead of the predicted zero. The discrepancy is primarily due to shear flow at the wall, not taken into account by these equations.

There is less information on the orientation of platelets. In converging flow these particles are less susceptible to orientation. In fact there is conflicting information on the alignment of mica particles in the extruded strands. Okuno and Woodhams[223] reported that, near the center-line, mica flakes in polypropylene are aligned perpendicularly to the flow direction, with a progressive change toward parallel orientation near the surface. More recently[9,51,55] the orientation of mica in HDPE and PP was shown to be uniform throughout the full cross-section of the extrudate; it seems that in this case the platelets aligned themselves in concentric circles, parallel to the capillary wall and to the direction of flow. The orientation improved with increase of $\dot{\gamma}$. Recent experiments on flow orientation of mica flakes in PP during extrusion reported by Remillard and Fisa[224] point out a surprisingly large effect of vapors and gases adsorbed on the filler surface.

By contrast with rods, platelets undergo a two-stage orientation. Upstream from the die they are randomly oriented. During the convergent flow into the die they orient with the flow. However, at that stage a cut perpendicular to the flow direction reveals a near-random orientation of the platelets in respect to the die wall. Thus, the second stage of orientation can only be accomplished during the residence time flow through a die (long die or slow flow).

Considering flow through a cone, Harris and Pittman[225] derived expressions for suspensions in Newtonian liquids, predicting that the alignment of rods should depend on the ratio of the initial and final position of the particle and be independent of convergence angle, flow rate, viscosity and aspect ratio. Takano reported[226] that for convergence angles larger than $120°$ there are stagnation regions. For $60°$ the alignment was observed to start upstream from the cone and achieve its limiting value Ω_{min} (where Ω is the average angle between the particle and cone axes) upstream from the cone end.[227]

The anisometric particle in shear flow rotates with the period given by eqn (15.17). Thus this flow was reported to have a disordering effect on particles aligned in the extensional flow field.[228-231] However, in Couette flow of dilute fiber suspensions there is preferential orientation on the central surface of the annulus.[14,82,221] At regular intervals fibers rapidly flip by $180°$, i.e. statistically, as shown in Fig. 15.5, they are preferentially aligned within the narrow portion of the annular gap.

To quantify the orientation of discontinuous fibers in composites, Pipes et al.[232] proposed the following relation between an effective elastic constant $\langle C_{ij} \rangle$ and orientation functions f_i and g_i:

$$\langle C_{ij} \rangle = C_{ij}^0 + f_i F(C_{ij}^0, \bar{C}_{ij}) + g_i G(C_{ij}^0, \bar{C}_{ij}) \qquad (15.86)$$

with functionals F and G depending on isotropic and combinatorial values of elastic constants. For $f_i = g_i = 0$ the isotropic value C^0 is recovered. For $f_i = g_i = 1$ a perfect alignment exists. In the case of planar orientation:

$$f_p = 2\langle \cos^2 \Psi \rangle - 1 \qquad (15.87)$$

$$g_p = (8\langle \cos^4 \Psi \rangle - 3)/5 \qquad (15.88)$$

with

$$\langle \cos^m \Psi \rangle = \int_0^{\pi/2} n_p(\Psi) \cos^m \Psi \, d\Psi \qquad (15.89)$$

Taking

$$n(\Psi) = k \cos \lambda \Psi: \qquad (15.90)$$

$$g_p = 2f_p(7 - 2f_p)/5(4 - 2f_p) \qquad (15.91)$$

with

$$0 \leqslant f_p, g_p \leqslant 1$$

Similarly, for axial orientation:

$$f_a = (3\langle\cos^2\Psi\rangle - 1)/2 \qquad (15.92)$$

$$g_a = (5\langle\cos^4\Psi\rangle - 1)/4 \qquad (15.93)$$

and assuming eqn (15.90)

$$g_a = 3f_a/(5 - 2f_a) \qquad (15.94)$$

Note that eqn (15.92) has a form proposed by Hermans and Platzek[233] to characterize molecular orientation in fibers from anisotropy of polarizability:

$$f_H = (\alpha_1 - \alpha_2)\Delta\alpha = (3\langle\cos^2\Psi_c\rangle - 1)/2 \qquad (15.95)$$

where α_1 and α_2 are polarizabilities in fiber axial and radial directions, $\Delta\alpha$ is the inherent polarizability difference and Ψ_c is the angle between the molecular backbone and fiber axis.

Menendez and White[234] measured, by X-ray diffraction, the orientation of chopped Kevlar fibers in a polymethylmethacrylate matrix during extrusion in a capillary rheometer. The authors calculated $\langle\cos^2\Psi\rangle$ and then, from eqn (15.95), $f_H = 0.154$ (reservoir), 0.455–0.488 (die) and 0.300 below the die.

The orientation has a profound effect on flow and hence processability.[177] Its effects on the performance of the finished product are even more dramatic.[235,236] Orientation plays an important role in injection molding where the anisometric particles may become oriented in a complex manner. Layered structures, weld lines, splice lines, swirls and surface blemishes are well known to practitioners. There is extensive literature on the subject. Mold geometry (e.g. inserts) and transient effects of the filled systems greatly complicate the predictive approach. The temperatures of the melt and the mold, as well as the mold geometry and injection rate, affect the shear and elongational fields,[228–230,237–247] leading to changes in orientation and performances of the moldings. At high injection rates, as the melt enters the cavity, there is a divergent flow and relatively slow solidification. This leads to a transverse alignment of fibers. At low injection rates, solidification reduces divergence so that fiber orientation, acquired upstream in the convergent part of the flow, is largely preserved. Theoretically and experimentally Vincent[221,248] demonstrated that, when designing a mold for composites with anisometric particles, the principles developed for simple melts should not be applied. The extent of divergence and convergence, length of flow channels, and selection of temperature profile must all be taken into account.

Due to reduced extrudate swell, gating must also be modified. As demonstrated by Crowson *et al.*[228-231] to prevent jetting (which leads to numerous weld lines and abominable mechanical performance), gate height should be equal to cavity depth. A review of processing of glass fiber filled melts has recently been published by Folkes.[249]

To close on an optimistic note, the sophistication of modern programs for computer simulation of injection molding already allows prediction, for simple geometries, of the distribution of residual stresses and of crystallinity.[250,251] In effect, the model predicts orientation on molecular (birefringence) and microstructural (crystallinity, tensile strength) levels. Hopefully the model will soon be extended to filled systems.

15.3. LIQUID-IN-LIQUID DISPERSIONS

Under this heading two types of system will be considered: those in which the Newtonian liquid forms the continuous phase, i.e. emulsions, and those where the viscoelastic liquid constitutes the matrix, i.e. polymeric alloys and blends.

15.3.1. Emulsion Rheology
Early works have been summarized by Sherman,[105,106] Barry[252] and Nielsen in his monograph.[253] The rheology of emulsions has also been discussed by Utracki *et al.*[11,254-257] as a model for flow of polymer blends and alloys.

15.3.1.1. Newtonian Flow
(a) *Infinite dilution.* Taylor extended Einstein's treatment to emulsions.[258] Neglecting the influence of the interphase, he expressed the intrinsic viscosity of the liquid droplets as

$$[\eta]_E = 2 \cdot 5(\eta_p + 2\eta_m/5)/(\eta_p + \eta_m) \qquad (15.96)$$

where subscripts E, p and m indicate respectively emulsion, droplet and medium. For $\eta_p \gg \eta_m$, Einstein's limit is recovered. At low concentration, and for $\eta_p \geqslant \eta_m$, eqn (15.96) is well obeyed.[259]

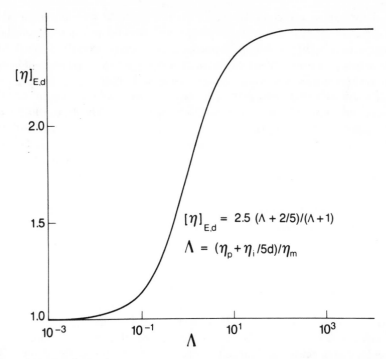

Fig. 15.22. Prediction by eqn (15.97) of the emulsion intrinsic viscosity versus Λ dependence, where Λ combines the influence of relative viscosity of the two liquids, droplet diameter and shear as well as extensional properties of the interface.

Droplet size, particle diameter and relative viscosity of the two phases, were considered by Oldroyd, who wrote[260]

$$[\eta]_{E,d} = 2 \cdot 5(\eta_p + 2\eta_m/5 + \eta_i/5d)/(\eta_p + \eta_m + \eta_i/5d) \quad (15.97)$$

where $\eta_i = 2\eta_{si} + 3\eta_{ei}$ expresses the shear, η_{si}, and extensional η_{ei}, viscosities of the interface. Defining the parameter Λ as

$$\Lambda = (\eta_p + \eta_i/5d)/\eta_m \quad (15.98)$$

the dependence $[\eta]_{E,d}$ versus Λ, shown in Fig. 15.22, was computed. For $\Lambda \to 0$ the solution value of the intrinsic viscosity is obtained, while for $\Lambda \to \infty$ the hard sphere suspension value is recovered. Equations (15.97) and (15.98) were found to be valid for a wide range of $\Lambda > 1 \cdot 3$.

(b) Dilute systems. For hard sphere suspensions, eqns (15.2) and (15.3) are valid in a full range of concentrations. For emulsions, in the absence

of deformation and coalescence, they can be used as well, provided $[\eta]_E$ and ϕ_m are treated as adjustable parameters, dependent primarily on the interphase.[261] This pragmatic approach has been successfully used to describe η versus ϕ variation for such complex systems as industrial latices (at various stages of conversion), plastisols and organosols.[40]

The emulsions are usually prepared as concentrated systems. In industrial emulsions containing $\phi \leqslant 0.99$ are being used. Owing to interface interactions and deformability of droplets, these systems behave rather like elastic, soft solids without any sign of Newtonian behavior. Between the highly concentrated and dilute regions there is a wide zone of structural change reflected in a spectrum of non-Newtonian behavior.

15.3.1.2. Non-Newtonian Flows

(a) Structures. Even in the dilute region, emulsion droplets rarely exist individually.[14] In most cases, droplets are polydispersed in size, forming structures or aggregates. Two types can be distinguished: (a) that formed by the shear field (e.g. skin–core structures in long tube flows); and (b) that formed by particle–particle interaction. Knowledge of type (a) structures is important for proper interpretation of the flow phenomena, as influenced by the flow profiles,[14,262–264] as well as of the shear coagulation.[265] Knowledge of type (b) structures is the key for utilization of suspension rheology in processing.[266] Since the effective volume fraction of dispersed particles increases with increase of association, the η_r is strongly affected. In general, η_r of these systems depends on shear history.[90]

By contrast with polymer blends (to be discussed in a later part of this chapter), emulsions are prepared by carefully designing the interface system and by sequential addition of ingredients. Both elements are essential when 99 vol% of one liquid must be dispersed in 1% of another. If, due to interactions of emulsifiers, the continuous phase becomes viscoelastic, the emulsion has high consistency or a 'body'. There is gradual passage of structures from rotating doublets in dilute systems to entrapment of the dispersed phase in a continuous network of interacting interphases. Consequently, emulsions do possess both a purely Newtonian character as well as a complex thixotropic and viscoelastic one.[252,253]

(b) Theoretical treatment. Cox and Mason[85] and Leal[87] reviewed the theoretical treatment of flow of two-phase systems.

The shear flow of dilute emulsions is controlled by two parameters:

$$\lambda \;\equiv\; \eta^{(1)}/\eta^{(2)} \tag{15.99}$$

$$\kappa \equiv \sigma_{12}/dv\eta^{(2)} \tag{15.100}$$

where the superscripts (1) and (2) indicate the dispersed and continuous phases, respectively, and v is the interfacial tension. The droplet deformability can be expressed as[258]

$$D \equiv (d_1 - d_2)/(d_1 + d_2) = (19\lambda/16 + 1)/\kappa(\lambda + 1) \tag{15.101}$$

where d_1 and d_2 are major and minor axes of the deformed ellipsoid. For small deformations eqn (15.101) predicts the conditions when the drop will burst[14]

$$\sigma_{12}/2dv\eta^{(2)} < (19\lambda/16 + 1)/(\lambda + 1) \tag{15.102}$$

(equivalent to $d_1 > 3d_2$), the rate of droplet migration away from the wall[85]

$$U = (33Dvd^3/4480y_0^2)(79\lambda^2 + \lambda + 54)/(\lambda + 1)^2 \tag{15.103}$$

(where y_0 is the distance of the droplet from the wall), or the first normal stress difference[267]

$$N_1 = \phi d(\sigma_{12}D\kappa)^2/40v \tag{15.104}$$

Equations (15.101)–(15.104) are strictly valid for dilute emulsions of monodispersed droplets with the interphase characterized only by the interfacial tension. On the basis of this simple model Oldroyd[260] derived an expression for the relaxation time:

$$\tau^* = d\eta^{(2)}D\kappa(2\lambda + 3)/40v \tag{15.105}$$

Two other models were considered, the first[260] where the interphase is characterized by four parameters (shear and tensile moduli and viscosities), and the second[268] in which the interphase is treated as the third component with two interfacial tension coefficients, v_1 and v_2, for the inner and outer interfaces. Both these models predict two relaxation times. Oosterbroek *et al.*[269] examined the problem experimentally. The authors noted that results can be equally well fitted to the first model with two sets of parameters describing very different physical situations, the first where the behavior is dominated by the interphase shear modulus, $G \gg v, E$ (E is the tensile modulus of the interphase), and the second where the interfacial tension dominates, $v \gg G, E$. This seems to put the first model in an ambiguous situation. Unfortunately the second model has not been experimentally tested. Its two relaxation times are given by

$$\tau_1^* = 5v_1v_2\eta^{(2)}d^3(\lambda + 1)/24\Delta^2(v_1 + v_2) \tag{15.106}$$

$$\tau_2^* = \eta^{(2)} dD\kappa(2\lambda + 3)/40(\nu_1 + \nu_2) \tag{15.107}$$

where Δ is the thickness of the interphase.

Acrivos and co-workers[270,271] theoretically studied deformation and breakup of single droplets suspended in another liquid under extensional, hyperbolic or shear fields. The theory leads to an integro-differential equation for the equilibrium shape of a drop which can be solved numerically. Approximate solutions for low and high deformation rates are respectively

$$\tilde{l} \simeq 3.50\tilde{G}^{1/2}; \quad \tilde{G} < 0.045 \tag{15.108}$$

$$\tilde{l} \simeq 261\tilde{G}^2 + 0.0231/\tilde{G}; \quad \tilde{G} > 0.05 \tag{15.109}$$

where $\tilde{l}$ and $\tilde{G}$ are the dimensionless half-length of a drop and non-dimensional shear rate, defined respectively as

$$\tilde{l} = 2L\lambda^{1/3}/d \tag{15.110}$$

$$\tilde{G} = \sigma_{12} d\lambda^{2/3}/2\nu \tag{15.111}$$

with L being the droplet length. The theoretical prediction for droplet breakup, $\tilde{G}_{\text{crit}} = 0.0541$, compared quite well with experimental data by Grace[272] for droplet breakup due to fracture

$$\sigma_{12} d\lambda^{0.55}/2\nu = 0.17 \tag{15.112}$$

Grace also reported that droplet breakup due to droplet tip streaming occurred at:

$$\sigma_{12} d/2\nu = 0.56 \tag{15.113}$$

The rate of shear dependence of dilute emulsion viscosity at small deformation was derived by Barthes-Biesel and Acrivos:[273]

$$\eta_r = 1 + [(5\lambda + 2)/2(\lambda + 1) - f(\lambda)(\sigma_{12}/E\Delta)^2 + 0(\sigma_{12}^3)]\phi \tag{15.114}$$

where $f(\lambda) > 0$ is a rational function of λ. The relation predicts a decrease of η_r with the square of the shear stress. The effect of stress is moderated by interphase elasticity expressed as $E\Delta$. The theory was experimentally verified using emulsions with a crosslinkable interphase; varying the degree of crosslinking changed the value of $E\Delta$.[274] The work of Barthes-Biesel is discussed fully in Chapter 16.

Esmukhanov *et al.*[275] examined the rheological behavior of dilute systems with dispersed deformable particles, characterized by viscoelastic memory functions. The theory, originally written for ellipsoidal molecular clusters of polymer chains in a poor solvent without Brownian motion, can easily be adapted to describe the rheological behavior of dilute emulsions.

The semi-concentrated emulsions in the linear viscoelastic region were examined both theoretically and experimentally by Mellema and co-workers[276–278] The work follows an earlier concept of rheologically complex behavior of the interphase developed by Oldroyd[260] or Sakanishi and Takano.[268] The authors considered two models: (i) a two-dimensional viscoelastic film; and (ii) the interphase of final thickness. Both models led to at least two relaxation times. The experimental results of dynamic testing in the kHz region for ionic emulsions[277] could be equally well interpreted in terms of either model. However, since the thickness of the interface was monomolecular, model (i) was considered a better reflection of the physical reality. The mechanism responsible for emulsion elasticity was found to originate in droplet deformation.

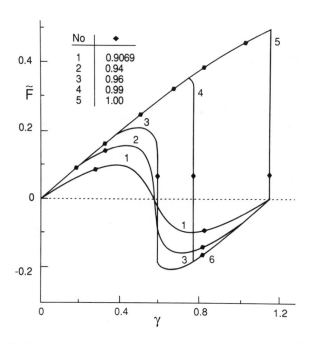

Fig. 15.23. Stress–strain master curves for concentrated two-dimensional emulsions with $0.9069 \leqslant \phi \leqslant 1.00$, where $\tilde{F}$ is the reduced stress per unit cell.[279]

For non-ionic emulsions[278] only one relaxation time was observed. These results were interpreted in terms of the second Oldroyd model[260] in which v is important rather than the viscoelasticity of the interphase. The steady state viscosities of both ionic and non-ionic systems for $\phi \leqslant 0.2$ were found to follow Simha's equation (15.2) fairly well.

Concentrated emulsions have been less frequently discussed. For emulsions and foams, Princen proposed a stress–strain theory based on a two-dimensional cell model;[279] its prediction is illustrated in Fig. 15.23. Initially, at small deformation, γ, the stress, σ, increases linearly with modulus, G. At higher values of γ, σ increases up to its maximum value at yield, $\sigma = \sigma_y$, then catastrophically drops to negative values. The reason for the latter behavior is the creation of an energetically unstable (at that γ) cell structure. The theory was evaluated using a concentrated oil-in-water system.[280] The predicted dependencies are

$$G = a_0 v \phi^{a_1}/d_{v/s} \tag{15.115}$$

$$\sigma_y = a_2 G \tilde{F}_{max}(\phi) \tag{15.116}$$

where a_i are numerical parameters, and $d_{v/s}$ is the average volume-to-surface diameter. For the three-dimensional case $a_1 = 1/3$. The function

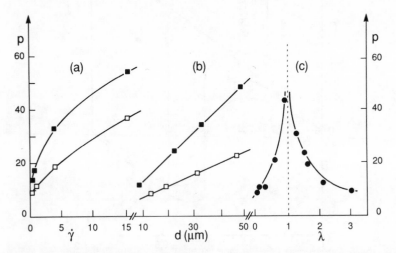

Fig. 15.24. Droplet axial ratio as a function of shear rate (a), initial diameter (b) and viscosity ratio (c), for polyvinyl alcohol/gelatine/H_2O (solid points) and dextran/gelatine/H_2O (open squares) systems at 32·5 °C.[281]

$\tilde{F}(\phi)$ is the concentration dependent dimensionless contribution to stress per drop; $\tilde{F}_{max}$ is taken at the yield point. Equations (15.115) and (15.116) can be used for foams as well.

(c) Experimental observations. In the flow of emulsions, three concentration regions can be identified: dilute with $\phi < 0.3$, characterized by nearly-Newtonian behavior; semi-concentrated at $0.3 \leqslant \phi < \phi_m$, with mainly pseudoplastic character; and concentrated at $\phi_m \leqslant \phi < 1.0$, exhibiting solid-like properties with modulus and yield.

The key condition for non-Newtonian flow is droplet deformation. Figure 15.24 illustrates the effect of $\dot{\gamma}$, d, and λ on the droplet axial ratio, p.[281] For low and high values of λ a pseudoplastic dependence has been observed. However, if the droplet is made of a viscoelastic liquid of relatively low viscosity, $\eta \simeq 4\,\mathrm{mPa\,s}$, a strongly dilatant effect at $\sigma_{12} > 0.8\,\mathrm{Pa}$ was reported.[282] The effect was observed for both low-conversion and plasticized PS latices.

The theoretical treatments assume monodispersity of droplet size. In experimental works the distribution was found to follow the gamma distribution relation[283] for surface distribution:

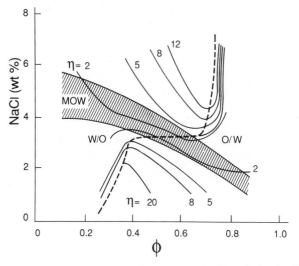

Fig. 15.25. Iso-viscosity contour map for oil/water/sodium dodecyl sulfate system at 25°C; MOW, W/O and O/W respectively stand for multiple oil in water microemulsion, water-in-oil and oil-in-water emulsions; the numbers refer to system viscosity in mPa s.[285]

$$n_i s_i / S = [a^{ad_i+3} / \Gamma(aD + 3)] x^{aD+2} \exp^{-aD} \tag{15.117}$$

where n_i is the number of particles each having surface s_i and diameter d_i, a is a characteristic parameter of the distribution and D is a characteristic diameter related to mean diameter by the dependence

$$\bar{d} = D + 3/a \tag{15.118}$$

and to specific surface

$$S = 6/\bar{d} \tag{15.119}$$

To express the average droplet diameter, the volume-to-surface ratio has been used:

$$d_{v/s} = \Sigma n_i d_i^3 / \Sigma n_i d_i^2 \tag{15.120}$$

For liquid–liquid systems with emulsifier, upon increase of ϕ a phase inversion is frequently observed; suddenly the dispersed and continuous liquids exchange roles. Salager *et al.*[284,285] reported two types of phase

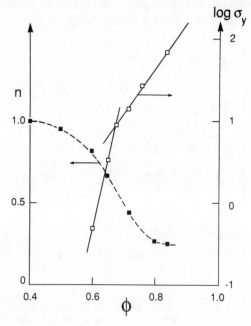

Fig. 15.26. The concentration dependence of the power-law exponent, n, and the yield stress for oil-in-water emulsion.[287]

transition in ionic emulsions: in the first, viscosity goes through a minimum; in the second it goes through a maximum. The transition map in Fig. 15.25 presents the observations. The first type of transition (normal) is associated with a decrease of v and formation of a micro-emulsion. The second (catastrophic) inversion is associated with an unstable-to-stable phase transition. It is not certain if both transition types can also take place in a non-ionic system such as a polymer blend.

Viscoelastic properties of oil-in-water emulsions at $\phi \leqslant 0.7$ were found[286] to follow a two-retardation time process

$$J(t) = J_0 + \sum_1^2 J_i \exp(-t/\tau_i^*) \qquad (15.121)$$

where J, J_0 and J_i are, respectively, compliance, its instantaneous and retarded values. All three constants J_0, J_1 and J_2 were found to decrease nearly linearly with ϕ on a log–log plot.

Highly concentrated oil-in-water emulsions, $0.4 \leqslant \phi \leqslant 0.86$, were measured in a cone-and-plate test geometry.[287] The data could be approximated by the power law model (at $\dot{\gamma} > 1\,\text{s}^{-1}$) with yield. Concentration dependence of σ_y and n is presented in Fig. 15.26.

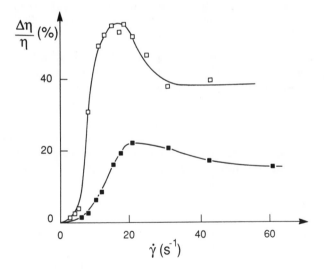

Fig. 15.27. Decrease of oil-in-water viscosity as a function of the average shear rate for $\phi = 0.65$ at frequency $10\,\text{Hz}$ and ratio of dynamic to steady state deformation rate $\beta = 1$ (bottom) and 2 (top).[288]

TABLE 15.7
Polymer Alloys and Blends: Basic Terms

Polymer blends (PB)	Mixtures of different polymers and/or co-polymers
Polymer alloys (PA)	Polymer blends with modified interfacial properties and/or morphology
Miscible PB	PB behaving as a single-phase system down to molecular level of dispersion, usually associated with $\Delta H_m < 0$
Compatible PB	Utilitarian term indicating commercially attractive PB or PA; usually homogeneous to the eye with enhanced physical properties
Compatibilization	Any physical or chemical action which results in stabilization (prevention of separation) of PB
Engineering polymer (EP)	Processable polymeric material, capable of being formed to precise and stable dimensions, exhibiting high mechanical properties at continuous use temperatures ($T > 100\,°C$), and having a tensile strength in excess of 40 MPa (6 kpsi)
Engineering PB (EPB)	PA or PB exhibiting properties and/or containing EP as at least one component of the blend

Quemada *et al.*[120,288] theoretically and experimentally investigated the rheological behavior of concentrated crude oil emulsions at $\phi = 0\cdot65$ under combined steady state, $\dot{\gamma}_{ss}$, and oscillatory shear rate, $\dot{\gamma}_{osc}$:

$$\dot{\gamma} = \dot{\gamma}_{ss} + \dot{\gamma}_{osc}\cos\omega t = \dot{\gamma}_{ss}(1 + \beta\cos\omega t) \qquad (15.122)$$

The effect of the oscillatory component on the average pressure loss in pipe flow was reported[288] to depend on both β and ω. This is expressed in Fig. 15.27 as a relative reduction of shear viscosity at frequency 10 Hz.

15.3.2. Polymer Alloys and Blends (PAB)
The basic terms are defined in Table 15.7. The technology of polymer alloys and blends is developing very rapidly. In 1986, polymer alloys and blends (PAB) constituted 16% of plastics consumption. The average growth rate of PAB is twice as high as that of all plastics and, for high performance engineering PAB, three times as high.[289]

Alloying polymer blends involves many operations, leading to *stable* and *reproducible* properties. Alloying may provide stabilization of the

interphase by the addition of a compatibilizer, just as a surfactant sta-
bilizes an emulsion, but this may be done equally well through a chemical
reaction or by high shear mechanical re-entanglement. About 60–70% of
polyethylene (PE) is used in producing PAB. In most cases blends of
different types of polyethylene with polypropylene (PP) are being
prepared. In these cases a compatibilizer is seldom required.[290-297] Blending
linear low density PE with PP seems to be particularly interesting.

15.3.2.1. Basic Concepts

Thermodynamics is the key to understanding the behavior and properties
of PAB. Miscibility defines the flow behavior, morphology and performance of the finished product.

Huggins[298] and Flory[299] derived the relation describing the concentration dependence of the free energy of mixing:

$$\Delta G_m/RTV = \Sigma(\phi_i/V_i)\ln\phi_i + \Sigma\chi'_{ij}\phi_i\phi_j \qquad (15.123)$$

where V and V_i are, respectively, volume of the mixture and molar volume
of species i, and χ'_{ij} is the binary interaction parameter. To achieve miscibility in a two-component system

$$2\chi'_{12} < (V_1^{-1/2} + V_2^{-1/2})^2 \qquad (15.124)$$

The first term on the right-hand side of eqn (15.123) expresses the combinatorial entropy of mixing. For polymer blends, the V_i are large and this
contribution can usually be neglected. The second term was originally
identified with Van Laar's enthalpy of mixing. Over the years it came to
be recognized that there are two non-combinatorial contributions in the
second term: energetic and volumetric[300]

$$\chi'_{12}RT_1^*/P_1^*V_1^* = X_{12}v/P_1^*(v-1) + \tau^2v/2(4/3-v) \qquad (15.125)$$

where

$$1 < v \equiv (V_1/V_1^*)^{1/3} < 4/3$$

$$\tau = 1 - T_1^*/T_2^* \qquad (15.126)$$

and P_1^*, V_1^* and T_1^* are the reducing parameters of pressure, volume and
temperature for liquid 1. According to eqn (15.125) the interactions are
characterized by two terms: the energetic interaction parameter,
$X_{12} \equiv X_{12}^L + X_{12}^S$; and the free volume contribution, $\tau^2 > 0$. The parameter X_{12} can be treated as originating from Van Laar's term, $X_{12}^L > 0$,
and from specific interactions, $X_{12}^S < 0$.

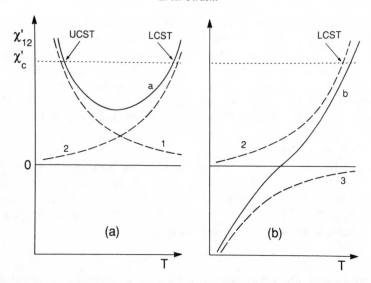

Fig. 15.28. Schematic χ'_{12} versus T dependence indicating contributions from (1) dispersion forces, (2) free volume and (3) specific interactions; solid curves 'a' and 'b' represent respectively χ'_{12} versus T dependence for dispersion and specific force dominated system with two and one critical solution temperatures, respectively.

Their relative contributions are plotted in Fig. 15.28. The resulting χ'_{12} versus T plot is parabolic with two intercepts with the line $\chi'_{12} = 2/V_1$ according to eqn (15.124) expressing the critical miscibility condition for a system with $V_1 \simeq V_2$ existing in polymer blends. The two intercepts result in two critical miscibility temperatures: lower critical solution temperature (LCST) and upper critical solution temperature (UCST). According to definition, LCST > UCST! The schematic phase diagram for a system with both critical temperatures in Fig. 15.29 explains the origin of these terms. In the case where $|X^L_{12}| \ll |X^S_{12}|$ only LCST is possible.

In Fig. 15.29 the pair of lines, binodal and spinodal, is marked, the first indicating incipient phase separation, the second a limit of the unstable region.[301] The binodals and spinodals provide boundaries for three regions of polymer blends: miscible, unstable (or metastable) and immiscible. The equilibrium thermodynamics, by definition, is not concerned with time effects or size of the dispersed phase (provided the interfacial energy is insignificant!). The newer works on phase separation dynamics distinguish two types of mechanism:[302-305] nucleation and growth (NG) and spinodal decomposition (SD). NG is associated with shallow quenching into the

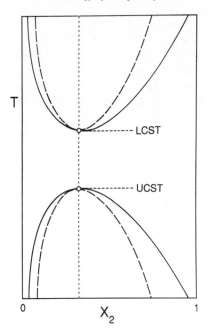

Fig. 15.29. Lower (LCST) and upper (UCST) critical solution temperature; solid and broken lines indicate binodal and spinodal, respectively; X_2 is the mole fraction.

unstable region and rapid molecular segregation into droplet/matrix type morphology. SD is observed for deep-quenched systems into the immiscible region. Owing to relative time scales for the molecular diffusion and kinetics of phase separation, SD leads to an interpenetrating network morphology even at low loading, $\phi \simeq 0.1$. Both these morphologies are unstable, observed in dynamic light scattering or in samples quenched below the melting point, T_m, or glass transition temperature, T_g. From a theoretical point of view both NG and SD result from different degrees of supercooling but are not due to different molecular processes, and both can be described by the same set of equations. Their initial phase separation sizes are similar (1–9 nm).[305] At the later stage, Ostwald ripening (OR) and coalescence result in coarsening toward the morphology determined by equilibrium thermodynamics.

Owing to the dynamic nature of phase separation, the definition of miscibility in Table 15.7 is not always easy to follow. The pragmatic test for miscibility is to measure T_g versus ϕ. If only one $T_g = T_g(\phi)$ is observed the system is functionally miscible; if two T_g, nearly independent of ϕ, are recorded, the system is considered immiscible. This practical definition leads to highly ambiguous results if the difference between T_g of the two polymers is small *and* when the samples did not reach their equilibrium morphology. T_g is not a measure of miscibility but of dispersed phase size, and if domain size d_d is less than 10–15 nm a single T_g is observed.[306-310] Shultz and Young[311] demonstrated that single or double T_g can be recorded for a PS/PMMA system depending upon whether the freeze dried sample is annealed or not.

When PAB undergo deformation under stress, the free energy of the system can be written as

$$\Delta G = \Delta G_m + \Delta G_{el} \tag{15.127}$$

where ΔG_{el} expresses the contribution originating in elastic deformation of polymer molecules. For constant stress experiments Lyngaae-Jorgensen and Sondergaard[312] proposed

$$\Delta G_{el}/RT = N\alpha_x^2/2 \tag{15.128}$$

where N is the number of entanglements per unit volume and α_x is the degree of orientation under stress, σ. Since α_x decreases with increase of N, the contribution of ΔG_{el} to χ'_{12} is negative, forcing the LCST to occur at higher temperature. For systems at processing temperatures near phase separation, NG or SD morphology can be generated at will by judiciously selecting the processing temperature, stress level and cooling procedure.

In short, the morphology of PAB depends on equilibrium thermodynamics, phase separation dynamics and on the stress history imposed on the thermodynamically controlled structures during processing and/or rheological testing. The latter effects will be discussed in Section 15.3.2.4.

15.3.2.2. Rheology of Miscible PAB

By definition, miscible PAB are single-phase mixtures and as such do not qualify to be included in this chapter on rheology of two-phase flows. On the other hand it would be illogical to neglect the flows of miscible blends. Miscibility depends on molecular weight, concentration, temperature, pressure, deformation rate, etc.

It is instructive to look for simple model systems; for miscible blends these are (i) solutions, and (ii) homologous polymer blends.

For solutions[313,314]

$$\log(V\eta_0) = \sum_i x_i \log(V_i\eta_{0_i}) + \log(V\eta)^E \qquad (15.129)$$

where V is the specific volume, x_i is the mole fraction, and the 'excess' term can be written as

$$\log(V\eta)^E = - \prod_i x_i \Delta H_m / 2 \cdot 45 R^* T \qquad (15.130)$$

For miscible PAB, $\Delta H_m < 0$ and the above relations predict a positive deviation from the log-additivity rule (PDB) in a $\eta = \eta(\phi)$ plot. This indeed has been reported for poly(2,6-dimethylphenyl ether)/polystyrene (PPE/PS),[315] polypropylene/poly(butene-1) (PP/PB-1)[316] or high density polyethylene/poly(ethylene-r-vinyl acetate) (HDPE/EVA)[317] blends. In the case of the last system, the $\log \eta_0$ versus composition plot was irregular, with deviations of less than 30% from the smooth curve due to clustering of the acetate groups in the PE matrix. The first normal stress coefficient, ψ_1, for these blends was also found to show positive deviations. The 50/50 blend of HDPE/EVA showed a 4-fold higher value of ψ_1 than that predicted by the additivity rule, indicating associative crosslinking.

Several blending rules for solution viscosity have been proposed.[314] Recently the one derived by McAllister[318] enjoyed enthusiastic but somewhat confused[319,320] attention:

$$\ln v_B = x_1^3 \ln v_1 + x_2^3 \ln v_2 + 3x_1^2 x_2 \ln v_{12} + 3x_1 x_2^2 \ln v_{21}$$
$$+ 3x_1^2 x_2 \ln[(2M_1 + M_2)/3] + 3x_1 x_2^2 \ln[(M_1 + 2M_2)/3]$$
$$+ x_1^3 \ln M_1 + x_2^3 \ln M_2 - \ln(x_1 M_1 + x_2 M_2) \quad (15.131)$$

where v_i is the kinematic viscosity, x_i is the mole fraction, M_i is the molecular weight, and the two kinematic viscosities with double subscripts are the empirical interaction viscosities. Equation (15.131) was derived from a three-body model of a miscible mixture of two low molecular weight liquids with two interaction viscosities. Use of this formula for immiscible systems negates the physical sense of its parameters, and reduces its significance to an empirical one. As indicated by Carley and Crossan,[319] a third order polynomial

$$y = \sum_{n=0}^{3} a_n x^n \qquad (15.132)$$

with $y = \log \eta$ versus $x = \phi$, provides at least as good a description of $\eta = \eta(\phi)$ dependence as eqn (15.131).

The zero-shear viscosity for narrow molecular weight distribution samples can be expressed as

$$\eta_0 = KM_w^a \qquad (15.133)$$

where K and a are parameters: for $M_w < M_e$ $a \simeq 1$, for $M_w > M_e a \simeq 3\cdot4$, M_e being the entanglement molecular weight. Since

$$M_w = \Sigma w_i M_{wi} \qquad (15.134)$$

where w_i is the weight fraction of polymer with M_{wi}, from eqns (15.133) and (15.134)[321-323]

$$\eta_0 = (\Sigma w_i \eta_{0i}^{1/a})^a \qquad (15.135)$$

For two-component systems with $a = $ const, it can be easily demonstrated that

$$d^2 \ln \eta_0 / dw_2^2 = -a(\eta_{02}^{1/a} - \eta_{01}^{1/a})^2 / \eta_0^{2/a} < 0 \qquad (15.136)$$

i.e. binary mixture viscosity should also show a positive deviation from the log-additivity rule (PDB). Experimentally the data for homologous polymer blends have been fitted[321-323] with the parameter $1\cdot75 \leqslant a \leqslant 100$.

Another method of predicting $\eta_0 = \eta_0(\phi)$ dependence for a miscible system was proposed by Wisniewski et al.[324] The authors started from Doolittle's equation

$$\ln \eta_0 = \ln a_0 + a_1/f \qquad (15.137)$$

where the a_i are parameters, and f is the free volume fraction, proportional to T. Assuming additivity of a_0 and f, the predictive relation is

$$\ln \eta_0 = \ln\Sigma a_{0i}\phi_i + a_1/\Sigma\phi_i f_i \qquad (15.138)$$

with (from eqn (15.137))

$$a_{0i} = \eta_{0i}\exp(-a_1/f_i) \qquad (15.139)$$

For a two-component system, assuming[324] that $a_1 \simeq 1$

$$\partial^2\ln\eta_0/\partial\phi_2^2 = -[(a_{02} - a_{01})/(\phi_2 a_{02} + \phi_1 a_{01})]^2$$
$$+ 2(f_2 - f_1)^2/(f_2\phi_2 + f_1\phi_1)^3 \qquad (15.140)$$

predicting PDB for most cases with a possibility of small negative deviation from the log-additivity rule (NDB).

There is a mounting evidence that PDB is far from the rule for miscible PAB. Depending on the system and method of preparation,[325] $\eta_0 = \eta_0(\phi)$ can be PDB, additive or NDB.[326-328]

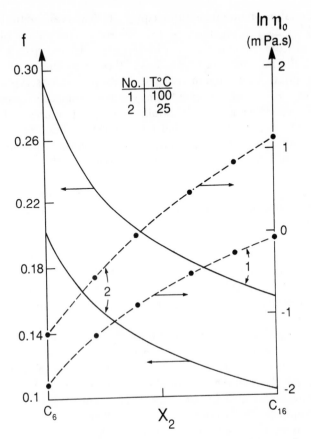

Fig. 15.30. Computed free volume fraction, f, and $\ln\eta_0$ of hexene/hexadecane mixture of 25 and 100 °C plotted versus mole fraction of hexadecane; the points are from experimental data.[341]

During the last few years the experimental data on the pressure and temperature dependence of zero-shear viscosity, $\eta_0(P, T)$, of liquids and their mixtures have been analyzed[329-333] by means of the free volume fraction, computed from Simha's statistical theory.[334-340] The analysis indicated that

$$\ln\eta_0 = a_0 + a_1/(f + a_2) \qquad (15.141)$$

with $a_0 = \ln\eta_0^*$, where η_0^* is the iso-free-volume viscosity, a_1 depends on molecular branching and polydispersity, and $a_2 \simeq 0.07$ is the linearization parameter. For n-paraffin mixtures, eqn (15.141) was valid in the full range of ϕ, $T = 25–100\,°C$ and $P = 0·1–500\,MPa$. The values of f were computed from the coupled equations of state derived from a cell/hole model.[334] For mixtures, the parameters of these two equations were taken as appropriate mol-fraction averages.[338–340] It was observed that, at $f = \text{const}$, $a_0 = \ln\eta_0^*$ increased linearly with molecular weight and $a_1 = 0·79$ was constant for all n-paraffins and their mixtures. In Fig. 15.30 the theoretical variation of F and $\ln\eta_0$ for hexane/hexadecane blend is shown by solid and broken lines, respectively. Points indicate the variation of the system viscosity as reported by Dymond et al.[341]

It has been reported[342,343] that η_0 versus ϕ dependence increases sharply as ϕ and T approach the critical condition of phase separation. However, once the separation has occurred, upon further change in ϕ, the viscosity decreases. Interestingly, the activation energy of flow undergoes discontinuity at the critical concentration, but its slope, $dE_\eta/d\phi$, is nearly identical on both sides of this concentration.[343] This behavior has been noted for low molecular weight liquids, oligomers and PAB. In the latter case a decrease of ΔH_m or ΔG_m resulted in a local increase of viscosity, followed by a sometimes sharp decrease in η once the separation had taken place.[344–348]

15.3.2.3. Melt Flow of Block Copolymers

The subject has been well discussed in numerous books and reviews.[349–352] In particular, the melt rheology of block copolymers was recently discussed by Lyngaae-Jorgensen,[353] and that for copolymer solutions by Kotaka and Watanabe.[354] The following summary will be an attempt to stress the common aspects of block copolymer flow behavior with other two-phase systems, especially PAB.

Very rarely the components of a block copolymer (BC) are soluble in one another. BC is purposely designed as a two-phase system with 'rigid' and 'soft' domains, and the concentration and molecular weights are purposely selected to provide interconnection between the domains. The existence of a dispersed rigid phase in an elastomeric matrix is responsible for its 'thermoplastic elastomer' behavior.

Considering melt flow of BC, it is usually assumed that test temperature, $T > T_{gc}$, where T_{gc} stands for glass transition temperature (T_g) of the continuous phase. However, at $T_{gc} < T < T_{gd}$ (T_{gd} is T_g of the dispersed phase) the system behaves as a crosslinked rubber with strong viscoelastic character. At $T > T_{gd}$ the viscosity of BC is much greater than would be expected on the basis of the total molecular weight and composition.[355–361]

The reason for this behavior is a need to deform the domain structure and pull filaments of one polymer through domains of the other. Viscosity increases with incompatibility of the BC components,[362,363] in a manner similar to the way in which the increase of the interfacial tension coefficient in concentrated emulsions causes η to rise.

Also BC exhibits yield stress[364]

$$\sigma_{12} = \sigma_y + \eta_0\dot{\gamma}(1 + \beta b\dot{\gamma}^m)/(1 + b\dot{\gamma}^m) \qquad (15.142)$$

where β represents the relative residual viscous dissipation parameter, and b and m are parameters originating from the structural breakdown and reformation of structure. Note that, for $\dot{\gamma} \to \infty$, $\sigma_{12}/\dot{\gamma} \to \eta_0\beta = \eta_\infty$. The five-parameter eqn (15.142) can be extended to include the transient effects:

$$\sigma_{12}(t) = \sigma_y + \eta_0\dot{\gamma}\{\beta + [(1 - \beta)/(1 + b\dot{\gamma}^m)]$$
$$\times [1 + b\dot{\gamma}^m \exp(- kt(1 + b\dot{\gamma}^m)/b)]\} \qquad (15.143)$$

where k is the loss-rate constant. For $t \to \infty$, eqn (15.143) reduces to eqn (15.142). Equations (15.142) and (15.143) are capable of describing multiple phenomena: yield, upper and lower Newtonian plateaux, pseudo-plasticity, stress growth and overshoot, thixotropy, hysteresis, etc.

The multiplicity of rheological phenomena observed in BC is related to sensitivity of the melt structure to independent molecular and rheological variables. The structure, as indicated in eqn (15.143), is time and rate of deformation dependent, varying with molecular weight, macromolecular architecture and concentration. For example, for styrene–butadiene–styrene (SBS) the activation energy of flow $\Delta E_\eta = 80$ or $160\,\text{kJ}\,\text{mol}^{-1}$ for compositions containing less or more that 31 vol% of styrene.[358] The difference originates in the structure; it is dispersed below 31% and interconnected above.

Effects of molecular parameters and composition were reviewed by Holden[365] who expressed the temperature dependence of shear viscosity for BC in terms of a relation similar to eqn (15.137)

$$\ln\eta = a_0 + a_1/(T - T_\infty) \qquad (15.144)$$

where, by definition, T_∞ is the temperature at which $\eta \to \infty$. Differentiating eqn (15.144) one obtains an expression for the temperature dependent activation energy for flow:

$$\Delta E_\eta = a_1 R[T/(T - T_\infty)]^2 \qquad (15.145)$$

Experimentally, T_∞ is not far away from the glass transition temperature, but the curvature in the ΔE_η versus T plot is frequently much greater than would be expected from WLF theory.[366] An explanation for this effect is the temperature dependent solubility of the components (Fig. 15.29). On the basis of statistical thermodynamics, Leary and Williams[367] introduced a concept of a separation temperature, T_s, at which $\Delta G_m = 0$. Since, in the model, the volume of the interphase depends on geometry (spheres, cylinders, lamellae), T_s also depends on morphology. At $T > T_s$, BC is a homogeneous liquid; below T_s, two phases coexist. However, it follows from Lyngaae-Jorgensen's work[353] that at $T \leqslant T_s$ a possibility of homogenization exists if $\sigma_{12} > \sigma_{cr}$, where

$$\sigma_{cr}^2 = a_0 T(T_s - T); \qquad T \leqslant T_s \tag{15.146}$$

For SBS, $T_s \simeq 425\,K$ and at $396\,K$ $\sigma_{cr} \simeq 55\,kPa$ which gives the value of the proportionality factor: $a_0 = 0\cdot263$.

The BC structure depends on the nature of the casting solvent. Correspondingly, the rheological response as well as T_s are affected. SBS structure breakup was studied by Sivashinsky *et al.*[368] by stress growth and relaxation methods. Detailed studies on the nature of structural changes introduced by solvent nature, concentration, temperature and deformation were carried out by Kotaka and Watanabe.[354,369] The authors found the dynamic tests to be particularly suitable. The storage and loss moduli, G' and G'', versus frequency, ω, as well as the relaxation spectrum, provided a detailed image of structural changes. The results were interpreted in terms of the 'tube renewal' model.

Block polymers, owing to the tendency for formation of regular structures tailored by molecular design, are ideal models for PAB. As will be evident later, PAB show similar rheological phenomena, e.g. yield, pseudoplasticity, thixotropy, structural rearrangements, etc., but since the morphology is more difficult to control the interpretation of data may present serious problems. Comparison with better understoood systems (solutions, suspensions, emulsions and block copolymers) frequently serves as a guide.

15.3.2.4. *Rheology of Immiscible PAB*

Over the years, in several publications from Kiev,[348,370–376] the relation between thermodynamics and rheology for miscible and immiscible PAB has been examined. In most cases ΔH_m (or ΔG_m) versus ϕ were compared with η versus ϕ graphs. The equilibrium thermodynamic functions were measured by inverse gas chromatography (IGC), and η in a capillary viscometer.

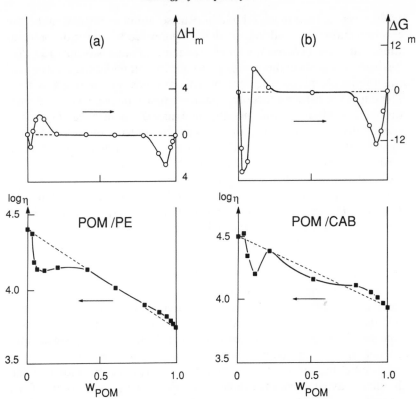

Fig. 15.31. Correlation between ΔH_m (or ΔG_m) and $\log\eta$ plotted versus weight fraction of POM for its blends with PE (a) or with cellulose acetate butyrate (CAB) (b).[348]

On the basis of discussion on the relation between thermodynamics and rheology for low molecular weight mixtures[313,314] summarized in eqns (15.129) and (15.130) in miscible PAB, Eyring's 'mirror image' can be expected: when ΔH_m decreases, the excess viscosity, η^E, should increase, and vice versa. When critical concentration is approached, by analogy to low molecular weight mixtures[342] or with oligomeric systems,[343] the viscosity is expected to increase sharply *before* phase separation occurs. When the concentration exceeds the critical value, the flow becomes controlled mainly by the structure: η will increase further if a dispersion with rigid ellipsoids is created; it will stabilize for an emulsion-type system or decrease for lamellar morphology with interlayer slip. One cannot expect that, for immiscible systems, there will be a relation between ΔG_m and η^E.

However, a falsehood is built into these arguments. In view of the experimentally observed and theoretically derived[312,353] relation between stress and critical conditions for phase separation (e.g. see eqn (15.146)), it is apparent that conditions for phase separation under thermodynamic equilibrium conditions, ϕ_{ceq}, do not represent those in flow; $\phi_{cflow} \neq \phi_{ceq}$. The difference between these two parameters will increase with stress. In short, for immiscible blends, the thermodynamic argument can be used as a qualitative tool to explain concentration dependence of the rheological function at vanishingly small deformation rates, but not as a quantitative predicting tool. Much more work must be done on the non-equilibrium thermodynamics of PAB before it can be used as a predictive tool.

An example of experimental correlation between concentration dependence of ΔH_m (or ΔG_m) and η is presented in Fig. 15.31. There is a degree of symmetry in the thermodynamic functions: addition of a small amount of polymer A to B or B to A causes a similar initial decrease of ΔG_m or ΔH_m toward minima defining the binodal concentration. By contrast, the plot of η versus ϕ is not symmetrical; addition of a small amount of low viscosity component causes a sharp reduction of blend viscosity at about binodal concentration. On the other hand, addition of high viscosity polymer causes increase of blend viscosity above the log-additivity prediction. This asymmetry can be explained by the concept of 'complementary morphologies' proposed by Van Oene,[377] to be discussed later.

For PAB the authors[370-376] concluded that there is a correlation between the thermodynamic and rheological functions: the positive value of the heat of mixing, $\Delta H_m > 0$, indicating immiscibility, was paralleled by NDB behavior. For $\Delta H_m < 0$, in most cases additivity of η was observed. This behavior is similar to that of low molecular weight liquids. However, for PS/polycarbonate (PS/PC) blends a reverse situation was reported.

Manevich et al.,[378] considering Onsager's density fluctuation near the spinodal region, derived the following relation for binary blends of components 1 and 2, each with its degree of polymerization, n_i, molar fraction, x_i, and segmental relaxation time τ_i^*:

$$\eta^E = 2 \cdot 0937 \delta \beta^2 R^* T (\Sigma n_i x_i \tau_i^*)(n_1 n_2)^{1/2}/n_e (\Sigma n_i x_i - 2\chi'_{12} x_1 x_2 n_1 n_2)^{1/2}$$

$$(15.147)$$

where δ is the segmental density, β is the Onsager coefficient, n_e is the entanglement degree of polymerization and R^* is the gas constant. The η^E expresses the excess viscosity term due to segmental fluctuation near phase separation. Excepting blends with high polymer–polymer interactions,

$\chi'_{12} < 0$, the relation predicts an increase of η in the vicinity of the phase separation, in accord with observations for low molecular weight mixtures.[342,343]

Structure of PAB melts. In immiscible PAB the properties are strongly related to the interface as well as to the size and shape of the dispersed phase. The morphology is controlled by equilibrium and non-equilibrium thermodynamics as well as by the flow fields. At equilibrium, for low volume fraction of dispersed phase, $\phi \leqslant 0.12$, droplets are expected; above this value fibers and lamellae are usually found.[349-352,379,380] If the polymers are miscible under one set of pressure (P) and temperature (T) conditions but immiscible under another, the non-equilibrium morphology depends on the quench depth and time scale (see Section 15.3.2.1).

15.3.2.5. Flow Imposed Morphology
The flow conditions superimpose another set of morphologies. Flow encapsulation of one phase by another, deformation leading to fiber or platelet formation due to shear or extensional field, shear induced coalescence, interlayer slip and shear controlled SD or NG are well documented.[147,292,381-383]

Several relations between flow conditions and resulting morphology have been proposed. These can be grouped into two sets of criteria: purely rheological and those coupled with the interfacial tension coefficient. In Section 15.3.1.2 the pertinent information for stress deformations in emulsions was discussed.

(a) Rheological criteria.[384-387]. In order to achieve maximum dispersion at minimum expended energy in a steady-state shear flow, η and N_1 of the two immiscible polymers should be the same. This statement is valid only if η and N_1 are compared in the full range of shear stress generated during dispersing and processing stages. Two other factors complicate the phenomenon. It was shown[388] that co-continuous structures are generated when

$$\phi_1/\phi_2 = \eta_1/\eta_2 \equiv \lambda \qquad (15.148)$$

where the subscripts 1 and 2 indicate respectively the dispersed phase and the matrix. On the other hand, at $\phi = $ const in capillary as well as in rotational shear field (cone-and-plate), droplets were formed[389] at shear stress

$$\phi_{12,c} < a\lambda^b \qquad (15.149)$$

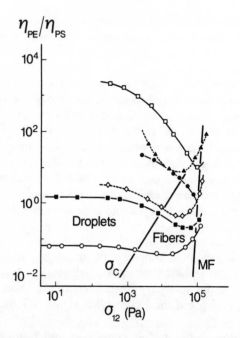

Fig. 15.32. Shear viscosity ratio of polyethylene (PE) (minor phase, 30%) to polystyrene (PS) versus shear stress, σ_{12}, at 180 °C for six PE/PS blends; lines indicated σ_c and MF represent the limiting values for droplet formation and melt fracture, respectively (data valid for capillary *and* rotational shear field).[389]

where a and b are constants dependent on ϕ and the type of blend, and the subscript c indicates a critical value. As shown in Fig. 15.32, at $\sigma_{12} > \sigma_{12,c}$, up to the melt fracture region, formation of fibers was observed for PS/PE containing 1, 10 or 30 wt% of PE.

It has been reported[147,386,390] that in shear flow (for both Newtonian and pseudoplastic liquids) droplets can form only if $\lambda < 4$; above this limit, fibers were obtained. These observations do not agree with data in Fig. 15.32, where droplets are reported for $0.04 \leqslant \lambda \leqslant 2000$.

(b) Rheological–interfacial criteria. The dependencies in which the interfacial tension coefficient, v, is taken into account belong to the second group of criteria. Van Oene derived[377]

$$v = v_0 + (d/12)(N_{1,1} - N_{1,2}) \qquad (15.150)$$

In the relation, d stands for the diameter of droplet (polymer 1) and $N_{1,i}$

for N_i of liquid $i = 1$ or 2. At equilibrium $v = v_0$. The relation has three interesting features: (i) for $N_{1,1} > N_{1,2}$ the interfacial tension increases with shear stress, i.e. droplets are becoming more difficult to break; (ii) for $N_{1,1} < N_{1,2}$ there is a reduction of the interfacial tension and enhancement for generation of fine dispersion at high shear stress; (iii) as $v \geqslant 0$ a conversion from droplet to continuous morphology is predicted at

$$N_{1,2} = N_{1,1} + 12v_0/d \qquad (15.151)$$

The above features lead to complementarity of polymer blend pairs: if, at low content of polymer A in B, a droplet dispersion is observed, at low content of B in A a continuous (fibers or lamellae) morphology is to be expected. Equation (15.150) neglects numerous aspects influencing PAB morphology. It is, however, a valuable tool directing development of structured PAB when the other factors are kept constant.

The conditions for single Newtonian liquid droplet breakup were discussed by Acrivos and co-workers.[270,271] A summary of this work was presented earlier in eqns (15.107)–(15.112). In particular, eqn (15.110) predicts that, if in a given range of shear stress $\lambda = const$ and $v = v_0$ is assumed, then d should be inversely proportional to σ_{12}. For a series of different PABs processed under similar conditions, d should be proportional to v. The latter correlation was experimentally verified by Wu.[391]

Use of the rheological–interfacial criteria is difficult due to lack of simple and rapid methods for v determination. In commercial polymers, due to presence of additives (lubricants, processing aids, stabilizers, antioxidants, etc.), the use of a general value is meaningless. There is a desperate need for a reliable experimental method of measurement of the interfacial tension using the actual resins to be blended.

The 'predictive' relations are valid only for steady state flow of specified nature. The parameters used in these relations must be valid under the full range of flow conditions. The conditions are assumed to be uniform within the sample, i.e. they may not hold for die or capillary flow. The morphology must not be affected by other factors, i.e. phase ripening or crystallization. The derived equations are valid at low concentration $\phi \leqslant 0.3$. Above this limit, co-continuous structures predominate.

Furthermore, it is worth stressing the dynamic character of the flow induced morphologies. It is not only important to generate the desired structure but also to preserve it. The rate of reverting to equilibrium depends on the magnitude of the driving forces (mainly v_0) and the barrier heights (e.g. the diffusion constant D). To stabilize the structure, both factors, reduction of v_0 and increase of D, must be considered. It has been demonstrated[195,292] that in semi-crystalline polymer blends there is a possibility of generating fibrillar morphology at T well below the melting point of dispersed polymer. Owing to the presence of crystallinity, once formed the structure remains stable.

(c) Shear flows. Owing to the variability of PAB structure with flow conditions, the rheological responses must be sensitive to the way they are measured. As for the emulsions, PABs show yield stress.[392] At higher stress or strain further structural changes occur. For this reason the selected type of test procedure should reflect the final use of the data; when simulation of flow through a die is attempted, the large strain capillary flow is useful, but if the material characterization is important the low strain dynamic testing should be preferred.

During the capillary flow the maximum extensional velocity gradient is located upstream from the entrance to the capillary and the minimum is downstream from the capillary exit where the extrudate swell predominates. Cogswell derived the following correlation between the extensional viscosity at the entrance to the die and the shear viscosity on the die wall:[393]

$$\eta_E/\eta \; = \; 2\tan^{-2}\alpha \tag{15.152}$$

where α is the half-angle of convergence given by the ratio of the respective deformation rates

$$\alpha \; = \; \arctan(2\dot{\varepsilon}/\dot{\gamma}) \tag{15.153}$$

It is interesting to note that, from eqns (15.152) and (15.153), it follows that the energy dissipated in shear $\eta\dot{\gamma}^2 = 2\eta_E\dot{\varepsilon}^2$, i.e. the entrance pressure loss due to extensional flow is a significant part of the total effect. Recently[394] $\alpha = 20\cdot6 \pm 1\cdot6°$ was computed for HDPE. Using this value, one finds $\dot{\varepsilon} = 0\cdot188\dot{\gamma}$, $\eta_e = 14\cdot156\eta$ and $\sigma_{11} = 2\cdot660\sigma_{12}$. A theory of free convergenece for multiphase systems has not been developed. However, it is accepted that the shear stress is the same across the interphase, whereas the deformation rate changes inversely with viscosity.

It has been reported[195] that blends of commercial high density polyethylene and polyamide-6 resins (HDPE/PA-6) containing up to 30 wt% of PA-6 and extruded in a capillary viscometer at 150, 200 and 250 °C show fibrillation of the PA-6 phase at all temperatures, below and above the melting point of this polymer, $T_m = 219$ °C. The fibrillation was found to be associated with a shear-induced coalescence. During capillary flow at 150 °C, the shear stress of the matrix varied from 20 to 300 Pa, i.e. the available extensional stress calculated from eqns (15.152) and (15.153) was

was $\sigma_{11} = 50$–$800\,kPa$. The tensile yield stress for PA-6 at $150\,°C$ was found to be only $15\,kPa$, independent of the rate of straining. In short, the extensional stress in the capillary entrance was more than enough to deform the amorphous part of 'solid' PA-6. The fibrils, once created, could not elastically return to their undeformed state. The following three other flow-induced morphological changes were reported:

(i) A shear-induced segregation of polymer domains, related to encapsulation in flow.

(ii) Dynamic dispersion/coalescence. For low concentrations of dispersed phases, it was observed that the average diameter of droplets decreased with σ_{12} from its value in the pre-blend. These dimensions are *not* related to equilibrium conditions determined by the thermodynamic interactions. Similar observations were reported by Min.[395]

(iii) The shear-induced interlayer slip was theoretically predicted by Lin[396] who derived the following relation for immiscible blend with interlayer slip factor β_1:

$$1/\eta = \beta_1 \Sigma w_i/\eta_i; \qquad i = 1, 2 \qquad (15.154)$$

$$\beta_1 = 1 - (\beta_{12}/\sigma_{12})(\Pi w_i)^{1/2} \qquad (15.155)$$

and w_i stands for weight fraction. These dependencies predict a negative deviation from the log additivity rule. Interlayer slip creates a tree-ring structure in the extruded strands readily observed for samples containing $30\,wt\%$ of PA-6 in HDPE matrix at $T > T_m$.[397] The HDPE/PA-6 capillary viscosities at $250\,°C$ followed eqn (15.154) quite well.

There is a reciprocal relation between morphology and flow behavior. Plochocki[384,385,398,399] defined the 'particular rheological composition' (PRC) most frequently reported for polyolefin blends. At PRC the $\eta = \eta(\phi)$ function reaches a local maximum or minimum. The existence of the maximum is related to a change of the dispersed phase, from spherical to fibrillar, while that of the minimum is related to a reciprocal change. Plochocki[398–400] also demonstrated that reduction of η in incompatible polymer blends is associated with an increase of specific volume. The origin of this phenomenon is not known, but since the blends are immiscible the locus must be associated with the interphase. Bye and Miles[401] reported on capillary flow of PS/PMMA and polyethylene terephthalate/polyamide-6,6 (PET/PA-66) blends. For the first system the fluidity additivity equation (15.154) with $\beta_1 = 1$ and w_i replaced by

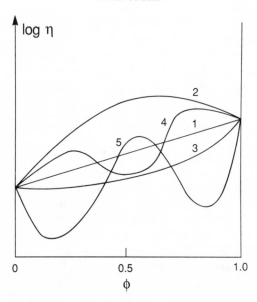

Fig. 15.33. Summary of viscosity–concentration dependence for PAB as expected on the basis of morphological argument. 1. Log-additivity. 2. Emulsion/suspension flow. 3. Stratified flow with interlayer slip. 4. Co-continuous morphology at $\phi \simeq 0.5$ and dispersed morphology at other values. 5. Limited miscibility at low concentrations, discontinuous near $\phi \simeq 0.5$.[401]

ϕ_i worked very well. For the second system 'as expected for these reactive polymers' the rheological responses were found to depend on history. The authors summarized the literature information on the influence of morphology on shear viscosity as in Fig. 15.33.

Tsebrenko *et al.*[402] reported on fibrillation of poly(oxymethylene (POM)) in a copolyamide (CPA) matrix as a result of flow through a capillary. As for PA-6 in an HDPE matrix,[195] here also the droplets undergo coalescence and stretching in the entrance zone. Very fine fibrils with diameters of about $20\,\mu$m and length $3200\,\mu$m were obtained during extrusion at $177\,°$C, i.e. $6\,°$C above the POM melting point. In the later publication[382] the authors reported PDB behavior of η and the extrudate swell, B (see Fig. 15.34). It is apparent that PDB behavior, illustrated as curve 2 in Fig. 15.33, can be observed for systems in which the morphology changes during the flow from droplets to fibers. This type of behavior has been reported frequently for systems in which droplets were observed before and after test (e.g. see reference 403).

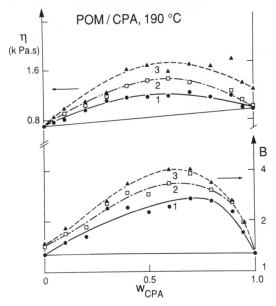

Fig. 15.34. Viscosity, η, and extrudate swell, B, of poly(oxymethylene)/copolyamide blends as a function of concentration; the number of times the sample was extruded is indicated.[382]

(d)   Relation between steady state (η) and dynamic (η') viscosities. This is illustrated in Fig. 15.35. An HDPE blend with 10 wt% of PA-6 was measured at 150, 200 and 250 °C in the capillary viscometer and mechanical spectrometer.[195,397] The data were superimposed on a master curve with the reference temperature $T_R = 250$ °C, using a modified Vinogradov–Malkin method. While η'/a_T versus ωa_T show a reasonable superposition, the high strain η/a_T versus $\dot{\gamma} a_T$ results do not. Since there was no slip on the die, the lower η/a_T values are $T < T_R$ are related to strain induced morphological changes.

Chuang and Han[404] reported that for miscible and immiscible blends at $\phi =$ const the plots of N_1 versus σ_{12} and G' versus G'' are independent of T. However, while for single phase systems the two dependencies are more or less parallel, for immiscible blends, such as PS/PMMA the steady state relation may be quite different from the dynamic one.

Probably the most dramatic example of different shear behavior between capillary and dynamic flow is that reported for the blend of ethylene–propylene–1,4-hexadiene terpolymer (EPDM) with poly(vinylidene-co-hexafluoropropylene), Viton. While Shih[405,406] for capillary flow reported a six-fold reduction of shear viscosity upon addition of about 2%

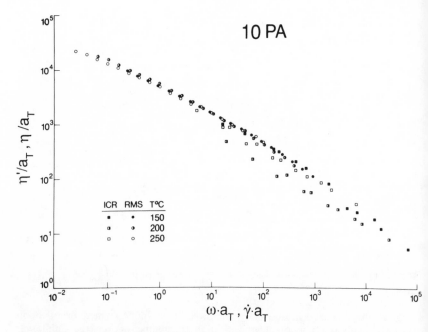

Fig. 15.35. Reduced shear and dynamic viscosities versus reduced shear rate for polyethylene containing 10% polyamide-6.[195]

of the other component, Kanu and Shaw[407] demonstrated that in dynamic test the complex viscosity of EPDM and EPDM with 5% Viton gave a very similar response in a wide range of frequency and strain. The latter authors postulated accumulation of the second component at the capillary entrance, which periodically feeds into the capillary, lubricating the main stream by a sort of roll bearing effect. In this particular case the difference is related not only to material properties but also to a flow segregation enhanced by the geometry of the measuring device. Since the effect is strongly affected by flow geometry, the data obtained in capillary flow have little value for process line design requirements.

Over the years the value of dynamic testing has been increasingly appreciated. It has been extensively used in testing of multiphase systems in Japan (Kyoto, Osaka), France (Pau) and Canada (Montreal, Toronto). Numerous reports from these centres have already been cited. Here two additional ones will only be mentioned.

Nishi *et al.*[408] carried out careful studies on the dynamic behavior of cast specimens of PS/polyvinylmethylether (PVME) at temperatures below

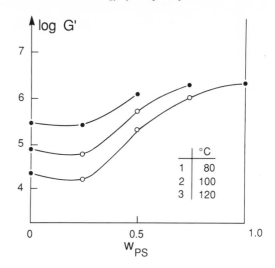

Fig. 15.36. Compositional dependence of loss modulus for PS/PVME at frequency $\omega = 37.7\,\mathrm{s}^{-1}$ and at three temperatures; solid points indicate homogeneous system.[408]

and above LCST $\simeq 95\,^{\circ}\mathrm{C}$, as well as for polyvinylidene fluoride $(\mathrm{PVF_2})/$ polyethylmethacrylate below its LCST $\simeq 200\,^{\circ}\mathrm{C}$. As shown in Fig. 15.36 for PS/PVME within the range $T < \mathrm{LCST}$, G' versus ω shows a usual pattern suggesting superposition onto a master curve, but this is not possible at $T > \mathrm{LCST}$. The plot of isochronal G' or G'' versus w_2 at 80, 100 and 120 °C has a very similar sigmoidal shape, as the phase separation had little bearing on the rheological response (see Fig. 15.36).

The group in Pau studied the dynamic properties of polycarbonate (PC) blend with PS,[409] with tetramethyl polycarbonate (TMPC) and with both PS and TMPC.[410] The zero shear viscosity versus $\phi(\mathrm{PC})$ for the binary blends is shown in Fig. 15.37, the broken line indicating immiscibility. For PS/PC at very low loading $\phi \simeq 0.01$ and 0.99, a sharp local minimum was obtained. The effect is related to partial miscibility (the 'mirror image' in Eyring's concept). Since neither the reproducibility nor the error of measurements is mentioned, it is difficult to be certain how to draw the curve through the data points. However, it is apparent that NDB behavior is obtained for blends, suggesting interlayer slip. For partially miscible TMPC/PC blends the solid curve indicates the miscible and the broken curve the immiscible region. In the latter case slight NDB behavior is noted. The authors reported that for immiscible blends two relaxation

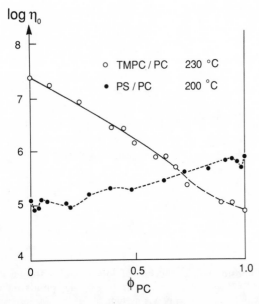

Fig. 15.37. Zero-shear viscosity versus volume fraction of polycarbonate in blends with tetramethyl polycarbonate (TMPC) and with polystyrene (PS); broken lines indicate immiscibility, and points are experimental values.[409,410]

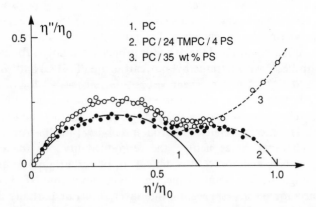

Fig. 15.38. Cole–Cole plot for three systems. 1. PC (solid line) adjusted to coincide with high frequency data of system 2, PC with 24 wt% of TMPC and 4% PS (solid points), and 3. PC with 35 wt% PS (open points).[409,410]

processes can be identified. In Fig. 15.38 the data for PC (system 1) gave a perfect semicircle, indicating a simple liquid structure. Upon addition of 35 wt% of PS (system 3) the spectrum can be decomposed into three parts: PC phase (the high frequency, low η' data), PS (mid-range) and an interphase or interface interaction. In the latter case yield behavior is suspected. The three-component system 2 containing 72% PC, 24% TMPC and 4% PS is significantly simpler. Owing to partial miscibility of PC/TMPC blend, two phases again coexist, but by contrast with system 3 there is no evidence of yield at low frequencies. Defining the main relaxation time as $\tau_i^* = 1/\omega_i$ (ω_i being the frequency corresponding to a local maximum in the $\eta'' = \eta''(\eta')$ plot), two relaxation times can be

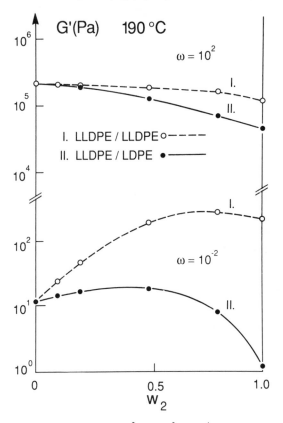

Fig. 15.39. Isochronal G' (at $\omega = 10^{-2}$ and $10^2 \, \mathrm{rad\,s^{-1}}$) versus weight fraction of the second component for linear low density polyethylene (LLDPE) blended with another LLDPE or with low density polyethylene (LDPE).[428]

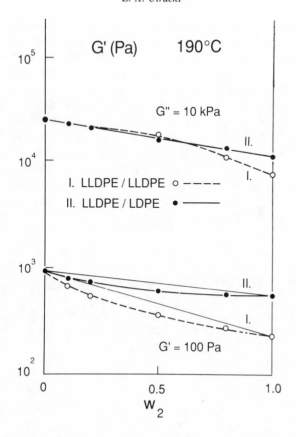

Fig. 15.40. G' of linear low density polyethylene (LLDPE) blends with another LLDPE or with low density polyethylene (LDPE); the data taken at 190 °C and constant $G'' = 10^2$ (bottom) and 10^4 Pa (top) (same data as shown in Fig. 15.39).

defined; both follow the Arrhenius dependence, with the activation energy for τ_2^* about 2·5 times as high as that for τ_1^*.

(e) Blend elasticity. Four measures of melt elasticity are commonly used: in steady state shearing, the first normal stress difference, N_1; in dynamic tests, the storage modulus, G'; and the two indirect and controversial ones, namely entrance–exit pressure drop (Bagley correction), P_e, and the extrudate swell, B. In homogeneous melts the four measures are in qualitative agreement. More complex behavior is expected for blends. If the blend can be regarded as an emulsion, in the absence of

interlayer slip the PDB behavior for the elastic measurements is to be expected. In the case where the dispersed phase is difficult to deform (as in suspensions) the extrudate swell should be small. Deformation-and-recovery of the dispersed phase provides a potent mechanism for energy storage leading to an elastic response.

The direct measurements of N_1[384,395,411–413] indicate a parallel dependence on ϕ for both η and N_1 even when these have a sigmoidal form. In dynamic testing, isochronal G' measurements primarily show PDB behavior,[292,414,415] although NDB, parallel to η, was also reported.[345]

Considering the steady shear flow of a two-phase system, it is generally accepted that the rate of deformation may be discontinuous at the interface, and it is more appropriate to consider constant stress variation of various rheological functions than constant rate.[147] Using a similar argument for the dynamic functions, it should be concluded that G' at constant G'' should be used. To illustrate the point, in Fig. 15.39 the isochronal G' is plotted versus weight fraction of the second component for linear low density polyethylene (LLDPE) blends with another LLDPE or with low density polyethylene (LDPE), whereas in Fig. 15.40 the same data are plotted at $G'' = $ const rather than at $\omega = $ const. While in Fig.

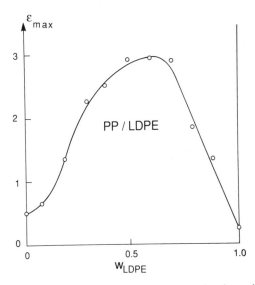

Fig. 15.41. Maximum shrinkage of polypropylene/low density polyethylene (PP/LDPE) blend extrudates after 60 min in silicone oil at 180 °C; W_{LDPE} is the weight fraction of LDPE.[427]

15.39 strong PDB is observed, in Fig. 15.40 the data show either additivity or NDB, a behavior similar to that of η versus w_2.

Another method of estimating the elasticity contribution is via the Bagley entrance–exit pressure drop correction, P_e. The plot of P_e versus σ_{12} for single-phase systems is independent of capillary diameter, temperature and molecular weight, but rather sensitive to changes in flow profile.[290] Furthermore, for a series of polymers with an increasing degree of branching, P_e (at $\sigma_{12} = $ const) increases as expected from the network model. The plot was found to be quite useful for interpretation of the stress, temperature and composition dependent morphological changes in immiscible polymer blends.[195,397] At low $\phi \leqslant 0.1$, P_e was found to be independent of T, and at constant shear stress it increased with loading. At higher concentrations P_e behaved in a complex manner, dependent on ϕ, T and σ_{12}.

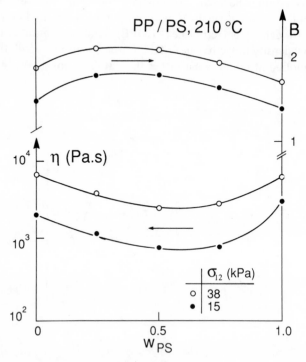

Fig. 15.42. Extrudate swell (top) and shear viscosity at 210 °C and shear stress $\sigma_{12} = 15$ and 38 kPa as a function of weight fraction of polystyrene in blends with polypropylene.[426]

The extrudate swell, B, has been used to calculate the recoverable shear strain, γ_R, for single-phase materials.[416,417] Introduction of the interface negates the basic theoretical assumptions on which the calculation of γ_R was based. In addition, presence of the yield stress, frequently observed in multiphase systems, prevents B from reaching its equilibrium value required to calculate γ_R and then N_1. Nevertheless, B is used as a qualitative measure of blend elasticity.[418] Extrudate swell for rubber compounds was reviewed by Leblanc.[419] In several papers the maximum of B was observed for approximate 1:1 mixtures.[420–427] It seems that the presence of the second deformable phase leads to the enhancement of B. This phenomenon may originate in the elastic recovery of domains extended during the convergent flow in the capillary entrance. In Fig. 15.41 the shrinkage, defined as

$$\varepsilon_{max} = \lim_{t \to \infty} \ln(L_0/L) \tag{15.156}$$

is presented for polypropylene/low density polyethylene blends (PP/LDPE).[427] In eqn (15.156) L_0 and L stand for the initial and final lengths

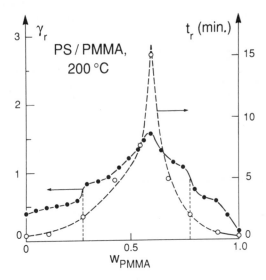

Fig. 15.43. Strain recovery of polystyrene/polymethylmethacrylate blends at 200 °C; the total recoverable strain, γ_r, and the time of recovery, t_r, are plotted versus the weight fraction of the second component; the concentrations of morphological changes are indicated.[413]

of the extrudate kept in a silicone oil bath at 180 °C; $\varepsilon_{max} = 3$ means that $L_0 \simeq 20L$ or $D \simeq 4.5D_0$. Directly measured extrudate swell for ribbons (die width six times larger than height) gave $B_{width} \simeq 1.5$, $B_{height} \simeq 3.7$. These large swells and shrinkages are related to fibrillation of the dispersed phase and subsequent tendency to contract into spherical domains. As demonstrated in Fig. 15.42, even when $\eta = \eta(\phi)$ shows NDB, B versus ϕ may show PDB.[426]

Similar information was obtained from measurements of strain recovery, γ_r, for PS/PMMA blends.[413] A maximum of γ_r was reported at $w_{PMMA} = 0.58$, coinciding with the longest recovery time. The plot of γ_r versus w_2 (see Fig. 15.43) indicated two steps at $w_2 \simeq 0.27$ and 0.78, interpreted by the authors as evidence of the boundary concentration at which the dispersed and co-continuous morphologies meet. It is unfortunate that this test procedure is not more widely used in research on PAB.

(f) Elongational flows. Owing to experimental difficulties there are only a few publications on uniaxial deformation of PAB. To prepare specimens for testing, samples usually have to be transfer molded and relaxed, both operations requiring the blend to be kept molten for a relatively long time (up to an hour). During this period only well stabilized blends will not coarsen.

It is convenient to distinguish two contributions to the tensile stress growth function, η_E^+, one due to the linear viscoelastic response, η_{EL}^+, and the other originating in the structural change of the specimen during deformation, η_{ES}^+. The first can be calculated from any linear viscoelastic response, e.g. in shear[428,429]

$$\eta_{EL}^+(t) = 3\eta_L^+(t) = 3\eta_0 \int_{-\infty}^{\infty} \tilde{H}_G[1 - \exp(\omega t)] \, d\ln\omega \quad (15.157)$$

where $\tilde{H}_G$ is the frequency relaxation spectrum

$$\tilde{H}_G = (2/\pi) r_h^{-m_2} \sin(m_2 \theta_h) \quad (15.158)$$

with the parameters r_h and θ_h given by

$$r_h = [1 + 2(\omega\tau^*)^{m_1} \cos(m_1 \pi/2) + (\omega\tau^*)^{2m_1}]^{1/2} \quad (15.159)$$

$$\theta_h = \arcsin[(\omega\tau^*)^{m_1} r_h^{-1} \sin(m\pi/2)] \quad (15.160)$$

with η_0, τ^*, m_1 and m_2 being the parameters of eqn (15.46).

The second component, η_{ES}, depends on the intermolecular interactions or entanglements, and its value depends on both the total strain, $\varepsilon = \dot{\varepsilon}t$,

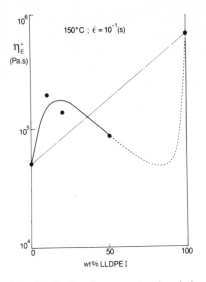

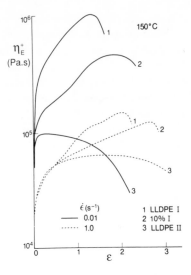

Fig. 15.44. Steady state extensional viscosity of two different linear low density polyethylene blends as a function of composition; points are experimental, and the curve is from eqn (15.132).

Fig. 15.45. Log η_E versus ε for LLDPE-I (showing the strain hardening behavior), LLDPE-II (a standard resin), and their blend containing 10% of LLDPE-I; 150 °C, $\dot{\varepsilon} = 0.01$ and $1\,\text{s}^{-1}$.[290]

and either strain rate $\dot{\varepsilon}$ or straining time t. Owing to the industrial importance of strain hardening (SH), a large body of literature focuses on the optimization of PAB composition to maximize SH. Since SH depends on the entanglement, blending branched polymers usually affects SH even in a low concentration range.

In homologous polymer blends,[323] plots of the zero-extension rate, Troutonian viscosity, $\eta_{E,0}$, versus ϕ indicate PDB behavior in agreement with the prediction of the statistical thermodynamic theory discussed in Section 15.3.2.2. The creep curves for these blends were very similar.

Most of the work on uniaxial extensional flow of immiscible polymer blends has focused on the behavior of systems containing polyethylene. The main reason is the need for better, easier-to-process film resins, and also for a relative stability of polyolefin blend morphology. The film blowing conceptually involves two different engineering operations: extrusion and blowing. For most production lines the latter limits productivity. For the low density resins (LDPE), the strain hardening provides a self-regulating, self-healing mechanism. For high density (HDPE) and the newest, linear low density (LLDPE) polyethylenes, some strain hardening can be obtained for the high MW and MWD resins. As a result, 60–70% of LLDPE on the market are blends. For film blowing the LLDPE is blended with LDPE, rubbers, copolymers, or another type of LLDPE resin. In all cases improvement in strain hardening has been observed. Examples of uniaxial extensional behavior of LLDPE-I/LLDPE-II[290,429] are shown in Figs. 15.44 and 15.45. The obtained strain hardening translated directly into improved bubble stability and increased output. SH was also found to be an important resin characteristic in wire coating.[293] Here the surface finish and uniformity of the deposited layer were superior for blends with high strain hardening and low shear viscosity.

LaMantia et al.[430] calculated η_E from the entrance–exit pressure drop in capillary flow. The method did not allow control of the straining time, and the results represent neither equilibrium nor constant strain values. Nevertheless the method allows gradation of relative performance. The authors reported that for a series of HDPE blends with LDPE, η_E varies systematically with composition: 'When the shear viscosity of the LDPE is much higher than that of HDPE all blends show a behavior very similar to that of LDPE . . .'. The miscibility of the system was not discussed.

Min[395] reported η_E versus w_2 dependence for blends of HDPE with PS, polyamide-6, PA-6, and polycarbonate (PC). Three HDPE samples of different molecular weight (MW) blended with PS showed either positive or negative deviation from the log-additivity rule (PDB or NDB); the blend with PA-6 showed NDB, that with PC a PDB behavior. Min reported that increase of steady state shear stress viscosity occurred when droplet formation was observed; it decreased when layered ones were present.

The 50:50 LLDPE/PP blend, with or without compatibilizing ethylene–propylene copolymer (EPR), was studied by Dumoulin et al.[292] The rheological behaviors under extensional, dynamic and steady state shear flow fields were compared. In spite of the expected immiscibility, the blends showed additivity of properties with good superposition of the stress growth functions in shear and elongation as well as with the zero deformation rate Trouton ratio $R_T^0 \simeq 1$. In the earlier work,[431] blends of medium density PE (MDPE; of the LLDPE type) with small quantities, $w_2 \leqslant 0.06$, of ultra-high molecular weight polyethylene (UHMWPE) were studied in shear and extension. Owing to only partial dissolution of UHMWPE, the blends had the character of a miscible blend with compatible filler particles. Again $R_T^0 \simeq 1$ was observed, but upon increase of UHMWPE content a strain hardening in extension took place.

It has been shown[290,291] that the stress growth function in uniaxial extension provides three important pieces of information on the polymer. The initial slope

$$S_i = \lim_{t \to 0} (d \ln \eta_E^+ / d \ln t) \tag{15.161}$$

correlates with the polydispersity index M_z/M_n as measured by size exclusion chromatography (SEC); M_z and M_n are respectively z- and n-average molecular weight. The plateau or equilibrium value

$$\eta_E^0 = \lim_{t, \dot{\varepsilon} \to 0} \eta_E^+ (\dot{\varepsilon}, t) \tag{15.162}$$

provides information on the weight average molecular weight, and the stress hardening part, η_{ES}, on entanglement, i.e. branching, association, etc.

The S_i defined in eqn (15.161) can provide an indication of miscibility in PAB. Solubility usually broadens the width of the MW distribution (MWD) and S_i value increases; by contrast, immiscibility causes separation of high molecular weight fractions, narrowing MWD and decreasing S_i. The sigmoidal curve in Fig. 15.44 was found to be paralleled by S_i

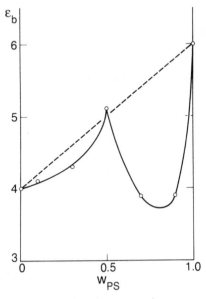

Fig. 15.46. The maximum strain at break versus polystyrene content for PS/PE-2 blends.[395]

versus w_2 dependence. Knowing the relation between S_i and M_z/M_n allowed postulation of partial miscibility in the molten LLDPE blends at the $w_2 < 0.25$ limit.

The miscibility can also be reflected in a maximum strain at break, ε_b, versus w_2 dependence. In 'antagonistically' immiscible blends of PA-6 in LLDPE, a sharp decrease of ε_b in the investigated range of $w_{PA} \leqslant 0.35$ was observed. In some blends the presence of co-continuous structures around the 50:50 composition allows ε_b to increase to an average value, with negative deviations on both sides. This is illustrated in Fig. 15.46 with data for PS/PE blends.[395]

The convergent flow at the die entrance provides a powerful means of droplet deformation, leading to modification of properties. These effects have been reported for PE with PS, PC, and PA-6,[387,395,432] for HDPE with PA-6,[195,397] or blends containing polymeric liquid crystals (LCP).[433,434]

As in emulsions, in PAB the low frequency dynamic data as well as the uniaxial extension allow measurement of the apparent yield stress. In extension, the operational definition for the yield stress is lack of detectable deformation during a 30 min test under constant stress conditions when the set stress level is $\sigma_{11} < \sigma_y$. Interestingly, it was observed for PP/LLDPE blends;[392] σ_y was detected in blends of polymer A dispersed in B, but absent for blends of B dispersed in A. Obviously, in this case the Trouton ratio $R_T^0 > 1$.

Finally, it is worth mentioning the fine studies on extensional properties of acrylonitrile–butadiene–styrene terpolymer (ABS) by Saito.[435] Several resins of different morphology and composition were studied. The results provide an excellent basis for interpretation of extensional behavior of compatibilized polymer alloys, such as PS/LDPE containing poly(hydrogenated butadiene-b-styrene) as the interface modifier.[436]

15.4. CONCLUSIONS

In this chapter an attempt has been made to underline the common features of multiphase flows. It is shown that to obtain non-Newtonian behavior one does not have to have systems containing non-Newtonian liquids. Strong interparticle interactions, generated by interface modification or concentration, provide sufficient conditions for the complex rheological behavior of suspensions or emulsions based on simple fluids. As an example, apparent yield stresses exist not only in suspensions but also in emulsions and foams.

TABLE 15.8
Summary of Rheological Responses of Polymer Composites and Blends

No.	Property	Condition	Responses	
			Composites	*Blends*
1.	Newtonian	$\eta_r = \eta_r(\phi)$	Increases as a function of ϕ and p	Increases in most cases, decreases in the case of morphological change or interlayer slip
2.	Non-Newtonian	Yield stress	Prevalent for small particles, high p and ϕ	Observed for 'compatibilized' blends at higher ϕ
		$\eta = \eta(\dot\gamma)$	Discontinuities occuring at $\dot\gamma$ motivated morphological rearrangements of liquids	
		G', G''	Secondary plateau at high ϕ strain sensitivity	Secondary plateau and high ϕ strain sensitivity seldom observed
		$N_1 = N_1(\phi)$	Signal dependent on orientation and morphology; yield in G' and G'' Increases with ϕ	
		N_1 vs σ_{12}	Do not superimpose for different ϕ	
		G' vs G''	Superimpose for $\phi < \phi_m$ then decreases with ϕ	Superimposes for different ϕ

TABLE 15.8—*contd.*
Summary of Rheological Responses of Polymer Composites and Blends

No.	Property	Condition	Responses	
			Composites	*Blends*
		$B = B(\phi)$	Decreases	Increases for most (except rigid droplet dispersion) up to maximum near 1:1: composition
3.	Extensional	η_{E}^{+} vs t	Yield stress, orientation; does not superimpose at different $\dot{\varepsilon}$	Strong effect of constituents with strain hardening; at low $\dot{\varepsilon}$ usually $\eta_{E}^{+} = 3\eta^{+}$
		$\eta_{E}/3\eta$	Increases with ϕ	Complex, dependent on strain hardening, morphology, ...
		Orientation	Orientation with stress field	Deformation and orientation may lead to dramatic morphological changes

These simpler systems provide an excellent introduction to the rheology of polymer alloys, blends and composites (PABC). Here the flow is not only controlled by the interphase conditions, but also by the viscoelastic properties inside each phase. Because of significant commercial interest in PABC, publications dealing mainly with experimental evaluation of these complex systems have been rapidly increasing. A summary is provided in Table 15.8.

In any multiphase system there is an inherent, reciprocal relation between structure and rheology. Depending on the interface properties and concentration, straining changes the system morphology, inflicting various rheological responses, such as normal stress in Newtonian liquid emulsions. The most efficient method of structure modification is extensional flow, but large strain Couette or Poiseuille flow also affect the morphology. To study material behavior with well defined structure only low strain dynamic methods may provide the answer. For generating data to be used in modeling or interpretation of die flow, one must simulate not only flow conditions but also the system's past history as well as the geometry to scale. Since miscibility changes with temperature and pressure, flow of some PABs may be very sensitive to these variables.

There is a growing need for accelerated, dedicated, multidisciplinary research on flow, thermodynamics, processability and properties of multiphase systems. This domain of science lags behind industrial progress not only for predicting, but frequently for explaining, the observed facts.

REFERENCES

1. R. Darby, *Viscoelastic Fluid*, Marcel Dekker, New York, 1976.
2. R. B. Bird, R. C. Armstrong and O. Hassager, *Dynamics of Polymeric Liquids*, Vol. 1, Wiley, New York, 1977.
3. R. B. Bird, O. Hassager, R. C. Armstrong and C. F. Curtiss, *Dynamics of Polymeric Liquids*, Vol. 2, Wiley, New York, 1976.
4. C. J. S. Petrie, *Elongational Flows*, Pitman, London, 1979.
5. R. I. Tanner, *Engineering Rheology*, Clarendon Press, Oxford, 1985.
6. H. L. Frish and R. Simha, in *Rheology*, Vol. 1, F. R. Eirich (Ed.), Academic Press, New York, 1956.
7. R. Rutgers, *Rheol. Acta*, 1962, **2**, 305.
8. D. G. Thomas, *J. Colloid Sci.*, 1965, **20**, 267.
9. L. A. Utracki and B. Fisa, *Polymer Comp.*, 1982, **3**, 193.
10. L. A. Utracki, Proc. 74th AIChE meeting, Los Angeles, Nov. 15–18, 1982.
11. L. A. Utracki, in *Current Topics in Polymer Science*, R. M. Ottenbrite, L. A. Utracki and S. Inoue (Eds), Hanser, München, 1987.

12. J. Mewis, in *Rheology*, G. Astarita, G. Marrucci and L. Nicolais (Eds). Vol. 1, Plenum Press, New York, 1980, pp. 149–68.
13. A. B. Metzner, *J. Rheol.*, 1985, **29**, 739.
14. H. L. Goldsmith and S. G. Mason, in *Rheology*, F. R. Eirich (Ed.), Vol. 4, Academic Press, New York, 1967.
15. R. Simha, *J. Appl. Phys.*, 1952, **23**, 1020.
16. M. Mooney, *J. Colloid Sci.*, 1951, **6**, 162.
17. L. A. Utracki, *J. Macromol. Sci. Phys.*, 1980, **B18**, 725.
18. L. A. Utracki and R. Simha, *J. Rheol.*, 1981, **25**, 329.
19. A. Einstein, *Ann. Phys.*, 1906, **19**, 289; 1911, **34**, 591.
20. A. Einstein, *Kolloid-Z.*, 1920, **27**, 137.
21. W. R. Hess, *Kolloid-Z.*, 1920, **27**, 1.
22. W. Vand, *Nature*, 1954, **155**, 364.
23. H. De Bruyn, *Rec. Trav. Chim. Pays-Bas*, 1942, **61**, 863.
24. S. H. Maron and P. E. Pierce, *J. Colloid Sci.*, 1956, **11**, 80.
25. D. Quemada, *Rheol. Acta*, 1977, **16**, 82.
26. H. C. Brinkman, *J. Chem. Phys.*, 1952, **20**, 571.
27. R. F. Landel, B. G. Moser and A. Bauman, Proc. 4th Int. Congr. Rheol., USA, 1963.
28. R. Roscoe, *Brit. J. Appl. Phys.*, 1952, **3**, 267.
29. I. M. Krieger and T. J. Dougherty, *Trans. Soc. Rheol.*, 1959, **3**, 137.
30. H. E. White and S. F. Walton, *J. Amer. Ceram. Soc.*, 1937, **20**, 155.
31. C. D. Scott, *Nature,* 1960, **188**, 908.
32. R. Rutgers, *Rheol. Acta*, 1962, **2**, 202, 305.
33. D. I. Lee, *J. Paint Technol.*, 1970, **42**, 579.
34. M. Smoluchowski, *Kolloid-Z.*, 1916, **18**, 190.
35. H. de Bruijn, *Discuss. Faraday Soc.*, 1951, **11**, 86.
36. R. S. J. Manley and S. G. Mason, *J. Colloid Sci.*, 1952, **7**, 354.
37. G. F. Eveson, in *Rheology of Dispersed Systems*, C. C. Mill (Ed.), Pergamon Press, London, 1959.
38. H. Goto and H. Kuno, *J. Rheol.*, 1982, **26**, 387; 1984, **28**, 197.
39. R. K. McGeary, *J. Amer. Ceram. Soc.*, 1961, **44**, 513.
40. L. A. Utracki, Gulf Oil Corp., Internal Reports, 1970, 1971.
41. H. T. Horsfield, *J. Soc. Chem. Ind.*, 1934, 107T–115T.
42. J. Ritter, *Appl. Polym. Symp.*, 1971, **15**, 239.
43. F. W. Lord, UK Patent Appl. No. 51292, 1971.
44. R. J. Farris, *Trans. Soc. Rheol.*, 1968, **12**, 281.
45. C. Parkinson, S. Matsumoto and P. Sherman, *J. Colloid Interface Sci.*, 1970, **33**, 150.
46. J. S. Chong, E. B. Christiansen and A. D. Baer, *J. Appl. Polym. Sci.*, 1971, **15**, 2007.
47. T. G. M. van de Ven, NRCC/IMRI symposium, Composites '84, Boucherville, Quebec, Canada, Nov. 20, 1984; *Polym. Compos.*, 1985, **6**, 209.
48. R. Simha, *J. Res. Nat. Bur. Stand.*, 1949, **42**, 409; *J. Colloid Sci.*, 1950, **5**, 386.
49. R. Simha, *J. Phys. Chem.*, 1960, **44**, 25; *J. Chem. Phys.*, 1945, **13**, 188.
50. S. Haber and H. Brenner, *J. Colloid Interface Sci.*, 1984, **97**, 496.
51. B. Fisa and L. A. Utracki, *Polym. Compos.*, 1984, **5**, 36.
52. L. A. Utracki, *Rubber Chem. Technol.*, 1984, **57**, 507.

53. H. Brenner and D. W. Condiff, *J. Colloid Interface Sci.*, 1979, **47**, 199.
54. M. Doi and S. F. Edwards, *J. Chem. Soc., Faraday Trans. II*, 1978, **74**, 560, 918.
55. L. A. Utracki, B. D. Favis and B. Fisa, NRCC/IMRI symposium Composites '83, Boucherville, Quebec, Canada, Nov. 29, 1983; *Polym. Compos.*, 1984, **5**, 277.
56. M. M. Cross, A. Kaye, J. L. Stanford and R. F. T. Stepto, *ACS Polym. Mater. Sci. Eng. Div., Preprints*, 1983, **49**, 531.
57. R. O. Maschmeyer and C. T. Hill, *Adv. Chem.*, 1974, **134**, 95.
58. R. O. Maschmeyer and C. T. Hill, *Trans. Soc. Rheol.*, 1977, **21**, 183, 195.
59. H. Brenner, *J. Fluid Mech.*, 1970, **4**, 641.
60. G. K. Batchelor, *J. Fluid Mech.*, 1970, **44**, 419; 1971, **46**, 813.
61. R. Patzold, *Rheol. Acta*, 1980, **19**, 322.
62. T. E. Kizior and F. A. Seyer, *Trans. Soc. Rheol.*, 1974, **18**, 271.
63. G. B. Weinberger and J. D. Goddard, *Int. J. Multiphase Flow*, 1974, **1**, 465.
64. J. Mewis and A. B. Metzner, *J. Fluid Mech.*, 1974, **62**, 593.
65. A. Karnis, H. L. Goldsmith and S. G. Mason, *J. Colloid Interface Sci.*, 1966, **22**, 531.
66. E. B. Vadas, H. L. Goldsmith and S. G. Mason, *J. Colloid Interface Sci.*, 1973, **43**, 630.
67. R. L. Hoffman, *Trans. Soc. Rheol.*, 1972, **16**, 155.
68. R. L. Hoffman, *J. Colloid Interface Sci.*, 1974, **46**, 491.
69. T. A. Strivens, *J. Colloid Interface Sci.*, 1976, **57**, 476.
70. I. M. Krieger and G. N. Choi, Proc. IX Int. Congr. Rheol., Mexico, 1984; *Advances in Rheology*, B. Mena, A. Garcia-Rejon and C. Rangel-Nafaile (Eds), Univ. Nat. Auton. Mexico, 1984, **2**, 641.
71. M. Tomita and T. G. M. van de Ven, *J. Colloid Interface Sci.*, 1984, **49**, 374.
72. M. Tomita, K. Takano and T. G. M. van de Ven, *J. Colloid Interface Sci.*, 1982, **92**, 367.
73. A. Karnis, PhD thesis, McGill University, 1966.
74. F. Gauthier, H. L. Goldsmith and S. G. Mason, *Rheol. Acta*, 1971, **10**, 344.
75. E. Bartram, H. L. Goldsmith and S. G. Mason, *Rheol. Acta*, 1975, **14**, 776.
76. H. Giesekus, private communication, 1981.
77. D. C. Prieve, M. S. John and T. L. Koenig, *J. Rheol.*, 1985, **29**, 639.
78. T. E. Karis, D. C. Prieve and S. L. Rosen, *J. Rheol.*, 1984, **28**, 381.
79. T. Matsumoto, S. Yao and S. Onogi, *J. Rheol.*, 1986, **30**, 509.
80. S. Onogi and T. Matsumoto, *Polym. Eng. Rev.*, 1981, **1**, 45.
81. K. N. Murty and G. F. Modlen, *Polym. Eng. Sci.*, 1977, **17**, 848.
82. F. Folgar and C. L. Tucker III, *J. Reinf. Plast. Compos.*, 1984, **3**, 98.
83. A. Salinas and J. F. T. Pittman, *Polym. Eng. Sci.*, 1981, **21**, 23.
84. L. A. Utracki, Proc. NRCC/IMRI Symp., Composites '85, Boucherville Quebec, Canada, Nov. 19 and 20, 1985; *Polym. Compos.*, 1986, **5**, 274.
85. R. G. Cox and S. G. Mason, *Ann. Rev. Fluid Mech.*, 1971, **3**, 291.
86. G. K. Batchelor, *Ann. Rev. Fluid Mech.*, 1974, **6**, 227.
87. L. G. Leal, *Ann. Rev. Fluid Mech.*, 1980, **12**, 435.
88. T. Sato, *J. Coat. Technol.*, 1979, **51**, 79.
89. T. L. Smith and C. A. Bruce, *J. Colloid Interface Sci.*, 1979, **72**, 13.
90. A. Zosel, *Rheol. Acta*, 1982, **21**, 72.

91. R. J. Hunter, R. Matarese and D. H. Napper, *Colloid Surf.*, 1983, **7**, 1.
92. C. R. Wildemuth and M. C. Williams, *Rheol. Acta*, 1984, **23**, 627.
93. J. T. Lin, M. S. El-Aasser, C. A. Silebi and J. W. Vanderhoff, *J. Colloid Interface Sci.*, 1986, **110**, 305.
94. Y. Mikami, *Nihon Reor. Gakk.*, 1980, **8**, 137.
95. Y. Mikami, *Nihon Reor. Gakk.*, 1980, **8**, 3.
96. I. E. Denisov, A. I. Krasheninnikov and V. G. Chervin, *Kolloid. Zhurn.*, 1985, **47**, 790.
97. J. F. Brady and G. Bossis, *J. Fluid Mech.*, 1985, **155**, 105.
98. J. D. Goddard, *S. M. Archives*, 1977, **2**, 403.
99. J. Mewis, *J. Non-Newtonian Fluid Mech.*, 1979, **6**, 1.
100. W. B. Russel, *J. Rheol.*, 1980, **24**, 287.
101. W. B. Russel, in *Theory of Dispersed Multiphase Flow*, R. E. Meyer (Ed.), Academic Press, New York, 1983.
102. D. D. Joye and G. W. Pohlein, *Trans. Soc. Rheol.*, 1971, **15**, 51.
103. C. C. Mill (Ed.), *Rheology of Dispersed Systems*, Pergamon Press, London, 1959.
104. J. R. Van Wazer, J. W. Lyons, K. Y. Kim and R. E. Colwell, *Viscosity and Flow Measurements*, Interscience, New York, 1963.
105. P. Sherman, in *Rheology of Emulsions*, P. Sherman (Ed.), Pergamon Press, Oxford, 1963.
106. P. Sherman, in *Emulsion Science*, P. Sherman (Ed.), Academic Press, London, 1968.
107. W. A. Bauer and E. A. Collins, Thixotropy and dilatancy, in *Rheology*, Vol. 4, F. R. Eirich (Ed.), Academic Press, New York, 1968.
108. D. J. Jeffrey and A. Acrivos, *AIChE J.*, 1976, **22**, 417.
109. A. I. Leonov, in *Progress in Heat and Mass Transfer*, W. R. Showalter (Ed.), Pergamon Press, Oxford, 1972.
110. O. V. Voinov and A. A. Trapeznikov, *Dokl. Akad. Nauk SSSR*, 1972, **202**, 1049.
111. T. Matsumoto, A. Takashima, T. Masuda and S. Onogi, *Trans. Soc. Rheol.*, 1970, **14**, 617.
112. T. Kataoka, T. Kitano, M. Sasahara and K. Nishijima, *Rheol. Acta*, 1978, **17**, 149.
113. L. A. Utracki and B. Schlund, *Polym. Eng. Sci.*, 1987, **27**, 367.
114. L. A. Utracki, *S.P.E. Techn. Pap.*, 1985, **31**, 1024; *J. Vinyl Technol.*, 1985, **7**, 142.
115. T. Amari and K. Watanabe, *Polym. Eng. Rev.*, 1983, **3**, 277.
116. N. Q. Dzuy and D. V. Boger, *J. Rheol.*, 1983, **27**, 321; 1985, **29**, 335.
117. M. M. Cross, *J. Colloid Sci.*, 1965, **20**, 417; 1970, **33**, 30; 1973, **44**, 175.
118. R. V. Williamson, *J. Rheol.*, 1930, **1**, 283.
119. L. Nicodemo, L. Nicolais and R. F. Landel, *J. Eng. Sci.*, 1974, **29**, 729.
120. D. Quemada, P. Flaud and P. H. Jezequel, *Chem. Eng. Comm.*, 1985, **32**, 61.
121. G. N. Choi and I. M. Krieger, *J. Colloid. Interface Sci.*, 1986, **113**, 101.
122. E. J. Hinch and L. G. Leal, *J. Fluid Mech.*, 1972, **52**, 683.
123. W. E. VanArsdale, *J. Rheol.*, 1982, **26**, 477.
124. C. N. De Silva, *Acta Mech.*, 1982, **47**, 7; 1983, **49**, 221.
125. S. M. Dinh and R. C. Armstrong, *J. Rheol.*, 1984, **28**, 207.

126. M. A. Bibbo, S. M. Dinh and R. C. Armstrong, *J. Rheol.*, 1985, **29**, 905.
127. G. J. Lin, J. H. Perry and W. R. Schowalter, *J. Fluid Mech.*, 1970, **44**, 1.
128. D. Chan and R. L. Powell, *J. Non-Newtonian Fluid Mech.*, 1984, **15**, 165.
129. K.-W. Lem and C. D. Han, *J. Rheol.*, 1983, **27**, 263.
130. G. K. Batchelor, *J. Fluid Mech.*, 1977, **83**, 97.
131. F. A. Gadala-Maria, PhD thesis, Stanford University, 1979.
132. F. A. Gadala-Maria and A. Acrivos, *J. Rheol.*, 1980, **24**, 799.
133. L. Carter and J. Goddard, NASA Report N67-30073, 1967.
134. T. Kitano and T. Kataoka, *Rheol. Acta*, 1981, **20**, 390.
135. C. D. Han and R. G. King, *J. Rheol.*, 1980, **24**, 213.
136. S. Goto, H. Nagazono and H. Kato, *Rheol. Acta*, 1986, **25**, 119, 246.
137. K. D. Roberts, MSc thesis, Washington University, St. Louis, 1973.
138. K. D. Roberts and C. T. Hill, *S.P.E. Techn. Pap.*, 1973, **19**, 563.
139. M. A. Newab and S. G. Mason, *J. Phys. Chem.*, 1958, **62**, 1248.
140. E. Ganani and R. L. Powell, *J. Comp. Mater.*, 1985, **19**, 194.
141. K. Watanabe and T. Amari, *Rep. Progr. Polym. Phys. Japan*, 1984, **27**, 123.
142. M. Doi, *Adv. Colloid Interface Sci.*, 1982, **17**, 233.
143. Y. Ivanov, T. G. M. van de Ven and S. G. Mason, *J. Rheol.*, 1982, **26**, 213.
144. Y. Ivanov and T. G. M. van de Ven, *J. Rheol.*, 1982, **26**, 231.
145. A. Okagawa, R. G. Cox and S. G. Mason, *J. Colloid Interface Sci.*, 1973, **45**, 303.
146. M. Zuzovsky, Z. Priel and S. G. Mason, *J. Rheol.*, 1980, **24**, 705.
147. C. D. Han, *Multiphase Flow in Polymer Processing*, Academic Press, New York, 1981.
148. L. A. Faitelson, *Int. J. Polym. Mater.*, 1980, **8**, 207.
149. J. L. White, *Plast. Comp.*, 1982, **5**, 47.
150. C. E. Chaffey, *Ann. Rev. Mater. Sci.*, 1983, **13**, 43.
151. L. A. Goettler and K. S. Shen, *Rubber Chem. Technol.*, 1983, **56**, 619.
152. L. A. Goettler, NRCC/IMRI symposium Composites '82, Montreal, Quebec, Canada, Nov. 30, 1982; *Polym. Compos.*, 1984, **5**, 60.
153. H. G. Bundenberg de Jong, H. R. Kruyt and J. Lens, *Kolloid-Beth*, 1932, **36**, 429.
154. A. F. Martin, Proc. A.C.S. Meeting, Memphis Tennessee, 1942.
155. F. M. Chapman and T. S. Lee, *S.P.E. Techn. Pap.*, 1969, **15**, 293.
156. G. V. Vinogradov, A. Ya Malkin, E. P. Plotnikova, O. Yu. Sabsai and N. E. Nikolayeva, *Int. J. Polym. Mater.*, 1972, **2**, 1.
157. L. Nicodemo and L. Nicolais, *J. Appl. Polym. Sci.*, 1974, **18**, 2809.
158. K. Iwakura and T. Fujimura, *J. Appl. Polym. Sci.*, 1979, **24**, 975.
159. W. M. Lobe and J. L. White, *S.P.E. Techn. Pap.*, 1979, **25**, 575: *Polym. Eng. Sci.*, 1979, **19**, 617.
160. G. Menges, P. Geisbuesch and U. Zingel, *Kautsch. Gummi Kunst.*, 1979, **32**, 485.
161. T. Matsumoto, O. Yamamoto and S. Onogi, *J. Rheol.*, 1980, **24**, 379.
162. H. Tanaka and J. L. White, *Polym. Eng. Sci.*, 1980, **20**, 949.
163. J. L. White and H. Tanaka, *J. Appl. Polym. Sci.*, 1981, **26**, 576.
164. H. Münstedt, Proc. 7th Int. Congr. Rheology, Gothenburg, Sweden, Aug. 23–27, 1976.
165. J. E. Stamhuis and J. P. A. Loppé, *Rheol. Acta*, 1982, **21**, 103.

166. D. M. Bigg, *Polym. Eng. Sci.*, 1982, **22**, 512; 1983, **23**, 206.
167. T. S. Cantu and J. M. Caruthers, *J. Appl. Polym. Sci.*, 1982, **27**, 3079.
168. R. S. Ziegelbaur and J. M. Caruthers, *J. Non-Newtonian Fluid Mech.*, 1985, **17**, 45.
169. L. E. Kosinski and J. M. Caruthers, *J. Non-Newtonian Fluid Mech.*, 1985, **17**, 69; *J. Appl. Polym. Sci.*, 1986, **32**, 3393.
170. R. E. S. Bretas and R. L. Powell, *Rheol. Acta*, 1985, **24**, 69.
171. D. R. Saini, A. V. Shenoy and V. M. Nadkarni, *Polym. Compos.*, 1986, **7**, 193.
172. B. Fisa and L. A. Utracki, S.P.E.-NATEC, Detroit, Michigan, Sept. 20–22, 1983.
173. L. A. Utracki and J. Lara, Proc. NRCC/IMRI symposium Composites '82, Montreal, Quebec, Canada, Nov. 30, 1982; *Polym. Compos.*, 1984, **5**, 44.
174. T. Kitano, T. Kataoka, T. Nishimura and T. Sakai, *Rheol. Acta*, 1980, **19**, 764.
175. T. Kitano, T. Nishimura, T. Kataoka and T. Sakai, *Rheol. Acta*, 1980, **19**, 671.
176. T. Kitano and T. Kataoka, *Rheol. Acta*, 1980, **19**, 753.
177. H. M. Laun, *Colloid Polym. Sci.*, 1984, **262**, 257.
178. A. T. Mutel and M. R. Kamal, NRCC/IMRI symposium Composites '82, Montreal, Quebec, Canada, Nov. 30, 1982; *Polym. Compos.*, 1984, **5**, 29.
179. M. R. Kamal, A. T. Mutel and L. A. Utracki, NRCC/IMRI symposium Composites '83, Boucherville, Quebec, Canada, Nov. 29, 1983; *Polym. Compos.*, 1984, **5**, 289.
180. J. L. White, L. Czarnecki and H. Tanaka, *Rubber Chem. Technol.*, 1980, **53**, 823.
181. B. A. Knutsson, J. L. White and K. B. Abbas, in *Rheology*, G. Astarita, G. Marrucci and L. Nicolais (Eds), Vol. 3, Plenum Press, New York, 1980, p. 83; *J. Appl. Polym. Sci.*, 1981, **26**, 2347.
182. T. Kitano, T. Kataoka and Y. Nagatsuka, *Rheol. Acta*, 1984, **23**, 20.
183. C. D. Han, *J. Appl. Polym. Sci.*, 1974, **18**, 821.
184. F.-D. Martischius, *Rheol. Acta*, 1982, **21**, 311.
185. P. K. Agarwal, E. B. Bagley and C. T. Hill, *Polym. Eng. Sci.*, 1978, **18**, 282.
186. D. C. Goel, *Polym. Eng. Sci.*, 1980, **20**, 198.
187. A. K. Bagchi and K. Sirkar, *J. Appl. Polym. Sci.*, 1979, **23**, 1653.
188. R. J. Crowson and M. J. Folkes, *Polym. Eng. Sci.*, 1980, **20**, 934.
189. W.-K. Lee and H. H. George, *Polym. Eng. Sci.*, 1978, **18**, 146.
190. E. B. Bagley, *Trans. Soc. Rheol.*, 1961, **5**, 355.
191. J. S. Vrentas and C. M. Vrentas, *J. Non-Newtonian Fluid Mech.*, 1983, **12**, 211.
192. E. Mitsoulis, J. Vlachopoulos and F. A. Mirza, NRCC/IMRI symposium Modeling '84, Boucherville, Quebec, Canada, Jan. 24, 1984; *Polym. Eng. Sci.*, 1985, **25**, 677.
193. G. Chauvetau, M. Moan and A. Maguer, *J. Non-Newtonian Fluid Mech.*, 1984, **16**, 315.
194. F. N. Cogswell, *Polym. Eng. Sci.*, 1972, **12**, 69.
195. L. A. Utracki, M. M. Dumoulin and P. Toma, NRCC/IMRI symposium

Polyblends '85, Boucherville, Quebec, Canada, Apr. 16–17, 1985; *Polym. Eng. Sci.*, 1986, **26**, 37.

196. Y. Suetsugu and J. L. White, The influence of particle size and surface coating of calcium carbonate on the rheological properties of its suspensions in molten polystyrene, PATRA Report No. 186, June 1982.

197. Y. Chan, J. L. White and Y. Oyanagi, *J. Rheol.*, 1978, **22**, 507.

198. F. Nazem and C. T. Hill, *Trans. Soc. Rheol.*, 1974, **18**, 87.

199. L. Nicodemo, B. De Cindo and L. Nicolais, *Polym. Eng. Sci.*, 1975, **15**, 679.

200. N. Minagawa and J. L. White, *J. Appl. Polym. Sci.*, 1976, **20**, 501.

201. Y. Kawase and J. J. Ulbrecht, *Chem. Eng. Commun.*, 1983, **20**, 127.

202. J. D. Goddard, *J. Rheol.*, 1978, **22**, 615.

203. Y. Suetsugu and J. L. White, *J. Non-Newtonian Fluid Mech.*, 1984, **14**, 121.

204. J. V. Milewski, A.C.S., Div. Org. Coat. Plast. Chem. Prepr., 1977, **38**, 127; *Ind. Eng. Chem. Prod. Res. Dev.*, 1978, **17**, 363.

205. B. W. Sands and C. G. Smith, Proc. 34th Ann. Techn. Conf. Reinf. Plast./ Compos. Inst., Soc. Plast. Inc., S19-B1, 1979.

206. K. D. Roberts and C. T. Hill, Report HPC-72-159, 1974.

207. B. Fisa, B. Sanschagrin and B. D. Favis, NRCC/IMRI symposium Composites '83, Boucherville, Quebec, Canada, Nov. 29, 1983; *Polym. Compos.*, 1984, **5**, 264.

208. B. Fisa, NRCC/IMRI symposium Composites '84, Boucherville, Quebec, Canada, Nov. 20, 1984; *Polym. Compos.*, 1985, **6**, 232.

209. L. R. Daley and F. Rodriguez, *Ind. Eng. Chem. Prod. Dev.*, 1983, **22**, 695.

210. L. A. Utracki and R. Gendron, *J. Rheol.*, 1984, **28**, 601.

211. G. Akay, *J. Non-Newtonian Fluid Mech.*, 1983, **13**, 309.

212. S. Wu, *Polym. Eng. Sci.*, 1979, **19**, 638.

213. V. V. Prokopenko, O. K. Titova, N. S. Fesik, Yu. M. Malinskii and N. F. Bakeyev, *Vysokomol. Soed.*, 1977, **A19**, 95.

214. M. Mansuripur, *Int. J. Multiphase Flow*, 1983, **9**, 299.

215. J. L. White, *J. Appl. Polym. Sci., Appl. Polym. Symp.*, 1985, **41**, 241.

216. P. D. Patel and D. C. Bogue, *Polym. Eng. Sci.*, 1981, **21**, 449.

217. M. R. Kamal and F. H. Moy, *J. Appl. Polym. Sci.*, 1983, **28**, 1787.

218. M. R. Kamal and V. Tan, *Polym. Eng. Sci.*, 1979, **19**, 558.

219. J. L. White and J. E. Spruiell, *Polym. Eng. Sci.*, 1983, **23**, 247.

220. A. I. Isayev, *Polym. Eng. Sci.*, 1983, **23**, 271.

221. M. Vincent, Dr Eng thesis, École Nationale Supérieure des Mines de Paris, Sophia Antipolis, France, 1984.

222. R. Takeserman-Krozer and A. Ziabicki, *J. Polym. Sci.*, 1963, **A1**, 491.

223. K. Okuno and R. T. Woodhams, *Polym. Eng. Sci.*, 1975, **15**, 308.

224. B. Remillard and B. Fisa, 68th Canadian Chemical Conference, 2–5 June 1985, Kingston, Ontario, Canada; *J. Polym. Eng.*, 1986, **6**, 135.

225. J. B. Harris and J. F. T. Pittman, *Trans. Inst. Chem. Eng.*, 1977, **54**, 73.

226. M. Takano, A.R.P.A. Report HPC-73-165; AD-774 968, 1973.

227. K. N. Murty and G. F. Modlen, *Polym. Eng. Sci.*, 1977, **17**, 848.

228. P. F. Bright, R. J. Crowson and M. J. Folkes, *J. Mater. Sci.*, 1978, **13**, 2497.

229. R. J. Crowson, M. J. Folkes and P. F. Bright, *Polym. Eng. Sci.*, 1980, **20**, 925.

230. R. J. Crowson and M. J. Folkes, *Polym. Eng. Sci.*, 1980, **20**, 934.
231. R. J. Crowson, A. J. Scott and D. W. Saunders, *Polym. Eng. Sci.*, 1981, **21**, 1014.
232. R. B. Pipes, R. L. McCullough and D. G. Taggart, *Polym. Compos.*, 1982, **3**, 34.
233. P. H. Hermans and P. Platzek, *Kolloid-Z.*, 1939, **88**, 68.
234. H. Menendez and J. L. White, *Polym. Eng. Sci.*, 1984, **24**, 1051.
235. L. A. Goettler, A. J. Lambright, R. I. Leib and P. J. DiMauro, *Rubber Chem. Technol.*, 1981, **54**, 277.
236. P. D. Patel and D. C. Bogue, *Polym. Eng. Sci.*, 1981, **21**, 449.
237. L. R. Schmidt, *Adv. Chem. Ser.*, 1975, **142**, 415.
238. Y. Chan, J. L. White and Y. Oyanagi, *Polym. Eng. Sci.*, 1978, **18**, 268.
239. G. Akay, *Polym. Eng. Sci.*, 1982, **22**, 1027.
240. G. Akay, *Polym. Compos.*, 1983, **4**, 256.
241. M. J. Folkes and D. A. M. Russell, *Polymer*, 1980, **21**, 1252.
242. A. G. Gibson and G. A. Williamson, *Polym. Eng. Sci.*, 1985, **25**, 968, 980.
243. A. G. Gibson, *Plast. Rubb. Proces. Appl.*, 1985, **5**, 95.
244. D. M. Bigg, *Polym. Compos.*, 1985, **6**, 20.
245. B. Chung and C. Cohen, *Polym. Eng. Sci.*, 1985, **25**, 1001.
246. M. Sanou, B. Chung and C. Cohen, *Polym. Eng. Sci.*, 1985, **25**, 1008.
247. S. Kenig, *Polym. Compos.*, 1986, **7**, 50.
248. M. Vincent and J. F. Agassant, *Polym. Compos.*, 1986, **7**, 76.
249. M. J. Folkes, *Short Fibre Reinforced Thermoplastics*, Wiley, R.S.P. Div., New York, 1982.
250. P. G. Lafleur and M. R. Kamal, *Polym. Eng. Sci.*, 1986, **26**, 92.
251. M. R. Kamal and P. G. Lafleur, *Polym. Eng. Sci.*, 1986, **26**, 103.
252. B. W. Barry, *Adv. Colloid Interface Sci.*, 1977, **5**, 37.
253. L. E. Nielsen, *Polymer Rheology*, Dekker, New York, 1977.
254. L. A. Utracki and G. L. Bata, Polymer alloys, paper presented at CANPLAST meeting, Montreal, Oct. 25, 1981; *Matériaux Techn.*, 1982, **70**, 223, 290.
255. L. A. Utracki and M. R. Kamal, Polyblends '81 symposium, NRCC/IMRI, Montreal, April 1981; *Polym. Eng. Sci.*, 1982, **22**, 96.
256. L. A. Utracki, Proc. NATEC, Bal Harbour, Florida, October 25–27, 1982; *Polym. Eng. Sci.*, 1983, **23**, 602.
257. L. A. Utracki, *Polym-Plast. Technol. Eng.*, 1984, **22**, 27.
258. G. I. Taylor, *Proc. Roy. Soc.*, 1932, **A138**, 41; 1934, **A146**, 501.
259. M. A. Nawab and S. G. Mason, *Trans. Faraday Soc.*, 1985, **54**, 1712.
260. J. C. Oldroyd, *Proc. Roy. Soc.*, 1953, **A218**, 122; 1955, **A232**, 567.
261. S. Matsumoto and P. Sherman, *J. Colloid Interface Sci.*, 1969, **30**, 525.
262. A. Brandt and G. Bugliarello, *Trans. Soc. Rheol.*, 1966, **10**, 229.
263. O. Okagawa and S. G. Mason, *Can. J. Chem.*, 1975, **53**, 2689.
264. J. B. Harris and J. F. T. Pittman, *Trans. Inst. Chem. Eng.*, 1976, **54**, 73.
265. L. A. Utracki, *J. Colloid Interface Sci.*, 1973, **42**, 185.
266. T. L. Smith, *J. Paint Technol.*, 1972, **44**, 71.
267. W. R. Schowalter, C. E. Chaffey and H. Brenner, *J. Colloid Interface Sci.*, 1968, **26**, 152.

268. A. Sakanishi and Y. Takano, *Jap. J. Appl. Phys.*, 1974, **13**, 882.
269. M. Oosterbroek, J. S. Lopulissa and J. Mellema, in *Rheology*, G. Astarita, G. Marrucci and L. Nicolais (Eds), Vol. 2, Plenum Press, New York, 1980, p. 601.
270. A. Acrivos and T. S. Lo, *J. Fluid Mech.*, 1978, **86**, 641.
271. E. J. Hinch and A. Acrivos, *J. Fluid Mech.*, 1979, **91**, 401.
272. H. P. Grace, Eng. Found. 3rd Res. Conf. Mixing, Andover, New Hampshire, 1971.
273. D. Barthes-Biesel and A. Acrivos, *Int. J. Multiphase Flow*, 1973, **1**, 1.
274. M. Bredimas, M. Veyssie, D. Barthes-Biesel and V. Chhim, *J. Colloid Interface Sci.*, 1983, **93**, 513.
275. M. M. Esmukhanov, Yu V. Pridatchenko and Yu. I. Shmakov, *Priklad. Mekh.*, 1985, **21**, 110.
276. M. Oosterbroek and J. Mellema, *J. Colloid Interface Sci.*, 1981, **84**, 14.
277. M. Oosterbroek, J. Mellema and J. S. Lopulissa, *J. Colloid Interface Sci.*, 1981, **84**, 27.
278. A. Eshuis and J. Mellema, *Colloid Polym. Sci.*, 1984, **262**, 159.
279. H. M. Princen, *J. Colloid Interface Sci.*, 1983, **91**, 160.
280. H. M. Princen, *J. Colloid Interface Sci.*, 1985, **105**, 150.
281. V. B. Talstoguzov, A. I. Mzhel'sky and V. Ya. Gulov, *Colloid Polym. Sci.*, 1974, **252**, 124.
282. V. L. Kuznetsov, E. A. Dorokhova, V. Yu. Erofeev and B. K. Basov, *Kolloid, Zhur.*, 1985, **47**, 806.
283. L. Djakovic, P. Dokic, P. Radivojevic and V. Kler, *Colloid Polym. Sci.*, 1976, **254**, 907.
284. J. L. Salager, M. Minana-Perez, J. M. Anderez, J. L. Grosso and C. I. Rojas, *J. Disp. Sci. Technol.*, 1983, **4**, 161.
285. M. Minana-Perez, P. Jarry, M. Perez-Sanchez, M. Ramirez-Gouveia and J. L. Salager, *J. Disp. Sci. Technol.*, 1986, **7**, 331.
286. N. Gladwell, R. R. Rahalkar and P. Richmond, *Rheol. Acta*, 1986, **25**, 55.
287. R. Pal, S. N. Bhattacharya and E. Rhodes, *Canad. J. Chem. Eng.*, 1986, **64**, 3.
288. P. H. Jezequel, P. Flaud and D. Quemada, *Chem. Eng. Commun.*, 1985, **32**, 85.
289. M. S. Rappaport and S. N. Curry, *Modified Plastics: Speciality Polymer Blends and Alloys 1984*, Survey Analysis Report, Klein & Co., Fairfield, New Jersey, 1984.
290. L. A. Utracki, *Adv. Polym. Technol.*, 1985, **5**, 41.
291. B. Schlund and L. A. Utracki, *Polym. Eng. Sci.*, 1987, **27**, 359, 380.
292. M. M. Dumoulin, C. Farha and L. A. Utracki, NRCC/IMRI symposium Polymer Blends '84, Boucherville, Quebec, Canada, April 17, 1984; *Polym. Eng. Sci.*, 1984, **24**, 1319.
293. L. A. Utracki, M. R. Kamal and N. M. Al-Bastaki, *SPE-Techn. Pap.*, 1984, **30**, 417.
294. M. M. Dumoulin and L. A. Utracki, Proc. CRG/MSD symposium Quantitative Characterization of Plastics and Rubber, June 21–22, 1984, Hamilton, Ontario.

295. L. A. Utracki, IX Int. Congr. Rheology, Acapulco, Mexico, 8–13 Oct. 1984; *Advances in Rheology*, B. Mena, A. Garcia-Rejon and C. Rangel-Nafaile (Eds), Univ. Nat. Autonom. Mexico, 1984, **3**, 567.
296. W. E. Baker and A. M. Catani, NRCC/IMRI symposium Polyblends '84, Boucherville, Quebec, Canada, April 17, 1984; *Polym. Eng. Sci.*, 1984, **24**, 1348.
297. L. A. Utracki and B. Schlund, *S.P.E. Techn. Pap.*, 1986, **32**, 737.
298. M. L. Huggins, *J. Chem. Phys.*, 1941, **9**, 440.
299. P. J. Flory, *J. Chem. Phys.*, 1941, **9**, 660.
300. D. D. Patterson and A. Robard, *Macromolecules*, 1978, **11**, 690.
301. H. Tompa, *Polymer Solutions*, Butterworths, London, 1956.
302. J. S. Langer, in *Fluctuations, Instabilities and Phase Transitions*, T. Riste (Ed.), Plenum Press, New York, 1977.
303. H. L. Snyder, P. Meaking and S. Reich, *Macromolecules*, 1983, **16**, 757.
304. H. L. Snyder and P. Meakin, *J. Chem. Phys.*, 1983, **79**, 5588.
305. I. G. Voigt-Martin, K.-H. Leister, R. Rosenau and R. Koningsveld, *J. Polym. Sci., Polym. Phys. Ed.*, 1986, **24**, 723.
306. R. F. Boyer, *J. Polym. Sci.*, 1966, **C14**, 267.
307. R. W. Warfield and B. Hartmann, *Polymer*, 1980, **21**, 31.
308. D. S. Kaplan, *J. Appl. Polym. Sci.*, 1976, **20**, 2615.
309. H. E. Bair and P. C. Warren, *J. Macromol. Sci. Phys.*, 1981, **B20**, 381.
310. K. C. Frisch, D. Klempner and H. L. Frisch, NRCC/IMRI symposium Polyblends '82, Montreal, Quebec, Canada, April 20, 1982; *Polym. Eng. Sci.*, 1982, **22**, 1143.
311. A. R. Shultz and A. L. Young, *Macromolecules*, 1980, **13**, 663.
312. J. Lyngaae-Jorgensen and K. Sondergaard, NRCC/IMRI symposium Polyblends '86, Montreal, Canada, April 4, 1986; *Polym. Eng. Sci.*, 1987, **27**, 344, 351.
313. S. Glasstone, K. L. Laidler and H. Eyring, *Theory of Rate Processes*, McGraw-Hill, New York, 1941.
314. A. Bondi, in *Rheology, Theory and Applications*, Vol. 4, F. R. Eirich (Ed.), Academic Press, New York, 1967.
315. W. M. Prest, Jr and R. S. Porter, *J. Polym. Sci., A-2*, 1972, **10**, 1639.
316. R. Genillon and J. F. May, 5th Conf. Europ. Plast. Caoutch., Paris, 1978, paper E-12.
317. T. Fujimura and K. Iwakura, *Int. Chem. Eng.*, 1970, **10**, 683; *Kobunshi Ronbunshu*, 1974, **31**, 617.
318. R. A. McAllister, *AIChE J.*, 1960, **6**, 427.
319. J. F. Carley and S. C. Crossan, *S.P.E. ANTEC Tech. Papers*, 1980, **26**, 285; *Polym. Eng. Sci.*, 1981, **21**, 249.
320. A. P. Plochocki, NRCC/IMRI symposium Polyblends '85, Boucherville, Quebec, Canada, April 16–17, 1985; *Polym. Eng. Sci.*, 1986, **26**, 82.
321. J. P. Monfort, G. Marin, J. Arman and Ph. Monge, *Polymer*, 1978, **19**, 277.
322. S. F. Christov, I. I. Skorokhodov and Z. V. Shuralava, *Vysokomol. Soed.*, 1978, **A20**, 1699.
323. A Franck and J. Meissner, *Rheol. Acta*, 1984, **23**, 117.
324. C. Wisniewski, G. Marin and P. Monge, *Eur. Polym. J.*, 1984, **20**, 691.
325. N. P. Suprun and O. V. Romankevich, *Khim. Tekhnol.* (Kiev), 1984, **2**, 29.

326. E. Martuscelli, *Macromol. Chem., Rapid Commun.*, 1984, **5**, 255.
327. Y. P. Singh and R. P. Singh, *J. Appl. Polym. Sci.*, 1984, **29**, 1653.
328. Y. Aoki, *Polym. J.*, 1984, **16**, 431.
329. L. A. Utracki, *J. Rheol.*, 1986, **30**, 829.
330. L. A. Utracki, *Canad. J. Chem. Eng.*, 1983, **61**, 753.
331. L. A. Utracki, *Polym. Eng. Sci.*, 1983, **23**, 446.
332. L. A. Utracki, *ACS Polym. Prepr.*, 1983, **24**(2), 113.
333. L. A. Utracki, Paper No. 2, NRCC/IMRI symposium on mathematical modeling of plastics processing and properties, Modeling '84, Boucherville, Quebec, Canada, Jan. 24, 1984; *Polym. Eng. Sci.*, 1985, **25**, 655.
334. R. Simha and T. Somcynsky, *Macromolecules*, 1969, **2**, 342.
335. J. E. McKinney and R. Simha, *Macromolecules*, 1976, **9**, 430.
336. O. Olabisi and R. Simha, *J. Appl. Polym. Sci.*, 1977, **21**, 149.
337. R. K. Jain and R. Simha, *J. Chem. Phys.*, 1980, **72**, 4909.
338. R. K. Jain and R. Simha, *Macromolecules*, 1980, **13**, 1501.
339. R. Simha, *Polym. Eng. Sci.*, 1982, **22**, 74.
340. R. Simha and R. K. Jain, *Polym. Eng. Sci.*, 1984, **24**, 1284.
341. J. H. Dymond, K. J. Young and J. D. Isdale, *Int. J. Thermophys.*, 1980, **1**, 345.
342. M. H. Doan and J. Brunet, *Ind. Eng. Chem. Fund.*, 1972, **11**, 356; J. Brunet and K. E. Gubbins, *Trans. Faraday Soc.*, 1969, **65**, 1255.
343. G. D. Kirianov, R. M. Vasenin and B. N. Dinzburg, *Vysokomol. Soed.*, 1975, **B17**, 492.
344. L. A. Utracki and G. L. Bata, Am. Chem. Soc., *Prepr. Org. Coatings Plastics Chem.*, 1981, **45**, 180.
345. L. A. Utracki and G. L. Bata, *Polymer Alloys*, Vol. III, D. Klemper and K. C. Frisch (Eds), Plenum Press, New York, 1982.
346. L. A. Utracki, M. R. Kamal, V. Tan, A. Catani and G. L. Bata, *J. Appl. Polym. Sci.*, 1982, **27**, 1913.
347. L. A. Utracki and G. L. Bata, *SPE ANTEC Tech. Papers*, 1982, **28**, 84.
348. Yu S. Lipatov, E. V. Lebedev and V. F. Shumskii, *Dopov. Akad. Nauk URSR*, Ser. B, 1983(9), 39.
349. D. C. Allport and W. H. Jones (Eds), *Block Copolymers*, Applied Science, London, 1973.
350. R. J. Ceresa (Ed.), *Block and Graft Copolymerization*, Wiley, London, 1973.
351. A. Noshay and J. E. McGrath, *Block Copolymers: Overview and Critical Survey*, Academic Press, New York, 1977.
352. M. J. Folkes (Ed.), *Processing, Structure and Properties of Block Copolymers*, Elsevier Applied Science, London, 1985.
353. J. Lyngaae-Jorgensen, Chapter 3 in reference 352.
354. T. Kotaka and H. Watanabe, in *Current Topics in Polymer Science*, R. M. Ottenbrite, L. A. Utracki and S. Inoue (Eds), Hanser, München, 1987.
355. G. Kraus and J. T. Gruver, *J. Appl. Polym. Sci.*, 1967, **11**, 2121.
356. G. Holden, E. T. Bishop and N. R. Legge, *J. Polym. Sci.*, 1969, **C26**, 37.
357. G. M. Estes, S. L. Cooper and A. V. Tobolsky, *J. Macromol. Chem.*, 1970, **C4**, 313.
358. K. R. Arnold and D. J. Meier, *J. Appl. Polym. Sci.*, 1970, **14**, 427.
359. F. N. Cogswell and D. E. Hanson, *Polymer*, 1975, **16**, 936.

360. C. I. Chung and J. C. Gale, *J. Polym. Sci., Phys. Ed.*, 1976, **14**, 1149.
361. N. V. Chii, A. I. Isayev, A. Ya. Malkin, G. V. Vinogradov and I. Yu. Kirchevskaya, *Polym. Sci.* (USSR), 1975, **17**, 983.
362. E. R. Pico and M. C. Williams, *Nature*, 1976, **259**, 388.
363. C. P. Henderson and M. C. Williams, *J. Polym. Sci., Polym. Lett. Ed.*, 1979, **17**, 257.
364. T. Y. Liu, D. S. Soong and D. DeKee, *Chem. Eng. Commun.*, 1983, **22**, 273.
365. G. Holden, Chapter 6 in reference 350.
366. M. L. Williams, R. F. Landel and J. D. Ferry, *J. Am. Chem. Soc.*, 1955, **77**, 3701.
367. D. F. Leary and M. C. Williams, *J. Polym. Sci.*, 1970, **B8**, 335; *J. Polym. Sci., Phys. Ed.*, 1973, **11**, 345; 1974, **12**, 265.
368. N. Sivashinsky, T. J. Moon and D. S. Soong, *J. Macromol. Sci., Phys.*, 1983, **B22**, 213.
369. H. Watanabe and T. Kotaka, *Macromolecules*, 1983, **16**, 769; 1984, **17**, 342.
370. Yu. S. Lipatov, A. Ye. Nesterov and T. D. Ignatova, *Vysokomol. Soed.*, 1979, **A21**, 2659.
371. V. D. Klykova, *Mash. Tekhnolk. Pererab. Kauch. Polim. Rezin. Smesei*, 1981, 15.
372. A. N. Gorbatenko, T. D. Ignatova, V. G. Shumskii, A. Ye. Nesterov, Yu. S. Lipatov, L. S. Bolotnikova and Yu. N. Panov, *Kompoz. Polim. Mater.*, 1982, **15**, 18.
373. Yu. S. Lipatov, A. Ye. Nesterov, T. D. Ignatova, V. F. Shumskii and A. N. Gorbatenko, *Vysokomol. Soed.*, 1982, **A24**, 549.
374. Yu. S. Lipatov, V. F. Shumskii, A. N. Gorbatenko and I. P. Gietmanchuk, *Fiz. Khim. Mekh. Disp. Strukt.*, 1983, 117.
375. Yu. S. Lipatov, *Mekh. Kompoz. Mater.*, 1983, **3**, 499.
376. Yu. S. Lipatov, V. P. Shumskii, Ye. V. Lebedev and A. Ye. Nesterov,*Dokl. Akad. Nauk SSSR*, 1979, **244**, 148.
377. H. Van Oene, *J. Colloid. Interface Sci.*, 1972, **40**, 448.
378. L. I. Manevich, V. S. Mitlin and Sh. A. Shaginyan, *Khim. Fiz.*, 1984, **3**, 283.
379. A. Skoulios, in *Advances in Liquid Crystals*, G. H. Brown (Ed.), Academic Press, New York, 1975.
380. T. Soen, M. Shimomura, T. Uchida and H. Kawai, *Kolloid-Z., Z. Polym.*, 1974, **252**, 933.
381. T. I. Ablazova, M. V. Tsebrenko, A. B. V. Yudin, G. V. Vinogradov and B. V. Yarlykov, *J. Appl. Polym. Sci.*, 1975, **19**, 1781.
382. M. V. Tsebrenko, A. I. Benzar, A. V. Yudin and G. V. Vinogradov, *Vysokomol. Soed.*, 1979, **A21**, 830.
383. N. M. Rezanova and M. V. Tsebrenko, *Kampoz. Polym. Materialy*, 1981, **11**, 47.
384. A. P. Plochocki, NRCC/IMRI symposium Polyblends '82, Montreal, Quebec, Canada, April 20, 1982; *Polym. Eng. Sci.*, 1982, **22**, 1153.
385. A. P. Plochocki, NRCC/IMRI symposium Polyblends '85, Boucherville, Quebec, Canada, April 16–17, 1985; *Polym. Eng. Sci.*, 1985, **25**, 82.
386. T. Tavgac, PhD thesis, University of Houston, 1972.
387. S. Endo, K. Min., J. L. White and T. Kyu, NRCC/IMRI symposium Polyblends '85, Boucherville, Quebec, Canada, April 16 and 17, 1985; *Polym. Eng. Sci.*, 1986, **26**, 45.

388. G. M. Jordhamo, J. A. Manson and L. H. Sperling, *Polym. Eng. Sci.*, 1986, **26**, 517.
389. N. P. Krasnikova, E. V. Kotova, E. P. Plotnikova, M. P. Zabugina, G. V. Vinogradov, V. E. Dreval and Z. Pelzbauer, *Kompoz. Polim. Mater.*, 1984, **21**, 37.
390. W. Berger, H. W. Kammer and C. Kummerlöwe, *Makromol. Chem. Suppl.*, 1984, **8**, 101.
391. S. Wu, NRCC/IMRI symposium Polyblends '86, Montreal, Canada, April 4, 1986; *Polym. Eng. Sci.*, 1987, **27**, 335.
392. M. M. Dumoulin, L. A. Utracki and P. J. Carreau, Paper No. 186, at 36th Conf. Canad. Soc. Chem. Eng., Sarnia, Ontario, Oct. 5–8, 1986.
393. F. N. Cogswell, *Polym. Eng. Sci.*, 1972, **12**, 69.
394. A. M. Catani and L. A. Utracki, Proc. Ann. Meet. Polymer Processing Society, Akron, Ohio, March 28–29, 1985; *J. Polym. Eng.*, 1986, **6**, 23.
395. K. Min, PhD thesis, University of Tennessee, Knoxville, 1984.
396. C.-C. Lin, *Polym. J.*, 1979, **11**, 185.
397. M. M. Dumoulin, P. Toma, L. A. Utracki, I. Jinnah and M. R. Kamal, *S.P.E. Techn. Papers*, 1985, **31**, 534.
398. A. P. Plochocki, *Polym. Eng. Sci.*, 1983, **23**, 618.
399. A. P. Plochocki, S. S. Dagli and H. Emmanuilides, *Am. Chem. Soc., Polym. Prepr.*, 1985, **26**, 288.
400. A. P. Plochocki, in *Polymer Blends*, D. R. Paul and S. Newman (Eds), Academic Press, New York, 1978.
401. D. J. Bye and I. S. Miles, paper presented at 2nd Conf. Europ. Rheol., Prague, CSSR, 1986; *Eur. Polym. J.*, 1986, **22**, 185.
402. M. V. Tsebrenko, A. V. Yudin, T. I. Ablazova and G. A. Vinogradov, *Polymer*, 1976, **17**, 831.
403. A. A. Gerasimchuk, O. V. Romankevich and E. M. Aizenshtein, *Khim. Volok.*, 1986, **2**, 21.
404. H.-K. Chuang and C. D. Han, *J. Appl. Polym. Sci.*, 1984, **29**, 2205.
405. C. K. Shih, *Polym. Eng. Sci.*, 1976, **16**, 198.
406. C. K. Shih, in *Science and Technology of Polymer Processing*, N. P. Suh and N.-H. Sung (Eds), MIT Press, Cambridge, Massachusetts, 1979.
407. R. C. Kanu and M. T. Shaw, *Polym. Eng. Sci.*, 1982, **22**, 507.
408. M. Nishi, H. Watanabe and T. Kotaka, *Nihon Reor. Gak.*, 1981, **9**, 23.
409. C. Wisniewski, G. Marin and Ph. Monge, *Eur. Polym. J.*, 1985, **21**, 479.
410. C. Belaribi, G. Marin and Ph. Monge, *Eur. Polym. J.*, 1986, **22**, 481, 487.
411. L. A. Utracki, G. L. Bata, V. Tan and M. R. Kamal, 2nd World Congr. Chem. Eng., Montreal, Quebec, Oct. 5, 1981, Proceeding Preprints, 1981, **6**, 428.
412. V. Ye. Dreval, A. Kassa, Ye. K. Borisenkova, M. L. Kerber, G. V. Vinogradov and M. S. Akutin, *Vysokomol. Soed.*, 1983, **A25**, 156.
413. B. A. Thornton, R. G. Villasenor and B. Maxwell, *J. Appl. Polym. Sci.*, 1980, **25**, 653.
414. L. S. Bolotnikova, A. K. Evseer, Yu. N. Panov and S. Ya. Frenkel, *Vysokomol. Soed.*, 1982, **B24**, 154.
415. Y. Lipatov, *J. Appl. Polym. Sci.*, 1978, **22**, 1895.
416. L. A. Utracki, M. R. Kamal and Z. Bakerdjian, *J. Appl. Polym. Sci.*, 1975, **19**, 487.

417. R. I. Tanner, *J. Polym. Sci., A-2*, 1970, **8**, 2067.
418. M. V. Tsebrenko, A. I. Benzar, A. V. Yudin and G. V. Vinogradov, *Vysokomol. Soed.*, 1979, **A21**, 830.
419. J. L. Leblanc, *Rubber Chem. Technol.*, 1981, **54**, 905.
420. O. V. Romakevich, T. I. Zhila, S. E. Zabello, N. A. Sklyar and S. Ya. Frenkel, *Vysokomol. Soed.*, 1982, **A24**, 2282.
421. T. I. Zhila, V. I. Mazurenko, O. V. Romankevich, S. E. Zabello and V. V. Anokhin, *Khim. Tekhnol.* (Kiev), 1980, **5**, 37.
422. O. V. Romankevich and S. Y. Frenekl, *Kompoz. Polim. Mater.*, 1982, **14**, 6.
423. O. V. Romankevich, K. V. Yakovlev, S. E. Zabello, T. I. Zhila and V. S. Rudchuk, *Khim. Volokna*, 1984, **1**, 21.
424. F. P. LaMantia, D. Curto and D. Acierno, *Acta Polym.*, 1984, **35**, 71.
425. D. Acierno, D. Curto, F. P. LaMantia and A. Valenza, NRCC/IMRI symposium Polyblends '85, Boucherville, Quebec, Canada, April 16–17, 1985; *Polym. Eng. Sci.*, 1986, **26**, 28.
426. F. Deri, R. Genillon and J. F. May, *Angew. Makromol. Chem.*, 1985, **134**, 11.
427. A. Santamaria, M. E. Munoz, J. J. Pena and P. Remiro, *Angew. Makromol. Chem.*, 1985, **134**, 63.
428. L. A. Utracki and B. Schlund, NRCC/IMRI symposium Polyblends '87, Boucherville, Quebec, Canada, April 28–29, 1987; *Polym. Eng. Sci.*, 1987, **27**, 1512.
429. B. Schlund and L. A. Utracki, NRCC/IMRI symposium Polyblends '87, Boucherville, Quebec, Canada, April 28–29, 1987; *Polym. Eng. Sci.*, 1987, **27**, 1523.
430. F. P. LaMantia, D. Acierno and D. Curto, *Rheol. Acta*, 1982, **21**, 452.
431. M. M. Dumoulin, L. A. Utracki and J. Lara, NRCC/IMRI symposium Polyblends '83, Montreal, Quebec, Canada, April 12, 1983; *Polym. Eng. Sci.*, 1984, **24**, 117.
432. K. Min, J. L. White and J. F. Fellers, NRCC/IMRI symposium Polyblends '84, Boucherville, Quebec, Canada, April 17, 1984; *Polym. Eng. Sci.*, 1984, **24**, 1327.
433. H. Sugiyama, D. N. Lewis, J. L. White and J. F. Fellers, *ACS Polym. Prepr.*, 1985, **26**(1), 255.
434. G. Kiss, NRCC/IMRI symposium Polyblends '86, Montreal, Quebec, Canada, April 4, 1986; *Polym. Eng. Sci.*, 1987, **27**, 410.
435. Y. Saito, *Nihon Reor. Gakk.*, 1982, **10**, 123, 128, 135.
436. R. Fayt, R. Jerome and Ph. Teyssié, *J. Polym. Sci., Polym. Lett. Ed.*, 1986, **24**, 25.

Chapter 16

Mathematical Modelling of Two-Phase Flows

D. BARTHES-BIESEL

Université de Technologie de Compiègne, Division de Biomécanique et Instrumentation Médicale, Compiègne, France

NOTATION

$\langle \ \rangle$	bulk value of enclosed quantity
*	superscript for bulk particle properties
s	superscript for interfacial particle properties
—	superscript bar denoting symmetric deviatoric part, defined in eqn (16.45)
$\partial/\partial t$	partial derivative with respect to time

$\mathcal{D}/\mathcal{D}t$	corotational derivative with respect to time, defined in eqn (16.43)
a	characteristic length scale for incompressible particles
n_i	outer unit vector normal to particle surface, Fig. 16.1
N	number density of particles
ϕ	volume fraction of particles
d	mean particle spacing
η	viscosity of suspending medium
ρ	density of suspending medium
$\dot{\gamma}$	shear rate
ω	bulk vorticity intensity
$P(C, t)$	joint probability density function of finding particles in configuration C
x_i^m	position of particle m between times t and $t + \mathrm{d}t$
f_i	constant body force per unit volume
δ_{ij}	Kronecker delta
ΔV	representative volume of suspension
ΔL	length scale of ΔV
e_{ij}	SS local rate of strain tensor
σ_{ij}	local stress tensor
v_i	local velocity
v_i'	deviation from mean velocity
p	pressure, eqn (16.5)
p_{ij}	particle stress
α	denotes a generic particle of ΔV, eqn (16.6)
V^α, S^α	volume and surface area of a generic particle of ΔV, eqn (16.6).
f_i'	inertia effect for particle motion, eqn (16.6)
$\mathrm{Re_p}$	microscopic Reynolds number, eqn (16.7)
S_{ij}^α	deviatoric dipole strength due to one particle, eqns (16.8) and (16.9)
F_j^α	non-hydrodynamic resultant force on a particle at x_i^α, eqn (16.10)
kT	Boltzmann temperature, eqn (16.11)
$\langle S_{ij} \rangle$	bulk particle stress tensor, eqn (16.12)
$P_{\mathrm{c}}(C|x_i^0)$	normalized conditional probability density, eqn (16.13)
C_{ij}	measure of particle anisotropy and orientation
P'	conditional probability of finding one particle at x_i^0 with orientation C_{ij}
v_i^∞	undisturbed bulk velocity field, eqn (16.16)
Ω_{ij}	vorticity tensor, eqn (16.16)

λ	viscosity ratio of dispersed fluid to bulk fluid, eqn (16.21)
E^*	elastic bulk modulus of particles
η^s, E^s	viscosity and elastic modulus of particle interface
X_i, x_i	position of given point in reference state at time t
x	distance from particle surface to centre of mass
$f(x_i, t)$	equation of deformed particle surface
F_i^s	force exerted by interface, eqns (16.25) and (16.26)
λ^s	viscosity ratio between interface and bulk fluid
k	capillary number, eqns (16.27) and (16.28)
p'	deviation from main pressure, eqn (16.30)
T_{ij}	symmetric and traceless coefficient, eqn (16.30)
η_r	relative viscosity of suspension
A_{ijkl}	expression dependent on instantaneous orientation of an ellipsoid, eqn (16.37)
Pe_B	Brownian motion Peclet number, eqns (16.38), (16.39) and (16.41)
D	rotation diffusion coefficient, eqn (16.38)
α	particle axis ratio, eqn (16.40)
u_i	unit vector oriented along axis of a spheroid, eqn (16.40)
$P_o(u_i, t)$	orientation probability density
A, B, C, F	shape factors, eqn (16.42)
A', B'	shape factors, eqn (16.44)
$[\eta]$	intrinsic viscosity
N_1, N_2	normal stress differences
ε	measures deviation from sphericity, eqns (16.47)–(16.49)
ψ	local electric potential, eqns (16.50)–(16.52)
q	local charge density, eqn (16.50)
ε	$1/4\pi$ (dielectric constant of suspending medium)
w_i	ion velocity, eqn (16.51)
μ	ion mobility, eqn (16.51)
z	ion valence, eqns (16.51) and (16.53)
n	ion number density, eqn (16.51)
e	electronic charge, eqn (16.51)
κ	reciprocal Debye length, eqn (16.53)
n_∞	equilibrium ion number density, eqn (16.53)
ζ	particle potential
Pe_E	electrical Peclet number
H	electrical Hartmann number
β	first-order electroviscous correction to Einstein equation, eqn (16.54)
τ	suspension characteristic response time

D_f	capsule deformation, eqn (16.63)
τ_1, τ_2	relaxation times
C'_{ij}	measure of in-plane interface deformation
L_{ij}, M_{ij}	two linear combinations of deformation tensors C_{ij}, C'_{ij}, eqns (16.67) and (16.68)
ψ'	measure of non-linearity of an elastic membrane constitutive law
K	constant, eqn (16.71)
P_2	pair density, eqn (16.72)
r_i	distance of two spheres, eqn (16.72)
v_{ri}	relative velocity of two spheres, eqn (16.72)
D_{ij}	Brownian diffusion tensor, eqn (16.72)
F_i^α	electrostatic force between charged spheres, eqn (16.77)
U_2	electrostatic pair potential, eqn (16.77)
L	characteristic particle separation, eqn (16.80)
b	measures ratio of electrical to thermal forces, eqn (16.81)
P'	defined in eqn (16.85)
β_1	coefficient, eqn (16.85)
ϕ_m	maximum concentration, eqn (16.87)
C'	constant, eqn (16.87)
d'	interparticle distance
L_c	cluster size

16.1. INTRODUCTION

When the size of the suspended particles is much smaller than the length scale of the flow, or equivalently the characteristic dimensions of the device in which the suspension is flowing, it is possible to treat the suspension as a homogeneous fluid having specific rheological properties, which can be investigated with classical experimental means. Owing to the number of parameters that may influence the rheology (particle concentration, size, geometry, deformability, type of flow, colloidal forces, etc.), it is usually extremely difficult, if not outright impossible, unambiguously to relate the few experimental rheological parameters (shear viscosity, normal stresses, elastic modulus, etc.) to the numerous intrinsic physical properties of the particulate fluid. It is thus the aim of suspension theory to establish a relationship between the microscopic parameters of the suspension and the measurable bulk properties.

Initially it was also hoped to be able to derive a general constitutive equation, giving explicitly the non-Newtonian behaviour of the corresponding homogeneous fluid, since standard rheometric measurements only give partial information about the fluid behaviour. However, it was soon realized that, except in special cases, the fluid mechanical problems to be solved are so complex that it is necessary to seek particular solutions for specific flow types.

In the second section the theoretical background for the proper formulation of a constitutive law is established. The special case of dilute suspensions, for which there are many available results, is then presented in the third section. The eventual non-Newtonian features of such dilute suspensions are investigated in detail and related to the microstructure properties. In the fourth section, non-dilute suspensions are studied, and the first corrective term to the dilute constitutive equation is sought. The limiting case of a very concentrated suspension is also treated. Some recent advances in the numerical simulation of the flow of particulate systems are presented.

16.2. GENERAL FORMULATION OF A CONSTITUTIVE EQUATION

16.2.1. Statement of the Problem
Consider a suspension of incompressible particles having a characteristic length scale denoted a, and otherwise known physical properties (internal viscosity, elasticity, etc.). The outer unit vector normal to the particle surface is n_i (Fig. 16.1). The number density of particles and the corresponding volume fraction are respectively N and ϕ. The mean particle spacing is d. The suspending fluid is incompressible and Newtonian with a viscosity η and a density ρ. The suspension is subjected to a bulk flow, with shear and vorticity intensities denoted respectively $\dot{\gamma}$ and ω. Temperature gradients are ignored. The configuration of particles is represented by a joint probability density function $P(C, t)$ which gives the probability of finding m particles in configuration C, i.e. at positions $x_i^1, \ldots,$ x_i^m, between time t and $t + dt$. The suspension is assumed to be statistically homogeneous, which means that P is invariant under translation. The analysis is thus valid for suspensions where sedimentation may be neglected. The suspending fluid and the particles are acted upon by the same constant body force per unit volume f_i.

The Cartesian notation with implicit summation on repeated indices is

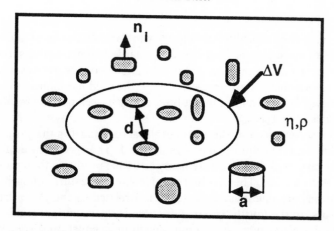

Fig. 16.1. A suspension is treated as a homogeneous fluid if there exists a characteristic volume, ΔV, containing many particles, but small with respect to the flow scale.

used throughout. The identity matrix is represented by the Kronecker symbol

$$\delta_{ij} = 1, \qquad i = j$$
$$= 0, \qquad i \neq j$$

It is assumed that the suspension may be treated as a homogeneous fluid. This means that the particle size is much smaller than the flow length scale, or more specifically, that it is possible to find a representative volume ΔV, containing many particles, but with dimensions small compared to the characteristic scale of variation of the bulk quantities. The objective is to define the bulk properties of the equivalent continuum as averages of the corresponding microscopic properties. Consequently, the determination of the rheology of a multiphase fluid may be broken down into two steps. The first one consists in calculating the bulk stress at a given time, as a function of the instantaneous state of the suspension (and thus as a function of parameters such as the position of the particles, their velocities, deformation, etc.). The second step consists in determining the time evolution of the suspension configuration. Thus, in principle, the velocity and stress fields both in the continuous liquid and in the particles must be computed. It is clear then that there is in general a strong interaction between the motion and deformation of the microstructure, and the bulk rheology of the suspension. One should expect time dependent phenomena, as well as a possibility of memory effects.

The theoretical framework for the proper formulation of the constitutive equation of a suspension has been established by Batchelor[1] in the case where all the above hypotheses are fulfilled.

16.2.2. Definition of Bulk Quantities

The definition of the bulk quantities follows the concepts of statistical mechanics or thermodynamics. For a given set of macroscopic boundary conditions, there are many different possible configurations of the suspension. Following Hashin,[2] a bulk quantity is defined as an ensemble average over a number of possible realizations. If the suspension is statistically homogeneous, there exists a length scale ΔL, large with respect to the particle spacing, d, and such that the statistical properties of the suspension do not vary over ΔL. Then the different bulk quantities are stationary random functions of position over distances of order ΔL. The volume average of a quantity over an elementary volume ΔV of characteristic dimension ΔL is equivalent to the ensemble average (this, of course, is not true near solid boundaries).

Correspondingly, a bulk velocity gradient or, similarly, a bulk rate of strain tensor may defined as

$$\left\langle \frac{\partial v_i}{\partial x_j} \right\rangle = \frac{1}{\Delta V} \int_{\Delta V} \frac{\partial v_i}{\partial x_j} \, dV \tag{16.1}$$

$$\langle e_{ij} \rangle = \frac{1}{2} \left(\left\langle \frac{\partial v_i}{\partial x_j} \right\rangle + \left\langle \frac{\partial v_j}{\partial x_i} \right\rangle \right) = \frac{1}{\Delta V} \int_{\Delta V} e_{ij} \, dV \tag{16.2}$$

where bulk quantities are enclosed in brackets.

The bulk stress is similarly given by

$$\langle \sigma_{ij} \rangle = \frac{1}{\Delta V} \int_{\Delta V} (\sigma_{ij} - \rho v_i' v_j') dV \tag{16.3}$$

where a primed quantity represents the deviation of the corresponding local quantity from its mean value, e.g.

$$v_i' = v_i - \langle v_i \rangle \tag{16.4}$$

The momentum flux in eqn (16.3) is added to the definition of $\langle \sigma_{ij} \rangle$ to ensure that the bulk quantities do satisfy the equations of motion.

The correspondence between the bulk and measured quantities cannot be established in general for any type of flow. However, for a simple shear flow, Batchelor shows that $\langle \sigma_{ij} \rangle$ defined by eqn (16.3) is identical to the measured average stress over a solid boundary. He also proves that $\langle e_{ij} \rangle$

is identical to the rate of strain that would be computed from the motion of the boundaries, assuming a homogeneous velocity gradient.

From eqn (16.3), the bulk stress may be rewritten as

$$\langle \sigma_{ij} \rangle = -p\delta_{ij} + 2\eta \langle e_{ij} \rangle + \Sigma p_{ij} \qquad (16.5)$$

The first two terms represent the constitutive equation of the pure suspending liquid, where p is the pressure. The contributions of the particles are all contained in the last term, which is given by Batchelor as

$$\Sigma p_{ij} = \frac{1}{\Delta V} \sum_{\alpha} \left\{ \int_{S^{\alpha}} [(1/2)(\sigma_{ik}x_j + \sigma_{jk}x_i)n_k - \eta(v_i n_j + v_j n_i)]\mathrm{d}S \right.$$
$$\left. - \int_{V^{\alpha}} (1/2)\rho(f_i'x_j + f_j'x_i)\mathrm{d}V \right\} - \frac{1}{\Delta V} \int_{\Delta V} \rho v_i' v_j' \mathrm{d}V \qquad (16.6)$$

where α denotes a generic particle of ΔV, with volume and surface area respectively V^{α} and S^{α}. The summation is taken over all the particles present in ΔV. Inertia effects for the particle motion are represented by f_i'. The relative importance of inertia forces and of viscous forces on the particle scale may be evaluated by the microscopic Reynolds number

$$\mathrm{Re}_p = \frac{\rho \dot{\gamma} a^2}{\eta} \qquad (16.7)$$

In suspensions, Re_p is usually much smaller than unity, owing to the very small size of the particles. When this is the case, the contribution of the particles reduces to a sum of deviatoric dipole strengths S_{ij}^{α}

$$\langle \sigma_{ij} \rangle = -p\delta_{ij} + 2\eta \langle e_{ij} \rangle + \frac{1}{\Delta V} \sum_{\alpha} S_{ij}^{\alpha} \qquad (16.8)$$

where

$$S_{ij}^{\alpha} = \int_{S^{\alpha}} [(\sigma_{ik}x_j - (1/3)\sigma_{lk}x_l\delta_{ij})n_k - \eta(v_i n_j + v_j n_i)]\mathrm{d}s \qquad (16.9)$$

The surface integral should be taken over the external fluid layer immediately adjacent to the particle surface. Consequently, the flow around the particle must first be computed. In the absence of inertia forces, this is a Stokes flow problem for which analytical solutions can be found only in some simple cases. For solid particles, a further simplification occurs since the contributions of the velocity terms in eqn (16.9) identically vanish. The expression of S_{ij}^{α} may be completed by the addition of terms due to the effect of an externally imposed couple acting on the particles.[1]

Equation (16.9) gives the bulk stress in a suspension of particles submitted to hydrodynamic interactions only. However, colloidal size particles may be subjected to other forces such as thermal diffusion, electrostatic or steric repulsions. In order to account for such effects, eqn (16.9) must be modified by the addition of an interaction term (Batchelor[3,4]):

$$\langle \sigma_{ij} \rangle = -p\delta_{ij} + 2\eta \langle e_{ij} \rangle + \frac{1}{\Delta V} \Sigma(S_{ij}^{\alpha} - x_i^{\alpha} F_j^{\alpha}) \qquad (16.10)$$

where F_j^{α} represents the non-hydrodynamic resultant force on a particle located on x_i^{α}. For example, in the case of thermal diffusion, the force term is related to the probability density by

$$F_i^{\alpha} = kT \frac{\partial \log P}{\partial x_i^{\alpha}} \qquad (16.11)$$

The expression of S_{ij}^{α} is still given by eqn (16.9) but, of course, the stress and velocity fields are affected by the colloidal forces. However, in view of the linearity of the Stokes equations which describe the microscopic problem, the contributions to S_{ij}^{α} of hydrodynamic forces and of colloidal forces may be decoupled, and this simplifies somewhat the solution of the problem.

When the particles are identical, the summation in eqn (16.8) over all the particles present in ΔV is equivalent to an ensemble average, thus

$$\frac{1}{\Delta V} \sum_{\alpha} S_{ij}^{\alpha} = N \langle S_{ij} \rangle \qquad (16.12)$$

The ensemble average is defined in terms of the normalized conditional probability density $P_c(C|x_i^0)$ which expresses the probability of finding the other particles in configuration C (i.e. at positions x_i^1, x_i^2, . . .) when one of them is located at position x_i^0. Then

$$\langle S_{ij} \rangle = \int S_{ij}(x_k^0, C) P_c(C|x_k^0) dC \qquad (16.13)$$

Thus, in order to find the bulk stress, information about the configuration of the suspension is needed. The determination of P is a very difficult problem which can be solved analytically only in simple situations, or otherwise, which necessitates a numerical simulation. It is however obvious that $P_c(C|x_i^0)$ depends not only on the nature of the particles but also on the type and intensity of the flow imposed on the suspension. As a consequence, non-Newtonian effects may be expected to occur. Finally, for a given configuration, the tensor S_{ij} may also depend on the orientation of the particles if they are not isotropic. This orientation can be measured by a second-order tensor C_{ij}, corresponding for example to the ellipsoid of inertia of the particle profile at time t. In this case, the bulk particle stress becomes

$$\langle S_{ij} \rangle = \int S_{ij}(x_k^0, C_{ij}, C)P'(C_{ij}, C|x_i^0)dCdC_{ij} \qquad (16.14)$$

where now P' is the conditional probability of finding one particle at x_i^0, with orientation C_{ij}, while the other particles are in configuration C. The time evolution of C_{ij} and its dependency on the bulk flow are obtained from the solution of the microscopic problem. It is clear that this is also a difficult task. Consequently, the available results in the literature deal essentially either with solid spheres for which C_{ij} is irrelevant, or with anisotropic particles, but in the limiting case where the suspension is very dilute.

16.2.3. Case of Dilute Suspensions

The dilute-suspension hypothesis implies that there are so few particles present that they are far apart and thus do not interact with one another. As a consequence, each particle behaves as if it were immersed in an infinite fluid subjected to bulk flow. It follows that the bulk value of S_{ij} cannot depend on the configuration and that the contributions of all the particles in ΔV (if identical) simply add up:

$$\langle S_{ij} \rangle = S_{ij} \qquad (16.15)$$

This greatly simplifies the determination of the bulk properties. Furthermore, the microscopic problem also becomes much simpler to solve, since it is reduced to the computation of a creeping flow field around an isolated particle. This may explain the interest that dilute suspensions have attracted in the past. Indeed, although they are not of great practical importance, they provide a good model of the main physical phenomena which act on the microscale.

16.3. DILUTE SUSPENSIONS

16.3.1. General Formulation of the Microscale Flow Problem

Since interparticle forces are neglected, the microscale flow problem consists in determining the motion of a single representative particle suspended in an infinite fluid domain undergoing the bulk motion of the suspension. The aim is, of course, to calculate the velocity and stress fields around the particle profile in order to deduce the contribution to the bulk stress, given by the surface integral in eqn (16.9).

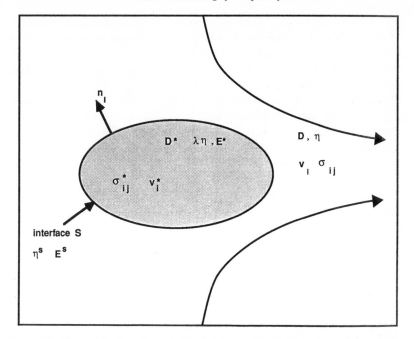

Fig. 16.2. The suspending liquid is Newtonian and incompressible, with viscosity η. The particle is incompressible, with internal viscosity $\lambda\eta$ and elastic modulus E^*. The interface has viscosity η^s and elastic modulus E^s.

The undisturbed bulk velocity field v_i^∞ is usually taken to be a linear shear flow. This restriction actually does not exclude quadratic flows, because, on the particle scale, they can usually be considered as locally linear. Consequently, far from the particle, the fluid velocity is assumed to be given by

$$v_i^\infty = e_{ik}x_k + \Omega_{ik}x_k \tag{16.16}$$

For dilute suspensions, the bulk velocity gradient and the undisturbed velocity gradient are identical, and consequently the brackets are dropped to simplify notations. The rate of strain e_{ij} and the vorticity tensor Ω_{ij} both depend only on time.

The suspended particles are incompressible, have a known stress-free geometry, and their density is equal to that of the suspending liquid. The internal medium is incompressible and has otherwise known physical properties: these are a viscosity $\lambda\eta$ and/or an elastic bulk modulus E^*.

Similarly the interface of the particle has also known properties, such as a viscosity η^s and an elasticity E^s (which can be simply a surface tension). Internal and surface variables are respectively denoted by a star (*) or by the superscript s (see Fig. 16.2). For the sake of simplicity, it is assumed that there are no colloidal forces acting on the particle or in the fluid. These effects will be examined later. A key procedure of the analysis consists in non-dimensionalizing the microscale equations. This provides the main dimensionless parameters of the problem; from the experimentalist's point of view, this indicates useful combinations of parameters to analyse the data. Lengths are scaled with a, time with $\dot\gamma^{-1}$, stresses with $\eta\dot\gamma$. Inertia effects are neglected, and thus the particle Reynolds number given by eqn (16.7) is assumed to be much smaller than unity. Unless otherwise stated, all microscale equations are written in non-dimensional form, whereas the resulting bulk constitutive equations will be cast back in dimensional form.

The fluid motions are referred to a frame with the origin at the center of mass of the particle. The latter may be deformable; consequently, material points which were at position X_i in some reference state (corresponding for example to time $t = 0$) are displaced to position x_i at time t. The equation of the deformed particle surface is

$$x = (x_i x_i)^{1/2} = f(x_1, x_2, x_3, t) \tag{16.17}$$

where f must be determined as part of the solution of the problem. The equations of the suspending liquid are thus the Stokes equations

$$\frac{\partial^2 v_i}{\partial x_j \partial x_j} = -\frac{\partial p}{\partial x_i}, \qquad \frac{\partial v_i}{\partial x_i} = 0 \tag{16.18}$$

For the particle, the equations of motion are

$$\frac{\partial}{\partial x_i} \sigma_{ij}^* = 0, \qquad \frac{\partial v_i^*}{\partial x_i} = 0 \tag{16.19}$$

The first equation indicates that the particle dynamics are inertialess, while the second is the incompressibility condition.

The particle stress σ_{ij}^* is determined by the specific constitutive law of the internal medium, for example:

Solid particle

$$\sigma_{ij}^* = -p^* \delta_{ij} \tag{16.20}$$

Newtonian viscous liquid

$$\sigma_{ij}^* = -p^*\delta_{ij} + \lambda\left(\frac{\partial v_i^*}{\partial x_j} + \frac{\partial v_j^*}{\partial x_i}\right) \tag{16.21}$$

Hookean incompressible elastic solid

$$\sigma_{ij}^* = E^*/3\eta\dot{\gamma}\left(\frac{\partial x_i}{\partial X_j} + \frac{\partial x_j}{\partial X_i}\right) \tag{16.22}$$

A linear viscoelastic solid may be obtained by adding eqns (16.21) and (16.22).

The associated boundary conditions are the following:

Far from the particle

$$v_i \to v_i^\infty \text{ as } x \to \infty \tag{16.23}$$

On the surface of the particle

—continuity of velocity

$$v_i^* = v_i^s = v_i \text{ at } x = f \tag{16.24}$$

—equilibrium of the interface

$$(\sigma_{ij} - \sigma_{ij}^*)n_j + F_i^s = 0 \tag{16.25}$$

The force exerted by the interface on the fluid is denoted F_i^s, and takes different forms depending on the surface behaviour. For example, a liquid interface is governed by the Laplace law

$$F_i^s = -\frac{E^s}{\eta\dot{\gamma}a}n_i\frac{\partial n_j}{\partial x_j} \tag{16.26}$$

More elaborate constitutive laws may be imagined, such as the ones describing an elastic or a viscoelastic membrane. They are however quite complicated, and thus are not included here. They have been derived for the specific case of capsules, and are given by Barthes-Biesel and Rallison[5] and by Barthes-Biesel and Sgaier.[6]

Dimensional analysis indicates that, in general, the problem depends on several parameters:

λ: the viscosity ratio between the internal and external liquids;
$\lambda^s = \eta^s/a\eta$: the viscosity ratio between the interface and the external liquid;
k: the capillary number representing the ratio between viscous deforming forces and elastic shape restoring forces. Depending on the origin of the latter forces, k is defined as

$$k = \eta \dot{\gamma} a / E^s, \text{ for an elastic interface;} \quad (16.27)$$

$$k = \eta \dot{\gamma} / E^*, \text{ for a homogeneous elastic particle.} \quad (16.28)$$

It is very difficult to find a general solution of eqns (16.17)–(16.26), because the problem being of the free surface type, is non-linear. The presently available analytical solutions have been obtained for solid spherical or ellipsoidal particles, or for initially spherical particles subjected to moderate deformations. However, some common features of the solutions can be found as shown by Batchelor.[1] Indeed, the suspension liquid motion is described by the Stokes equations, and the general solution may thus be expanded as an infinite series of spherical harmonics, the first terms of which are

$$v_i' = T_{kj} \left(-\frac{3x_i x_j x_k}{2x^5} + \frac{x_j \delta_{ik} - x_k \delta_{ij}}{x^3} \right) + \dots \quad (16.29)$$

$$p' = -T_{jk} \left(\frac{3x_j x_k}{x^5} - \frac{\delta_{jk}}{x^3} \right) + \dots \quad (16.30)$$

where eqn (16.29) already satisfies eqn (16.23), and where the fact that no external net force acts upon the particle has been taken into account. The coefficient T_{ij} is symmetric and traceless; it depends only on time and must be determined from the other boundary conditions. It may be interpreted as the intensity of a force doublet located at the center of mass of the particle, and is dynamically equivalent to the effect of the presence of the particle on the surrounding fluid. The viscous stress in the suspension liquid follows from eqns (16.29) and (16.30):

$$\sigma_{ij} = -p\delta_{ij} + 2e_{ij} + T_{kl} \left[\frac{3x_k(x_i \delta_{jl} + x_j \delta_{il})}{x^5} + \frac{15 x_i x_j x_k x_l}{x^7} \right] + \dots$$

$$(16.31)$$

The above expressions of σ_{ij} and of v_i' may be used now to evaluate the particle contribution to the bulk stress of the suspension, as indicated by eqn (16.9). After noting that the integral over the particle surface may be replaced by an integral over another arbitrary surface enclosing the particle and intersecting no other, Batchelor shows that

$$S_{ij} = 4\pi \dot{\gamma} a^3 \eta T_{ij} \quad (16.32)$$

and thus the constitutive law of the suspension becomes

$$\langle \sigma_{ij} \rangle = -p\delta_{ij} + 2\eta e_{ij} + \frac{\eta \dot{\gamma}}{\Delta V} \sum_\alpha 4\pi a^3 T_{ij} \tag{16.33}$$

16.3.2. Suspensions of Solid Particles

16.3.2.1. Solid Spheres

In the case where the suspended particles are solid spheres, the flow field can be easily computed, and it follows that

$$T_{ij} = (5/3)e_{ij} \tag{16.34}$$

Consequently the constitutive equation of the suspension is

$$\langle \sigma_{ij} \rangle = -p\delta_{ij} + 2\eta[1 + (5/2)\phi]e_{ij} \tag{16.35}$$

This is the famous result obtained by Einstein[7] who showed that such a suspension is Newtonian, with a relative viscosity

$$\eta_r = 1 + (5/2)\phi \tag{16.36}$$

Comparison with experimental results indicates that this expression is valid in the absence of colloidal effects (Brownian motion, electrostatic or van der Waals forces), and for particle concentrations no larger than 5% (Fig. 16.4).

16.3.2.2. Ellipsoidal Particles

The case of ellipsoidal particles has received a lot of attention for two main reasons. Firstly, ellipsoids may be used as an approximation for a great variety of shapes ranging from flakes to rods. Secondly, the motion of an ellipsoid suspended in a shear flow has been completely determined by Jeffery[8] who gives the stress distribution on the surface of the particle, as a function of its instantaneous orientation. From these results, Batchelor[1] shows that the tensor T_{ij} is given by

$$T_{ij} = A_{ijkl}e_{kl} \tag{16.37}$$

where A_{ijkl} is a complicated expression which depends only on the geometry and on the instantaneous orientation of the ellipsoid. It follows that, in general, the suspension behaves as an anisotropic fluid. In order to obtain its constitutive equation, the contributions of all the ellipsoids present in the volume ΔV must be summed. However, Jeffery shows that, in general, an ellipsoid has a periodic rotational motion, with a time dependent angular velocity, which is a function of the principal axis ratios and of the initial position. In the absence of inertia effects, or of hydro-dynamic interactions with other particles, the ellipsoid remains indefinitely on its orbit. Consequently, in the case of flows with vorticity, it is first necessary to time-average the orientations for one particular orbit, and then to compute the probability density of the different orbits. The first step is straightforward, but the second is impossible to perform unless some further assumptions are made. Thus, in general, it is not possible to obtain the constitutive equation of a suspension of Jeffery ellipsoids except in two particular cases where the orientation distribution is known: nearly spherical particles (orientation is irrelevant) or a pure straining motion. In the latter situation, Jeffery shows that a particle orients itself so that its largest diameter is parallel to the principal rate of extension and its smallest diameter is parallel to the least principal rate of extension. Thus, for identical particles, the summation is easy to perform.

For anisotropic particles subjected to flows with vorticity, supple-mentary hypotheses can be made to remove the indeterminacy. For example, assuming that initially the orientation re-partition is isotropic, Okagawa *et al.*[9] have computed the orbit distribution of ellipsoids for a steady simple shear flow and conclude that it is a periodic function of time (as would also be the resulting shear viscosity). However, when they measure the time evolution of the orientation distribution of a dilute suspension of rods, they observe a kind of orbit drift of the particles towards a steady configuration. This phenomenon is not accounted for by Jeffery's theory, and is difficult to explain. It may be attributed to small differences in the shapes of the particles, to inertia effects, to particle interactions and/or to Brownian motion. It is clear then that quite dif-ferent physical phenomena are responsible for the loss of memory of the suspension, but so far neither inertia forces nor hydrodynamic particle interactions have been modelled. In contrast, the study of the effect of Brownian motion is tractable and thus has received a lot of attention. Also, particles of colloidal size (less than 1 μm) occur frequently, and it is well known that they can be affected by thermal agitation.

Suspensions of axisymmetric ellipsoids subjected to Brownian forces have been studied by Leal and Hinch in a series of papers.[10-15] The choice of spheroids suspended in a simple shear flow greatly simplifies the solution of the problem, without restricting the generality of the results too much. Indeed, Bretherton[16] shows that, for Stokes flow, the dynamics of any axisymmetric body are equivalent to those of a spheroid with a modified aspect ratio which depends on the geometry of the body. Furthermore, the simple shear results may be transposed to any two-dimensional flow with a rate of strain $\dot{\gamma}$ and a vorticity ω if the aspect ratio is also redefined.[12]

The spheroid is characterized by its aspect ratio α (defined as the axial diameter divided by the transverse diameter), and its position is specified by a unit vector u_i directed along the axis of revolution.

The relative intensity of convective and Brownian forces is measured by a Peclet number

$$\text{Pe}_\text{B} = \dot{\gamma}/D \qquad (16.38)$$

where D is the rotation diffusion coefficient which has a well defined expression for spheroids.[10] It is assumed that Brownian effects dominate over inertia forces or particle–particle interactions, correspondingly

$$\rho\dot{\gamma}a^2/\eta \ll \text{Pe}_\text{B}^{-1} \quad \text{(small inertia)}$$

$$(a/d)^3 \ll \text{Pe}_\text{B}^{-1} \quad \text{(no interactions)} \qquad (16.39)$$

When it is suspended in the linear shear flow, eqn (16.16), the ellipsoid rotates according to Jeffery's solution[14]

$$\frac{\mathrm{d}u_i}{\mathrm{d}t} = \Omega_{ik}u_k + G(e_{ik}u_k - u_i e_{km}u_k u_m) \qquad (16.40)$$

where $G = [(\alpha^2 - 1)/(\alpha^2 + 1)]$.

In the presence of Brownian motion, the orientation probability density $P_\text{o}(u_i, t)$ is defined as the probability of finding a particle with its major axis having an orientation between u_i and $u_i + \mathrm{d}u_i$, at a time between t and $t + \mathrm{d}t$. It must satisfy a Fokker–Planck equation

$$\frac{\partial P_\text{o}}{\partial t} + \frac{\partial}{\partial x_i}\left(P_\text{o}\frac{\mathrm{d}u_i}{\mathrm{d}t} - \text{Pe}_\text{B}^{-1}\frac{\partial P_\text{o}}{\partial x_i}\right) = 0 \qquad (16.41)$$

which states that the time evolution of P_o results from the effects of the normal Jeffery motion of the particle and of random Brownian rotations. The solution of eqns (16.41) and (16.40) thus gives in principle the configuration of the particles at any time. Then the constitutive equation of the suspension, obtained from eqns (16.10) and (16.14), may be written as[12]

$$\langle\sigma_{ij}\rangle = -p\delta_{ij} + 2\eta e_{ij} + 2\eta\phi[2A\langle u_i u_j u_k u_m\rangle e_{km} + 2B(\langle u_i u_k\rangle e_{kj}$$

$$+ \langle u_j u_k\rangle e_{ki}) + Ce_{ij} + FD\langle u_i u_j\rangle] \qquad (16.42)$$

where A, B, C, F are shape factors. The averages are taken in the sense of eqn (16.14). The main difficulty consists in evaluating the second and fourth moments of u_i. In principle they can be obtained from the solution of eqn (16.41), but no closed form solution for P_o has been found for flows with both vorticity and significant Brownian motion. It is usual to pre-average the Fokker–Planck equation to obtain directly the time evolution of $\langle u_i u_j \rangle$:

$$\frac{\mathscr{D}}{\mathscr{D}t} \langle u_i u_j \rangle = G[e_{ik}\langle u_k u_j \rangle + e_{jk}\langle u_k u_i \rangle - 2\langle u_i u_j u_k u_m \rangle e_{km}]$$

$$- 6D(\langle u_i u_j \rangle - \delta_{ij}/3) \qquad (16.43)$$

where the convected, corotational Jaumann derivative is defined for any tensor A_{ij} by

$$\frac{\mathscr{D}}{\mathscr{D}t} A_{ij} = \frac{\partial}{\partial t} A_{ij} + v_k \frac{\partial}{\partial x_k} A_{ij} - \Omega_{jk} A_{ki} - \Omega_{ik} A_{kj}$$

However, the resulting relation contains the fourth-order moment of u_i, and one is confronted with a classical closure problem frequently encountered in rheology. Analytical solutions can only be found in the two limiting cases where Brownian forces dominate ($Pe_B \ll 1$) or where Brownian motion is weak ($Pe_B \gg 1$). In the limit of strong Brownian agitation, the orientation distribution is nearly isotropic. The pure strain component of the bulk motion generates small perturbations from isotropy. For slow time variations, a second-order fluid constitutive law is found (Giesekus[17]):

$$\langle \sigma_{ij} \rangle = - p\delta_{ij} + 2\eta e_{ij} + 2\eta\phi \left[A'e_{ij} + B'\overline{e_{ik}e_{kj}} - \frac{GF}{90D} \frac{\mathscr{D}}{\mathscr{D}t} e_{ij} \right]$$

$$(16.44)$$

where A' and B' are known[15] and depend only on α, and where an overbar denotes a symmetric deviator defined by

$$\overline{A_{ij}} = (1/2)[A_{ij} + A_{ji} - (2/3)\delta_{ij}A_{kk}] \qquad (16.45)$$

It follows from eqn (16.44) that the suspension has a non-Newtonian time dependent behaviour with a characteristic time $O(D^{-1})$. In simple shear flow, a constant shear viscosity is predicted, with small normal stress differences which increase as $\dot{\gamma}^2$.

More interesting for practical applications is the case of relatively weak Brownian motion ($Pe_B \gg 1$). The easiest situation is encountered when the flow has no vorticity and tends to align the particles along a direction

TABLE 16.1

Rheological Functions for a Dilute Suspension of Axisymmetric Ellipsoids with Extreme Axis Ratios α and Subjected to Simple Shear Flow and Brownian Motion. Shear Thinning Behaviour is Predicted. (From Hinch and Leal[13])

	$[\eta]$	$N_1/\eta\phi\dot{\gamma}$	$N_2/\eta\phi\dot{\gamma}$
	$Pe_B \ll 1$ Strong Brownian motion		
Rod $(\alpha \gg 1)$	$4\alpha^2/15\log\alpha$	$2\alpha^2 Pe_B/35\log\alpha$	$-\alpha^2 Pe_B/105\log\alpha$
Disc $(\alpha \ll 1)$	$32/15\pi\alpha$	$4Pe_B/21\pi\alpha$	$-8Pe_B/105\pi\alpha$
	$(\alpha^3 + \alpha^{-3})Pe_B^{-1} \ll 1$ Weak Brownian motion		
Rod $(\alpha \gg 1)$	$0{\cdot}315\alpha/\log\alpha$	$\alpha^4 Pe_B^{-1}/4\log\alpha$	$\ll (Pe_B^{-1}\alpha^4/\log\alpha)$
Disc $(\alpha \ll 1)$	$3{\cdot}13$	$4Pe_B^{-1}/3\pi\alpha^3$	$-Pe_B^{-1}/3\pi\alpha^3$

u_i^O while thermal agitation creates a small spread of orientations around u_i^O, then

$$\langle u_i u_j \rangle = u_i^O u_j^O + \text{smaller terms} \qquad (16.46)$$

In the case of simple shear flow, Leal and Hinch[10,11] have solved eqn (16.41) up to terms of order Pe_B^{-2}. They find that, as time takes large values, a steady state orbit distribution is reached, which is independent of the initial particle orientation. Furthermore, for particles having an extreme axis ratio ($\alpha \gg 1$, rods; $\alpha \ll 1$, discs), the orientation distribution is sharply peaked, so that the alignment assumption, eqn (16.46), is a good approximation. In this case, it is possible to compute asymptotic values[10,11] for the orientation distributions, and for the shape factors appearing in eqn (16.42). The corresponding expressions of the intrinsic viscosity and of the two normal stress differences are given in Table 16.1 for weak and strong Brownian motion. It appears that, in both regimes, the predicted shear viscosity is Newtonian but the difference between the low and high shear limiting values of the viscosity indicates shear thinning. This effect may be quite significant since it is of order α (or α^{-1}). It is due to the fact that the hydrodynamic alignment of the particles is weakly disturbed by thermal agitation. Similarly the normal stress differences are much larger for high shears than for low ones.

The case of nearly spherical particles is also considered by Hinch and Leal[11,13] who find, for simple shear flow, the following expression for the rheological functions, valid for any Pe_B:

$$[\eta] = 5/2 + \delta^2\{26/147 + 3/[5(1 + Pe_B^2/36)]\} + \ldots \quad (16.47)$$

$$N_1/\eta\dot{\gamma}\phi = \frac{36}{35}\delta^2 \frac{6Pe_B^{-1}}{1 + (6Pe_B^{-1})^2} + \ldots \quad (16.48)$$

$$N_2/\eta\dot{\gamma}\phi = -\frac{6}{35}\delta^2 \frac{6Pe_B^{-1}}{1 + (6Pe_B^{-1})^2} + \ldots \quad (16.49)$$

where

$$\alpha = 1 + \delta, \quad \delta \ll 1$$

Consequently, shear thinning is also predicted, but this phenomenon is very small $(O(\phi\varepsilon^2))$. It is interesting to note that the above theoretical predictions for near spheres are in qualitative agreement with the experimental data of Krieger,[18] although the latter were obtained for suspensions of polystyrene latices, at concentrations which are too high for the dilution hypothesis to apply. For rods, the shear thinning behaviour predicted by the model is also in qualitative agreement with the experimental measurements of Chauveteau[19] on suspensions of rod-like xanthan macromolecules.

Since the orientation distribution is known exactly for weak flows and for strong flows, Hinch and Leal[15] suggest a closed form expression for the fourth-order moment $\langle u_i u_j u_k u_m \rangle$ as a function of $\langle u_i u_j \rangle$ which is simply an interpolation between the two relations found for the limiting cases $Pe_B \gg 1$ and $Pe_B \ll 1$. They thus obtain a general constitutive law which has a form suggested by Hand.[20] The rheological predictions of the model are studied for a number of flows: uniaxial or biaxial extension (shear thickening), two-dimensional straining motion (shear thickening), simple shear (shear thinning). The transient responses are also given. Frattini and Fuller[21] use an optical method to measure the average particle orientation and the average degree of alignment as a function of time and of Pe_B. They find that the interpolated orientation distribution of Hinch and Leal is in reasonable agreement with their experimental data, a result which gives support to the credibility of Hinch and Leal's constitutive law.

16.3.2.3. *Primary Electroviscous Effect*

The rheology of suspensions may be noticeably affected by electrostatic effects. Indeed when a charged particle is suspended in an electrolytic liquid, it is surrounded with a cloud of counter-ions. The corresponding local perturbation of the electric equilibrium has several rheological consequences. Firstly, strong repulsive long range forces may be created and may modify the particle distribution. This is the so-called 'secondary' effect which is investigated in Section 16.4. Secondly, the motion of the fluid tends to distort the charge cloud, and this gives rise to an additional energy dissipation or, equivalently, to an increased stress on the microscale. This is the 'primary' effect, outlined below.

The primary electroviscous effect for a dilute suspension of solid spheres was first studied by Booth,[22] and later in more generality by Sherwood.[23] They show that the electrostatic forces modify the microscale equations, which are given in dimensional form in the following. The suspending fluid is now locally characterized by the velocity and pressure (v_i, p) and also by an electric potential ψ and a charge density q, related by Poisson's equation:

$$\frac{\partial^2 \psi}{\partial x_i \partial x_i} = -q/\varepsilon \qquad (16.50)$$

where ε is the suspending liquid dielectric constant (divided by 4π). The ion conservation equation states that the ion velocity w_i is due to convective, electrical and thermal forces:

$$w_i = v_i + \mu\left(-ez\frac{\partial \psi}{\partial x_i} - kT\frac{\partial \log n}{\partial x_i}\right) \qquad (16.51)$$

where μ, z and n represent respectively the ion mobility, the valence and the number density, and e is the elementary charge. Equation (16.51) must be written for each ionic species present in the suspension. Finally the Stokes equations (16.18) for the liquid motion now include a new term due to the electrical force on the fluid particles:

$$\frac{\partial p}{\partial x_i} + \frac{q\partial \psi}{\partial x_i} = \eta \frac{\partial^2 v_i}{\partial x_j \partial x_j} \qquad (16.52)$$

Of course, the electrical phenomena are important only in the charge cloud since, far from the particle, the electrical equilibrium is restored, and the potential is constant. The thickness of the cloud is measured by the Debye length, κ^{-1}, defined by

$$\kappa^2 = \frac{e^2}{\varepsilon kT}\Sigma z^2 n_\infty \qquad (16.53)$$

where the summation is taken over each type of ion in the liquid, and where n_∞ represents the equilibrium number density of each species. Depending on the ionic strength of the suspension, the Debye length varies considerably from about $1\,\mu$m for distilled water to $1\cdot0$ nm for a solution of $1\,$mol$\,$l^{-1} of NaCl.

Equations (16.50)–(16.53) are written in dimensional form. If the electrical energy is scaled with $e\zeta$ (ζ is the particle potential) and lengths with κ^{-1}, the non-dimensionalization of the equations indicates that the main parameters of the microscale motion are the following:

$a\kappa$: ratio of the particle radius to the Debye layer thickness ($a\kappa \gg 1$, thin cloud; $a\kappa \ll 1$, thick cloud);

$e\zeta/kT$: ratio between the electrical and thermal energies of the ions; for weak surface potentials ($e\zeta/kT \ll 1$) the ion distribution near the particle is only slightly displaced from equilibrium;

$\mathrm{Pe_E} = \dot{\gamma}/\mu kT\kappa^2$; electrical Peclet number, ratio of diffusion to convection times (usually small);

$H = \varepsilon\zeta^2/\eta\mu kT$: electrical Hartmann number, representing the ratio of the electrical and viscous forces in the fluid.

Booth solves the problem for weak surface potentials ($e\zeta/kT \ll 1$), and for small Hartmann and Peclet numbers. He finds that the suspension is Newtonian with an apparent viscosity which differs from Einstein's formula:

$$\eta_r = 1 + (5/2)\beta\phi$$

$$\beta = 1 + Hf(a\kappa) \qquad (16.54)$$

where $f(a\kappa)$ is a dimensionless analytical function given by Booth. When the electrical layer is thin, Sherwood shows that β can be expanded in terms of H:

$$\beta = 1 + \frac{6H}{(a\kappa)^2}(1 - H/a\kappa + \ldots) \qquad (a\kappa \gg 1, H \ll 1, e\zeta/kT \ll 1)$$

$$(16.55)$$

The first term corresponds to Einstein's relation, the second is due to Booth and the last indicates that the electroviscous effect grows more slowly than Booth's linear prediction. For thick layers, Booth finds that

$$\beta \simeq 1 + H(\tfrac{1}{25})(a\kappa)^{-1} + O(a\kappa) \qquad (a\kappa \ll 1, H \ll 1, e\zeta/kT \ll 1)$$

$$(16.56)$$

The case of weak potentials and large Hartmann numbers has also been investigated by Sherwood, who points out that strong electric forces tend to slow down the fluid layer adjacent to the sphere. The electrical forces decay exponentially away from the sphere whereas the viscous forces decay algebraically. Consequently, in the far field, viscous forces dominate, while the equilibrium between viscous and electric forces is reached at distances of order κ^{-1}. A numerical model confirms these hypotheses, but shows that Booth's theory gives surprisingly good predictions for the intrinsic viscosity even when H is not very small. For example, for typical experimental values ($H = 6$, $a\kappa = 1$), eqn (16.55) overestimates by 3% the contribution to the viscosity from the electroviscous effect.

For high surface potentials and thin layers ($e\zeta/kT \gg 1$, $a\kappa \gg 1$), Sherwood shows that the intrinsic viscosity first increases with ζ, reaches a maximum which depends on $a\kappa$, and then decreases to a limiting value. For thick layers ($e\zeta/kT \gg 1$, $a\kappa \ll 1$) and large potentials, the viscosity is found to increase with ζ up to a limiting value. Booth's theory predicts results within 10% of the numerical solution up to values of $\zeta e/kT$ of order 2.

In conclusion, it appears that Booth's results may be used as a good estimate of the primary electroviscous effect provided the surface potential is not too high. Saville[24] gives a comparison between Booth's predictions for β and experimental results obtained by Stone-Masui and Watillon[25] for colloidal particles suspended in solutions of varying ionic strength. For Debye layers such that $a\kappa$ varies from 9 to 2, the agreement between experiment and theory is within the experimental errors (which are quite large). However, the same data indicate that the secondary electroviscous effect may also have been present, which might explain why the agreement between theory and experiment is only fair.

16.3.3. Suspensions of Deformable Particles

When the particles are deformable even when the suspension is quite dilute, one observes non-Newtonian properties such as a shear thinning viscosity and normal stress differences. These effects have been experimentally measured in solutions of entangled macromolecules, in suspensions of red blood cells or of capsules. The non-Newtonian behaviour may be attributed to the adaptation of the microstructure to the viscous forces exerted by the flow. This is of course very difficult to model and to predict, because the microscale flow problem is of the free surface type and thus very complex mathematically. At present there are only a few solutions available for the dilute case (see the review by Rallison[26]) but none for the more concentrated situation where particle–particle interactions and particle deformability are coupled. Results are presented for two types of deformable particle: homogeneous elastic spheres and capsules (i.e. a liquid drop enclosed by a deformable elastic membrane).

16.3.3.1. Suspensions of Homogeneous Elastic Spheres

The rheology of a dilute suspension of elastic spheres has been studied independently by Goddard and Miller[27] and by Roscoe.[28] The common assumption is that the particle is a viscoelastic solid, characterized by a bulk elastic modulus E^*. The microscale flow problem is defined by eqns (16.18), (16.19) and (16.22), with boundary conditions (16.23)–(16.25), where F_i^s is identically zero. The capillary number here is given by eqn (16.28). Since inertia forces are neglected, the internal stresses are homogeneous and the sphere deforms into an ellipsoid. Equation (16.17) of the surface may then be written as

$$x^2 = 1 + 2kC_{lm}x_l x_m \tag{16.57}$$

where the second-order tensor C_{lm} characterizes the deformation of the particle and has eigenvalues equal to the three principal diameters of the deformed profile. Jeffery's[8] solution may be adapted to ellipsoids with moving boundaries, and the microscopic problem is amenable to solution, once a constitutive law for the particle material has been postulated. It should be pointed out that, for this problem, the anisotropy of the microstructure is induced by the flow. Consequently, identical spheres all deform in the same fashion and their orientations with respect to stream lines are parallel. The contributions of all the particles in the elementary volume ΔV simply reduce to the contribution of one typical particle weighted with the volume fraction.

When deviations from sphericity are small, i.e. when $k \ll 1$, Goddard and Miller show that the rheology of the suspension is described by two equations, as suggested by Hand.[20] The first gives the time evolution of the deformed profile:

$$\frac{\mathscr{D}}{\mathscr{D}t}C_{ij} + \frac{2\dot{\gamma}}{3k}C_{ij} = \frac{5}{3k}e_{ij} + \frac{10}{7}\overline{e_{il}C_{lj}} - \frac{24}{7}k\overline{C_{il}(\mathscr{D}C_{lj}/\mathscr{D}t)} + O(\gamma k)$$

$$\tag{16.58}$$

The second relates the bulk stress to the bulk rate of strain and to the local anisotropy:

$$\langle \sigma_{ij} \rangle = -p\delta_{ij} + 2\eta\left(1 + \frac{5}{2}\phi\right)e_{ij} + 5\eta\phi k\left[-\frac{\mathscr{D}}{\mathscr{D}t}C_{ij} + \frac{6}{7}\overline{e_{il}C_{lj}}\right.$$

$$\left. - \frac{20}{7}k\overline{C_{il}(\mathscr{D}C_{lj}/\mathscr{D}t)} + O(\dot{\gamma}k^2)\right] \tag{16.59}$$

Consequently the suspension appears to be viscoelastic with a characteristic response time τ given by

$$\tau = 3\eta/2E^*$$ (16.60)

For small deformations eqn (16.58) may be solved by successive approximations and it becomes

$$\langle\sigma_{ij}\rangle + \tau\frac{\mathscr{D}}{\mathscr{D}t}\langle\sigma_{ij}\rangle = 2\eta\left[\left(1 + \frac{5}{2}\phi\right)e_{ij} + \left(1 - \frac{5}{3}\phi\right)\tau\frac{\mathscr{D}}{\mathscr{D}t}e_{ij}\right.$$

$$\left. + \frac{25}{7}\phi\tau\overline{e_{il}e_{lj}} + O(k^2\dot{\gamma})\right]$$ (16.61)

which is the second-order fluid equation. Consequently the shear viscosity is constant and given by Einstein's formula. However, normal stress differences are predicted:

$$N_1 = \frac{25}{2}E^*\phi[k^2 + O(k^2)]$$

$$N_2 = -\frac{275}{56}E^*\phi[k^2 + O(k^2)]$$ (16.62)

A shear dependent viscosity would be predicted if the next-order terms in particle deformation were included in eqns (16.58) and (16.59), but the analysis becomes quite complicated and has not been carried out. However, Roscoe has considered large deformations of a viscoelastic sphere made of a rubber-like material. He obtains a numerical solution to the problem for the case of simple shear flow and predicts shear thinning behaviour of the suspension, with a typical S-shaped viscosity curve showing Newtonian behaviour both in the low shear and high shear limits. The high-shear limit of $[\eta]$ is about half the Einstein value. The drawback is that the numerical solution must be sought for each specific system under consideration.

Furthermore, the elastic sphere model predicts shear thickening for pure straining flows, and viscoelastic behaviour for any unsteady linear shear flow. It can thus be used to analyse data in those situations. This model thus predicts qualitatively the rheological behaviour of solutions of coiled macromolecules.

16.3.3.2. Suspensions of Capsules

Capsules may be considered as generalized liquid droplets, since the only condition is that their interface be elastic. There has been long-standing research starting with Taylor's pioneering work to understand the deformation and bursting of liquid drops or of capsules suspended in shear flow, and tᴏ infer the rheological consequences for suspensions of such particles.

The microscale flow problem is described by eqns (16.18), (16.19) and (16.21), with boundary conditions (16.23)–(16.25), where the surface force is expressed either by eqn (16.26) for a liquid interface, or by a more general equation.[5,6] The capillary number is defined by eqn (16.27). Owing to the complexity of the problem, the only available analytical solutions apply to initially spherical capsules subjected to moderate deformations D_f ($D_f \ll 1$). The corresponding physical factors which prevent large deviations from sphericity are either high internal viscosity or large surface rigidity. Thus the solutions are valid when either of the two following conditions is fulfilled:

$$\lambda \gg 1 \quad \text{then } D_f = O(\lambda^{-1})$$
$$k \ll 1 \quad \text{then } D_f = O(k) \tag{16.63}$$

For liquid droplets the time dependent motion of the particle is given by Cox[30] and by Frankel and Acrivos[31] up to $O(D_f)$, and by Barthes-Biesel and Acrivos[32] up to $O(D_f^2)$. These authors also predict the burst of the drop when the capillary number is increased beyond a limit $k_c(\lambda)$ which depends on the viscosity ratio and on the flow type. It is thus possible to determine the maximum size of the drops under given flow conditions. The corresponding constitutive equations are obtained for identical particles, having a diameter small enough for bursting to be avoided. Then Barthes-Biesel and Acrivos[33] find that, up to $O(D_f^2)$, the deformation of the microstructure must be described with second- and fourth-order tensors C_{ij} and C_{ijkl} (higher order approximations would lead to still higher order tensors, corresponding to elongated drops);

$$x = 1 + D_f C_{lm} x_l x_m / x^2 + D_f^2 (R_0 + C_{lmpq} x_l x_m x_p x_q / x^4) + \ldots$$

where R_0 is computed from the requirement that the drop volume remains constant. The rheology of the emulsion is then determined by two time-evolution equations for C_{ij} and C_{ijkl} and by the equation relating the bulk stress to the rate of strain tensor and to the local anisotropy, as measured by C_{ij} and C_{ijkl}. These equations, being obviously very complicated, are not given here but can be found explicitly elsewhere.[33] The emulsion appears to have viscoelastic behaviour with a discrete spectrum of relaxation times corresponding to the different modes of deformation of the microstructure:

$$\tau_1 = (a_1 a_2/40a_0)\eta a/E^s \qquad (C_{ij} \text{ deformation})$$

$$\tau_2 = (a_3 a_4/360a_0)\eta a/E^s \qquad (C_{ijkl} \text{ deformation}) \qquad (16.64)$$

where

$$a_0 = \lambda + 1, \qquad a_1 = 2\lambda + 3, \qquad a_2 = 19\lambda + 16,$$

$$a_3 = 17\lambda + 16, \qquad a_4 = 10\lambda + 11$$

For weak flows ($k \ll 1$) and slow-time variations, the constitutive equation of the suspension simplifies and is found to be of the Rivlin–Eriksen type:

$$\langle \sigma_{ij} \rangle = -p\delta_{ij} + 2\eta e_{ij}\left[1 + \phi\left(\frac{5\lambda + 2}{2a_0} + \frac{k^2}{\dot{\gamma}^2}\frac{a_2 a_5}{a_1 a_3 a_4 a_0^5}e_{lm}e_{lm}\right)\right]$$

$$+ \eta\phi\frac{k}{\dot{\gamma}}\frac{a_2}{20a_0^2}\left[-\frac{a_2}{2}\frac{\mathscr{D}}{\mathscr{D}t}e_{ij} + \frac{3(25\lambda^2 + 41\lambda + 4)}{7a_0}\overline{e_{ik}e_{kj}}\right.$$

$$- \frac{k}{\dot{\gamma}}a_2\frac{150\lambda^3 + 2179\lambda^2 + 2897\lambda + 724}{280a_0^2}\overline{e_{ik}(\mathscr{D}e_{kj}/\mathscr{D}t)}$$

$$\left. + \frac{k}{\dot{\gamma}}\frac{a_2^2 a_1}{80a_0}\frac{\mathscr{D}^2}{\mathscr{D}t^2}e_{ij}\right] + O(\dot{\gamma}k^3\phi) \qquad (16.65)$$

where

$$a_5 = 422{\cdot}3\lambda^7 + 3208{\cdot}5\lambda^6 + 9960{\cdot}9\lambda^5 + 11053{\cdot}0\lambda^4 + 5115{\cdot}6\lambda^3$$

$$+ 2848{\cdot}1\lambda^2 + 1711{\cdot}7\lambda + 100{\cdot}9$$

It follows that the intrinsic viscosity is given by

$$[\eta] = \frac{5\lambda + 2}{2(\lambda + 1)} - \frac{k^2}{2}\left(\frac{a_2^3 a_1}{1600a_0^3} - \frac{a_2 a_5}{a_1 a_3 a_4 a_0^5}\right) \qquad (16.66)$$

The first term of eqn (16.66), obtained by Taylor,[29] indicates that the zero-shear viscosity depends on λ. The second term is always negative and thus predicts shear thinning behaviour, which is due to fairly large deformations of the drops (at least $O(D_f^2)$ or equivalently here $O(k^2)$), which cannot be obtained from an $O(D_f)$ analysis, such as that of Frankel and Acrivos[31] (the same remark also applies to the elastic spheres suspension, where shear thinning is predicted only numerically). Expression (16.66), being quadratic in k, does not predict a constant high-shear viscosity. It can only model the behaviour of the suspension for moderate shear rates.

When the drop deformation is limited by the high internal viscosity of the particle ($\lambda > 3$), the structure relaxation times τ_1 and τ_2 become very large too, and the resulting constitutive relations of the emulsion cannot be cast into an expression similar to eqn (16.65). The time evolution of the structure and the stress–structure relationship must then all be written explicitly.[33] In this case shear thinning behaviour and a constant high shear viscosity are predicted. The latter phenomenon may be attributed to the fact that highly viscous drops reach a limiting deformation and orientation with increasing shear rates.[32]

In both cases the shear thinning behaviour is due to the deformation and orientation of the droplets in shear flow. The computation of drop profiles[32] and recent experimental observations by Bentley and Leal[34] indicate that these phenomena should be expected for values of the capillary number greater than $0\cdot1$ for which the deformation of the drop is of the order of 10%. Furthermore, the emulsion is predicted to exhibit flow-induced anisotropy as well as normal stress effects which can be easily computed from eqn (16.65).

The case of capsules has been considered only recently. One important application is in the understanding of the phenomena encountered when blood is undergoing flow, whether it be *in vivo* or *in vitro* (e.g. extracorporeal circulation). There are essentially three main differences between a capsule and a liquid droplet:

—the interface of the capsule, being solid, can sustain shearing forces;
—a great variety of membrane constitutive behaviours may be imagined (e.g. viscoelastic, shear-strengthening, shear-softening, plastic, etc.);
—the reference rest shape of a capsule is not necessarily spherical (e.g. a red blood cell is a biconcave disc), and the deformability of the capsule may thus be increased.

The analysis of the microscale problem is complicated by the fact that the interface dynamics are no longer governed by the simple Laplace law, eqn (16.26), but by the complicated theory of large deformations of membranes. Up to now, there are very few available solutions, except for initially spherical capsules. The rheology of dilute suspensions of spherical capsules with an elastic membrane subjected to moderate deformations, D_f, has been studied up to $O(D_f^2)$ by Barthes-Biesel and Chhim[35] for weak slowly varying linear shear flows. The time dependent motion of such capsules has been obtained to $O(D_f)$ by Brunn[36] for a linearly elastic membrane and by Barthes-Biesel and Rallison[5] for a thin interface having arbitrary elastic properties. The importance of membrane viscoelasticity has been assessed by Barthes-Biesel and Sgaier.[6]

These studies show that the $O(D_f)$ distortion of the capsule must be specified by two second-order tensors C_{ij} and C'_{ij}. The first corresponds to the overall deformation of the sphere into an ellipsoid, whereas the second measures the in-plane deformation of membrane elements. Correspondingly, as shown by Barthes-Biesel and Rallison, the constitutive equation of the suspension is given by

$$\langle \sigma_{ij} \rangle = -p\delta_{ij} + 2\eta e_{ij} + \frac{2\eta\phi}{a_1}\left[5(\lambda - 1)e_{ij} \right.$$
$$\left. - \frac{D_f}{k}\left(\frac{5}{2} L_{ij} + M_{ij}\right) + O(D_f, D_f^2/k)\right] \quad (16.67)$$

where L_{ij} and M_{ij} are two linear combinations of the deformation tensors C_{ij} and C'_{ij}, the coefficients of which depend solely on the elastic properties of the membrane material (values of these coefficients have been given[5] for a very thin sheet of an isotropic incompressible elastomer, for a liquid interface, for an incompressible bilayer). The time evolution of the deformation is described by two differential equations analogous to those found for elastic homogeneous spheres:

$$D_f \frac{\mathscr{D}}{\mathscr{D}t} C_{ij} = (5/a_1)e_{ij} + D_f/k[L_{ij}/a_1 + (10a_0/a_1 a_2)M_{ij}]$$

$$D_f \frac{\mathscr{D}}{\mathscr{D}t} C'_{ij} = (5/a_1)e_{ij} + D_f/k[L_{ij}/a_1 + 2(3\lambda + 2)M_{ij}/a_1 a_2] \quad (16.68)$$

It thus appears that, in general, a suspension of capsules is viscoelastic with two time constants depending on k, λ and on the constitutive properties of the membrane material. For steady flows, Newtonian shear viscosity is predicted. However, for weak, slowly varying flows, Barthes-Biesel and Chhim have extended the analysis of the microscale problem to $O(D_f^2)$ terms. They obtain a constitutive equation of the Rivlin–Ericksen type, analogous to eqn (16.65):

$$\langle \sigma_{ij} \rangle = -p\delta_{ij} + 2\eta e_{ij} + 2\eta\phi\left\{(5/2)e_{ij} + (k/\dot{\gamma})\left(26\cdot8\,\overline{e_{il}e_{lj}} - 23\cdot75\frac{\mathscr{D}}{\mathscr{D}t}e_{ij}\right)\right.$$

$$- (k/\dot{\gamma})^2\left[(-22\cdot4 + 42\cdot0\psi')e_{ij}e_{lm}e_{lm}\right.$$

$$- (1377\cdot2 - 70\cdot0\lambda + 196\cdot4\psi')\overline{e_{il}(\mathscr{D}e_{lj}/\mathscr{D}t)}$$

$$\left.\left. - (79\cdot7 + 59\cdot4\lambda)\frac{\mathscr{D}^2}{\mathscr{D}t^2}e_{ij} + O(k^3\dot{\gamma})\right]\right\} \quad (16.69)$$

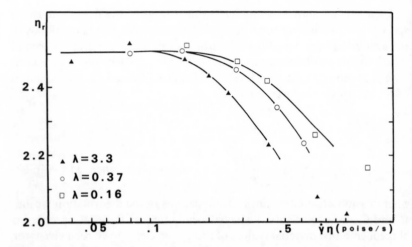

Fig. 16.3. Comparison between the experimental data of Bredimas *et al.*[38] and the theoretical value of the relative viscosity (full curves) predicted by eqn (16.70). For the same degree of interfacial polymerization, the fit between experiment and theory yields a unique value of E^s for the three values of λ.

This equation is established for a suspension of spherical capsules enclosed in an infinitely thin sheet of an incompressible isotropic elastic material characterized by ψ' ($\psi' \in [0, 1]$, a linear neo-Hookean material corresponds to $\psi' = 0$). The constitutive relation (16.69) thus predicts normal stress effects and shear thinning behaviour, since the intrinsic viscosity is given by

$$[\eta] = 5/2 - k^2(68{\cdot}5 + 21{\cdot}0\psi' + 59{\cdot}4\lambda) + O(k^3) \quad (16.70)$$

It is interesting to note that Bredimas and Veyssié[37] have measured the rheology of dilute suspension of spherical microcapsules obtained after interfacial polymerization of a dilute oil-in-water emulsion. They find shear thinning behaviour which may be interpreted by means of eqn (16.70) (where ψ' has been set to zero) as shown by Bredimas *et al.*[38] For a given λ, fitting the experimental intrinsic viscosity curve with eqn (16.70) yields a value of the elastic modulus E^s of the interface (Fig. 16.3). Repeating the process for different λ should result in the same value of E^s, as is indeed the case. Furthermore, the evolution of the corresponding values of E^s with the degree of polymerization correlates well with permeability measurements of the membrane, and with what is known about the polymerization process.

This example illustrates how an exact constitutive equation of a suspension can be used to analyse macroscopic measurements in terms of the microscopic properties of the microstructure and to infer information about the suspended particles from bulk rheological data.

16.4. NON-DILUTE SUSPENSIONS

The dilute suspensions results, although useful from the fundamental point of view, are of limited applicability for the interpretation of actual experimental data usually obtained at concentrations where particle interactions cannot be neglected. There have been in the past a number of attempts to derive constitutive laws valid at higher concentrations. The problem is of course very complex (see the review by Russel[39]) since the rheology of the suspension depends on both the motion and the deformation of the particles, and on the configuration of the suspension. The latter can be determined approximately when the suspension is still dilute enough for pair interactions to be dominant over multibody interactions or when the suspension is highly concentrated. Another approach consists in assuming *a priori* a given particle distribution, and this leads to the so-called spatially periodic suspensions. Recently, numerical models analogous to Monte Carlo simulations have yielded exact distribution functions for suspensions of spheres at any concentration.

16.4.1. $O(\phi^2)$ Interaction Effects

The results presented in Section 16.3 are valid only for extremely dilute situations, such that ϕ is less than 5%. Many attempts have been made to extend these results and to express the relative viscosity as a power series in ϕ:

$$\eta_r = 1 + (5/2)\phi + K\phi^2 + O(\phi^3) \tag{16.71}$$

This expansion is limited to sufficiently dilute suspensions of particles for which the pair interactions are dominant.

Then, as shown by Batchelor,[4] the Fokker–Planck equation reduces to a conservation equation for the pair density P_2:

$$\frac{\partial}{\partial t} P_2 + \frac{\partial}{\partial r_i} (v_{ri} P_2) - \frac{\partial}{\partial r_i} D_{ij} \frac{\partial}{\partial r_j} P_2 = 0 \tag{16.72}$$

where r_i and v_{ri} are respectively the distance and the relative velocity of the two spheres and D_{ij} is a Brownian diffusivity tensor including the competing effects of hydrodynamic interactions and of thermal diffusion. So far the only available results are derived for suspensions of identical hard spheres, for which the particle Reynolds number is infinitely small.

16.4.1.1. Purely Hydrodynamic Interaction

The determination of the microscopic flow field around two freely moving spheres in linear shear flow has been completely determined by Batchelor and Green[40] who give the expression of v_{ri} and of the corresponding dipole strengths. They then solve eqn (16.72) and deduce an expression for the pair density, valid for points that lie on trajectories, of one sphere center with respect to another, that extend to infinity. In the case of pure straining motion, any point in space lies on one such trajectory, and it is possible to complete the computation of the bulk stress. Batchelor and Green[41] then found that the coefficient K is given by

$$K = 7{\cdot}6 \qquad (16.73)$$

In the case of simple shearing motion, the pair probability cannot be determined, owing to the existence of closed trajectories. To remove this indeterminacy, it is necessary either to take into account higher order hydrodynamic interactions (3-body or more), which is at present done with numerical simulation, or to assume that the particles are subjected to other non-hydrodynamic forces, such as those due to Brownian motion, to electrostatic or steric effects. It is interesting that, if a homogeneous spatial distribution of spheres is arbitrarily assumed ($P_2 = N$), the coefficient K becomes

$$K = 5{\cdot}2 \qquad (16.74)$$

The difference between this value and that in eqn (16.73) is due to the distortion of the pair distribution by the flow which creates a pair density greater than N in the vicinity of one given sphere.

16.4.1.2. Effect of Brownian Motion

As for dilute suspensions of spheres, the respective effects of convection and of thermal agitation are measured by the Peclet number Pe_B defined by eqn (16.38). The results in Section 16.4.1.1 may thus be considered as the asymptotic form of the apparent viscosity when $Pe_B \gg 1$.

The case of strong Brownian agitation ($Pe_B \ll 1$) was considered by Batchelor[42] who calculated D_{ij}, solved eqn (16.72) and found that the pair density distribution is slightly displaced from uniformity by thermal diffusion:

$$P_2(r_i) = N[1 - (\text{Pe}_\text{B} e_{ij} r_i r_j / 6\pi r^2) f(r/a)] \qquad (16.75)$$

where f is a function tabulated by Batchelor. The shear increases P_2 in regions where $r_i v_{ri} > 0$. This creates Brownian forces which oppose the motion and thus increase the stress. The corresponding coefficient for the relative viscosity, for any linear flow, is then

$$K = 6\cdot2 \qquad (16.76)$$

A comparison between the value of the apparent shear viscosity obtained from eqns (16.71) and (16.76) and different experimental data[43-45] on suspensions of polystyrene latices is shown on Fig. 16.4 where it appears that there is reasonable agreement between theory and experiment up to concentrations of order 15–20%.

Owing to the departure from the isotropic particle distribution, the bulk stress in the suspension is non-Newtonian. In particular, normal stress differences are predicted. However, since they are of order $\text{Pe}_\text{B} \phi^2$, they are very small, unlikely to be measurable, and thus have not been computed explicitly. However, they can be determined from Batchelor's results.[4]

Finally, for pure straining motion, the evolution of K from $6\cdot2$ for $\text{Pe}_\text{B} \ll 1$ to $7\cdot6$ for $\text{Pe}_\text{B} \gg 1$ indicates shear thickening behaviour similar to that observed for dilute suspensions of spheroids. In the case of simple shear, the high Peclet value of K has not been obtained, but it is expected to lie between $6\cdot2$ and $5\cdot2$. Such a small shear thinning effect would be difficult to measure.

16.4.1.3. Secondary Electroviscous Effect

The rheology of a suspension of charged spheres has been studied to $O(\phi^2)$ by Russel,[46] who shows that the microscopic flow problem is described by equations identical to those of Section 16.3.2.3. The suspension is assumed to be sufficiently dilute for pair interaction to be the dominant effect. Then the bulk stress expression is given by eqn (16.10) where F_i^α now represents the electrostatic force exerted on one sphere by the other component of the pair, and is given in dimensional form by

$$F_i^\alpha = \frac{\partial U_2}{\partial r_i} \qquad (16.77)$$

where U_2 is the electrostatic pair potential. For low surface potential ($e\zeta/kT \ll 1$ and $r - 2a > \kappa^{-1}$), the charge distribution may be linearised and U_2 written as

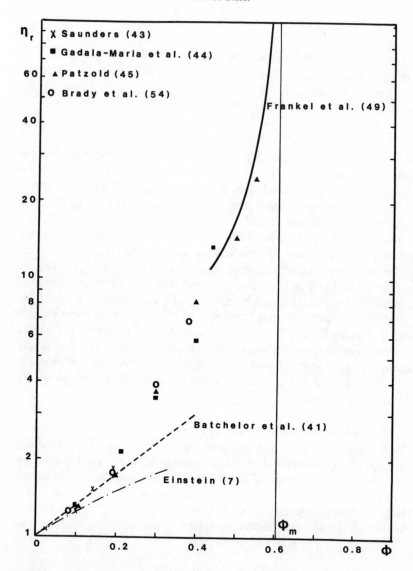

Fig. 16.4. Comparison between different experimental data and various theoretical models. The numerical predictions of Brady *et al.*, adapted to three-dimensional flows, are in excellent agreement with experiment. The maximum value $\phi_m = 0.605$ is the one computed for a cubic system.

$$U_2 = \frac{\varepsilon \zeta^2 a^2}{r} \exp\left[-\kappa(r - 2a)\right] \tag{16.78}$$

The pair distribution is then

$$P_2 = N \exp\left(-U_2/kT\right) \tag{16.79}$$

It follows that there exists a characteristic particle separation, L, at which the viscous force bringing together the two spheres is equal to the electric repulsive force. The expression for L is given by Russel as

$$\kappa L = \log[b/\log(b/\log b)] \tag{16.80}$$

where b measures the ratio of electrical to thermal forces and is here assumed to be much larger than unity, since electrostatic repulsion dominates over diffusion (otherwise, flocculation might occur):

$$b = \frac{4\pi\varepsilon\zeta^2 a}{kT} a\kappa \exp\left(2a\kappa\right) \tag{16.81}$$

The pair distribution thus varies sharply from $P_2 \simeq 0$, when $r < L$, to $P_2 \simeq N$ when $r > L$.

In the case of weak flows such that

$$Pe_B/(a\kappa)^2 \ll 1 \tag{16.82}$$

Russel found an exact solution to the full set of equations, valid for any $a\kappa$. He shows that, since convection is very small, the pair distribution is nearly isotropic, and the suspension is Newtonian, with a relative viscosity given by

$$\eta_r = 1 + \frac{5}{2}\beta\phi + \frac{5}{2}(\beta\phi)^2 + \frac{3}{40}\log\left(\frac{b}{\log b}\right)(\kappa L)^4 (a\kappa)^{-5}\phi^2 \tag{16.83}$$

The coefficient of the $O(\phi^2)$ term may be quite large, and thus may account for the large zero-shear viscosity measured in suspensions with a strong electroviscous effect. Indeed, Russel compares the predictions of eqn (16.83) with Stone-Masui and Watillon[25] data on polystyrene latices, and with Tanford and Buzzel[47] results with bovine serum albumin. He finds good agreement for $O(\phi^2)$ coefficients as large as 10^3.

The case of strong flows and thick double layers is also considered by Russel, who finds that the distortion of the isotropy of pair distribution by convection leads to non-Newtonian effects in the suspension. In particular, the shear viscosity becomes

$$\eta_r = 1 + (5/2)[\beta\phi + (\beta\phi)^2] + 0{\cdot}92\phi^2(a\kappa)^{-5}(P')^{5/3} \quad (16.84)$$

where

$$P' = \frac{4H}{Pe_E}\frac{a\kappa\exp(2a\kappa)}{3\beta_1} \quad (16.85)$$

The coefficient β_1 is given by Russel and is generally close to unity. Consequently, shear thinning behaviour is predicted, together with normal stress differences:

$$N_1/\varepsilon\zeta^2\kappa^2 = 20{\cdot}23\phi^2(a\kappa)^{-4}P'^{2/3}\log P'(1 - 1{\cdot}83/\log P')$$

$$N_2/\varepsilon\zeta^2\kappa^2 = -37.80\phi^2(a\kappa)^{-4}P'^{2/3} \quad (16.86)$$

The above results are obtained in the limiting case of thick double layers ($a\kappa \ll 1$), and for flows such that $1 < P' < (a\kappa)^{-3}$. They are in qualitative agreement with Fryling data[48] on suspensions of latex particles, which indicate a shear thinning viscosity for low solvent ionic strengths.

16.4.2. Very Concentrated Suspensions

A very concentrated suspension of identical solid spheres has been studied by Frankel and Acrivos.[49] They determined the steady shear viscosity by means of an asymptotic analysis, where they assumed that the leading contribution to energy dissipation arises in the lubrication layer between two spheres. Furthermore, the configuration of the suspension is approximately known at such high concentrations. Consequently, assuming the spheres to be in a periodic array, Frankel and Acrivos integrated the energy dissipation in a cell containing just one particle. They found that the relative viscosity behaves as

$$\eta_r = C'\frac{(\phi/\phi_m)^{1/3}}{1 - (\phi/\phi_m)^{1/3}} \quad \text{as } \phi/\phi_m \to 1 \quad (16.87)$$

where ϕ_m is the maximum attainable concentration and where the constant C' depends on the geometry of the integration cell and on the type of packing assumed for the spheres. A comparison with experimental data (Fig. 16.4) supports the prediction of eqn (16.87) with a constant C' equal to 9/8 (cubic array, spherical cell).

16.4.3. Spatially Periodic Suspensions

For suspensions which are neither very dilute nor very concentrated, prediction of the rheological properties implies the calculation of many body interactions, and the determination of the particle distribution function. A convenient way to solve these problems is to assume that the suspension has a spatially periodic structure.[50-52] The models available at present deal with identical spheres centred at the points of a periodic lattice. Then the volume of integration, ΔV, over which the bulk stress is computed, can be chosen to be simply a unit cell of the lattice, since all quantities are spatially periodic. Nunan and Keller[51] calculated the relative viscosity for instantaneous static configurations. They found that, as $\phi \to \phi_m$, η_r diverges as

$$\eta_r \sim (1 - \phi/\phi_m)^{-1/3}$$

which is identical to the Frankel and Acrivos result.

Adler *et al.*[52] studied the dynamics of a spatially periodic suspension, by averaging in time over many different configurations. They found that, as $\phi \to \phi_m$, the relative viscosity has a finite value. This is due to the fact that, in a dynamic situation, the interparticle distance d' may become small ($d' \ll 1$). This leads to large lubrication forces $O(d'^{-1})$, but which are applied for a short time $O(d')$, and thus the corresponding contribution to the bulk viscosity is $O(1)$. Conversely, in a static situation, the time of contact is implicitly assumed to be $O(1)$ and this gives rise to a contribution to the viscosity which is $O(d'^{-1})$. The conclusion is then that the asymptotic behaviour of the viscosity at high concentrations strongly depends on the microstructure dynamics.

Although periodic suspension models can be conveniently used to describe colloidal crystals subjected to small deformations, they are obviously a very rough approximation to what happens in a concentrated suspension, where flow tends to create clusters of particles (de Gennes[53]) rather than periodic arrays.

16.4.4. Numerical Simulations

Recently, Brady and Bossis[54] have developed a numerical method, using an approach similar to molecular dynamics, to follow the time evolution of the particle positions in a suspension, and to compute the corresponding flow field for any concentration. They assume that the many-body interactions are approximately equal to a sum of pair interactions. In the case of two identical spheres, the exact velocity and stress fields are known. Brady and Bossis use these results to simulate the flow of a suspension of identical spheres subjected to a simple shearing motion. Their computation is restricted to two-dimensional geometries (i.e. sheared monolayers) but can be interpreted to give a good insight into the corresponding phenomena occurring in three-dimensional situations. In particular, the model gives the time evolution of the particle configuration. In the absence of interparticle forces, the suspension exhibits a marked tendency to form clusters, the size of which, L_c, scales as $[1 - (\phi/\phi_m)^{1/3}]^{-1}$. The numerical simulation thus supports de Gennes' speculation[53] of the formation of an infinite cluster as $\phi \to \phi_m$, where ϕ_m acts as a percolation-like threshold.

The bulk rheological properties are determined from eqn (16.10) where the summation is taken over all the particles in the domain, and is then defined as an area average rather than a volume average. The rheological behaviour is Newtonian, with a viscosity that also scales as $[1 - (\phi/\phi_m)^{1/3}]^{-1}$ when ϕ/ϕ_m is nearly unity. Consequently the numerical simulation supports the results of Frankel and Acrivos. It would then seem that the finite viscosity for $\phi/\phi_m \simeq 1$, predicted by Adler *et al.*, is a consequence of the periodic suspension assumption. It may be explained by the fact that, in a periodic array, the time two particles spend nearby is short $O(d')$, whereas it is $O(1)$ in a cluster. A comparison with experimental data shows excellent agreement with the model over the full range of concentrations (see Fig. 16.4).

Brady and Bossis also consider the effect of colloidal interparticle forces of the DLVO type. Such forces have two effects on the rheology. Firstly, they modify the configuration; specifically, they reduce the tendency to cluster formation. Secondly, they influence directly the bulk stress through the force and stress terms in eqn (16.10). Then, marked non-Newtonian effects are predicted. The normal stress differences increase with ϕ and decrease linearly with $H/[\mathrm{Pe}_E(a\kappa)^2]$ as this quantity goes to zero. The shear viscosity is thickening. This behaviour is in contradiction to that predicted from the simple $O(\phi^2)$ pair interaction theory, which indicates shear thinning. It seems that this is due to the fact that shear thickening is the result of different coupled physical phenomena (microstructure, interparticle forces and cluster formation), not all taken into account in pair interaction theories.

16.5. CONCLUSIONS

Ever since the theoretical background for the proper formulation of constitutive laws for heterogeneous media was established, there has been considerable development of research on suspensions. At present there are many theoretical results predicting the rheological behaviour of suspensions of solid or deformable particles eventually subjected to colloidal forces. The advantage of such constitutive equations is that they relate *exactly* the measurable bulk properties to the physical parameters of the microstructure, and contain no adjustable parameter. Their disadvantage is that they often have a limited range of applicability, and cannot account for all the complexity of a real system.

They can also be used as a guide for the formulation of realistic phenomenological constitutive relations for a wide variety of fluids, since they exhibit many non-Newtonian properties.[33] Finally, suspension theory is based on an extensive analysis of the motion and the deformation of the microstructure. As such, it leads to the identification of the important microscale parameters, and provides experimentalists with proper dimensionless numbers with which they can analyse their data.

REFERENCES

1. G. K. Batchelor, *J. Fluid Mech.*, 1970, **41**, 545.
2. Z. Hashin, *Appl. Mech. Rev.*, 1964, **17**, 1.
3. G. K. Batchelor, *Ann. Rev. Fluid Mech.*, 1974, **6**,. 227.
4. G. K. Batchelor, *J. Fluid Mech.*, 1977, **83**, 97.
5. D. Barthes-Biesel and J. M. Rallison, *J. Fluid Mech.*, 1981, **113**, 251.
6. D. Barthes-Biesel and H. Sgaier, *J. Fluid Mech.*, 1985, **160** 119.
7. A. Einstein, *Ann. Phys.*, 1906, **19**, 289.
8. G. B. Jeffery, *Proc. Roy. Soc.*, 1922, **A102**, 161.
9. A. Okagawa, R. G. Cox and S. G. Mason, *J. Colloid Interface Sci*, 1973, **45**, 303.
10. L. G. Leal and E. J. Hinch, *J. Fluid Mech.*, 1971, **46**, 685.
11. L. G. Leal and E. J. Hinch, *J. Fluid Mech.*, 1972, **55**, 745.
12. L. G. Leal and E. J. Hinch, *Rheologica Acta*, 1973, **12**, 127.
13. E. J. Hinch and L. G. Leal, *J. Fluid Mech.*, 1972, **52**, 683.
14. E. J. Hinch and L. G. Leal, *J. Fluid Mech.*, 1973, **57**, 753.
15. E. J. Hinch and L. G. Leal, *J. Fluid Mech.*, 1976, **76**, 187.
16. F. P. Bretherton, *J. Fluid Mech.*, 1962, **14**, 284.
17. H. Giesekus, *Rheologica Acta*, 1962, **2**, 50.
18. I. M. Krieger, *Adv. Colloid Interface Sci.*, 1972, **3**, 111.
19. G. Chauveteau, *J. Rheology*, 1982, **26**, 111.
20. G. L. Hand, *J. Fluid Mech.*, 1962, **13**, 33.
21. P. L. Frattini and G. G. Fuller, *J. Fluid Mech.*, 1986, **168**, 119.
22. F. Booth, *Proc. Roy. Soc.*, 1950, **A203**, 533.
23. J. D. Sherwood, *J. Fluid Mech.*, 1980, **101**, 609.
24. D. A. Saville, *Ann. Rev. Fluid Mech.*, 1977, **9**, 321.
25. J. Stone-Masui and A. Watillon, *J. Colloid Interface Sci*, 1968, **28**, 187.
26. J. M. Rallison, *Ann. Rev. Fluid Mech.*, 1984, **16**, 45.
27. J. D. Goddard and C. Miller, *J. Fluid Mech.*, 1967, **28**, 657.
28. R. Roscoe, *J. Fluid Mech.*, 1967, **28**, 273.

29. G. I. Taylor, *Proc. Roy. Soc.*, 1934, **A146**, 501.
30. R. G. Cox, *J. Fluid Mech.* 1969, **37**, 601.
31. N. A. Frankel and A. Acrivos, *J. Fluid Mech.*, 1970, **44**, 65.
32. D. Barthes-Biesel and A. Acrivos, *J. Fluid Mech.*, 1973, **61**, 1.
33. D. Barthes-Biesel and A. Acrivos, *Int. J. Multiphase Flow*, 1973, **1**, 1.
34. B. J. Bentley and L. G. Leal, *J. Fluid Mech.*, 1986, **167**, 241.
35. D. Barthes-Biesel and V. Chhim, *Int. J. Multiphase Flow*, 1981, **7**, 493.
36. P. O. Brunn, *J. Fluid Mech.*, 1983, **126**, 533.
37. M. Bredimas and M. Veyssié, *J. Non-Newtonian Fluid Mech.*, 1983, **12**, 165.
38. M. Bredimas, M. Veyssié, D. Barthes-Biesel and V. Chhim, *J. Colloid Interface Sci.*, 1983, **93**, 513.
39. W. B. Russel, *J. Rheology,* 1980, **24**, 287.
40. G. K. Batchelor and J. T. Green, *J. Fluid Mech.*, 1972, **56**, 375.
41. G. K. Batchelor and J. T. Green, *J. Fluid Mech.*, 1972, **56**, 401.
42. G. K. Batchelor, *J. Fluid Mech.*, 1976, **74**, 1.
43. F. L. Saunders, *J. Colloid Sci.*, 1961, **16**, 13.
44. F. Gadala-Maria and A. Acrivos, *J. Rheology*, 1980, **24**, 799.
45. R. Patzold, *Rheologica Acta*, 1980, **19**, 322.
46. W. B. Russel, *J. Fluid Mech.*, 1978, **85**, 209.
47. C. F. Tanford and J. G. Buzzell, *J. Phys. Chem.*, 1956, **60**, 225.
48. C. F. Fryling, *J. Colloid Sci.*, 1963, **18**, 713.
49. N. A. Frankel and A. Acrivos, *Chem. Eng. Sci.*, 1967, **22**, 847.
50. M. Zuzovsky, P. M. Adler and H. Brenner, *Phys. Fluids*, 1983, **26**, 1714.
51. K. C. Nunan and J. B. Keller, *J. Fluid Mech.*, 1984, **142**, 269.
52. P. M. Adler, M. Zuzovsky and H. Brenner, *Int. J. Multiphase Flow*, 1985, **11**, 361.
53. P. G. de Gennes, *Physico-Chemical Hydrodynamics*, Vol. 2, Pergamon Press, 1981, p. 31.
54. J. F. Brady and G. Bossis, *J. Fluid Mech.*, 1985, **155**, 105.

Index